ETHNOPHARMACOLOGIC SEARCH *for* PSYCHOACTIVE DRUGS • 2022

55th Anniversary Symposium › May 23–26, 2022

Vol. III

55

ETHNOPHARMACOLOGIC SEARCH *for* PSYCHOACTIVE DRUGS • 2022

55th Anniversary Symposium › May 23–26, 2022 | Vol. III

PUBLISHED BY
SYNERGETIC PRESS

In association with the
McKenna Academy of Natural Philosophy

Published by Synergetic Press
1 Bluebird Court, Santa Fe, New Mexico 87508
& 24 Old Gloucester St., London WC1N 3AL, England

Published in Association with the McKenna Academy of Natural Philosophy

ISBN 978-1-957869-23-0 (paperback)
ISBN 978-1-957869-24-7 (ebook)

Book design and typesetting by Jon Hahn Design
Botanical illustrations on cover © Donna Torres

Printed by Versa Press, Inc
Display typeface: Dolly Pro
Body typeface: Adobe Caslon Pro

ACKNOWLEDGEMENTS

The 2022 ESPD Symposium Proceedings could not have been done without the generous support of our sponsors and donors. Additionally, the Symposium and the Proceedings reflect the hard work and dedication of many volunteers and support staff.

Individual Donors

Bohdana Tamas
David Petrou
Jeff Smith
James Velaise
Miranda Levine
O'Shaughnessy Family Partners LLC
Sea View Ranch Charities

Institutional Donors

1906
1906newhighs.com

Entheos
entheospsychedelics.com

Uniphi Studio
uniphi.studio

A.A Badenhorst Family Wines
aabadenhorst.com

Kosmicare
kosmicare.org

ATTMiND Podcast
jameswjesso.com

Fungi Academy
fungiacademy.com

Heroic Hearts Project
heroicheartsproject.org

Fantastic Fungi
fantasticfungi.com

Hefter Research Institute
heffter.org

Multidisciplinary Association for Psychedelic Studies
maps.org

ICEERS
iceers.org

St. Giles House
stgilesdorset.com

Resonant Mind Collective
resonantmindcollective.com

Entheogenesis Australis
entheogenesis.org

Ceruvia Life Sciences
ceruvialifesciences.com

Microdose
microdose.buzz

Jaguar Health
jaguar.health

Nachtschatten Verlag
nachtschatten.ch

Psygen
psygen.ca

Pretty Pictures
prettypictures.fr

VCENNA
vcenna.com

Woven Science
woven.science

Tyringham Initiative
tyringhaminitiative.com

Psychedelics.com
psychedelics.com

Beckley Foundation
beckleyfoundation.org

Synergetic Press
synergeticpress.com

Soltara Healing Centre
soltara.co

ESPD55 2022 SYMPOSIUM SPEAKERS

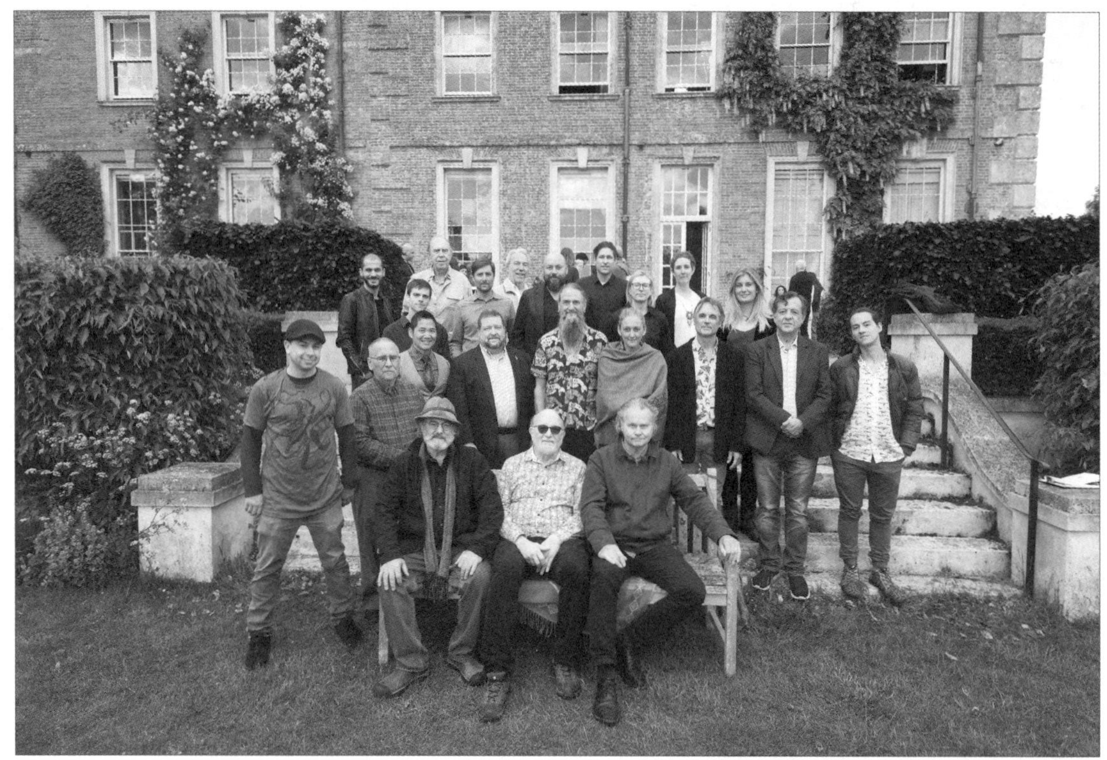

ABOVE: Conference Speakers at St. Giles House, Dorset, UK.

FRONT ROW, L TO R: Zak Kulberg, Professor Constantino Manuel Torres, Paul Stamets, Dr. Dennis McKenna, Professor Wade Davis.

SECOND ROW, L TO R: Jonathan Lu, Professor Chris McCurdy, Dr. Bruce Damer, Professor Monica Gagliano, Dr. Glenn H. Shepard Jr., Dr. Luis Eduardo Luna, David F. Rodriguez-Mora.

THIRD ROW, L TO R: Colin Domnauer, Dr. Bryn Dentinger, Josip Orlovac Del Río, Dr. Michelle St. Pierre, Laurel Sugden.

BACK ROW, L TO R: Dr. Shauheen Etminan, Professor Mark Merlin, Dr. Mark Plotkin, Barrett McBride, Andrea Langlois.

NOT SHOWN: Alexandre Tannous, Professor Andrew Weil, Carey Turnbull, Christina Chaya, Cody Swift, Dale Millard, Professor David Nutt, Professor Elaine Elisabetsky, Greg Hemmings, Jerónimo Mazarrasa, Dr. Michael Coe.

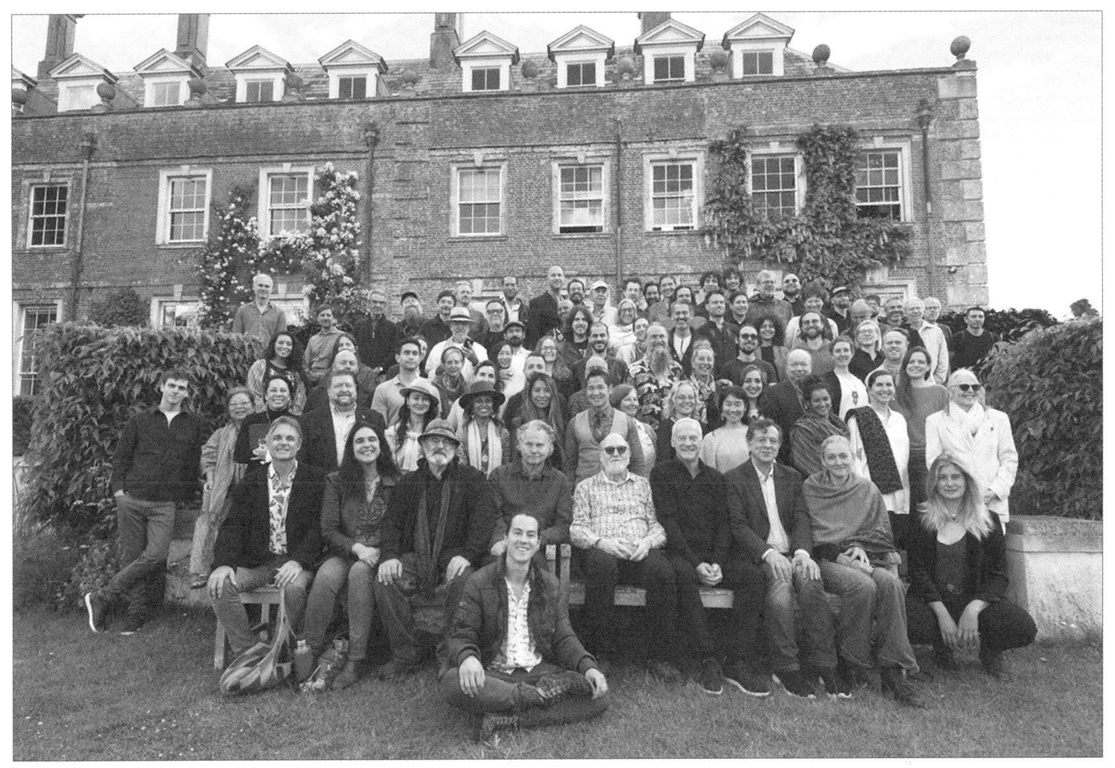

ABOVE: Conference Speakers, Organizers and Participants at St. Giles House, Dorset, UK.

Authors

Dennis J. McKenna, PhD
Director of Ethnopharmacology, Hefter Research Institute; Assistant Professor, University of Minnesota. He has studied the botany, chemistry and pharmacology of ayahuasca and other South American shamanic plants over the last forty years.

Andrea Langlois, MA
Andrea Langlois was the Director of Engagement for the International Center for Ethnobotanical Education Research and Service (ICEERS). She holds an MA in Communications from Concordia University, and is a community-based researcher, communicator, and trained facilitator with a passion for organizational development and systems change. Andrea is an advisor to the Conservation Committee of the Indigenous Medicine Conservation Fund.

Andy Weil, MD
Andrew Weil is a world-renowned leader and pioneer in the field of integrative medicine. Combining a Harvard education and a lifetime of practicing natural and preventive medicine, he is the founder and director of the Arizona Center for Integrative Medicine at the University of Arizona, where he is a clinical Professor of medicine and Professor of public health. He is also the editorial director of Dr.Weil.com, and a New York Times best-selling author.

Barrett McBride, Doctoral candidate
Barrett's current research for his PhD focuses on ethnopharmacology and comparative genomics, at the University of Reading Biological Sciences. Specifically he is investigating how phylogenetic studies and ethnobotany may provide context for phytochemical analysis and Drug discovery. Conservation of medicinal plants and respect for the people and places that have carried their knowledge is also a central emphasis of this research.

Brian Hettler
Brian Hettler is a geographer and cartographer with the Amazon Conservation Team (ACT) and works with indigenous communities in South America on participatory mapping initiatives that support indigenous land rights and rainforest conservation. He also partakes in a range of projects including monitoring forest cover using remote sensing techniques, designing maps in both static and interactive digital formats, and supporting ACT's field staff and indigenous partners in the innovative use of spatial data collection and monitoring tools. Brian also creates interactive, map-based digital stories designed to raise awareness of Amazonian cultures and ecosystems and the many external threats they face.

Bruce Damer, PhD
Dr. Bruce Damer is an astrobiologist who has spent his life pursuing two questions: how did life on Earth begin? And how can we give that life (and ourselves) a sustainable pathway into the future and a presence beyond the Earth? A decade of laboratory and field research with his collaborator Prof. David Deamer at UCSC and teams around the world resulted in the Hot Spring

Hypothesis for an Origin of Life published in the journal Astrobiology in 2020. Damer practices a form of visionary reverie described by Albert Einstein as his "thought experiments."

Bryn Dentinger, PhD

Bryn is a systematic mycologist who received his B.A. from Macalester College (St. Paul, MN) in 2000, and his PhD from the University of Minnesota in 2007. From 2010-2016 he worked as a senior scientist and Head of Mycology at the Royal Botanic Gardens, Kew in London, UK. He is currently the Curator of Mycology at the Natural History Museum of Utah and an Associate Professor in the School of Biological Sciences at the University of Utah.

Carey Turnbull

Carey Turnbull is Chair of the advisory board of the NYU Center for Psychedelic Medicine. He is a member of the Board and President of Heffter Research Institute and a past member of the Board of Usona Institute. He founded Ceruvia Lifesciences and B.More to transform psychedelic research into cutting edge medicine. Most recently he founded Freedom to Operate to protect psychedelic science and medical development for the public benefit. Mr. Turnbull provides time as an adjunct advisor to the legal defense of the Native American Church and other indigenous people's rights to the practice of their religion, ceremonies, and beliefs free from cultural, religious and legal pressure.

Chris McCurdy, PhD

Chris McCurdy is a Professor of Medicinal Chemistry, College of Pharmacy, University of Florida, Gainesville, FL. Professor McGurdy is Director of the UF Translational Drug Development Core and the 2017-2018 president of the American Association of Pharmaceutical Scientists. He is internationally recognized as an authority on Kratom, *Mitragyna speciosa.*

Colin Domnauer, Doctoral candidate

Colin Domnauer graduated from UC Berkeley, where he completed his thesis investigating the use of the psychoactive plant Vilca (*Anadenanthera spp.*) in pre-Columbian Andean cultures. He is now pursuing graduate research in Mycology at the University of Utah.

Dale Millard

Dale Millard is an ethnobotanist, naturalist and biodiversity explorer, with research interests ranging from herpetology to the study of plants used to treat tropical diseases and immune disorders. He has travelled and collected extensively in South Africa, Brazil and Indonesia.

David F. Rodriguez-Mora, Doctoral candidate

David F. Rodriguez-Mora is conducting his doctoral studies in environmental anthropology at the University of Texas at San Antonio. His doctoral research will expand the scope and geographic range of his master's research to better understand the Colombian Cofán territorial, cultural, and intellectual resources and help his Cofán colleagues protect them. David has also worked extensively on various interdisciplinary projects around biocultural preservation.

David Nutt, PhD

David Nutt is a psychiatrist and the Edmond J. Safra Professor of Neuropsychopharmacology in Imperial College London. He is currently Founding Chair of the charity DrugScience.org.uk and has been president of the European Brain Council, the BAP, BNA, and ECNP. David has published 35 books and over 1000 research papers that define his many landmark contributions to psychopharmacology.

Elaine Elisabetsky, PhD

Elaine Elisabetsky, PhD is a Professor of Pharmacology at the Federal University of Rio Grande do Sul (Porto Alegre, Brazil), and a member of the WHO Traditional, Complementary and Integrative Medicine advisory panel. Her research focuses on the identification and characterization of psychopharmacological properties of medicinal plant extracts and isolated compounds, as well as conservation, fair benefit sharing and indigenous rights. A founding member for the International Society of Ethnobiology (1988) and the International Society of Ethnopharmacology (1990), served as president for the latter as well as for the Brazilian Society of Ethnobiology and Ethnoecology.

Glenn Shepard, PhD

Glenn Shepard is a staff Researcher at Goeldi Museum, Belem, Brazil. His writing, research and photography on shamanism, traditional environmental knowledge and indigenous rights has appeared in *Nature*, *Science*, *National Geographic* and *The New York Review of Books*, among other prestigious publications. He has participated in several TV documentaries including an Emmy Award-winning Discovery Channel film.

Jerónimo Mazarrasa

Jerónimo Mazarrasa is an ayahuasca community activist. He works as Social Innovation Coordinator for ICEERS, and is a founding member of the Plantaforma (Platform for the Defense of Ayahuasca in Spain). Over the past 5 years he has devoted most of his energy to engaged research and innovation exploring how ceremonial plant practices can be integrated outside of their cultures of origin. Previously he wrote and produced four documentary films on various aspects of the encounters between the West and indigenous knowledge, from ayahuasca in the treatment of Drug addiction with Gabor Maté, to the Kogi Mamos, to the Brazilian ayahuasca religions.

Jonathan Lu, BS

Jonathan Lu is the co-founder of VCENNA, a CNS Drug discovery company focused on poly-pharmocology with naturally-extracted and purified alkaloid isolates. Jonathan is an expert generalist whose multidisciplinary career includes roles as a corporate manager, venture investor, and early stage operating executive. He is a graduate from Stanford University's Graduate School of Business, and received a BS in Chemical Engineering from Cornell University.

Josip Orlovac Del Río

Josip Orlovac Del Río is a maestro huachumero from coastal Peru with over 30 years of experience growing, cooking, drinking, and sharing the San Pedro cactus. He received his connection to the plant through his Andean grandfather, and from a young age studied traditional healing in a lineage of curanderos from the Río Santa. He co-founded Huachuma Collective, a nonprofit association in Peru which works with indigenous communities towards the biological and cultural sustainability of San Pedro. He has been planting San Pedro for 25 years, and collectively his gardens are home to nearly 6,000 individual cacti.

Laurel Sugden, Doctoral candidate
Laurel Anne Sugden is a PhD. candidate in Interdisciplinary Studies at the University of British Columbia. Her current work centers on the visionary San Pedro cactus (Huachuma), and its cultural and ecological roles in the Andes. Laurel co-founded Huachuma Collective, a nonprofit association in Peru which works with Indigenous communities towards the biological and cultural sustainability of San Pedro.

Luis Eduardo Luna, PhD
Dr. Luis Eduardo Luna is the director of Wasiwaska Research Center for the Study of Psychointegrator Plants, Visionary Art and Consciousness (wasiwaska.org). Dr. Luna is internationally recognized as an authority on the ethnography of ayahuasca.

Manuel Torres, PhD
Professor Emeritus, Art and Art History Department, Florida International University. Dr. Torres specializes in the art and iconography of ancient cultures of the Central Andes. He is recognized for his excavations of shamanic burial sites in the Atacama Desert, and is a recognized expert on the use of Anadenthera snuffs in ancient South America.

Mark Merlin, PhD
Professor Merlin is recognized as an authority on archaeological record and cultural biogeography of mind-altering Drug plants, and is highly regarded for his research and publications focused on traditional environmental knowledge of the societies in Remote Oceania. His research has focused on the cultural histories of human-plant interactions with special emphasis on the pan-global, traditional use of psychoactive species, including ancient cannabis and opium use.

Mark Plotkin, PhD
Dr. Mark Plotkin is an ethnobotanist, educator, filmmaker co-founder and President of the Amazon Conservation Team (ACT.org). He is widely recognized for his advocacy for the protection of indigenous knowledge and Amazonian ecosystems. Plotkin was a protégé of Richard Evans Schultes, and gave a unique and insightful look at his mentor as part of ESPD55.

Michael Coe, PhD
Michael A. Coe earned a bachelor's of science degree in ethnobotany from the University of Hawai'i at Mānoa in 2015 and was a recipient of the Richard Evans Schultes Research Award from the Society of Economic Botany in 2016 for his research on ayahuasca. In 2019, he received a PhD in botany with a focus on evolution, ecology and conservation biology from the same university. Michael's current research interests include the ritualistic and therapeutic use of ayahuasca and other teacher plants in ethnomedicinal contexts aimed at improving physiological, psychological, emotional, and spiritual well-being. Michael A. Coe, PhD, is currently an assistant

professor in the department of biological sciences at Tarleton State University. (www.drcoelab.com/research)

Michelle St. Pierre, PhD

Dr. Michelle St. Pierre received her doctorate in Clinical Psychology from The University of British Columbia (UBC), and was UBC's 2021 Researcher of the Year. Michelle's research broadly explores the use of cannabis and psychedelics for therapeutic purposes. She has published and presented nationally and internationally on these topics and had her research featured in outlets such as *Forbes*, *Time Magazine*, and *The Globe and Mail*. Her research is supported by a CIHR Vanier Canada Graduate Scholarship and Killam Doctoral Fellowship.

Nigel Gericke, MD

Dr. Nigel Gericke is a South African medical doctor, botanist, ethnopharmacologist and entrepreneur has published many peer-reviewed scientific papers on ethnobotany and ethnopharmacology; he is co-author of books on South African ethnobotany including *Medicinal Plants of South Africa* and *People's Plants: A Guide to Useful Plants of Southern Africa*. He is the world's foremost authority on Kanna, an indigenous psychoactive plant used by the San and Khoi peoples.

Orou Gaoue, PhD

Professor Orou Gaoue holds a PhD in ecology, evolution and conservation biology. He is an associate Professor at the University of Tennessee, and the research in his lab integrates population ecology and ethnobiology to study plant-human interactions in a changing world and how this informs the conservation of biodiversity and sustainable use of ecosystem services.

Pascual Gonzalez, MPhil

Pascual Gonzalez provides cartographic support to all of the Amazon Conservation Teams's programs, working jointly with the Senior Mapping Coordinator to produce, assemble, and visualize ACT's cartographic and GIS data. Pascual holds a B.A. in Geography and an MPhil in Development Studies from the University of Cambridge.

Paul Stamets

Paul Stamets is a speaker, author, mycologist, medical researcher and entrepreneur, is considered an intellectual and industry leader in fungi: habitat, medicinal use, and production. He lectures extensively to deepen the understanding and respect for the organisms that literally exist under every footstep taken on this path of life. Paul's philosophy is that "MycoDiversity is BioSecurity," and his passion is to preserve and protect as many ancestral strains of mushrooms as possible.

Shauheen Etminan, PhD

Dr. Shauheen Etminan is the founder of VCENNA, a CNS drug discovery biotech company focused on poly-pharmacology of natural neuro-pharmaceuticals for mental wellness. Shauheen is an inventor and repeat founder with a portfolio across multi-industries. He holds a PhD in chemical engineering from the University of Calgary.

Wade Davis, PhD

Professor Wade Davis is currently Professor of Anthropology and the BC Leadership Chair in Cultures and Ecosystems at Risk at the University of British Columbia. He is also an author a writer, photographer, and filmmaker whose work has taken him from the Amazon to Tibet, Africa to Australia, Polynesia to the Arctic. He was the explorer-in-Residence at the National Geographic Society from 2000 to 2013, and in 2016 he was made a Member of the Order of Canada.

Zach Walsh, PhD

Professor Zach Walsh is a Professor in the University of British Colombia Department of Psychology. He received a PhD in Clinical Psychology in 2008 from the Chicago Medical School, and his research topics span across cannabis use, psychedelics, harm reduction, drug policy and harm reduction.

Zak Kulberg

Zak completed a degree in Marine Toxicology, and then began work with Dutch sponge taxonomists in Indonesia. There he collected marine sponges, taking extracts, and tested them for bioactivity. He is now working on farming sponges on pearl farms across Indonesia to build biochemical libraries, and to transplant coral to grow for an ecological restoration program.

Contents

Foreword

Sir Ghillean Prance

Scientific Director of the Eden Project | Director (Ret.), Royal Botanic Gardens, Kew

On reading all of the papers in this book my greatest regret is that I did not attend the ESPD55 conference upon which it is based. This resulting book is a most important contribution to the study of psychedelic plants and fungi. It is full of good science and many interesting accounts of personal experiences of their use. The chapters here vary from descriptions of ritual and sacred ceremonies to DNA barcoding, the detailed molecular chemistry of sponges and neuroimaging. Many fascinating stories are told here, but this is not about the casual or tourist use of these compounds, rather it is a serious demonstration of the potential of these substances for medical uses based on good science. Something that immediately stood out to me is the great respect that the authors of each chapter have for the Indigenous Peoples with whom they associate or collaborate. This is a book in which the indigenous original discoverers of many of these chemical compounds are given due credit varying from the Matsigenka of southern Peru to the San people of Botswana. Richard Schultes who was one of the founding fathers of the ethnobotanical study of psychedelic plants is acknowledged in many chapters here. I am glad about this because, as Schultes was not present at the conference to write for himself, there is a chapter here about him and his huge contribution to research and teaching written by one of his former students Mark Plotkin. Two other people who are so frequently cited in the papers here for their contribution to the topic of this book are the McKenna brothers Terence and Dennis who really opened up this field of study. Dale Millard and Luis Eduardo Luna describe well the Wasiwaska Ethnobotanical Garden for medicinal plants that Terence helped them to set up in Florianopolis, Brazil. What a wonderful array of mind-altering plants are described here in some detail and that are cultivated in that garden. The existence of these species in this garden-preserve is increasingly important today as several of the psychedelic plant species are now seriously threatened by overharvesting.

In addition to accounts of contemporary research on psychedelics there is much interesting history of their uses given here which helps to put things into context and also helps us to understand the ancient uses of sacred plants. For example, we read about the uses of visionary plants by the ancient Tiwanaka and Wari people of Bolivia in 300-900 A.D. or the history of the sacred drink of the Zoroastrians of Iran. The use of the images depicted on ancient ceramics of the Pre-Columbian cultures Cupisnique, Paracas and Nazca clearly demonstrates the importance of the hallucinogenic *Anadenanthera* to them. Archeobotany has an important contribution to make about the ancient uses of psychedelic plants. Jonathan Lu in his chapter explains the long history of medicinal plants in China and shows that mind-altering substances from plants and fungi have played an important and often hidden role throughout the history of China. This chapter is an interesting comparison of the different attitudes to psychoactive substances between eastern and western cultures and it opens up a world that has been much neglected in the west. Another contribution from Asia is the chapter by Chris McCurdy on the alkaloid rich leaves of Kratom (*Mitragyna speciosa*) a popular stimulant tea in southeast Asia, and a possible alternative to opioids in the west.

As a botanist it impresses me to see the wide range of the plant kingdom and even beyond which is used in some way to stimulate or calm the brain. This varies from *Ephedra*, a conifer in Eurasia, a lily bulb (*Boophone disticha*) in South Africa for leshoma, to many higher plants, such as the San Pedro cactus (*Echinopsis* species) and the forest liana that is the source of ayahuasca (*Banisteriopsis caapi*). But in addition, here we also read about the fungi that produce psilocybin and the marine sponges that contain tryptamines. I am also glad to see a chapter about the hunting medicines of the Matsigenka, as this is an aspect I have come across several times in my ethnobotanical research, particularly with the Guaraní.

There is much about the use of medicinal plants here. Elaine Elizabetzky seeks to use her ethnopharmacological research to improve the discovery of new drugs. Michelle St. Pierre and Zach Walsh demonstrate the potential use of psychedelics for the reduction of interpersonal violence and other psychotic disorders following up on some of the original ideas of Timothy Leary. Andrew Weil gives a very personal account of his use of coca in therapeutics. Coca also features in a good review of the history of its uses by Wade Davis. Both authors make an important plea for the legalisation of coca. It is distressing that this mild stimulant and calmant that so many of us have used is so vilified outside its use by Indigenous Peoples. This is one of the sacred plants of the peoples of South America that could easily be produced sustainably and used more widely if its use were to become legal. Can we convince the world of the difference between using a whole entire coca leaf from the isolation of the cocaine molecule? The pathways toward the legalisation of prohibited substances are well covered here in the chapter by Carey Turnbull which also discusses the rash of unwarranted patents on these substances. I am glad to see a chapter on intellectual property rights covered by David Rodríguez-Mora using ayahuasca and the Kofán people as a fine example of Community-Based Participatory Research.

There are three things that particularly stand out to me. Firstly, is that most of the medicines and substances used are mixtures rather than a pure compound. So much of the effect produced is from the chemical interactions between a mixture of plant parts that occurs in the brew. Ayahuasca is not the same without chacruna (*Psychotria viridis*) and in coca it is the whole leaf that is used and not just pure isolated cocaine. Secondly the plant species involved do not always produce a consistent amount or quality of the compound involved. There are many genetic varieties of most plants that may have different levels of production. In addition, the production of a particular compound may be strongly influenced by the environment, the soil, or the climate conditions. Thirdly the authors here understand the magical and sacred nature of the plants that they are studying, and this is often through their own personal experience of their use in authentic ceremonies with the native peoples. Those of us who have been through various ceremonial plant practices with our indigenous friends are often concerned about the use of these plants outside their place of origin. Jeronimo Mazarrasa provides here a very astute and useful analysis of this indicating both the positive and negative aspects.

In these times of environmental crisis I am glad to see concern expressed in several chapters about the threats of extinction by over harvesting of some of these sacred plants. This generally happens when the use extends beyond that of the Indigenous Peoples who know how use them sustainably. There is a great need to promote sustainable production rather than the harvest of the last specimens from their natural habitats as is emphasised here both by Michael Coe and Barrett McBride for the case of ayahuasca. Laurel Sugden and Josip del Rio emphasise that the endangered San Pedro cactus (*Echinopsis*) of Peru is fast disappearing as a result of massive over-harvesting. These authors are even cautious not to mention exact location of the plants to protect them from harvest by tourist or commercial users rather than serious indigenous users. Andrea Langlois and Jeronimo Mazarrasa show how the commercialization of ayahuasca, iboga and magic mushrooms are all seriously overharvested due to their increasing popularity. They also address the important question of: What happens when the rituals become commercial products? In promoting the conservation of the species involved we also need to do as much as possible to preserve the cultural knowledge associated with them. Most of the writers here have experienced and understand the sacred nature of their use and this must not be lost amongst the creators of these rituals.

It is good to see that the study of psychedelic plants is continuing well as Sugden and some of the other authors, including Colin Domnauer, were doctoral candidates when they wrote their chapters for this book. The work of the pioneers such as Schultes, the McKenna brothers and Tim Plowman is continuing on in good hands for the benefit of future generations.

—Ghillean T. Prance FRS, FLS, VMH

Note from the Editor-in-Chief: A Continuing Legacy

Dennis J. McKenna, PhD

President and Principal Founder | Mckenna Academy of Natural Philosophy

In the summer of 1967, the counter-cultural movement was in full swing. Droves of Hippies and others identifying with the psychedelic revolution made pilgrimages to the enchanted city of San Francisco, the switched-on epicenter of the action, to participate in the 'Summer of Love.' It was widely thought to mark the emergence of a new cultural epoch of peace and love, free thought and free sex, enlightenment and self-transformation, driven largely by the powerful psychedelic, LSD. It didn't take long for disillusion to set in; the idealistic aspirations of the young counter-cultural revolutionaries soon crumbled under the onslaughts of a toxic culture that was anything but enlightened. While the impact of the countercultural movement continues to influence events and the cultural conversation even today, no one believes any more that the psychedelic revolution catalyzed a global shift in our collective consciousness. This perception may be incorrect, however.

The seeds of the psychedelic revolution did not take root in the streets of Haight-Ashbury in the Summer of Love. Instead, it originated in another event in San Francisco that took place several months earlier, in January 1967. In the final week of January that year, a three day symposium that was virtually secret at the time was held at the San Francisco Medical Center (which later became UCSF) under the sponsorship of the National Institute of Mental Health. The symposium was titled the Ethnopharmacologic Search for Psychoactive Drugs. It brought together the leading investigators in disparate related fields, and there were few at the time. The conference was a landmark event marking the current state of knowledge in the search for novel psychoactive drugs in nature. Apart from a few specialists, almost no one noticed. The conference was closed to the public. Although funded by taxpayers, their only benefit was the eventual publication of the proceedings by the U. S. Government Printing Office (US Public Health Service publication #1645).

Somehow a copy of the book fell into my hands at the age of 18. It changed my life. It made me aware that there even was such a thing as ethnopharmacology, and moreover, that much of the field was focused on novel or obscure psychedelics. The conference proceedings inspired me to pursue a career in this odd discipline, and it has defined the trajectory of my professional life for nearly 60 years.

Originally the US Government had planned to organize follow-up symposia to the original ESPD conference about every ten years or so. The War on Drugs came along and the idea was abandoned. That the government had even sponsored such a conference became an embarrassment for them.

Fifty years after the original conference, I joined forces with colleagues to organize a fifty year commemorative symposium. Everything came together to make it happen; proper venue, and funding to invite a variety of researchers in the field. We held the conference in the spring of 2017 at Tyringham Hall, a lovely country estate in the UK. Thanks to generous support, we were able to include the proceedings of the 1967 conference, together with the 2017 conference, in a beautiful boxed set. This was published by Synergetic Press in 2018, in partnership with the Heffter Research Institute.

Publication of this double volume set marked the start of a tradition. In 2022, we organized and presented ESPD55, this time under the imprimatur of the McKenna Academy of Natural Philosophy, published in 2025.

Plans are already underway to present ESPD60, the 60th anniversary of the original symposium, again in the UK, in the Spring of 2027.

The ethnopharmacologic search for psychoactive drugs continues with the quest more important than ever. In the interim between 1967 and 2025, psychedelics, once vilified, have now become recognized for their therapeutic applications. The potential for the discovery of novel psychoactive molecules in plants, fungi, and animals remains high. Discoveries stemming from this work may yield compounds capable of treating a variety of psychological and neurological disorders. And, in an era when species, indigenous knowledge, and habitats are disappearing, the mission is more important and more urgent than ever.

We are grateful for the careful work of the Managing Editor, Rebecca Lazarou, and the Associate Editors for this Volume, Gabrielle Bangay, Nigel Gericke, and Wade Davis, to bring these proceedings to you.

Abbotsford, British Columbia
September 2025

ARCHAEOSPHERE

Ancient Psychoactive Plant Use in Ethnobotanical Archaeology

Chemically-Induced Otherworldly Journeys of Zoroastrian Magi in Iran

Shauheen Etminan, PhD

Founder of VCENNA | Chemical engineer

> *"There have been several speculations about the botanical identity of haoma. Among these candidates, the only one that mysteriously has secured its place in the house of every Iranian, including today's population with 98% non-Zoroastrian, is Peganum Harmala!"*
>
> —SHAUHEEN ETMINAN

Iran holds many ancient spiritual traditions that have included psychoactive plants and fungi. In this essay the ethnopharmacology of psychoactive substances in Iran is explored.

Access to the invisible and intangible realm of Mēnôg (middle Persian - مینو) is mentioned in the Zarathustra's Gâthâ, the most ancient part of the Zoroastrian's holy book Avesta. The Gathas describe Mēnôg as a realm of pure thought and wisdom, beyond the physical world. The trance state of M'ana (معنا) is also referred to by renowned Persian mystics and poets Rumi and Hafez. These states are commonly described as a special illumination that transcends language and perception and allows access to a higher level of consciousness. The pursuit of the world of M'ana is deeply mystified in the Persian literature of post-Islam-occupation Iran. However, in these mystic traditions, a vision of the spirit world is not achieved through neurochemical intervention; rather, it is experienced by divine grace as a reward for saintliness. In contrast, ancient Zoroastrian priests gained their omniscient wisdom and knowledge of mēnôg existence before death by drinking an inebriating botanical liquid extract called *Haoma*. The sacred drink was believed to allow the priest to enter the spiritual realm and communicate with the divine entities residing there. This ritualistic use of Haoma is also described in the Avesta.

There have been multiple speculations about the botanical identity of Haoma, or its Vedic version *Soma* to be the fly agaric mushroom (*Amanita Muscaria)*, ephedra (*Ephedra sinica*), black henbane (*Hyoscyamus niger*), psilocybin mushroom (*Psilocybe stropharia cubensis*), bhang (*Cannabis indica*), and wild rue (*Peganum harmala*). However, among these candidates, the only one that has mysteriously secured its place in the house of every Iranian (including in today's population, which is 98% non-Zoroastrian) is *Peganum harmala*. Known as espand (اسپند) in Farsi, they burn the dry brown seeds of wild Rue for its purifying smoke and earthy scent. This ritual is said to avert the devil's eyes and keep negative energies away from their day-to-day lives, with many Iranians barely knowing that the seeds contain strong psychoactive compounds. Like Yaǵe

(*Banisteriopsis Caapi*) in the Amazonian shamanic brew Ayahuasca , *Peganum Harmala* is a rich source of psychoactive beta-carboline alkaloids, harmine, and harmaline. In their book *Haoma and Harmaline*, David Flattery and Martin Schwartz concluded that *Peganum Harmala* was the original intoxicating plant in the Iranian religious potion Haoma.

This article will review the most detailed Iranian accounts of hallucinogenic intoxication for religious purposes through four otherworldly journeys. The journey of Arda Viraz (Ardā Wirāz Nāmag) is also shared, and he is said to have a vision of the fate of souls after death. Astoundingly, in Arda Viraz's story, the hallucinogenic journey preparation protocols (set, setting, and dose) are described. This allowed him to safely transition to an otherworldly dreamlike state where visions of the other realm were illuminated. By investigating the quality of subjective experiences and the neuropharmacology of different plants on the body, the botanical nature of the Zoroastrians' Haoma was re-examined.

THE MAGIC OF IRAN

Iran and the West have not had friendly relations for the past four decades. The fall of Mohammad Reza Pahlavi, the last *Shah* of Iran, in 1979 was followed by the Iranian Revolution. The 1979 Revolution was supposedly a social movement to end political restraints and oppressions and bestow more freedom on Shah's criticizers, including Islamists, communists, and nationalists. Instead, the 8-year-long war imposed by Iraq on Iran and backed by Western countries, actually served the Islamist hardliners as their narrative was able to dominate. They suffocated and eliminated all the alternative voices who participated in the revolution's triumph. This derailed Iran from a path to democracy and flourishment in the international community for multiple decades.

For the past 45 years, Iran has been associated with Ayatollahs and their anti-West nuclear threats in the Western media. The crippling US and EU sanctions on the Iranian economy have not changed the hardliner's level of hostility but instead has enabled the militia cartels to take over the whole country, isolated the Iranian people from the rest of the world, and impoverished and humiliated the middle class significantly. This reductionist narrative of Iran, produced by Western politicians and media and consumed globally, is far from the true nature of this land. It does not portray this lands potential, its people's philosophies or their ways of life.

Unlike the hyper-masculine and cruel essence often portrayed in the media, Iran has actually been home to different people, ethnicities, and faiths for over three millennia. Iran's super diverse geographical and anthropological landscape is the foundation for a symbiotic life amongst its people. Additionally, the long history and blend of early and advanced civilizations have sculpted the people's collective mindset so that *moderation* remains the natural theme and sustainable way of life. Extremist movements in the history of Iran have been rejected by mass and were dampened to milder social activations and responses. This is an important note about Iran in Western Asia, which is vastly misunderstood in the West. This inherent moderative approach and natural sense of symbiosis arises from a collective wisdom that holds space for everyone. It reflects Iran's feminine face, which this author calls Iran's *Magic*. This Magic owes its existence to a collective *state of mind* that appreciates diversity and has shown its intricacies in Iranian mysticism, literature, arts, and architecture. Despite the internal Islamist hardliners' deculturalization, oppression and corruption, and external media's propaganda, this Magic has not lost its power. As a philosophy and state of mind, it is worth elucidating.

While this article was written, a new uprising was sparked in Iran after the death of Mahsa Amini, who was in the custody of the Islamic regime's morality police for not wearing a proper compulsory hijab. The revolt results from a nation entirely sick of a corrupted theocracy. This has summoned the feminine Magic of Iran, birthing one of the most progressive social movements seeking democracy with the powerful slogan "Woman- Life- Freedom". Let's hope Iranians reclaim their lost identity and freedom in this difficult historical moment.

TODAY'S IRAN AND ARYANS

Iran, known as Persia until 1935, is a nation located in a specific section of a broader cultural and linguistic realm belonging to the Iranian group. This region encompasses not only Iran but also Afghanistan and Tajikistan, and its inhabitants speak a variety of languages, including Persian (Farsi), Dari, Tajiki, Ossetian, Kurdish, Pashto, Baluchi, and Sogdian. In ancient times, the Iranian people comprised not only Persians, Medes, Sogdians, and Bactrians but also the Scythians, Sarmatians, and Alans (Flowers 2017).

Proto-Indo-Iranians, called Aryans, migrated from the Eurasian Steppes between 2500 and 2000 BC to present-day Afghanistan, Eastern Iran, and the Indus Valley. These Indo-Iranian speakers shared numerous cultural, mystic, and religious traits. The Persian term Iranshahr* refers roughly to the Iranian plateau and the adjacent plains, regions ruled by different Iranian dynasties for an extended period.

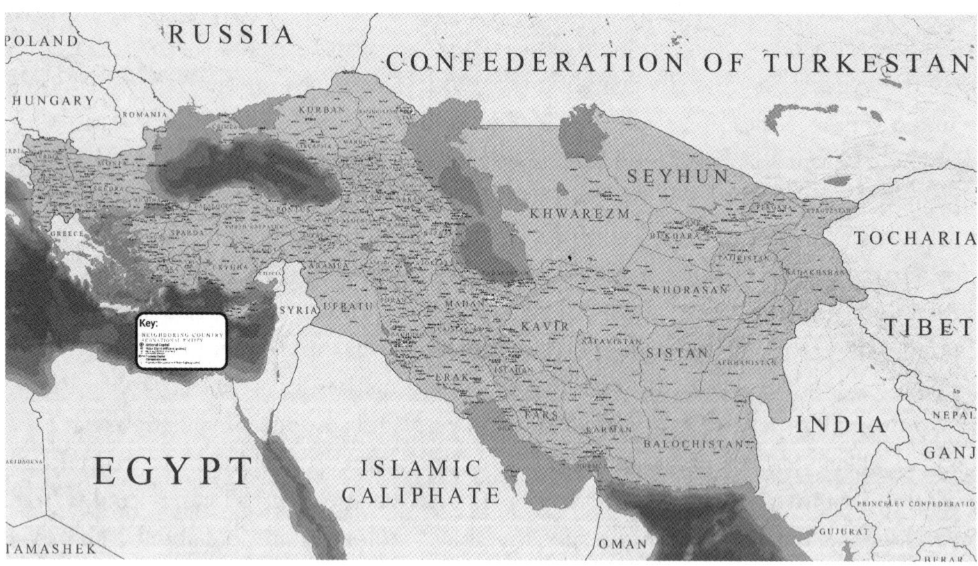

Fig. 1 An imaginative schematic of ancient Iranshahr on the Iranian Plateau (Nizam n.d.).

* Ērānšahr or Greater Iran

PAGANISM AND SHAMANISM IN IRAN AND THE USE OF CHEMICAL INTOXICANTS FOR OTHERWORLDLY JOURNEYS

Before the rise of Zarathustra and his first monotheistic philosophy, Zoroastrianism, pagan priests in the Iranshahr had legitimate offices (Karapan, Iranica Encyclopaedia 2012, 550) in society and promoted and worshiped multiple deities. These deities, gods, and demons were described as forces in nature (sun, wind, water, moon), human-related values (ethics, femininity) and misvalues (war, greed). Some of these deities were shared between Iranians and Indian Vedic daevas, like Asura/Ahura and Soma/Haoma, and some widely among Indo-Europeans, Mesopotamian and Greek deities, like Mithra. Moreover, rituals such as sacrificing animals to deities, and offering libations before the Gods, were heavily practiced in earnest by the Indo-Iranian religious groups.

These Pre-Zoroastrian Iranian religions were dominated by communities of priests and warriors who engaged in ecstatic practices. Based on ancient Indo-Iranian poems, certain classes of pagan priests, such as Usijs, Kawis, and Karapans, participated in the drinking and burning of sacred psychoactive and hallucinogenic natural extracts. Priests performed shamanic ecstasies and otherworldly journeys (Daryaee 2020, Nyberg 1938) to encounter deities and receive affirmations about the truth of their faiths. Warriors consumed these intoxicating drinks to provoke their sense of furiousness and bravery on the battlefields.

Indian Soma and its Iranian equivalent, Haoma, was identified in Vedic and Avestan poems as a deity and a psychoactive intoxicant. The presence of a psychoactive drink that facilitates access to after-death realms, is one of multiple indicators of the shamanic nature of the ancient religions in Iran. The concept of having a 'double soul' living in parallel with the intangible, invisible, and spiritual world is also shamanic (Ginoux 1979, Culiano 1990). This non-materialistic realm is referred to as *mēnôg* in the ancient Iranian religions. Based on David Flattery's research (Flattery and Schwartz 1989), in ancient Iranian religion visions into the spirit world were not thought to be attained by divine grace nor as a reward for saintliness; instead, it was achieved by priests as a result of haoma intoxication. This statement is in congruence with Mircea Eliade's view that the magico-religious value of intoxication for achieving ecstasy is of Iranian origin (Eliade 1951).

ZARATHUSTRA: A POET, REFORMING PRIEST & PHILOSOPHER

Zarathustra is primarily known to the West through the magnum opus of the German philosopher Friedrich Nietzche's, *Thus Spoke Zarathustra* (Nietzche 1883). He is widely regarded as the first teacher of wisdom who established a moral system. Known as *Zoroaster* in Greek, he is recognized as the prophet of ancient Iran, whose lifetime is estimated to be between 1400 to 1000 BCE. Born into a wealthy family of cattle runners, as a youth, he was trained as a *Zoatar*, which is a priest of ancient Iran. Zarathustra's reforms and the transformation of his pagan-shamanic inherited polytheistic religion(s) established a philosophical foundation that became the dominant religion in Iran until the conquest of Persia by Islam around 650 AD.

Through his revelations in a dreamy state, Zoroaster received omniscient wisdom that showed him an ultimate truth/order (*asha*), and the sovereignty of a supreme creator of the uni-

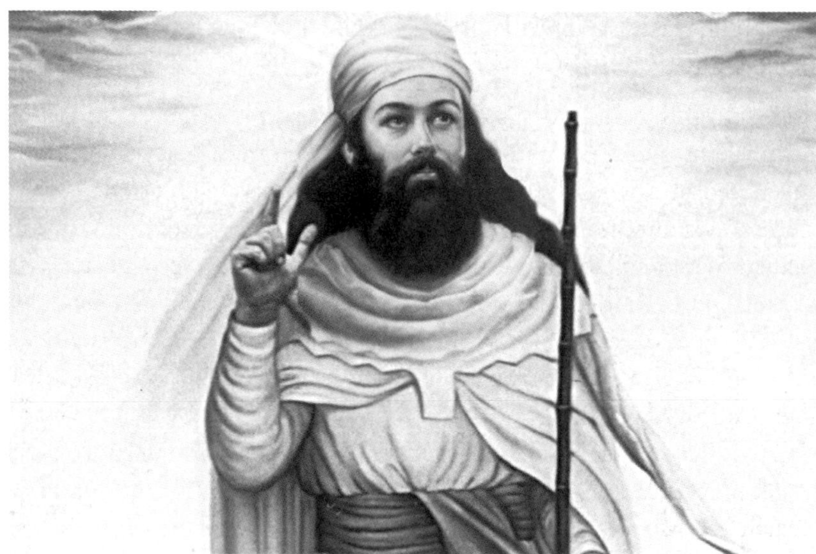

Fig. 2 Ancient Iranian Poet, Priest and Protagonist Philosopher, Zarathustra (~1700 BCE) (Zoroastrian Association of Metropolitan Washington Inc. 2023).

verse that he identified as the 'Lord of Wisdom' (*Ahura Mazda**). This is thought to have been illuminated by absolute focused consciousness. As a rebellious protagonist and priest, he revolutionized the polytheistic pantheon of his pagan precedents and established the first monotheistic philosophy based on the dominion of superior consciousness. The primary reforms ascribed to Zoroaster were ceasing from sacrificing animals for multiple pagan deities and his disapproval of the so-called Haoma-cult priests as wicked priests who misled their followers. Daryaee (2020) believes Zoroaster appears to have condemned Haoma intoxication practices because it promoted worshipping pagan deities, the most prominent being Mithra.

While Zoroaster's birthplace and time are not precisely known, a corpus of seventeen poems he composed in the Old Avestan language has survived. These are foundational documents of the Zoroastrian religion (Louchakova-Scgwartz 2018). The Gathas are Zarathustra's most profound contemplations and ideas that address moral choices and human's relationship with the divine. These poems were not transcribed until over a thousand years later and were transferred orally in the format of acrostics. Like Rumi and Hafez's poetry, Gatha's hymns are highly intellectual, esoteric, and linguistically super complex.†

Besides Ahura Mazda and Asha, the third element of Zarathustra's subjective triad is the Good Mind (*Vohu Manah*). Based on the Gatha, devotion and exercise of the following virtues;

---

* In Avestan, Maz is equivalent to brain and Ahura Mazda alleges the importance of thinking, thoughtfulness and contemplation.

† Prof. Martin Schwartz has dedicated close to half a century to decipher Gatha, and position Zarathustra's hymns as sophisticated metrical poetry with intentionally enigmatic lexical and synthetic ambiguities. They have coded alliterations and include a technique of scrambling critical words, ring-compositional generation of poems out of the sequential vocabulary of preceding poems, and quasi-spatial compositional patterns.

Good Thoughts, Good Words, and Good Deeds, can make an individual commune with the higher consciousness and receive insight through the Good Mind. Moral dualism posits itself firmly in Mazdaen's (Zoroastrian) philosophy and manifests as good and evil, constructive and destructive, orderly and chaotic, and most fundamentally, the conscious (wise) and un-conscious (ignorant) (Flowers 2017).

MAZDAYASNA, AVESTA AND ZOROASTRIANISM AS RELIGION

Besides Zoroastrianism, Zoroaster's philosophy was also known as the *Mazdayasna* religion. Two of the most glorious Iranian empires, the Achaemenids (559 to 330 BC) and Sasanids (224 to 651 AD) followed the Mazdaen religion. The former followed unofficially and the latter officially as its state religion. However, Zarathustra's reforms to the polytheistic pagan nature of the Iranian religion did not last long amongst his followers. Over time, other hymns ascribed to Zoroaster were added to Gatha through later Zoroastrian priests, *Magi** (plural of mogus). These sacred hymns, including Gatha, are called the Younger Avesta and reinstate some pagan gods, practices and rituals denounced by Zarathustra. For instance, while Zarathustra acknowledges Ahura Mazda as the only God and demonizes the other deities, one of the most extended hymns of Avesta, *Mithra (Mihr) Yasht*, states that Ahura Mazda created Mithra equal to himself† (Malandra 1983).

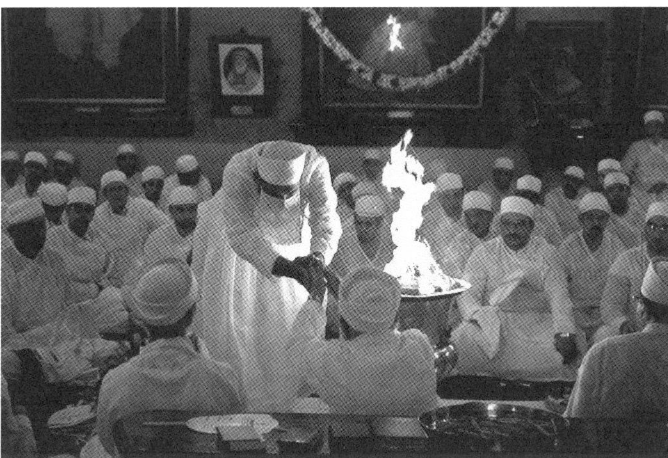

Fig. 3 Priests of Zoroastrian pantheon, Magi attending in Jashn ceremony in Mumbai in 2011 (Photo: Kainaz Amaria).

Zoroastrianism remained the official religion of Iranians until the invasion of Arab Muslims, the occupation of Iran, and the fall of the Sasanid dynasty. This was when Zoroastrian clergies had societal power, the religion had become ritual focused, and the priestly class had become oppressive towards the general laity (Eduljee 2005). Like other Indo-Europeans, the early Iranians had a social hierarchy and caste system for three social classes: warriors, clerics, and farmers. After the

---

* Plural of mogus, or مغ in Persian

† All stanzas of this Mithra Yasht hymns start with "We worship Mithra…"

conquest of Iran by the Islamic caliphate, Zoroastrians remained in Iran. Mistreated by the new theology and under coercion, they had three choices: death, conversion, or paying tax. Based on Boyce (Boyce 2001), there was a steady stream of converts, some willing, while for some, the new faith was enforced upon them. Sir Jean Chardin, a French traveler who visited Iran during the Safavid epoch, wrote that 40% of Iranians were Zoroastrians (Chardin 1711). Considering Iran's population to have been between 5 to 10 million in that era, 2 to 4 million Zoroastrians lived in Iran in the late Safavid time. Today's population of Zoroastrians is estimated to be 120,000 to 200,000, mainly residing in India and Iran (Riventa 2012).

HAOMA: ELIXIR OF TRUTH

One of the pagan/shamanic concepts reintroduced into the Zoroastrian religion in the Younger Avesta and imputed to Zarathustra is the use of the hallucinogenic intoxicant, Haoma. The Proto-Indo-Iranians who lived in the Eurasian Steppes as their early homeland sanctified Haoma/Soma at the center of their rituals. The preparation was said 'to press out', with both words inferring that they were not essentially a plant or fungal species but a juice or an aqueous extract. Later, Hôm/Haoma and Soma were recognized as the name of a plant whose identity has been the subject of research and speculation for over 200 years.

The use of Haoma/Soma by the Iranian and Indian ancestors returns to the same period. However, since Avesta was transcribed to text from verbal poems a thousand years later than Rigveda,* the allusions to the sacred intoxicant are considered more conservative. Rigveda has pointed to Soma both metaphorically and with extensive poetic elaboration. Therefore, the ethnopharmacological search for the intoxicating effect of *Haoma* in Zoroastrian texts is more likely to draw reliable and accurate conclusions. While the ritualistic intoxicant name remained unchanged, the botanical formulation used a variety of substitutes whose extracts could scarcely induce altered mental states written about in more genuine references (Malandra 1983). Therefore, it is unsurprising that due to the different flora of Iran and India, the psychoactive ingredient substitutes of Soma and Haoma have been dissimilar.

Most referrals to Haoma's psychoactive effect define it as the *Elixir of Truth*. Drinking Haoma evokes an altered state, like induced mindlessness, that enables the mind to grasp deep truths. This state is described as a special illumination and incorporeal psychic vision, a form of transcendental knowledge beyond language and perception (Culiano 1990). The Haoma experience facilitates a glimpse into after-death realms, but this is available only to righteous ones. A second

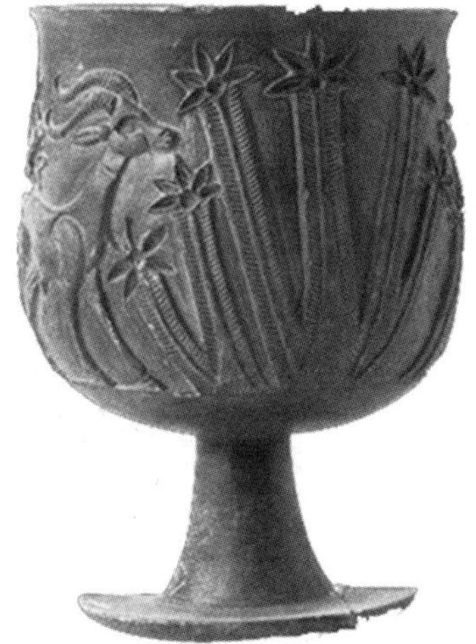

Fig. 4 A 5000-year Jiroft civilization object with plants similar to Peganum Harmala bush & flowers (Muscarella 2001).

* The Rigveda is the oldest known Vedic Sanskrit text.

allusion to the effect of the pressed-out extract is exhilaration, fury, and wrath, which aroused a warlike brotherhood among warriors. Haoma was consumed only in ritual settings, was charged with sacred power, and was infused with the divine essence.

HAOMA IN POST GATHA ZOROASTRIAN TEXTS

The contents of post-Gathic Avesta hymns and other Zoroastrian religious texts were devised by Magi and adherents of Zarathustra.

There are direct referrals and an entire hymn, Hôm Yasht (Yasna 9 -11), about Haoma in Younger Avesta. In these texts, there are a few referrals to the physical identity of Haoma. For instance, regardless of the type of plant, only its stems and stalks were pressed to yield Haoma. Also, the referral to the color ranges from brown to yellow (zairi/hari). Haoma's epithet is *radiant,* and Malandra (Malandra 1983) concludes it was yellow. Finally, it was alluded that the plant source was found in mountainous heights and that the juice had medicinal properties.

Hôm Yasht starts with a long conversation between Zarathustra and Haoma, where the prophet praises and reveres Haoma as he who keeps death away and grants health. These hymns seem like a dialogue ascribed to Zarathustra with Haoma's (plant) spirit while under its intoxicating psychoactive effect. He praises Haoma and asks for its protective power against death and daeva-created lies, jealousy, sorcery, and destructive people. Within these hymns, certain stanzas suggest that Zarathustra differentiated between the benevolent Haoma and the one accompanied by anger (possibly taken by warriors). The first endows blissful truth, and the horrible and bloody club used the latter. Stanza 17 of Yasna 9 says:

> *"I call down, O yellow (Haoma), your intoxicating power, strength, victoriousness, ability to grant health, curativeness, prosperity, growth, the force for the entire body, complete knowledge, (and) I call down this that I may go about among beings autonomously, overcoming hostility, defeating the lie." (Malandra, 1983)*

Referral to Haoma appears in *Zand-i-Wahman Yasht*, a late 9th-century Zoroastrian apocalyptic book indicating that based on Old Avesta, Zarathustra's revelation occurred through Haoma (Flattery and Schwartz 1989, 33).

HAOMA IN ZARATHUSTRA'S GATHA

Today's Zoroastrians dissociate their faith entirely from using hallucinogenic intoxicants. A majority firmly believe their prophet condemned the application of psychoactive drugs and the Haoma cult. The following allusions in Gatha are Zoroastrians' source of distancing from Haoma.

For decades, the only understanding of Gatha's referral to Haoma was limited to Yasna 48.10, where Zarathustra relates the use of an intoxication effect to the camp of his rivals *Karapan* priests, who were allegedly the misrulers of the lands. Karapans are described as wicked and false priests who misled people. The exact Old Avestan word for intoxication is *Madho* which in today's Farsi means 'drunk' or 'in a state of losing one's mind.'*

Through his advanced discovery of decrypting complex interrelated Gatha hymns, Schwartz (Schwartz 2022) has recently revealed that a direct mention of Haoma arises at the beginning of Yasna 32.10, related to the Zoroaster's rebuke of the mythical founder of the Haoma cult, mentioned earlier in Yasna 32.8.

An epithet of Haoma in Gatha is *dūraoša,* which refers to the burning of the intoxicating botanical source of Haoma used *to help* repel evil. This was interpreted to have been used for its apotropaic benefits.

MAGI AND THEIR OTHERWORLDLY JOURNEYS

Matthew's Bible (2:1-12) refers to *Magi* as Three Wise Men or Three Kings and noble pilgrims from the East who predicted the nativity of Jesus through their intricate knowledge of astrology. They followed a miraculous rising star to Bethlehem, where they paid homage to the newborn Jesus as the king of the Jewish people and brought him three gifts of gold, frankincense, and myrrh. When they learned that King Herod was after finding the infant Jesus to kill him, they returned to their land without disclosing the location of the newborn's nativity. In the Bible, there is no referral to the country of the Magi.

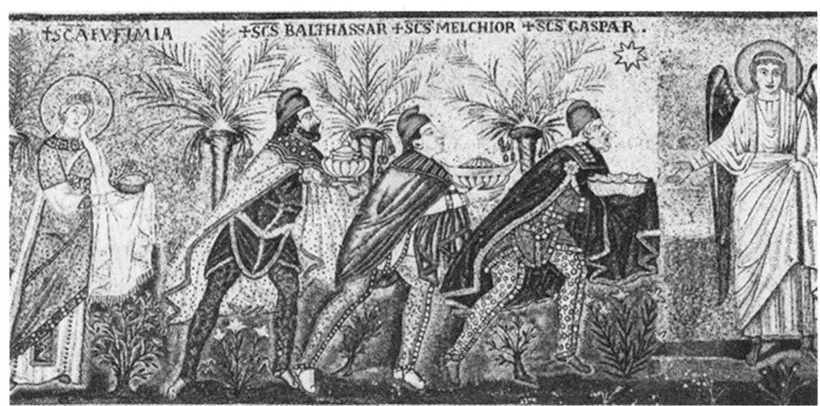

Fig. 5 The Three Wise Men, Magi, in Iranian costumes. Mosaic in the Basilica of Sant'Apollinare Nuovo, in Ravenna, Italy, completed within 526 AD by the so-called 'Master of Sant'Apollinare'.

In Gatha 29.11, Zarathustra asks Ahura Mazda when the society of his patrons accepts his teaching. Magi or *Magāi* †, was the title of Zoroastrian priests and sincere friends of Zarathustra who helped him effectively progress his new philosophy. Greeks called Persian priests Magi because they thought they were sorcerers with supernatural powers in their control. Etymologically, this is the root of the word *Magic*. Magic was the art of the Magi.

* There is an exact word in late Persian, today's Farsi "مدهش" defines as losing ones mind.

† In today's Farsi language: مغان

The art of ancient time Zoroastrian priests was their mastery of seeing into mēnôg existence and the spirit world before death, and making it visible to living people. Based on the Yasna rite, access to and seeing the visions of mēnôg, and the practice of dying before death must have been experienced and acquired as an initiation for Zoroastrian priests (Flattery and Schwartz, 1989). Based on Flattery (1989), in ancient Iranian religion, there was no substantial evidence of non-pharmacologically induced meditative practices for evoking visions of altered states. Also, these visions were not achieved due to divine grace or as a reward for saintliness. Instead, the consumption of Haoma facilitated the transition to the world of after-death.

The consumption of Haoma as an intoxicant was restricted to the caste of priests and those whom the Magi chose to enroll (priests, kings, righteous ones)*. Haoma extract was prepared in the Yasna ritual by a senior priest called *Raspi*. It was to be served to the priesthood candidate for an initiation, or another priest whose surrender to truth was the intention throughout the ceremony. Zoatar is the priest who drinks Haoma in the Yasna ceremony, and an extract prepared in his absence but must be ingested under the scrutiny of six additional priests. This assembly witnessed how Zoater responded to the elixir's hallucinogenic and intoxicating effects and, based on his level of surrendering to the truth, judged if he was one of the righteous. Based on Yasna 11.10, Zoatar must have surrendered his body to the intoxicant to be a follower of truth (Flattery and Schwartz 1989). Hence, the Yasna ritual, in its ancient form, must have been an ordeal. In Yasna 8.4, a punishment for sorcery was deemed for priests who falsely represented themselves. The first part of Stanza 10 of Yasna 11 says:

> *"O righteous Haoma, I dedicate to you this body of mine which seems to me well developed to swift Haoma for intoxication, beatitude, and possession of Truth."*

Today, the format of the Yasna rite has significantly changed. There is no sign of hallucinogenic intoxicants; instead, the liturgies' referral points to these "plants, waters and libation", which Flattery believes must have been referring to Haoma. This priestly ritual has allegedly not been conducted in Iran since 1962.† The Yasna rituals in the Zoroastrian Parsi community in India have been performed only symbolically and for its liturgical aspect, where the intoxicating property of Haoma is substituted with a mild relaxing effect.

Ancient Zoroastrian references describe the otherworldly journeys of Magi to occur in a dreamlike or sleep state called *xvafena*. This state is where the mystical voyager, Zarathustra, Zoroastrian priests, and other righteous candidates experienced a trance or hallucinogenic state (Culiano 1990, Daryayee 2020, Flattery and Schwartz 1989), cross-passed planes of meaning (Louchakova-Schwartz 2018), and instantly received awareness from the unknown and mēnôg. Four accounts of these dreamlike, otherworldly journeys are presented in the following, with documented references to drinking a mind-altering potion before the event.

* Rulers, kings and rightous candidates were among non-priesthood who drank an intoxicant as part of a religious practice.

† Based on Prof. Touraj Daryaee, the last Yasna Ceremony was held in Iran was in Sharif Abad of Yazd and conducted by Moubed Soroushian.

I. ZARATHUSTRA'S REVELATION

Being a Zoatar of ancient Iranian religion, it is expected that Zarathustra must have had an experience with Haoma. Based on *Zand-i-Wahman Yasht*, a 9th Pahlavi apocalyptic text of the Zoroastrian religion, Zoroaster's revelation was brought to him by Ahura Mazda and through Haoma. During a dream of seven days and nights, he received omniscient wisdom in the form of a liquid poured on his hands to drink. The induced dream, visions, and all-knowing wisdom allowed him to see the conditions of the righteous and unrighteous in the other world (Flattery and Schwartz 1989, 33). Based on Wahman Yasht (stanzas 12 and 13), when on day seven of the dream, the omniscient wisdom was taken back from Zoroaster, he reflected as:

> *"I saw something in the pleasant Ahura Mazda-created dream; I have not yet recovered from the dream. From the end of time I slept, I have not yet recovered from this pleasant Ahura Mazda-created dream."*

Besides, based on the nature of Zarathustra's poems, Louchakova-Schwartz phenomenologically elaborates on how Zarathustra achieved the consciousness of Gatha's hymn 30 through a dreamy state (Louchakova-Schwartz 2018).

II. JOURNEY OF KING WISHTASP, ZARATHUSTRA'S PATRON

Based on Denkird,* a 9th-century Pahlavi text, *Kay Wishtasp,* king of Zoroaster's time, accepted his teachings and philosophy by drinking hôm and *mang*. He received visions and saw into the mēnôg existence during the three-day and night near-death experience (Culiano 1990, Daryaee 2020) of *stardness. Stardīh,* in Pahlavi, is a state of mind equivalent to 'spreading out' into the broader consciousness, where the great mysteries are revealed. This state outwardly resembles sleep. Wishtasp journeyed through the upper paradise (Flattery and Schwartz 1989, 28-30), and when he came forth from stardīh , he called for Zoroaster and became his true patron. Other references this state out as the effect of haoma intoxication (Flattery and Schwartz 1989, 29).

The potion offered to King Wishtasp was called "*mang of Wishtasp*" and is speculated to be a combination of hôm and henbane.

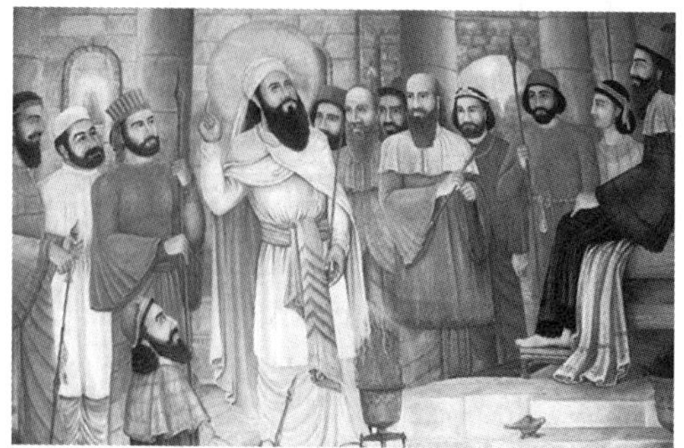

Fig. 6 Zarathustra sharing his teaching with Kay (King) Wishtasp—Painting from a Zoroastrian temple in Isfahan, Iran. Image by Ullstein blid-Vodjani

---

* A 9th century Pahlavi text, a summary from a lost Avestan source—BookVII, 4, 84-86

III. VISIONS OF PRIEST KERDIR

Kerdir was the most influential chief priest of the Sasanid epoch in the 3rd century BC. There are multiple inscriptions related to him in Fars province in Iran, narrating his otherworldly journey to the after-death realm, where he was taken to hell and heaven by his *daena* (the divine image of his faith) and his double. Kerdir's daena appeared as an indescribably beautiful woman, implying that he was one of the righteous, as otherwise, his daena would be ugly! (Culiano 1990).

In Kerdir's inscriptions, there is no referral to drinking Haoma, but from the context, it can be assumed he did so (Daryaee 2020).

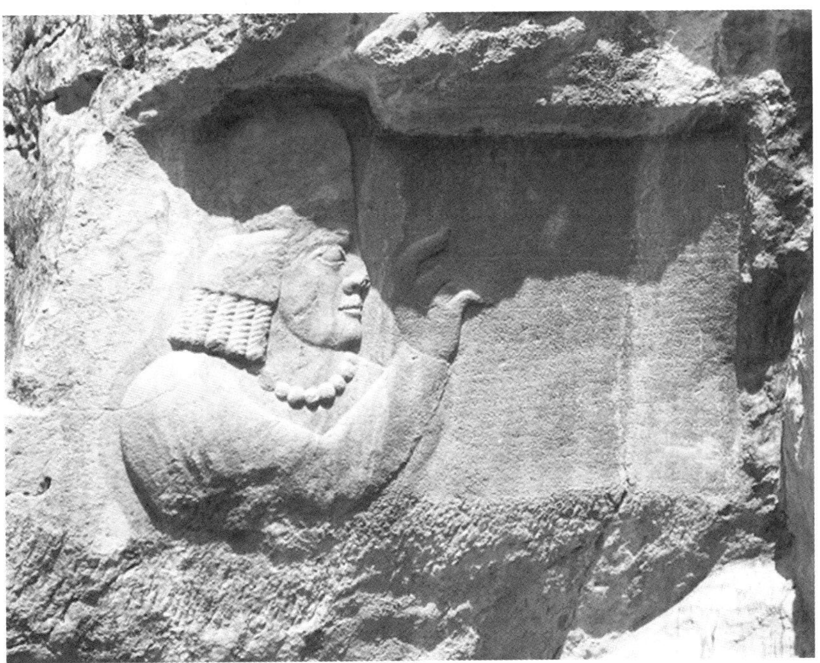

Fig.7 Chief priest Kerdir (Kartir) inscription at Naghshe-e-Rajab, Fars, Iran (5 kilometer North of Persepolis).

IV. JOURNEY OF ARDA VIRAZ

The most detailed and explicit Iranian account of mind-altering and hallucinogenic intoxication for religious purposes does not belong to castes of priests or kings but *Viraz*, who was an ordinary man known for his righteousness. *Arda Viraz Namag*, the Letter of Righteous Viraz, is an eight thousand words 9th century BC Pahlavi book of the Zoroastrian religion.

The narrative refers to a time when there was sedition and contention among the people of the Iranian Kingdom, their religion was in confusion, and people were in doubt (Belardi 1979). The Zoroastrian theologians had little authority left, and followers did not receive their teaching and liturgies. So, an assembly of Magi was summoned in the temple of the victorious Farrbāg fire (Figure 9.2) in Fars. After discussing a solution, they concluded they needed to seek means to their religious doctrines. So, they decided to send someone to go and bring information from the spirits to confirm if their liturgies and rituals were rightfully done and would come to help their soul on doomsday.

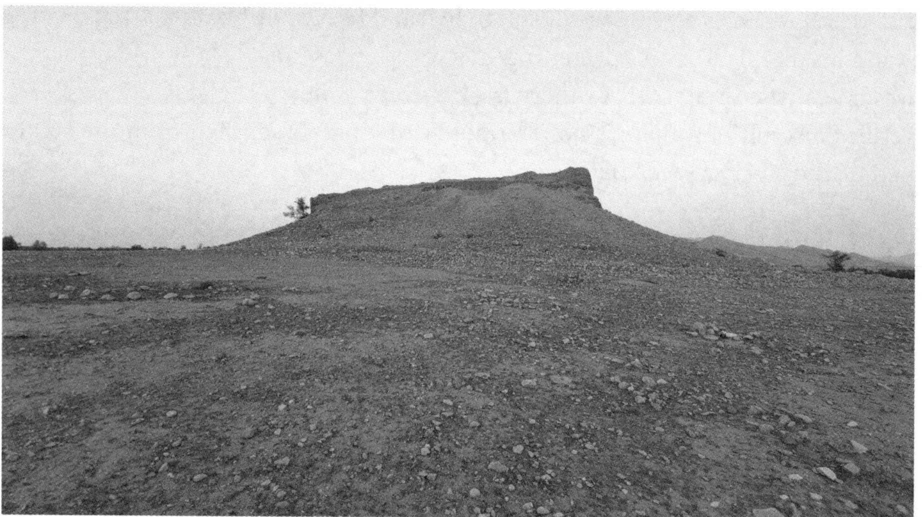

Fig.8 Ruins of Farrbāg fire temple or Adur Farnbag in Fars, Iran (Etminan 2025).

They called people to the fire temple and called on the most righteous to step forward for this ordeal. Among seven, they chose three, and they chose the most sinless and renowned person from the three. His name was Viraz.* At first, he was reluctant and did not desire to drink the intoxicating potion. His seven sisters weeping and crying, opposed the decision and were fearful of Viraz making it to the realm of the dead and not returning. But Mazdayasnean (Zoroastrian) Magi comforted and reassured them that they shall deliver Viraz back to his body, in perfection and with no harm after seven days as he was one of the righteous.

Viraz agreed with the order and asked for some leisure to set intentions by the fire, eat and put on his new garments and perfume. They set up a thirty-step wide stage with an appropriate board like a couch and clean blanket. He lay down on a blanket, ate some *dron* bread, and reminisced about the departed souls. Afterward, the theologians' assembly filled three cups of Mang of Whishtasp† and handed it to Viraz. He drank the mind-altering hallucinogenic potion, consciously said grace, and fell asleep on the blanket.

The Magi priests at the scene in Farrbāg temple and his seven sisters kept the fire burning for seven days, shed scent and recited liturgical poems from Avesta and Gatha. Viraz's body was protected with their care and prayers for seven days and nights with no neglect. When he awakened after day seven, he was cheerful and joyous and brought the greetings of Ahura Mazda, the archangels and Zarathustra to the assembly as the ratification of the righteousness of their rituals and liturgies. Then Viraz asked for some food and shared his visions for them to be written.

---

* Arda or Arday means righteous

† A combination of Haoma and Mang (Black Henbane)

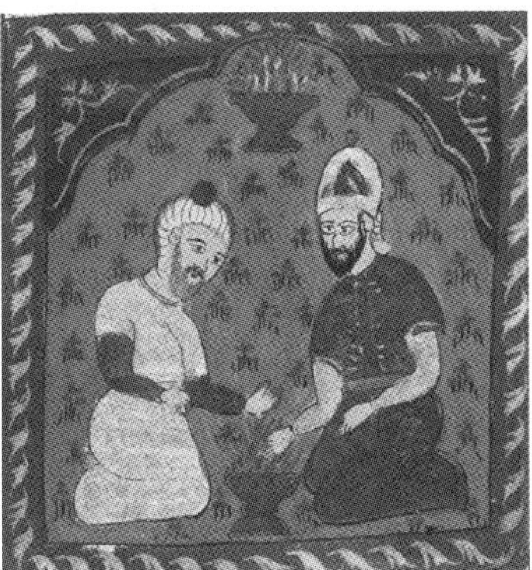

Fig. 9.1 Arda Viraz sitting by fire setting intention to embark on his chemically induced otherworldly journey.

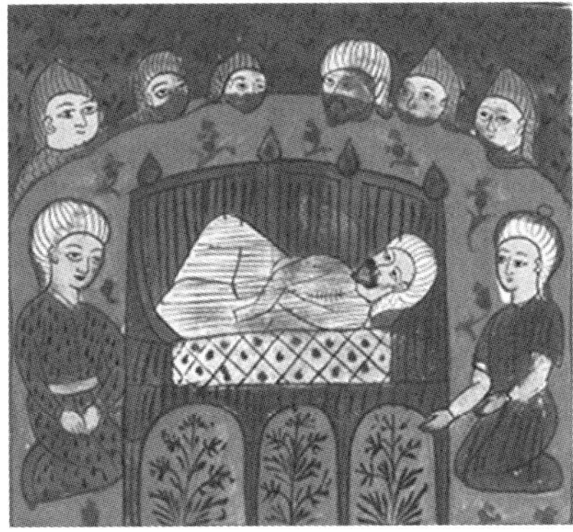

Fig. 9.2 Arda Viraz in Farrbag fire temple, surrounded by his seven sisters, after taking the Mang-e-Wishtasp potion (two types of plants in Homji's illustrations).

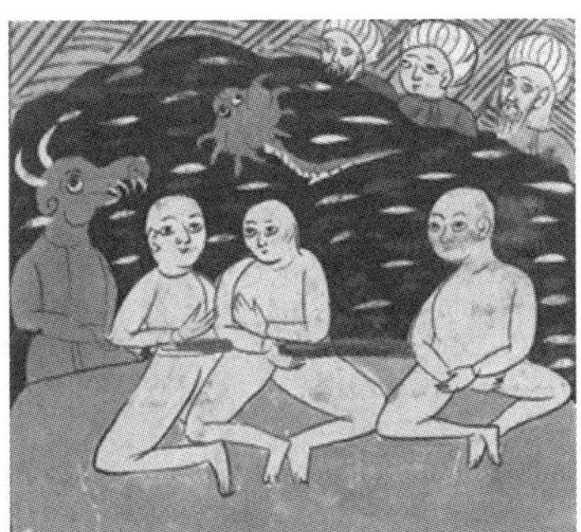

Fig. 9.3 Arda Viraz visiting the hell aided by Srosha & Adur angels.

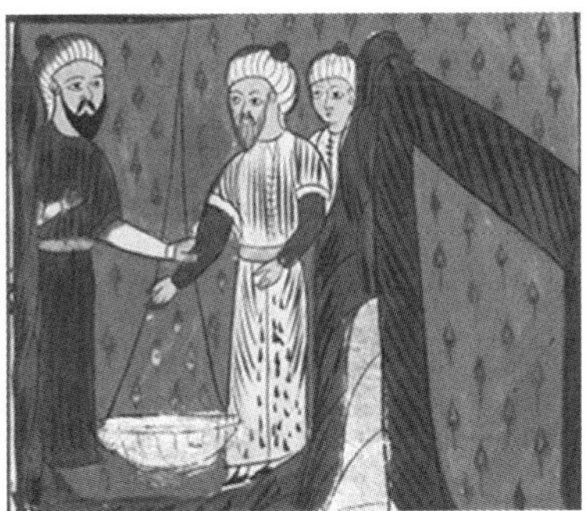

Fig. 9.4 Arda Viraz at Chinwad Bridge protected by god Mihr.

Illustrations credit: Homji 1789

The rest of the book describes Viraz's otherworldly journey to the realm of spirits and his visions of heaven and hell, where he was escorted by two spirit guides who interpreted what he saw. The reward of the good and retributions of the wicked souls in each stage of heaven and hell are delineated visually. Arda Viraz Namag is the apocalyptic Iranian Divine Comedy written a thousand years before Dante Alighieri's eponymous masterpiece.

Like King Wishtasp, Viraz drinks a psychoactive combination of plants referred to as a mixture of vine and mang, or hôm and mang. Some researchers have compared mang, also called bang/banj, with Sanskrit bhang, which primarily means hemp . However, until the 12th century, the word bang in Persian books means henbane (Belardi 1979).

HAOMA INTOXICATION

Haoma, the potent psychoactive drug that served as an Elixir of Truth, was eventually eliminated from the Zoroastrian pantheon. This was despite being used to test the righteousness of priests and rulers and to help unravel the mystery of life after death. The eponymous extract and liturgies, prepared and recited respectively as part of the Yasna rite, stayed in Zoroastrian rituals, but the subjective effect, hallucinogenic properties, and botanical identity of Haoma were substituted later. The exact date of the Haoma formulation substitution is not known. Unlike their ancient mythological ancestors, Zoroastrian priests and followers of today do not associate their faith with chemical intoxication. Instead, they refer to Zarathustra's disapproval of the Haoma cult in Gatha and barely know what Haoma's original subjective effect and use was.

Three main reasons are inferred for the disunification of Zoroastrians from Haoma (as a *potent* psychoactive intoxicant):

1. Haoma was only taken in priestly rituals, and its use and formulation stayed within the caste of elites (Magi and rulers) and never spread out. Hence, when its botanical identity was substituted and its use case changed, the original formulation was perhaps intentionally obscured, forgotten, and lost.
2. As people of the book, Zoroastrians did not want to associate their faith and liturgies to an intoxicating psychoactive drug.
3. After the conquest of Iran by Muslims, Zoroastrian priests, under pressure and attack, feared that Haoma intoxication might associate their faith with sorcery and witchcraft.

HAOMA: BOTANICAL IDENTITY, NEUROPHARMACOLOGY AND SUBJECTIVE EFFECT

Speculation about the botanical identity of Soma/Haoma has a long-standing history. Researchers have used different shreds of evidence to support their hypotheses, discovery, and conclusion on what sort of plant (extract) Haoma could have been. These indications range from metaphorical referrals to Soma/Haoma in Rigveda and Avesta, geography and flora, drugs' physiological symptoms and side effects, pharmacology, and subjective experiences. However, most of these studies have considered Haoma a single plant or fungus and justified their hypotheses around its proof.

Soma/Haoma as the Elixir of Truth had one botanical identity or formulation among Indo-Iranians before they separated in new geographical locations. However, after their migration and due to climate and flora change, and differences in the Iranian plateau and Indian plain, the Aryan settlers could not secure the exact same botanical or fungal source. As a result, from this period, Soma/Haoma terminology was attributed to any sacred ecstatic natural extract or concoction that was consumed in ritual settings and resembled the original subjective effect of these hallucinogenic intoxicants. As such, Haoma/Soma are thought to originate from the fly agaric mushroom (*Amanita Muscaria*), ephedra (*Ephedra sinica*), black henbane (*Hyoscyamus niger*), psilocybin mushroom (*Psilocybe stropharia cubensis*), bhang (*Cannabis indica*), and wild rue (*Peganum harmala*).

Among these speculative candidates, the most relevant choices for Haoma are ephedra and wild rue (*Peganum harmala).* They both fit the mountainous and dry flora of North East and East Iran. The ephedra plant is known as Hôm by the Irani and Parsi Zoroastrian communities in Iran and India. In India, Ephedra is also known as *Somalata.* There are reports that Zoroastrians of Iran have been collecting and shipping Ephedra to their Indian coreligionists. Moreover, *Peganum harmala*, is a sacred plant with numinous power which is wildly abundant in the Iranian plateau region. Two accounts (Wasson 1971, McKenna 1999) relate Soma, not precisely Haoma, to being a mushroom species because the growing criteria of *Amanita Muscaria* and *P. Stropharia Cubensis* are incompatible with the environment of Iranian territories of Indo-Iranian settlers. Nevertheless, *Amanita muscaria* aka *Fly Agaric* mushroom is presented here, as due to R. Gordon Wasson's theory many associate Haoma with *Amanita muscaria*.

SOMA AS A DELIRIANT: AMANITA MUSCARIA

R. Gordon Wasson, the former investment banker and ethnomycologist, played a major role in popularizing the psilocybin mushroom in the West. In exchange for secrecy, he partook in the Mexican curandera, Maria Sabina's underground mushroom healing ceremony. Instead, Wasson ultimately betrayed her and widely published her identity and ceremony photos, resulting in Sabina being jailed and her house being set on fire (Pollan 2018, Gerber et al. 2021, 573-577). In pursuit of other psychoactive mushrooms, in 1971, Wasson published "*Soma: Divine Mushroom of Immortality*" claiming that based on Vedic hymns, Soma was a mushroom, and it was *Amanita muscaria*. Siberian shamans had long used Fly Agaric mushrooms to induce shamanic journeys. Terence McKenna (McKenna 1999) found Wasson's reasoning weak as Fly Agaric did not induce strong visions, and Wasson himself never had an ecstatic experience with these mushrooms.

The known toxic and psychoactive compounds of *Amanita muscaria* are muscarine, muscimol, and ibotenic acids. Muscarine potency in Fly Agaric mushrooms is super low, a range of 0.0002–0.0003 wt % (Feeney 2010). It binds to the muscarinic sites of acetylcholine receptors as an acetylcholine agonist and stimulates the parasympathetic nervous system. Due to its molecular structure, muscarine is not counted as the primary psychoactive compound of *Amanita muscaria*. Muscimol is a $GABA_A$ agonist and a $GABA_C$ partial agonist linked to altered visual and auditory perception (Krogsgaard-Larsen et al 1981). This compound reduces neural excitability and is sedative, anxiolytic, and emetic. Ibotenic acid is the primary source of muscimol when it gets decarboxylated due to metabolism. It acts as an agonist for NMDA glutamate receptors, lowers the NMDA activation, and alters the memory recording of the experience, i.e., generates delirious psychoactive effects. Figure 10 depicts a relational presentation of the affinity of muscimol and ibotenic acid with the $GABA_A$ and glutamate receptors, respectively.

Most of the ibotenic acid is excreted in urine intact. Therefore, if the urine is drunk, it will still be inebriating. Urine drinking is associated with the practice of Siberian shamans. Wasson related the poetic referrals of Soma to urine (drinking) in Rig Veda (Crowley and Shulgin, 2019) and concluded that Soma was *Amanita muscaria*. The drawbacks to Wasson's hypothesis are that mushrooms could be eaten directly without needing to be pressed out. Besides, Flay Agaric mushrooms can't produce incense and do not provide reliable ecstasy. *Amanita muscaria* is recognized as a deliriant with psychoactive delusions and has been known to give an unfavorable mental state. Some people have had pleasant and meaningful experiences with this fungus; however, this is not what it is renowned for. The predominant experience does not match the Zoroastrian

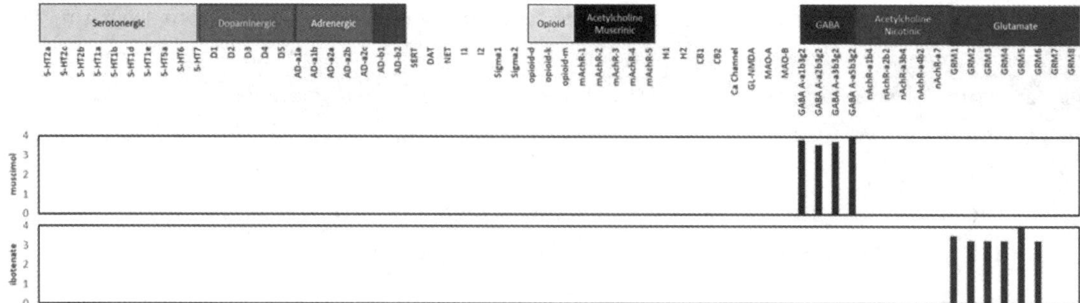

Fig.10 Relative selectivity of muscimol and ibotenic acid to GABA & Glutamate receptors, published inhibitory constant values from the University of North Carolina's Psychoactive Drug Screening Program Ki database (RRID n.d.).

Magi's dreamy state reports and otherworldly inner journeys, nor does it account for the fact that Iran's land in the northeast and East does not accommodate the growth of these mushrooms.

HAOMA AS AN ENTACTOGEN: EPHEDRA

Ephedra is a leafless plant that grows wild in the mountains and is abundant in the flora of Iran. Known as Hôm in Iran, it is the plant that present-day Zoroastrian priests press out with pomegranate twigs and offer as Haoma for drinking and libation. Ephedra was never sanctified, though, and nor was it an incense plant. Twigs of Ephedra are condensed and hard, and pressing them out with a pestle and mortar is cumbersome and relatively inefficient for extracting the active compounds. Flattery (Flattery and Schwartz 1989) believed that Ephedra was not a substitute for Haoma but originally an archaic additive as based on Avesta's Yasna 10.12, Haoma was made of many kinds of species.

Ephedrine is the main active compound in Ephedra, which is an entactogen and not a dream-inducing heavy entheogen. Ephedrine averts sleep and keeps the mind awake. There have been referrals to Haoma as an exhilarating compound taken by warriors for conjuring battle fury, which is consonant with the effect of Ephedrine. However, the otherworldly dreams of the Magi could not have been induced only by an extract mixture of Ephedrine and pomegranate twigs as the physiological impact and the subjective effect of the dreamy state do not pharmacologically match with that of Ephedrine.

Ephedrine is a sympathomimetic agonist at adrenergic receptors. It also displays indirect sympathetic activation, enhancing` the release of norepinephrine. The molecular structure of Ephedrine is comparable to that of methamphetamine, exhibiting less potent CNS effects with more prolonged effects (Soni et al 2004, Gad et al 2021). In Figure 11, the receptor binding profile of Ephedrine is compared with that of 3,4-methylenedioxy-methamphetamine (MDMA).

The receptor binding profiles relatively match, except that MDMA binds to 5HT-2a, 5HT-2b, and 5HT-2c serotonin sites, while Ephedrine does not. Instead, Ephedrine binds strongly to the opioid receptors, making Ephedrine an addictive substance.

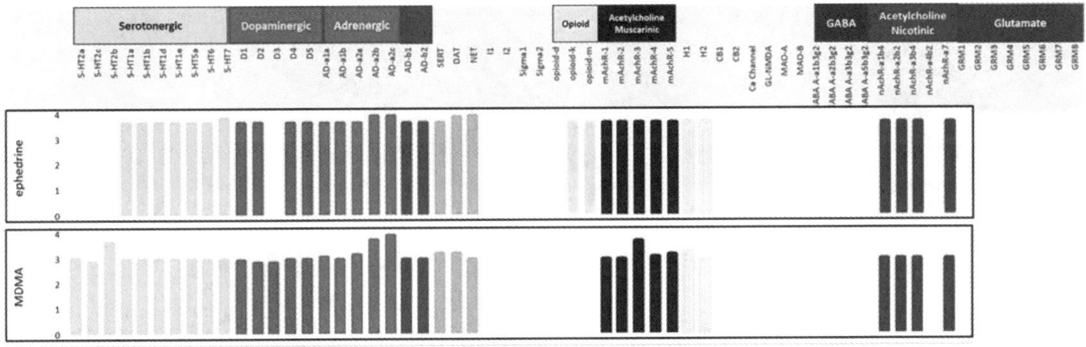

Fig.11 Relative selectivity of ephedrine and MDMA to multiple receptors, published inhibitory constant values from the University of North Carolina's Psychoactive Drug Screening Program Ki database (RRID n.d.).

Even though the entheogenic intoxication of Haoma was substituted with an entactogen within the Zoroastrian priestly pantheon, Flattery believed Ephedra was not the plant that replaced the intoxicating effect, but pomegranate twigs symbolically did.

HAOMA AS AN ONEIROPHERNIC: ESPAND

Among the different suspected botanical sources of the ancient intoxicating Haoma, espand (*Peganum harmala*), also known as Wild Rue is still revered as sacred in every Iranian household, including today's population of 98% non-Zoroastrians in mainland Iran and the diaspora. They burn espand seeds at their weddings, liturgical gatherings, and homes to avert and be protected from evil's eye and negative energies of jealousy and rivalries.

In their masterpiece, Haoma and Harmaline, a Western ethnopharmacologist and an Old Avestan linguist and Zoroastrian religion scholar, came together to unlock the mystery of the botanical identity of Haoma. Based on their evidence, Flattery and Schwartz (1989) declared that the intoxicating compound in Haoma responsible for inducing oneirophrenia and an entheogenic dreamlike state was *Peganum harmala*. The Farsi word "espand" is derived from Avestan Spənta, proto-Iranian *svanta*, meaning possessing productive numinous power (Flattery and Schwartz 1989, 59). It is consistent with espand being apotropaic and sacred (Flattery and Schwartz 1989, 63).

Espand grows uncultivated and widely spread over the Iranian plateau's flora. The brown plant seeds are a rich source of harmala compounds and burst over the fire, releasing a fragrant white smoke. The stem twigs of *Peganum harmala* and ephedra are similar. Espand's seeds are ground easily by pressing out in a pestle and mortar. Referral to Haoma color becomes relevant in the case of espand as the aqueous extract is predominantly yellow (harmaline fluoresce yellow). The dual application of Haoma as an inebriating elixir and apotropaic burning material is consistent with Gatha's referral (Yasna 32-14) and, among other botanical and fungal candidates, is only valid for espand.

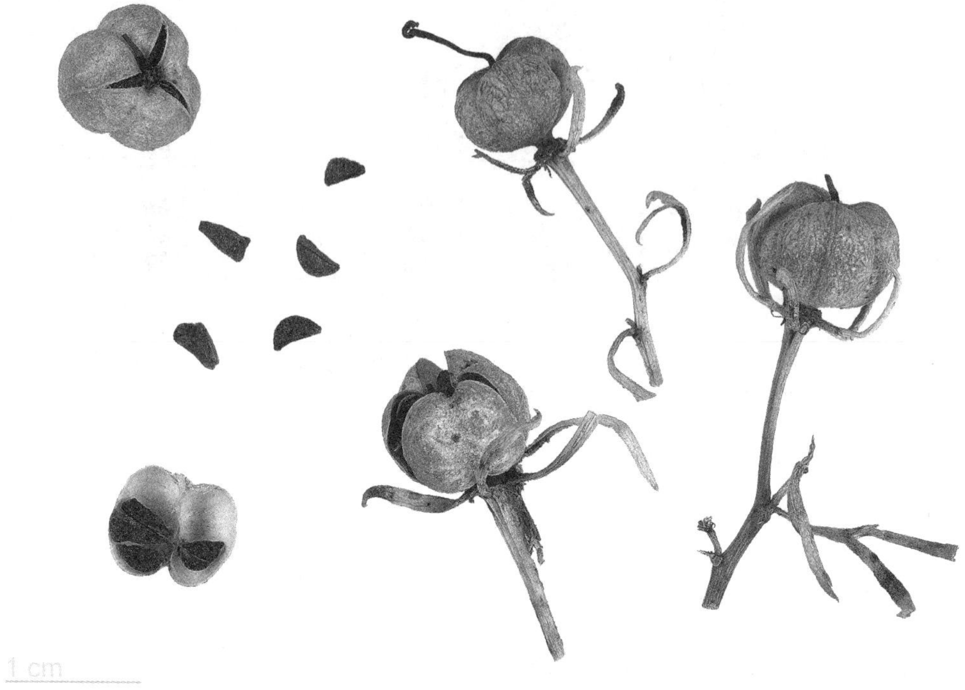

Fig. 12 Peganum Harmala (Espand) dried capsules and seeds. Photography by Roger Culos.

The psychoactive alkaloids in P. Harmala are ß-carbolines, including harmine, harmaline, and tetrahydroharmine (THH). While espand is a richer source of the first two compounds (Herraiz et al 2010), Ayahuasca's *Banisteriopsis caapi* bark has more Harmine and THH (Santos et al 2020). In general, seeds of espand contain around five times more ß-carbolines alkaloids than that of *Banisteriopsis caapi* (McKenna et al 1998). Harmine and harmaline are mainly recognized as monoamine oxidase inhibitors (MAOi). MAO metabolizes amine neurotransmitters in the pre-synaptic neurons and when blocked, the released neurotransmitters can be active in the synaptic cleft for longer. In the case of endogenous serotonin release or exogenous 5-hydroxytryptamine (5HT) intake, MAOi amplifies the serotonin's effect. Figure 13 depicts the receptor binding profiles for harmine and harmaline.

Both ß-carboline compounds have antidepressant benefits through their MAO inhibition effect. The other less-studied neuroreceptor with high binding affinity for harmine and harmaline is Imidazoline 1 and 2. The interaction of these compounds with I_2 binding sites may represent a unique mechanism for the putative hallucinogenic/oneirophrenic effect (Hamill et al 2019). Injection of Imidazoline 4-acetic acid (IMA) into rodents results in a hypnotic state resembling sleep with an accompanying seizure-type activity (Tunnicliff 1998). I_2 receptor agonists are effective analgesics and can modulate the monoamine system through inhibition (Bousquet 2020). The subjective effect due to the agonism of I_2 receptor sites, primarily by harmaline and then harmine, looks consistent with the outward dreamy state that, under Haoma intoxication, the Magi experienced in their otherworldly journeys.

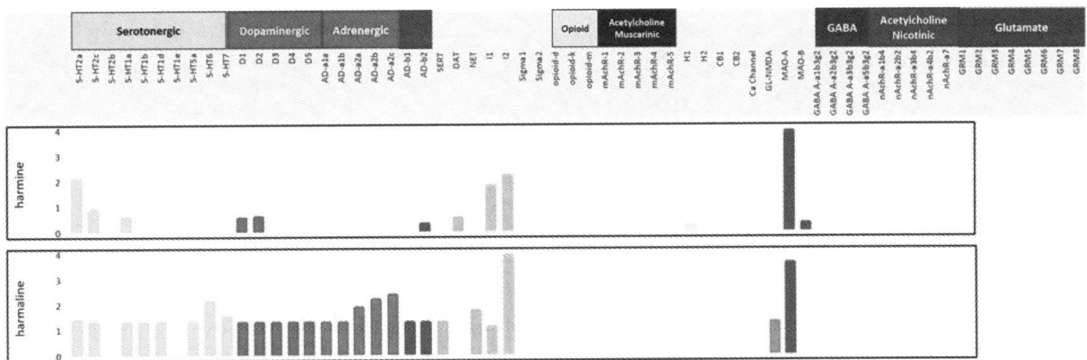

Fig. 13 Relative selectivity of harmine and harmaline to different receptors, published inhibitory constant values from the University of North Carolina's Psychoactive Drug Screening Program Ki database (Psychoactive Drug Screening Program Ki Database (RRID n.d.).

In his pioneering study in 1964 of the subjective effect of intravenous 10-methoxy-harmaline, Naranjo's patients described the effect as physical relaxation, a tendency to withdraw from the environment, a certain numbness to extremities and very visual images in the format of a meaningful dreamlike sequence (Naranjo 1973). His patients saw the same content in their visions, resembling those of Indians, birds, dark-skinned men, death, and circular patterns referring to the idea of centeredness/oneness. Naranjo concluded that harmaline evokes the connection into the consciousness of interpersonal experiences (the Jungian archetypes) and the collective unconscious. Under harmaline injection, patients experienced instantaneous improvements in the sense of proximity to their real *selves,* while their immediate epiphanies and insights were independent of their real-life stories and conditions.

Besides the subjective experience of Haoma that is coherent with that of Harmala compounds in espand, of the psychological side effects of ingesting ß-carbolines, we can refer to nausea, vomiting, diarrhea, headache, tremor, and body numbness (Djamshidian et al 2016). These body reactions are consistent with Schwartz's recent interpretation of Gatha's Yasna 48-10, which refers to the vomiting and diarrhea of Haoma-consuming priests (Schwartz 2022).

DISCUSSIONS

In this ethnopharmacological search for psychoactive drugs research, neuropharmacology from in-vitro assays and studies of subjective mind states from the most recent translations of Zoroastrians' Old Avestan ancient texts came together to reconfirm that the inebriating experience of Haoma was from *Peganum harmala* or espand. This conclusion is consonant with David Flattery and Martin Schwartz's hypothesis from 1989.

The revelation of Zarathustra and the otherwordly journey of Wishtasp refers to *Xvafena* and *Stard.* These are Old Avestan words describing a dream/sleep-like state as the subjective experience under the hallucinogenic intoxication of Haoma. This oneirophrenic state resembles outwardly sleep or the outspread of the mind to a broader consciousness. Naranjo's patients' anecdotes prove that under this state, one can instantaneously acquire knowledge from the pool of intersubjective consciousness. This experience is consistent with the revelation of Zoroaster. Under a dreamlike state, his mind crossed through planes of consciousness to immediately receive omniscient awareness. In phenomenology, this so-called instantaneous leap in self-awareness and state dream state mind is called a reduction, and revelations depend on the presence of reductions (Louchakova-Schwartz 2018). King Wishtasp seems to have had the same subjective experience. His deep-sleep dream under the effect of the potent, inebriating, intoxicant Mang and Haoma made him believe in the revelations and teachings of Zarathustra, such that he became his firm follower and patron.

Entheogenic plants, deep meditation (static and in motion), and lucid dreaming can cause immediate mind shifts and reductions. The denominator of all these states is the dreamlike state, at which the mind flows across consciousness planes while we are still awake. Amongst entheogenic plants, not all create this state of mind. For instance, tryptamines (strong 5HT-2a agonists) reinforce high entropic active thinking and heighten emotions. Their subjective cognitive effect is an interplay between conscious contemplation (sense of agency in introspection) and reminiscence from the subconscious, while brain regions are highly interconnected. Contrariwise, beta-carbolines hinder active thinking and induce lethargy, immobility, and a generalized sense of withdrawal from the environment (Naranjo 1967). Naranjo classifies harmala compounds as pure hallucinogens as they evoke a hypnotic, outwardly dreamlike state that involves delusions, depersonalization, and cognitive disturbances. These subjective effects are consistent with the documented dream reports of Zoroastrian Magi. Based on Yasna 30, Zoroaster's revelation occurred via a dream (Louchakova-Schwartz 2018), and the question remains whether Zarathustra's dream and revelation were attained through Haoma intoxication.

From translations and interpretations of Gatha, it is widely accepted that Zarathustra was against the Haoma *cult*. Nevertheless, it is known that he was a Zoater priest, meaning that he participated in Haoma rituals, prepared Haoma and served it to other priests. So, it is safe to assume that Zarathustra had experienced the subjective effect of intoxication under Haoma. In Gatha's Yasna 48-10, Zoroaster criticizes the Karpans, allegedly the Haoma cult, not necessarily Haoma. The decrying referral is to false priests who mislead people with wicked thoughts. Faulty and malicious metaphysics leads to false deification and worship (Louchakova-Schwartz 2018), which Zarathustra objected to by rebuking the Haoma cult. However, it does not seem he demonized Haoma itself, mainly the consumption context and the states of the minds at which Haoma should be consumed. The return of Haoma as a divine elixir in Hom Yasht (Yasna 9-11) can support this hypothesis. What if Haoma is only administered to righteous minds? That was the case of Viraz, who was chosen amongst the most virtuous and moral people.

Consequently, Zarathustra condemned the unrighteous people and the wrong way they used Haoma. In Viraz's mystical journey, the right person was chosen and guided by the Magi to take the hallucinogenic intoxicant. While journeying, his sisters and the Mazdaen were Viraz's sitters who cared for his body and chanted and prayed for him. As seen, the right person in the proper context was provided the potent hallucinogenic Wishtaspian Mang, and his journey has been honored as one of the apocalyptic religious stories among Zoroastrians. Remarkably, the three primary protocols of 21st-century psychedelic psychotherapy, i.e., set, setting, and dose, were accounted for in Viraz's otherwordly journey.

The Zoroastrian priests seem adept at formulating and dosing many kinds of Haoma for different rituals and purposes. Given that they were aware of the espand extract (beta-carbolines) as the dream-inducing potent intoxicating effect of Haoma, they mixed it with other psychoactive plants like black henbane (Mang) and ephedra to induce different subjective experiences. Besides, dosing was specified carefully at their discretion, as in the Arda Viraz journey, where he was offered three cups of Mang and Haoma. This hypothesis possibly explains how a psychotomimetic plant, ephedra replaced Haoma's hallucinogenic effect.

Most Iranians burn espand for its apotropaic effect, unaware that it contains the same strong psychoactive compounds as Amazonian *Yagé*. It is fascinating to see that both Ayahuasca and Haoma serve the consciousness of human beings in two very opposite geographies in the world.

ACKNOWLEDGEMENTS

First and foremost, the author would like to extend his utmost gratitude to David S. Flattery for his pioneering and unique ethnopharmacological study on the identity of Haoma within the Iranian Zoroastrian context. Analyzing these ancient texts and his work deserves unparalleled credit to the study of indigenous psychoactive drug use. Martin Schwartz, an Iranian Studies scholar and Old Avestan Linguist, takes this research to new heights, for which the author is deeply grateful. Through their ethnopharmacology masterpiece, Haoma and Harmaline, these two figures have preserved invaluable ancient Iranian knowledge.

The author would also like to express his gratitude to Dr. Dennis McKenna and the McKenna Academy of Natural Philosophy for their inspiration and trust in supporting the creation of this manuscript and presentation. The tireless efforts of the McKenna Academy team, especially Annette Badenhorst, created an unforgettable ESPD55 conference experience to which the author is indebted. Sincere thanks also go to Prof. Touraj Daryaee and Dr. Raheleh Hassani for their contributions. Final appreciation goes to Jonathan Lu, the author's friend and business partner at VCENNA.

Note: This author only used the chapter of the Haoma and Harmaline authored by David S. Flattery. However, Martin Schwartz, co-author of the book Haoma and Harmaline, would like to clarify that in the years since the book was published, his ideas expressed in that book have often substantially evolved.

BIBLIOGRAPHY

Belardi, Walter. 1979. *The Pahlavi Book of the Righteous Viraz. 1. Chapters I-Ii.* Univ. Department of Linguistics and Italo-Iranian Cultural Centre.

Bousquet, Pascal, Alan Hudson, Jesús A. García-Sevilla, and Jun-Xu Li. 2020. "Imidazoline receptor system: the past, the present, and the future." *Pharmacological reviews* 72, no. 1: 50-79.

Boyce, Mary. 2001. *Zoroastrians: Their Religious Beliefs and Practices.* Psychology Press.

Chardin, John. 1711.*Sir John Chardin's Travels in Persia.* Cosimo, Inc.

Callaway, Jace C. 1988. "A proposed mechanism for the visions of dream sleep." *Medical hypotheses* 26, no. 2: 119-124.

Clark, Matthew. 2019. "Soma and Haoma: Ayahuasca Analogues from the Late Bronze Age." *Journal of Psychedelic Studies* 3, no. 2: 104-16.

Culianu, Ioan P. 1990. *Out of This World: Otherworldly Journeys from Gilgamesh to Albert Einstein.* Shambala.

Crowley, Mike, and Ann Shulgin. 2019. *Secret drugs of Buddhism: Psychedelic sacraments and the origins of the Vajrayana.* Synergetic Press.

Daryaee, Touraj. 2020. "Shamanistic Elements in Zoroastrianism: The Pagan Past and Modern Reaction." *Pomegranate*: 31-37.

Djamshidian, Atbin, Sabine Bernschneider-Reif, Werner Poewe, and Andrew J. Lees. 2016. "Banisteriopsis caapi, a Forgotten Potential Therapy for Parkinson's Disease?." *Movement Disorders Clinical Practice* 3, no. 1: 19-26.

Doniger, Wendy, M Eliade, and W Trask. 2004. "Shamanism: Archaic Techniques of Ecstasy." Princeton: Princeton University Press.

Eduljee, K.E. 2005. "Zoroastrian Heritage".https://www.heritageinstitute.com/zoroastrianism/sects/index.htm

Eliade, Mircea. 2020. *Shamanism: Archaic Techniques of Ecstasy.* Vol. 76: Princeton University Press/

Feeney, Kevin. 2010. "Revisiting Wasson's Soma: exploring the effects of preparation on the chemistry of Amanita muscaria." *Journal of psychoactive drugs* 42, no. 4: 499-506.

Flattery, David Stophlet, and Martin Schwartz. 1989. *Haoma and Harmaline: The Botanical Identity of the Indo-Iranian Sacred Hallucinogen" Soma" and Its Legacy in Religion, Language, and Middle-Eastern Folklore.* Vol. 21: Univ of California Press.

Flowers, Stephen E. 2017. *Original Magic: The Rituals and Initiations of the Persian Magi.* Simon and Schuster.

Gad, Mohamed Z., Samar S. Azab, Amira R. Khattab, and Mohamed A. Farag. 2021. "Over a century since ephedrine discovery: an updated revisit to its pharmacological aspects, functionality and toxicity in comparison to its herbal extracts." *Food & Function* 12, no. 20: 9563-9582.

Gerber, Konstantin, Inti García Flores, Angela Christina Ruiz, Ismail Ali, Natalie Lyla Ginsberg, and Eduardo E. Schenberg. 2021. "Ethical concerns about psilocybin intellectual property." *ACS pharmacology & translational science* 4, no. 2: 573-577.

Ghadrdan M. 2015. "Zoroastrians—Social Life & Customs", Faravahr publication p. 250

Gignoux, Ph. 1987. "Apocalypses Et Voyages Extra-Terrestres Dans L'iran Mazdéen, Apocalypses Et Voyages Dans L'au-Delà, Ed." C. Kappler, Paris.

Gignoux, Philippe. 1979. "Corps Osseux Et Âme Osseuse: Essai Sur Le Chamanisme Dans L'iran Ancien." *Journal Asiatique Paris* 267, no. 1-2 : 41-79.

Hamill, Jonathan, Jaime Hallak, Serdar M. Dursun, and Glen Baker. 2019. "Ayahuasca: psychological and physiologic effects, pharmacology and potential uses in addiction and mental illness." *Current neuropharmacology* 17, no. 2: 108-128.

Haug, Martin, and Edward William West. 1872. *The Book of Arda Viraf: The Pahlavi Text Prepared by Destur Hoshangji Jamaspji Asa.* Vol. 1: Government Central Book Depot.

Herraiz, T., D. González, C. Ancín-Azpilicueta, Vicente J. Arán, and H. Guillén. 2010. "β-Carboline alkaloids in Peganum harmala and inhibition of human monoamine oxidase (MAO)." *Food and Chemical Toxicology* 48, no. 3: 839-845.

Homji, Peshotan Jiv Hirji. 1789. *Arda Viraf Namah: Ardāvirāfnāmah* The University of Manchester Library.

Iranica, Encyclopaedia. 2019. "Encyclopaedia Iranica." *Center for Iranian Studies-Columbia University* 7, no. 08 (1985): 2019.

Iranica, Encyclopaedia. 2012. "Karapan, Encyclopaedia Iranica." Vol. XV, Fasc. 5: p.550

Krogsgaard-Larsen, P. O. V. L., L. Brehm, and K. Schaumburg. 1981. "Muscimol, a psychoactive constituent of Amanita muscaria, as a medicinal chemical model structure." *Acta Chemica Scandinavica* 35, no. 5: 311-234.

Louchakova-Schwartz, Olga. 2018. "Intersubjectivity and Multiple Realities in Zarathushtra's Gathas." *Open Theology* 4, no. 1: 471-88.

Malandra, William W. 1983. *An Introduction to Ancient Iranian Religion: Readings from the Avesta and Achaemenid Inscriptions.* Vol. 2: U of Minnesota Press.

McKenna, Dennis J., James C. Callaway, and Charles S. Grob. 1998. "The scientific investigation of Ayahuasca: a review of past and current research." *The Heffter Review of Psychedelic Research* 1, no. 65-77 : 195-223.

McKenna, Terence. 1999. *Food of the Gods: The Search for the Original Tree of Knowledge: A Radical History of Plants, Drugs and Human Evolution.* Random House.

Muscarella, Oscar White. 2001."Jiroft and" Jiroft-Aratta" A Review Article of Yousef Madjidzadeh," Jiroft: The Earliest Oriental Civilization".":173-198.

Naranjo, C. 1973."The Healing Journey: Pioneering Approaches to Psychedelic Therapy." *Santa Cruz, CA: Multidisciplinary Association for Psychedelic Studies (MAPS).(Original work published 1973 by Pantheon Books, New York, under the title The Healing Journey: New Approaches to Consciousness).*

Naranjo, Claudio. 1967. "Psychotropic properties of the harmala alkaloids." *Ethnopharmacologic search for psychoactive drugs* 1645: 385-391.

Nizam. n.d. "The Sublime Republic of Iranshahr." Dropbox. Accessed June 5, 2023. https://www.dropbox.com/s/z15kx802fp0xnrd/Iranshahr.pdf?dl=0.

Nietzsche, Friedrich. 2008.*Thus Spoke Zarathustra: A Book for Everyone and Nobody.* Oxford University Press.

Nyberg, Henrik S. 1938. "Die Religionen Des Alten Iran." *Mitteilungen der vorderasiatisch-aegyptischen Gesellschaft.*

Pollan, Michael. 2018. "How to Change Your Mind: What the New Science of Psychedelics Teaches Us About Consciousness, Dying." *Addiction, Depression, and Transcendence.*

Rivetna, R. 2012." The Zarathushti World—A Demographic Picture" Federation of Zoroastrian Associations of North America (FAZENA).

RRID. n.d. "RESEARCH RESOURCE IDENTIFICATION PORTAL." Sci Crunch. Accessed June 5, 2023. https://scicrunch.org/resources/Tools/record/nlx_144509-1/SCR_003281/resolver.

Santos, Beatriz Werneck Lopes, Regina Célia de Oliveira, Julia Sonsin-Oliveira, Christopher William Fagg, José Beethoven Figueiredo Barbosa, and Eloisa Dutra Caldas. 2020. "Biodiversity of β-Carboline Profile of Banisteriopsis caapi and Ayahuasca, a Plant and a Brew with Neuropharmacological Potential." *Plants* 9, no. 7: 870.

Shulgin, Alexander Theodore, and Ann Shulgin. 1997. *TIHKAL: the continuation.* Vol. 546. Berkeley: Transform press.

Schwartz, Martin. 2022."Gathic Manarois: A Hapax Expatiated Compositionally."

Schwartz, Martin. 2018. "A Preliterate Acrostic in the Gathas: Crosstextual and Compositional Evidence." *for DABIR* 6.

Soni, Madhusudan G., Ioana G. Carabin, James C. Griffiths, and George A. Burdock. 2004. "Safety of ephedra: lessons learned." *Toxicology letters* 150, no. 1: 97-110.

Taillieu, Dieter, and Mary Boyce. 2014. "Haoma." In *Encyclopaedia Iranica Online*: Brill.

Tunnicliff, G. 1998. "Pharmacology and function of imidazole 4-acetic acid in brain." *General Pharmacology: The Vascular System* 31, no. 4: 503-509.

Wasson, R Gordon. 1971. "Soma: Divine Mushroom of Immortality."

Zoroastrian Association of Metropolitan Washington Inc. 2023."Zoroastrian Association of Metropolitan Washington Inc." Zamwi. May 18, 2023. https://zamwi.org/.

Ancient Psychoactive Drug Plant Use in Eurasia: A Case Study of *Ephedra* Species

Mark D. Merlin, PhD

Ethnobotanist | Archaeobotanist | Author

"From ancient times, plant and fungi sources of psychoactive substances have been used by humans. Shining some light on archaeobotanical evidence of their past use and status may alleviate some unwarranted disrespect or demonization." —Mark D. Merlin

This paper shares interdisciplinary insight on ancient psychoactive plant use in Europe, with a focus on the Ephedra species. Ephedra is commonly used by herbalists today, but research shows it was also used for its psychoactive properties across the globe for millennia.

INTRODUCTION

In most of the current world today, some parts of plants are used for psychoactive purposes; the herbaceous tobacco (*Nicotiana* spp.) plant, coffee shrubs (*Coffea arabica* L.), and betel nut palm tree (*Areca catechu* L.) are three prime examples of species that produce plant parts used very widely today to produce a variety of altered states of consciousness. However, from ancient times, plant and fungi sources of psychoactive substances have been used by humans (e.g., see Schultes et al. 2002, Merlin 2003, Fitzpatrick 2018, Samorini 2019, Guerra-Doce et al. 2023).

Motivations for such use have included desires to heal or provide support in daily work, as well as to escape from life's harsh realities, and inspire the ritualized development of spiritual beliefs. Although there are a relatively large number of drug plants and fungi that are regarded as having had ancient mind-altering relationships with humans, only a few have been well or even somewhat documented in the archaeological and/or the archaeobotanical record of the Eurasia; examples include: (1) *Cannabis* L., a genus of closely related multipurpose plants that are sometimes classified as hallucinogenic or entheogenic (e.g., see Clarke and Merlin 2018, Small 2016, and Long et al. 2017); (2) *Papaver somniferum* L., the opium poppy species, classified as an archetypical narcotic and pain suppressor (e.g., see Merlin 1984, Kritikos and Papadaki 1967, Chovanic et al. 2012, 2015); and (3) species in *Ephedra* Desf., a genus generally categorized as comprised of stimulant plants which is discussed in more detail below.

All of these three groups of plants (and other lesser known ones, or their psychoactive secondary metabolites), have drug use histories of varying adulation and condemnation. However, their traditional and modern use patterns of ethnopharmacological and medicinal importance should not be obscured by their shifting status from the sacred to the profane. Shining some light on archaeological and archaeobotanical evidence of their past use and status may alleviate some unwarranted disrespect or demonization.

This interdisciplinary essay reviews the ancient customary and more recent very widespread recreational uses of *Ephedra* in Eurasia, with special attention directed at botanical, ethnobotanical, archaeological and historical evidence of long-lasting psychoactive and medicinal use in Eurasia.

Old World Archaeological Evidence for Traditional of Psychoactive Drug Use

In the more modern or recent human societies, people's divine visionary experiences are often dismissed as hallucinations; furthermore, a desire to experience a direct communication with god is often interpreted as a sign of mental illness or false belief. However, a growing number of scholars and scientists contend that such visions and interpretations of them are fundamentally derived from an ancient and, in some situations, enduring traditional customs. Evidence presented in this study focused on *Ephedra* species suggests that the use of mind-altering experiences to produce insightful, cultural personal understanding is a very ancient widespread tradition involving humans, and often associated with improving health.

More than a half century ago a cross-cultural meta-study surveyed relevant ethnographic literature from 488 societies regarding the use of psychoactive substances designed to alter human consciousness (Bourguignon 1973). That study indicated that 90% of these societies had developed ritualized forms of "altered state of consciousness" (ASC). The highest percentages of customary consumption of parts or products of mind-altering substances were among the societies of "Aboriginal North America" (97%) and the lowest in the "Circum-Mediterranean region" (80%), including "North Africa, the Near East, and southern and western Europe as well as overseas Europeans." A large majority of these ASC rituals have been, and still are in many societies, produced through the consumption of psychoactive drug plant substances. This supports the idea that "the ubiquity of mind-altering agents in traditional societies cannot be doubted—just as the moods of industrial societies are set by a balance of caffeine, nicotine and alcohol, among many others" (Sherratt 1995a, also see Merlin 2003, Crocq 2003).

Among traditional societies, most use of psychoactive drug plant substances has been deeply connected with ceremonial and/or spiritual activity. As Sherratt (1995b) pointed out, ritualized consumption of several types, may be clearly spiritual, "as in the Christian Eucharist or the complex wine-offerings to the ancestors in the elaborate bronze vessels of Shang and Zhou dynasty China" (together these two dynasties reigned from *ca.* 1600-256 BCE).

In a 1970 journal article in Economic Botany (La Barre 1970), the ethnobotanist Richard Evans Schultes asked the anthropologist Weston La Barre a rhetorical question regarding the known distribution of traditional psychoactive drug plant use in the Old and New Worlds: why only relatively few known psychoactive drug plants are linked with traditional cultural use in the Old World. Schultes noted that there is much greater ecological diversity in the Old World than in the New World, and a much longer history of human occupation, but has many fewer of these known culturally associated "plants of the gods."

La Barre contended that there must have been many other psychoactive species that were utilized ritually in the Old World, but the advance of Western civilization, and in particular monotheistic religions eradicated most of these traditions. This included ritualized usage involving altered states of consciousness associated with direct encounters with divinities via use of psychoactive drug species in the Old World, and in many places throughout much of the New World, where European religious impact has eradicated traditional uses of such species.

More profoundly, La Barre suggested that humans, at least in pre-industrial contexts, have been "culturally programmed" to discover plants (or fungi) in their ecological environments that enable communication with the respective ancestors (i.e., their spirit world). La Barre proposed that this tradition goes far back into the Old Stone Age (i.e., before the invention of agriculture when people were all hunters and gatherers). According to his scenario, as bands of humans spread out into new regions, including new environments, they brought with them a culturally inspired motivation to find and use species of plants or fungi that would allow them to transcend their "normal" consciousness and enable them to communicate with their ancestors or gods—in essence, their spirit world.

The archaeological and paleobotanical records offer evidence for these assertions, albeit they are somewhat fragmentary now. However, with the powerful tools of modern science and human imagination, our understanding of our deep-rooted desire to experience ecstasy in the original sense of the word (to break the mind free from the body and communicate with the "gods" or the ancestors) may become more apparent with time. This interdisciplinary review documents the antiquity of a widespread ritualistic and therapeutic tradition of human use of a variety of *Ephedra* species in Eurasia.

In modern societies, psychoactive materials are used in a variety of ways. These include religious, medical, and secular applications, which in ancient times may or may not have been viewed as separate. For example, in the case of Neolithic Europe, Sherratt (1991) argued that psychoactive ("narcotic") substances were consumed in a ritualistic context: "Such 'religious' uses would no doubt have included 'medicinal' uses as well, since it would be artificial to separate physical healing from ritual observance." Sherratt (1995b) also suggested "that evidence for the employment of substances such as opium [or *Ephedra*,] at various times in the past should not immediately be interpreted as an indication either of profound ritual significance or of widespread employment for largely hedonistic purposes: they may simply belong to the material medica."

Under most conditions, in non-industrial societies, psychoactive substances were often, if not always used in ritualistic, religious contexts. It is generally assumed that that mind-altering plant species, including those in the genus *Ephedra* discussed below, can produce a variable altered state of consciousness depending upon the quality and quantity of the psychoactive chemicals ingested, as well as the psychological set of the user and the social-environmental setting in which the substance is consumed (e.g., see Advokat et al. 2018).

METHODOLOGY

Documentation of ancient human ingestion of psychoactive drug plants in several world regions is based on a multi-disciplinary methodology that combines various fields of study including, for example, archaeology, archaeobotany, anthropology, ethnobotany, chemistry, pharmacology, iconography, and written records. This documentation can be generally robust but mostly consists of indirect evidence of ancient human ingestion of psychoactive drug plants.

> "As mind-altering substances are usually invisible in the archaeological record, their presence used to be inferred from *indirect evidence*, such as the typology and function of certain artefacts possibly related to their preparation or consumption (pottery vessels, stone mortars, snuffing kits, smoking pipes, and enema syringes, among others) and botanical remains (macro and microfossils) of drug plants. Also, since psychoactive agents can remain preserved for millennia, chemical analysis of archaeological residues may provide indirect evidence of the consumption of drugs in the past" (Guerra-Doce et al. 2023, italics added for emphasis).

Examples of indirect evidence of ancient psychoactive plant use include chemical detection of opium alkaloids in Late Bronze Age containers putatively resembling inverted opium poppy capsules shaped so as "to advertise their contents" which were discovered in the eastern Mediterranean region (e.g., see Merrillees 1962, Smith et al. 2018, Linares et al. 2022). as well as the discovery in ancient burial contexts northwestern China of psychoactive compounds of *Cannabis* in ancient woven containers (Jiang et al. 2006) and in wooden braziers discovered in southwestern China (Ren et al. 2019).

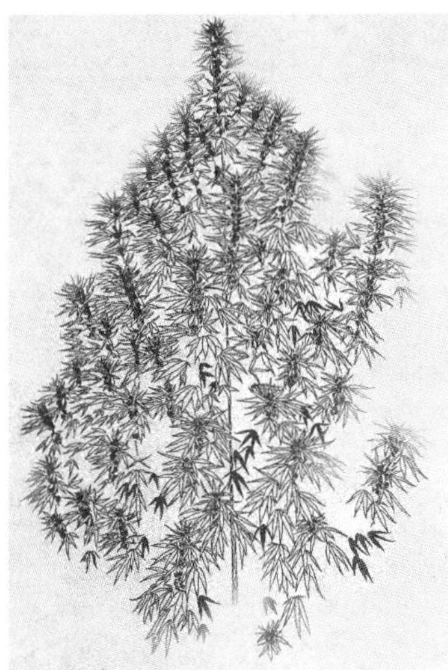

Fig.1 Drawing of flowering female Cannabis plant. *Courtesy of Robert Connell Clarke*

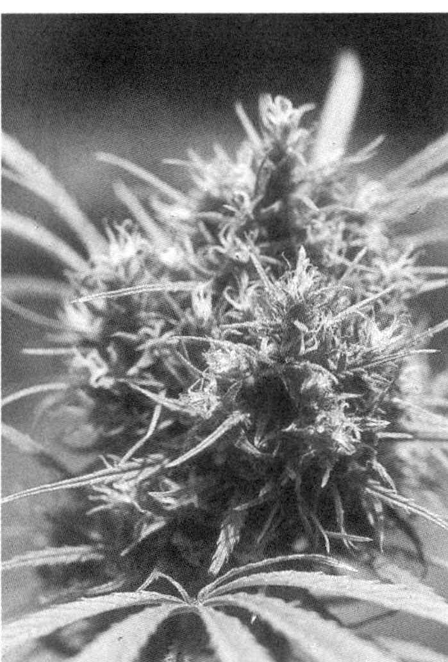

Fig. 2 Female flowers of Cannabis plant. *Courtesy of Robert Connell Clarke*

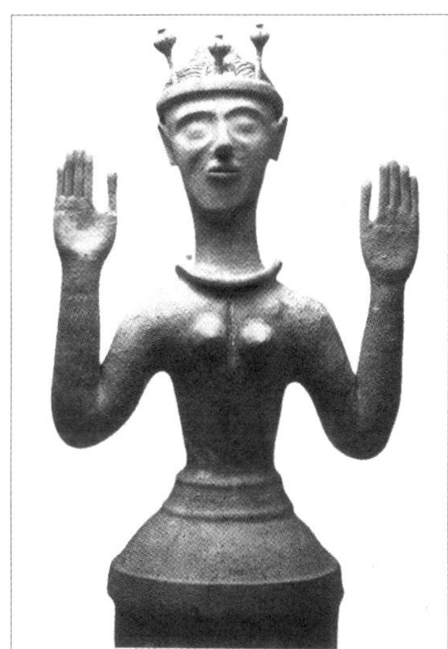

Fig. 3 Terracotta goddess figurine (ht. 80 cm) recovered from a subterranean "cult" chamber in Gazi, Crete (near Knossos). This "Poppy Goddess" is dated to Late Minoan III (1450-1100 B.C). *Photograph by Mark Merlin*

Direct evidence of the intake of drugs by ancient people, which is derived from chemical analysis of human remains, has been quite rare. However, Guerra-Doce and her colleagues (2023). have recently reported the detection of direct evidence of human ingestion of psychoactive plant substances from Solanaceae species, and from "*Ephedra fragilis*" in a dry cave on the western Mediterranean island of Menorca:

> "The recovery of human hair in a Late Bronze Age burial cave in Menorca, in the Balearic Islands, provided a unique opportunity to further probe into the medicinal and ritual realms of indigenous inhabitants of the Western Mediterranean as early as 3,000 years ago through the analysis of its alkaloid content. The results furnish direct evidence of the consumption of plant drugs and, more interestingly, they reveal the use of multiple psychoactive species".

This remarkable discovery and analysis of ancient psychoactive drug plant use, including *Ephedra* is discussed in more detail below along with various forms of ancient indirect evidence.*

TAXONOMIC, BIOGEOGRAPHIC AND BIOCHEMICAL PERSPECTIVES OF *EPHEDRA* SPECIES

The genus *Ephedra* L. is the type and sole genus in the family Ephedraceae. It belongs to the open seed-producing plants (gymnosperms; class Gymnospermae) that includes conifers, cycads, ginkgo, and three unique genera in the very small order Gnetales, comprised of only three genera, *Gnetum* L., *Welwitschia* Hook.f., and *Ephedra*. The life form of *Ephedra* plants varies, producing small trees, shrubs, subshrubs or herb-like subshrubs and infrequently lianas or vine-like shrubs; stems are generally branched profusely, producing green branchlets arranged opposite or in whorls at the nodes.

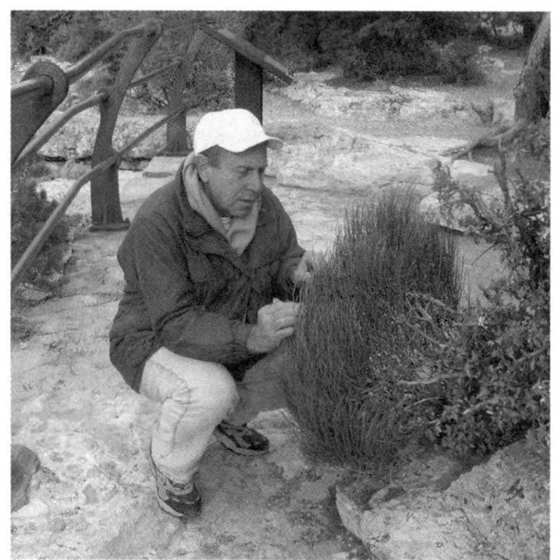

Fig.4 For a variety of uses, including psychoactive and medicinal, humans have developed very lengthy and diverse relationships with *Ephedra* species across much of Eurasia, and in some arid temperate areas of North and South America as well; the photograph shows author of this paper near *Ephedra viridis* plant in Northern Arizona at the edge of the Grand Canyon.

Key characteristics of *Ephedra* species are their greatly reduced leaves which resemble bracts and their evergreen, relatively thin, broom-like photosynthetic stems. In English, one of the most common names used for many *Ephedra* species is "jointfir" because plants in this genus have long slender branches, which have tiny scale-like leaves at their nodes. *Ephedra*

* See Merlin 2003 and Guerra-Doce et al. 2023 for more discussion of general methodologies used to gather relevant indirect data and dating of evidence used to support the hypothetical, widespread, ancient use of psychoactive drug species.

plants are dioecious (rarely monoecious) and their growth habit also varies, even within some species, from erect, ground sprawling, or climbing shrubs to vines; consequently, distinguishing among them requires close inspection. As a result, the number of recognized species in *Ephedra* is still unclear with totals ranging from approximately 35 to about 70 (e.g., see Stapf 1889, *Kubitzki* 1990, Stevenson 1993, Price 1996, Huang and Price 2003, Huang et al. 2005, Yang et al. 2005, Rydin and Korall 2009, Sharma et al. 2010, Ickert-Bond et al. 2016). This ambiguity is especially pronounced for the Old World species (Yang 2010). For example, based on a study of morphological, molecular, ecological and biogeographical evidence for the *E. distachya*/*E. sinica* complex, Kakiuchi et al. (2011), argued that *E. sinica* should be reduced to a subspecies of *E. dahurica*.

Today, *Ephedra* species are ecologically distributed in a variety of warm-temperate to subtropical environments and are adapted to dry, rocky or sandy semiarid and arid regions, with a few species occurring in grasslands; geographically, these species are found in North America, Mexico, South America, Europe, Asia, and North and East Africa, including the Canary Islands (Kubitzki 1990; Stevenson 1993; Fu et al. 1999; Yang 2010, Ickert-Bond and Renner 2016).

PHARMACOLOGY: A BRIEF OVERVIEW OF A KEY COMPOUND IN SOME *EPHEDRA* SPECIES

Ephedrine is the main active compound in the *Ephedra* species found within some Old World species, primarily in Central Asia. Although curiously ephedrine is not present in the New World species, the *Ephedra* species native in the Western Hemisphere do produce "other nitrogen-containing secondary metabolites with known neuropharmacological activity"* (e.g., Caveney et al. 2001).

The amount of ephedrine in any given Old World *Ephedra* plant can be anywhere from 30-90% of the plant's total alkaloids depending on the species of *Ephedra*. Ephedrine acts to release norepinephrine from the sympathetic nerves, causing stimulation of adrenergic activity. Ephedrine is in fact a potent sympathomimetic exciting the central nervous system and heart, as well as affecting the diameter of blood vessels. Ephedrine and some its analogues (phenylethylamine alkaloids), such as pseudoephedrine, methylephedrine, and methylpseudoephedrine, are used therapeutically today as decongestants and to alleviate bronchial asthma; and because they inhibit the production of the body substance histamine, they are also prescribed for allergic conditions along with antihistamines.

However, in the modern context of psychoactive substance use and abuse, these alkaloids along with norephedrine and norpseudoephedrine "can serve as the starting point for the manufacture of the semisynthetic compounds methamphetamine, amphetamine, and N,N-dimethlamphetamine respectively" (Kennedy 2004). Makino et al. (2005) referred to three methods by which "commercial ephedrine" can be produced: "(a) extraction from *Ephedra* plants, (b) full chemical synthesis or (c) via a semi-synthetic process involving the fermentation of sugar,

* To learn more about the medicinal use and history of *Ephedra* see: https://www.herbalreality.com/herbalism/western-herbal-medicine/history-ephedra-powerful-long-medicine-from-china/ and https://www.herbalreality.com/herbalism/western-herbal-medicine/ephedra-ephedrine-lesson-herbal-practitioners/ To learn more about herbal medicines go to https://www.herbalreality.com/

followed by amination; these authors also pointed out that "crystalline ethamphetamine can be synthesized from either natural or semi-synthetic ephedrine but not from synthetic ephedrine" (also see Andrews 1995).

Ephedrine has the same basic properties of naturally occurring epinephrine though ephedrine has certain advantages. For example, ephedrine lasts much longer and can pass readily through the blood-brain barrier to create an amphetamine-like condition. Ephedrine is metabolized to norephedrine which is responsible for the central nervous system stimulating effects of the drug. After making its rapid passage through the blood-brain barrier, ephedrine acts as a central nervous excitant. This excites neurons in the limbic system of the brain which also control a portion of the hypothalamus and therefore affect a variety of functions including emotions (Lee 2011).

ANCIENT USE OF *EPHEDRA* SPECIES IN EURASIA

Anatomically modern humans are now believed to have arrived in Eurasia as much as 80,000–120,000 years ago (e.g., see Callaway 2015), and in bands of hunters and gatherers these early people moved east and west progressively across the massive Eurasian landmass. In the process of spreading out over this vast continental region, they developed very ancient and long-lasting paleoethnobotanical relationships with numerous species; the more significant of these prehistoric relationships in Eurasia included a number of medicinally and psychoactively important genera such as *Cannabis*, *Papaver* and *Ephedra*.

Here we focus on *Ephedra* species that have ancient histories of use in Eurasia, especially but not entirely in the arid areas of this huge region. More recently, indirect and remarkable direct archaeological and archaeobotanical evidence, along with deeper understanding of relevant written records, have provided us with additional insight into the traditional utilization of this of genus of unusual plants with very special alkaloids. *Ephedra* plants have long served as a stimulant and therapeutic medicine for people, producing many tonic benefits because of their ability to serve as a bronchodilator and decongestant in addition to other significant effects on the central nervous system. Furthermore, given the appropriate set and setting, *Ephedra* combined with other substances in the past, as perhaps in the case of haoma and/or soma, can have potent psychoactive and physiological effects.

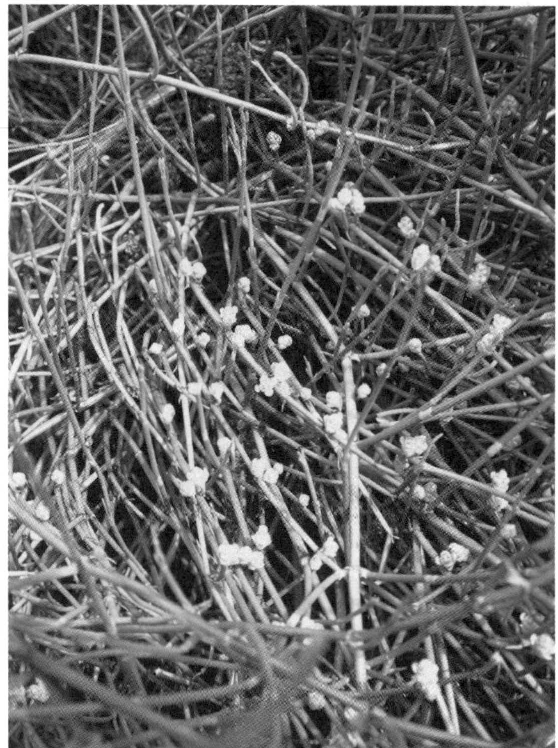

Fig.5 *Ephedra sinica* plant showing stems and fruits. *Photo by Alex Lomas licensed by Creative Commons Attribution 2.0 Generic license*

TRADITIONAL REFERENCES TO ANCIENT USE OF *EPHEDRA* IN CHINA

Plants in the genus *Ephedra* L. are commonly referred to in the literature as having been used by humans in China for medicinal or ritualistic purposes for 5,000 years or more (e.g., Chen 1974; Blumenthal and King 1995; Blumenthal 2003; Lee 2011; Eng et al. 2019). According to the flora of China there are nine *Ephedra* species in China, six of which are endemic (Fu et al. 1999). The *Ephedra* species referred to as having ancient relationships in China are primarily *E. sinica* Stapf, and to a lesser extent others such as *E. intermedia* Schrenk et C. A. Mey and *E. equisetina* Burge (syn. *E. shennungiana* T.H. Tang), all of which grow in the northern and western parts of China (Long et al. 2004).

In some areas of East Asia, the dry stems (haulms) of these *Ephedra* spp. are traditionally harvested in the fall and dried; these stems, the whole plant and medicines prepared from the plant parts are commonly known in China as *ma huang* (pinyin: *má huáng*) which can be literally translated as yellow or astringent hemp (e.g., see Bensky and Gamble 1993; Lee 2011). Officially listed in the Chinese Pharmacopoeia, *ma huang* is indeed among the oldest and most widely known traditional Chinese herbal medicines, having been used as an analeptic, antiasthmatic, antiallergenic, diaphoretic, antipyretic, and diuretic (e.g., see Chen 1974; Tang and Eisenbrand 1992; Tang et al. 2023; Zheng et al. 2023).

There is an oral tradition in China dating back several thousand years which is associated with the legendary herbalist or shaman Shennong (or Shennung). This famous, fabled Chinese leader probably lived sometime between 3,494 and 2,857 BCE (Chang 1962) and is traditionally credited with inventing agriculture and introducing medicines to Chinese culture. He has also been credited with compiling the oldest known medical text which contained descriptions of hundreds of medicines from natural sources. This legendary collection of traditional Chinese herbal treatments by Shennong was eventually written down. Flaws (1998) tells us that the first written record of *ma huang* use in Chinese literature can be found in the ancient text entitled "Shennong Bencao Jing" (pinyin: Shénnóng Běncǎo Jīng = "Divine Farmer's Materia Medica") which dates back to the first century A.D. (approximately at the end of the Han dynasty). This early, scholarly treatise, supposedly based on the medicinal tradition of Shennong, includes a large percentage of the knowledge about herbal medicine recorded before the rise of the Han dynasty. In total, this ancient treatise discusses the uses of 365 ancient medicinal plants, including some in the genus *Ephedra*.*

Shennong is said to have referred to the medicinal use of the dried stems of *ma huang* to cure multiple ailments such as the common cold, coughs, asthma, headaches, and hay fever; in fact, it is well known that *ma huang* has long been used to treat bronchial asthma and hay fever as well as both a spinal anesthesia and an analeptic agent in East Asia (Chen 1974).

More recently, in the 16th century A.D., Li Shih-Chen described *ma huang* (*E. sinica*) as "a circulatory stimulant, a diaphoretic and an antipyretic" which was considered to be effective in the treatment of cough. As a result, the stem of this *Ephedra* species "became an important ingredient of many antitussive preparations" (Lee 2011).

---

* For more information on Chinese medicines and psychedelics see our paper "Ethnopharmacology of Psychoactive Substances in Chinese Culture" by Jonathan Lu in this ESPD55 edition.

LITERARY REFERENCES TO ANCIENT *EPHEDRA* USE IN CENTRAL AND SOUTH ASIA

Through the ages, *ma huang*, the most famous and commercially valuable of the *Ephedra* species, has been used predominantly in East Asia as source of effective medication. However, it has also been suggested that *E. sinica* and other species of *Ephedra* may have been utilized in a variety of areas in Eurasia as mind-altering substances which have helped allow people to transcend normal consciousness, often to facilitate cognitive communication with their ancestors or deities (e.g., see Madhihassan 1963, 1978, 1981, 1982, 1983a/b, 1987a/b/c, 1990; Madhihassan and Mehdi 1989; Merlin 2003; Abdullaev 2010; Lee 2011; Dannaway 2011). In both cross-cultural healing and ritualistic use, the alkaloid-rich *Ephedra* species are emblematic of what the "Father of Ethnobotany," the late Richard Evans Schultes, along with some of his colleagues and students, have referred to as "plants of the gods" (e.g., see Schultes et al. 1979; Rätsch 1998).

When we look more closely at their natural distribution and customary usage, both in the present and the past, *Ephedra* species worldwide are among the most widely used traditional medicinal plants. Although the alkaloid production of *Ephedra* species varies, *Ephedra* plants have long served as a stimulant and therapeutic medicine for people, producing many tonic benefits because of their use as a bronchodilator and decongestant in addition to other significant therapeutic applications effecting the central nervous system. Furthermore, given the appropriate psychological set and environmental setting, when combined with other substances, as perhaps in the case of haoma or even soma, *Ephedra* alkaloids can have potent psychoactive as well as physiological effects: "Various religious groups, including Hindus and Parsees, used [*Ephedra* spp.] in their ceremonies to produce feelings of exhilaration" (Lee 2011).

ARCHAEBOTANICAL AND ARCHAEOBOTANICAL AND ARCHAEOLOGICAL EVIDENCE OF USE OF EPHEDRA IN EURASIA

The antiquity of *Ephedra* use for medicinal, psychoactive and other purposes does have an ancient history, which varies in time depth and ethnobotanical relationships for each species across its respective arid region distribution in both the Old and New Worlds. Some of the reputed evidence of the antiquity of *Ephedra* use is very old indeed. For example, pollen of *Ephedra* was reportedly discovered in a Neanderthal burial site of Shanidar Cave in northern Iraq that dates back more than 50,000 years (Solecki 1975; also see Lietava 1992; Sommer 1999, Merlin 2003). If this remarkable although controversial Pleistocene evidence and its age are comprehensively verified, it would represent the earliest probable human use of *Ephedra* for medicinal, ritualistic, or other purposes (Merlin 2018).

THE PUTATIVE EVIDENCE OF NEANDERTHAL OFFERINGS OF *EPHEDRA* IN SHANIDAR CAVE

Pollen of an *Ephedra* species (*E. altissima* Willk., cf. Leroi-Gourhan 1975; Solecki 1971) dated to more than 50,000 BCE was recovered from this Neanderthal burial site at Shanidar Cave, located in the Zagros Mountains of northern Iraq. Now located over 700 meters above sea level, the Shanidar limestone cave is well known because of the male Neanderthal burial known as Shanidar IV around which soil samples were extracted for palynological analysis. Two of these samples yielded a large amount of pollen grains from a variety of plant species which are still found in the surrounding region of the cave site. "This evidence has been used to support the hypothesis that the hominid body was deliberately, and perhaps ritualistically buried on a bed of woody branches and flowers sometime between May and July, when the flowers of many of the species were in bloom" (Merlin 2003). Pollen examination recognized many species including *Achillea*-type, *Centaurea solstitialis, Senecio*-type, *Muscari*-type, *Althea*-type, *Ephedra altissima* and others (Leroi-Gourhan 1975); this analysis was followed by a pharmacological assessment of the healing potential of the plants represented by the pollen. The subsequent study supported the hypothesis that these species possess objective therapeutic potential (Lietava 1992; also see Langley et al. 2008, Hardy et al. 2012, Monnier 2012 and the discussion below for relevant newer evidence about Neanderthal symbolic thought and the use of medicinal plants). The medical utility of these plants could have stimulated the deliberate use of these species by the Paleolithic Shanidar Neanderthals. Since *E. altissima* yields ephedrine, an alkaloid that produces sympatomimetic and amphetamine-like effects, as well as euphoria (Wenke 1986; Teuscher 1979, Taffe 2000), it may have served as an entheogen (spiritually stimulating plant) for ritualistic, spiritual and/or medicinal purposes. The pollen of *Ephedra* may also have become deposited in the burial as the result of its woody branches along with parts of other plants being laid down as bedding (Leroi-Gourhan 1975).

Some scientists and scholars have challenged the hypothesis that the placement of the flowering plant offerings at the burial site was a conscious choice of the Neanderthals, and instead suggest the presence of the aforementioned pollen might have become lodged in the soil around the ancient Neanderthal burial due to the activity of the "Persian jird" (*Meriones persicus* Blanford). This rodent species is known to have occurred in the area contemporaneously with the Neanderthals and is also known to store large amounts of seeds and flowers in its burrows such those from

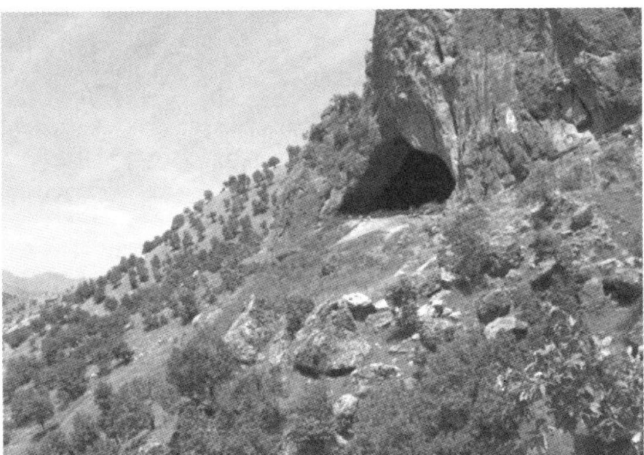

Fig.6 This image shows the exterior of the Shanidar IV Neanderthal burial cave site in the Zagros Mountains of northern Iraq. The photograph was taken during the summer of 2005. *Wikimedia Commons 2006*

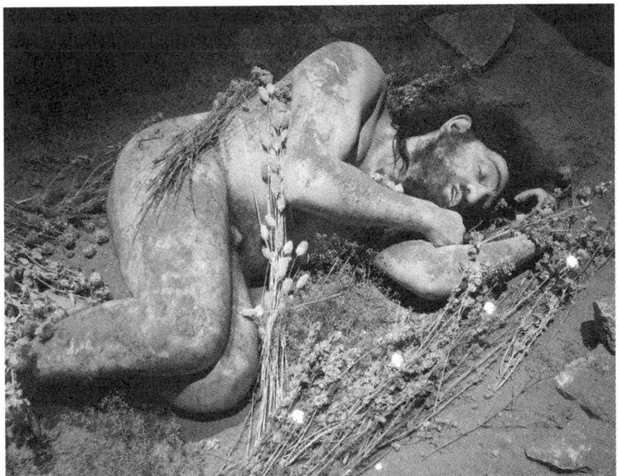

Fig.7 Life-size model of Shanidar burial with flowers and other plant material deposited around the young dead man more than 50,000 years ago in northern Iraq. *Courtesy of the National Anthropological Museum of Mexico*

the species identified via the pollen remains (e.g., see Sommer 1999). In any case, the ancient, tantalizing evidence of possibly very ancient medicinal, even ritualistic psychoactive use by our Neanderthal relatives about 50,000 years ago does need further study (e.g., see Hardy 2021).

However, there are indications that Neanderthals had developed some degree of symbolic thought which became more common after about 60,000 years ago (e.g., see Langley et al. 2008; Shipley and Kindscher 2016). This included the utilization of mineral pigments, the burials themselves, and additional evidence of behavioral complexity. Both symbolic thought and behavioral complexity could have developed "as a component of Neanderthal adaptations towards the end of their existence as a species" (Monnier 2012).

Furthermore, relevant ancient evidence has been provided more recently by a large, multi-national research team that "combined sequential thermal desorption-gas chromatography-mass spectrometry (TD-GC-MS) and pyrolysis-gas chromatography, mass spectrometry (Py-GC-MS) with morphological analysis of plant microfossilsto to identify material entrapped in dental calculus from five Neanderthal individuals found in the north Spanish site of El Sidrón" (Hardy et al. 2012). This ancient dental plaque evidence supports the hypothesis that Neanderthal diet was not necessarily only (or predominantly) based on meat but also included plant material. In addition, the remains from the El Sidrón site, offer the initial molecular evidence for smoke inhalation from fossil fuel and wood fires, ingestion of various cooked plant foods, and very early use of medicinal plants by a Neanderthal individual. Indeed, suggesting overall that "the Neanderthal occupants of El Sidrón had a sophisticated knowledge of their natural surroundings which included the ability to select and use certain plants". For example, when this new molecular archaeological evidence is combined with previous research that demonstrated the presence of the "bitter taste perception gene" in the ancient Neanderthals found in the El Sidrón site, it leads to the conclusion that at least one individual had even ingested bitter tasting plants most likely as a form of self-medication. In sum, The evidence from the El Sidrón site tends to support earlier suppositions about the use of medicinal plants by Neanderthals about 50,000 years ago (also see Weyrich et al. 2017; Morales et al. 2024).

ARCHAEOBOTANICAL EVIDENCE OF ANCIENT *EPHEDRA* USE IN CHINA

Many thousands of years after the extinction of the Neanderthals, but still far back in Holocene, we have evidence that *Ephedra* use in China has been a very long-lasting tradition (e.g., see Tang et al. 2023). The oral and written history in China provides special insight into the ancient relationships between Ephedrae Herba (*Ephedra*) and humans in East Asia. This type of evidence is supported by recent archaeological discoveries in western China. Many of the 12-14 or more *Ephedra* species native to China appear to have been used medicinally for hundreds, even thousands of years in the regions where they grow. Among those species known generally in China as *ma huang* is *E. sinica*, a shrub, 30 to 50 cm in height that is native to East Asia (see Ross 2001 for a brief but useful botanical description of *E. sinica*, which is one of the most medicinally significant of the widespread *Ephedra* species in the world).

In the early part of the 20th century, Sir Aurel Stein discovered burials in the Lop Nur desert (Tarim basin), where the extreme dryness of the climate preserved some organic items as well as the remains of the deceased. Among these objects were fibrous sacks containing twigs of *Ephedra* (Stein 1931); however, Stein did not draw any definitive conclusions on the significance of this discovery, even though the presence of *Ephedra* "at the burial site could indicate that it was used for its cultic and religious qualities or as an embalming plant" (Abdullaev 2010). Recent archaeobotanical research indicates that medicinal and other uses of *E. sinica* or additional species of *Ephedra* may well have had ancient significance, especially early on in their native regions of arid western and northwestern China. This includes Xinjiang and nearby regions beyond China.

Evidence of human presence and activity in Xinjiang traces back at least 10,000 years (Jiang et al. 2013); for example, stone artifacts have been recovered from the ancient site of Astana, Xinjiang that date back about 5,000 years (Wang 1993). For many centuries, if not millennia, Xinjiang served as an important area of passage linking the cultures of eastern and western Eurasia. Eventually it became well-known as the ancient "Silk Road" connecting Europe via Central Asia all the way to China. As a result, archaeological and archaeobotanical discoveries in Xinjiang, such as Loulan City in the Lop Nor area where *Ephedra* was discovered and connected to funeral ceremony, and the Yanghai Tombs in the Turpan Basin dated ca. 2,800 B.P. (Jiang et al. 2007), are studied today with significant interest (Xia 1997; see also Li et al. 2013).

Over the past 40 years or so, many cemeteries have been discovered in Xinjiang, in some cases with large numbers of tombs. Relevant ones for this *Ephedra* study include the Xiaohe Cemetery, dated ca. 3,980 to 3,540 years B.P. (Li et al 2013), the Gumugou Cemetery, dated ca. 3,800 B.P. (Wang 1983) and the Yuergou Site dated ca. 2,400-2,300 B.P. (Jiang et al. 2013); these archaeological sites as well as many much younger sites, reveal much about the lives and beliefs of these peoples living in ancient Xinjiang.

The Cemetery at the "well-developed oasis" of Xiaohe, with its mound shape forms a distinct landmark on the flat desert. Located near the downstream branch of Kongque River in Lop Nor Desert about 175 km east of the ancient Loulan city in Xinjiang, this archaeological site was initially exposed in 1911, excavated to some degree at that time, and then forgotten until the past decade or so (Bergman 1938; Li et al. 2013). Approximately 170 tombs have now been excavated, although many of these were devastated by "treasure hunters." Palynological and archaeobotanical evidence from the archaeological site of Xiaohe Cemetery dating back between ca. 3,500 and 4,000 years ago indicates that *Ephedra* was among the dominant native plants in the area and probably had relatively important uses, including ritualistic and spiritual significance; according to Li et al. (2013):

> "*Ephedra* was considered as a magic plant by the Lop people. Also, it is very common to find *Ephedra* branches in most of the graves of the ancient Lop people in the Lop Nur area, such as LF, LS and LD graveyards, Cemetery 36, Gumugou cemetery, and graveyards around Loulan ancient city [see Hedin and Bergman 1944; Wang 1983; Xia 1997]. Some Chinese archaeologists suggest that this phenomenon is a kind of plant worship and call it *Ephedra* worship [see Wang 1983; Xia 1997]. The medical use of *Ephedra* has been known for several thousand years in China. As a central nervous excitant, *Ephedra* was also used in ceremonies to produce feelings of exhilaration by various religious groups including Hindus [see Lee 2011; Xie et

> al. 2013]. As an ingredient of Haoma or Soma, *Ephedra* has been used for millennia in both Iran and India as a beverage to achieve longevity and immortality" [see also references authored by Madhihassan, e.g., 1987a]*.

At the Gumugou archaeological site and ancient community graveyard in the Lop Nor region of northwestern China, remarkable archaeobotanical evidence in the form of *Ephedra* twigs dated around 1,800 BCE has been recovered:

> "The macro-remains were first examined by scanning electron microscope (SEM) and then by gas chromatography-mass spectrometry (GC-MS) for traits of residual biomarkers under the reference of modern *Ephedra* samples. The GC-MS result of chemical analysis presents the existence of *Ephedra*-featured compounds, several of which, including benzaldehyde, tetramethyl-pyrazine, and phenmetrazine, are found in the chromatograph of both the ancient and modern sample. These results confirm that the discovered plant remains are *Ephedra* twigs. Although there is no direct archaeological evidence for the indication of medicinal use of this *Ephedra*, the unified burial deposit in which the *Ephedra* was discovered is a strong indication of the religious and medicinal awareness of the human inhabitants of Gumugou towards this plant" (Xie et al. 2013; also see Wang 1983).

The interpretation quoted above is supported by the ancient traditions of people living in the dry temperate regions of the northern hemisphere where a series of native shrub species of *Ephedra* occur. This traditional association with *Ephedra* species is "a cumulative application history reaching back well over 2,000 years for the treatment of asthma, cold, fever, as well as many respiratory system diseases, especially in China," and is further supported by "ethnological and philological evidence of *Ephedra* worship and utilization in many Eurasia Steppe cultures" (Xie et al. 2013).

In another ancient Xinjiang archaeological site, in this case at the Yuergou site in the Turpan basin, three species of cereals and two twigs of *Ephedra* dated to around 2,300–2,400 years B.P. were recently reported among the 21 taxa of plant species recovered as micro and macrofossils, and found in association with ancient human inhabitants (Jiang et al. 2013). Although the archaeobotanists and Paleoanthropologists who excavated at the site suggest that *Ephedra* may have been used here over two thousand years ago as a "medicine," it could also have been utilized for ritualistic psychoactive purposes.

In a related study, Wang et al. (2010) investigated the anatomy and biochemistry of *E. sinica*, the main Ephedra source of the Chinese herbal drug *ma huang*, sampling specimens from areas in eastern China, Mongolia, and Buryatia (north of Mongolia in Russia); the purpose of this study was to better understand biogeographical, functional, and alkaloid content relationships

---

* For more information about Haoma and Iranian psychedelic traditions see the paper "Chemically-Induced Otherworldly Journeys of Zoroastrian Magi in Iran" by Shauheen Etminan, in this ESPD55 publication.

among populations of *E. sinica*. The results of this study indicate that *E. sinica* grown in more arid conditions tend to have identifiable anatomical similarities and produce more total ephedrine alkaloids as well as high pseudoephedrine content; this suggests that high quality *ma huang* "should be collected from arid fields, and the chemical quality can be estimated by observing the anatomical characteristics". In addition to the climatic conditions, time of the year the plant is harvested, and the altitude at which the plant is growing, alkaloidal content is also affected according to whether it is being farmed or collected from the wild. For instance, another biochemical study using high performance liquid chromatography (HPLC) to measure the alkaloid content of ephedrine, pseudoephedrine, norephedrine, norpseudoephedrine, methylephedrine and methylpseudoephedrine among 12 native species in China collected in 24 districts indicated "that the cultivated *Ephedra sinica* showed lower alkaloids content compared with that growing wild" (Zhang et al. 1989). Our survey of ancient use of *Ephedra* now shifts beyond the boundaries of China and focuses on other parts of Central Asia and South Asia, as well as Western Europe. Note: much of what follows has been published previously by this author in an overview of traditional use of *Ephedra* species in eastern Eurasia (Merlin 2013), and in a more geographically extensive discussion of ancient use of *Ephedra* species in Eurasia and in the Western Hemisphere (Merlin 2018); the review presented here compliments and updates these publications with more recent remarkable discoveries and further interpretations relating to the ancient ethnopharmacology and sacred use of *Ephedra*.

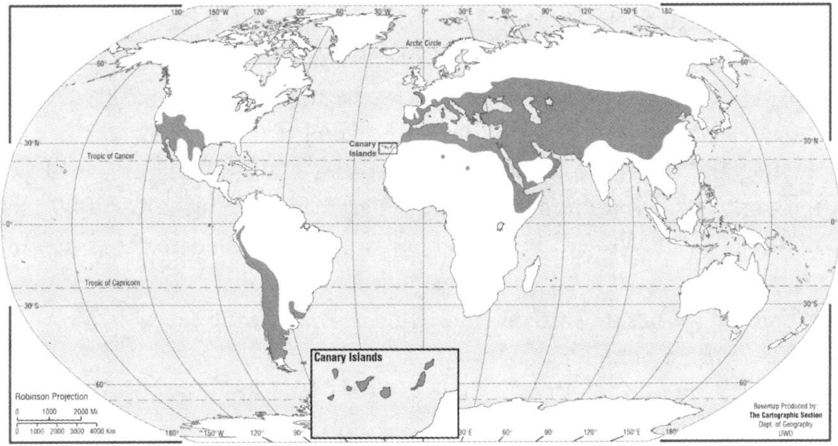

Fig.8 World distribution of Ephedra species. Shaded areas show regions where these species occur, based on data from Hunziker 1949; Freitag and Maire Stolte 1989, 1996; Zhang et al. 1989; and Stevenson 1993. *Map shown here based on map from Caveney et al.*

ANCIENT *EPHEDRA* IN THE NEAR EAST AND SOUTH ASIA

The most common scholarly psychoactive associations that *Ephedra* has in parts of Central and South Asia are with its putative cultural connection to the famous mind-altering *soma* (plant/

drink/god). However, along with ongoing debates regarding the alleged identification with such an important historic ethnobotanical relationship, *Ephedra* species occurring in the arid regions of the southern Eurasia presumably have had long standing customary use for therapeutic and other purposes. One early published example of direct observation comes from James E.T. Aitchison (1835-1898), a medical doctor who collected plants for many years in Northern India, Pakistan and Afghanistan during the latter part of the 19th century. Aitchison reported in his treatise on *The Botany of the Afghan Delimitation Commission* (1988) that *E. pachyclada* Boiss. (or another closely related *Ephedra* species) was a very common plant all along his travel paths from "northern Baluchistan, through the Hari-rud valley, the Dadghis district, and Persia" where this plant was called "*hum, huma, yehma*" and was used in the "tanning the skins of goats and water-bottles, and their ashes, when burnt, mixed with, or employed in lieu of snuff" (Aitchison 1888:111-112).

Ephedra species are used to varying degrees by native cultures for an assortment of medicinal purposes. This ethnopharmacological association applies throughout their native biogeographic distribution within and far beyond China in parts other parts of the Old and New Worlds. These therapeutic applications of *Ephedra* species include use as a cough medicine, an antipyretic, an antisyphilitic, a stimulant for poor circulation and as an antihistamine; the medicinal efficacy of *Ephedra* species for such uses is generally based on the presence of tannins and alkaloids, particularly ephedrine (e.g., Stevenson 1993).

In India, nine species of *Ephedra* distributed in the hot desert area of Arawali as well the cold deserts Western Himalaya have been identified, including "*E. foliata* Boiss, *E. gerardiana* Wall. ex Stapf, *E. intermedia* Schr. & Meyer, *E. nebrodensis* Tineo, *E. pachyclada* Boiss, *E. saxatilis* (Stapf) Royle ex Florin, *E. regeliana* Florin, *E. przewalskii* Stapf, and *E. sumlingensis* Sharma & Uniyal" (Sharma et al. 2010; Singh et al. 2007; Sharma and Uniyal 2008, 2009; Chopra et al. 1982). Although *Ephedra* has been the focus of several taxonomic surveys (e.g., Stapf 1889; Florin 1933; Freitag and Maire-Stolte 2003; Ickert-Bond et al. 2003; Huang et al. 2005; Yang et al. 2000, 2005; Yang, 2007; Motomura et al. 2007; Sharma and Uniyal 2008, 2009), species found in extreme conditions in the Western Himalaya had not been studied until recently in the Lahaul and Spiti districts of Himachal Pradesh where Sharma et al. (2010) identified isolated populations two new *Ephedra* species in Kardang and Khurik which "were found to be morphologically distinct from *E. intermedia* Schrenk & Meyer."

Sir Ram Nath Chopra (1882-1973)* made some of most important 20th century contributions to our knowledge about indigenous drugs, traditional medicine and modern pharmacology in India. Here we refer to some of his remarks regarding the traditional use of *Ephedra* species in South Asia. Although Chopra (1982:145) pointed out that the rhizomes of *E. gerardiana* produce large knobs "the size of footballs and are used as fuel by the Tibetans," he indicated that *Ephedra* was not used traditionally as a form of indigenous medicine throughout almost all of India even if species of this genus were present. Chopra referred to *E. major* (syn. *E. nebrodensis*)

* Chopra has been referred to as one who "sowed the seeds of self-reliance and triggered the movement of scientific research on traditional 'Indian medicine" (Ramalingaswami and Satyavati 1982; also see Mukerji 1973); as a result, Chopra became known as the "Father of Indian Pharmacology."

as "the richest source of ephedrine" among the Indian species of *Ephedra* and tells us that the 19th century botanical collector Aitchson reported the medicinal use of *E. vulgaris* in "Lahoul," but went on to tell us that "the drug [*Ephedra*] is not mentioned in the Ayurvedic (Hinda) or Tibbi (Mohammedan) medicine". Chorpa (1982:145) also refers to the belief that "one variety of *Ephedra*, probably *E. intermedia*, is the famous 'soma' plant from which the favorite drink of the Rishis (ascetics) of the vedic period was prepared," but he argued that "there is little evidence to support this statement" (Chopra 1982: 145). We will return to the putative association of *Ephedra* with the famous *soma* of the Indians and *haoma* of the Iranians later in this paper.

South of Xinjiang province of China lies Ladakh, one of the most sparsely populated regions of India (State of Jammu and Kashmir) between the Kunlun mountain range in the north and the main Great Himalayas to the south which is also an area inhabited by people of Indo-Aryan and Tibetan descent. In this area, Angmo et.al. (2012) reported that a species of *Ephedra* along with other plants "are ground crushed and boiled together in a big pot of water to make medicinal water" and that in Ladakh this "medicinal hydrotherapy" is used to treat "people suffering from paralysis, rheumatoid arthritis, acid peptic disease or movement disorders." Angmo et.al. (2012) also reported that the "medicinal properties of *E. gerardiana* Wall. ex Stapf" (a low lying *Ephedra* species) are used to treat "asthma, rheumatism and [as a] heart stimulant" in Ladakh.

Manandhar (1980) referred to the use of tea or incense including *E. gerardiana* in Nepal as an herbal medicine for colds, coughs, bronchitis, asthma, other bronchial troubles as well as arthritis and hay fever; and, according to Manandhar, in Tibetan medicine, a preparation including *E. gerardiana* has been utilized for rejuvenation. According to Rätsch (1998, 226-227), *E. gerardiana* occurs in various areas of the Himalayan Mountains from Bhutan to Afghanistan preferring arid uplands and high mountain deserts because it requires a minimum amount of water to survive, even persisting in soils with high saline content and also may be grown from seed in rocky soil. In these mountains during the winter, Rätsch also tells that the *Ephedra* plants serve as a significant source of sustenance for yaks and goats, which also apparently delight in the stimulating effects of these plants. In addition, according to Rätsch, during cremation ceremonies in Nepal, dried bundles of *E. gerardiana* are burned as incense producing a pleasant and spicy smoke that can be compared to the aroma of a forest fire. Rätsch also indicated that the remaining ashes may also be used as a snuff, but only powerful shamans and high lamas consume parts of this *Ephedra*, which is treated with much respect and reverence.

In Bhutan areas of Lingshi, Bumthang and Dagala, Wangchuk et al. (2008) carried out a field study of about 125 high altitude plants which they identified as being used "for day to day formulations in Bhutanese traditional medicine known as *gSp-ba-rig-pa*," Wangchuk et al. listed *E. gerardiana* Stapf ("Mtshe-idum" = Bhutanese name) as a plant whose aerial parts are "Used for wounds, injury, fever, liver inflammation, stopping bleeding and as a rejuvenator".

Chopra's extensive research notwithstanding, the 19th century reports of Aitchson and the recent research by others (discussed above) along with the variety of *Ephedra* species present in the remote Himalayan uplands, suggests strongly that more ethnobotanical research needs to be carried out in these mountainous, arid areas to determine if current or past traditional uses of these plants did and perhaps still do occur).

EPHEDRA AS THE PUTATIVE SOURCE OF SOMA AND HAOMA

We continue our overview of the ancient and more modern use of *Ephedra* species by focusing on their hypothetical usage in important religious contexts which continues to be debated due to their psychoactive potential, especially in reference to their putative connection to the ancient *soma/haoma* plant/drug of Indo-Iranian religion (e.g., see Stein 1931, Wasson 1968; Madhihassan, 1978, 1982, 1983a/b, 1987a/b/c, 1990; Madhihassan and Medhi 1989; Nyberg 1995; Kellen 1995, Abullaev 2010; Dannaway 2010; Shah 2015). Although this paper focuses on the case supporting one or more species of *Ephedra* as the ancient source of *soma* and *haoma*, the true identity of the original, sacred, mind-altering species has remained a mystery for at least two centuries. Although Bowman (1970) indicated that "most modern scholars assume that *Ephedra* was the ancient haoma plant," a large number of other species have been put forward during 19th and 20th centuries as putative candidates for the source of the active ingredient in the highly significant ancient *soma* and *haoma*—beverages that were used for ritualistic and religious purposes over a wide region Eurasia (e.g. see Hummel 1959 for association with *Rheum* L., a species of wild rhubarb; see Wasson 1968 for association with the fungus *Amanita muscaria* L.; see Flattery and Schwartz 1989 for association with *Peganum harmala* L; and see Mukerjee 1922, Merlin 1972, Bennett 2010, and Clarke and Merlin 2013 for association with *Cannabis*).

Whatever species or combination of species has been used (including perhaps *Ephedra*) to produce the famous *soma/haoma* beverage, it has been closely identified with the Indo-Iranians, people whose ancient home land was apparently located somewhere in Central Asia*. According to most archaeological interpretations, this early culture divided into two separate groups approximately 4,000 years ago. One group became the ancient Iranian peoples, and the other developed into the Indo-Aryans who migrated south into what is now Afghanistan and the Indus Valley and eventually influenced much of South Asia. These two groups of people preserved extensive, religious oral traditions that were subsequently rendered in written form as the Avesta of the Iranians and the Rig Veda of the Indians. Central rituals in both of these ancient cultural traditions involved consumption of an entheogenic plant and/or fungus. This psychoactive species (or mixture of species) became known as *haoma* among the Iranians and *soma* among the Indians (for some relevant discussion of Indo-Iranian linguistic and archaeological origins see Bryant 2001; Lubotsky 2001; Witzel 2005).

Similar rituals are performed by some of the descendants of these peoples who now use substitutes for *soma* or *haoma* that are not mind-altering or different species within the same genus. For example, Bowman (1970) points out that "In India the Brahmans now use the stalks of the Pitica [or Putika] plant [*Sarcostemma brevistigma* W. & A. in the family Asclepiadaceae] to produce their *soma* and the Parsis in India, who believe that they are importing the original plant from Persia, now use the *Ephedra gerardiana* (Gnetaceae), which is found in Baluchistan, Afghanistan, Kashmir, and western Tibet". Bowman argued that "this plant" is very similar to the Avestan description of the ancient *haoma* plant; when it is in bloom "the bush appears golden and it often bears the name zairi-gaona" (golden color), and indeed the pressed juice from its twigs

* To read more about haoma/soma and ancient Iranian psychoactive substances see our paper "Chemically-Induced Otherworldly Journeys of Zoroastrian Magi in Iran" by Dr Shauheen Etminan.

produces "a golden color, and it has an intoxicating and narcotic effect on the drinker." Bowman further suggests that "People have been reluctant to surrender the precious substance which has long been believed to promote health and promise immortality."

Madhihassan, a strong and persistent advocate for recognizing *Ephedra* as the original source of *soma/haoma*, referred to *E. gerardiana* as very likely having been used in India since the Vedic period as a substitute for *soma*:

> "There came a time when the Aryans were no longer able to find the original psychoactive plant known as soma, perhaps because the identity of that plant was kept so secret or perhaps because it had been lost, and so it was that many people took to preparing the sacred soma beverage with substitute plants, one of which was *E. gerardiana*. This is how the plant received the name *somalata*, 'plant of the moon'. The effects of *E. gerardiana* are more stimulating than visionary, however, suggesting that this plant is likely not the original soma of the Vedas" (Mahdihassan 1963).

Madhihassin (1990) also referred to what he considered to be "the importance of etymology which guides us to the original species [of *Ephedra* as the original source] of soma" which comes from Boyce (1975), a scholar of the Avesta and therefore also a very competent student of Sanskrit:

> "She [Boyce] transliterates soma as Sauma which as sound comes close enough Haoma. The original Chinese term appears to be Hau-Ma, Ma = Hemp fibre and Hau = Fire coloured or yellow, with trace of brown tinge. The stems of *Ephedra* are thus described long and thin like fibres of hemp and also approaching the latter in colour. Thus that plant has been named in Chinese according to its main appearance discussed in [Madhihassan's 1978 paper; also see Kellen 1995]."

After many decades of debate about the identity of the psychoactive substance in the *soma/haoma* drink, R. Gordon Wasson's (1968) publication of *Soma: Divine Mushroom of Immortality,* contended very persuasively at the time, that the fly-agaric mushroom, *Amanita muscaria* (L.) Lam. is the species in question. Wasson's argument was based mainly on ancient Indian sources, and many scholars accepted his thesis. However, a couple of decades later, Flattery and Schwartz (1989) argued strongly for a perennial dicot flowering species, Syrian rue or harmal rue (*Peganum harmala* in the family Zygophyllaceae), which was originally identified as the source of *soma* by Sir William Jones in 1794. Flattery and Schwartz relied primarily upon Iranian evidence to support their assertion that *soma* should be identified with *P. harmala* since this species is still well-known for its psychoactive effects in the home land region of the Indo-Iranians.

Evidence that human used *P. harmala* in the fifth millennium BCE has been recovered from the Caucasus region (Lisitsyna and Prishcepenko 1977); and according to Miller (2003), *P. harmala* "becomes more common in the third millennium [BCE] archaeobotanical samples in the Near East, and is therefore likely to be associated with overgrazing". However, it may have been used for religious purposes, or, as it is employed today in some areas of this region, simply to ward off evil spirits or as a "good luck charm".

As noted above, a number of scholars in modern times have asserted their case for *Ephedra* as the source of *soma/haoma*, including, for example, many publications by Madhihassan. The remarkable, relatively recent archaeological evidence recovered from Russian excavations at Gonur depe again suggested that perhaps *Ephedra* was the source (or part) of the *soma* drug. Gonur depe, in the Kara Kum desert of Turkmenistan, has been interpreted as the 4,000-year-old "Zoroastrian capital," known in ancient times as Margiana. The archaeological complex, now referred to as the Bactria-Margiana Archaeological Complex (BMAC), is part of the previously unknown Bronze Age civilization in Bactria (northern Afghanistan) and Margiana (Turkmenistan) which had was reported to have had two distinct cultural periods, the first between 1,900 and 1,700 BCE and the second between 1,700 and 1,500 BCE (Parpola 1994; these dates have been challenged by further archaeological dating, but the new dates are nevertheless very old, especially in terms of the microfossil and macrofossil evidence for *Ephedra* in the ancient BMAC complex; e.g., see Houben 2003; note Kufterin and Dubova (2013) provided approximate dates for occupation of the BMAC complex as 2,300–1,500 BCE).

At Gonur depe, archaeologists found monumental sites originally dated to the first half of the second millennium BCE (Sarianidi 1994). The Gonur South area of this site is comprised of a fortified compound of buildings. A large "sacred fire temple" situated within this compound has two parts; one appears to have been used for public worship, but the other was a hidden "inner sanctum of the priesthood" which contained private rooms. The discovery of ancient ritual vessels with the remains of mind-altering drug plants in at least one of these private rooms by Meier-Melikyan (1990) has been said to "show that *soma* in its Iranian form *haoma* may be considered as a composite psychoactive substance comprising of *Ephedra* and *Cannabis* in one instance and *Ephedra* and opium (*Papaver somniferum* L.) in another." (Rudgley 1998; cf. Parpola 1994; also see McGovern 2008). Thus, it has been suggested that both of these psychoactive substances had been used in conjunction in the making of psychoactive drinks. Chris Bennett (2010) published a very lengthy discussion and thought-provoking argument suggesting *Cannabis* as the true source of *soma* and *haoma* which is also discussed by Clarke and Merlin (2013) in their book on the evolution and ethnobotany of *Cannabis*.

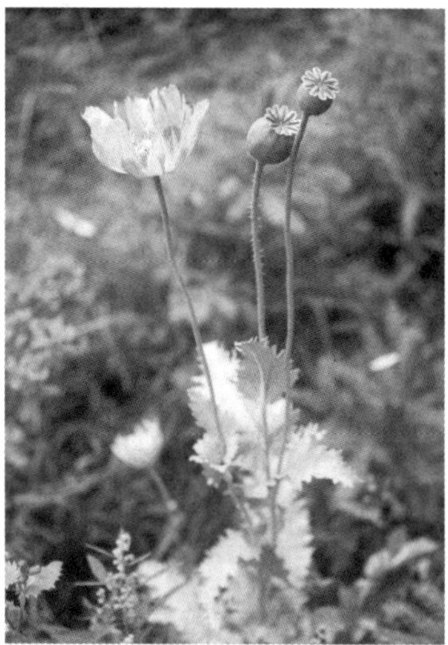

Fig.9 Semi-wild opium poppy, *Papaver somniferum*. *Photograph taken near Brussels, Belgium by Mark Merlin.*

According to Miller (2003), photographs of the *Ephedra, Cannabis,* and *Papaver,* and archaeological specimens presented in the Togolok-21 report by Meier-Melikyan (1990) appear to be consistent with the respective species; however, the determination of the *Papaver* species needs further study to confirm that it is *P. somniferum.* Indeed, Miller suggested that the poppy seeds could have come from field weeds or have been used as a food plant rather than as an opiate source for medicine or ritual. Miller also pointed out that in an arid climate, the woody parts of *Ephedra* could have been burned for fuel rather than for medicine or ritual; as noted earlier, Chopra (1982) referred to the use large rhizomes of *E. gerardiana* for fuel among Tibetans. Other scientists, who have critically reviewed the evidence for *Cannabis* in the Central Asian BMAC sites, concluded that the clay impressions from Gonur Temenos which are claimed to have been made with hemp (*Cannabis*) by Sarianidi (in Appendix I of 'Margiana and protozorastrism') "are clearly of [Millet] *Panicum miliaceum*" (Bakels 2003; Nesbitt 2002).

In any case, the remarkable discoveries at the BMAC continue to focus on a cult beverage, which theoretically can be identified as *haoma* or *haoma*-like drinks and whose use in cult ceremonies and rituals appears to have been relatively common in ancient Central Asia. Pertinent evidence from our perspective are the ancient microscopic twigs of *Ephedra* found in large vats in the Gonur depe complex of the BMAC. Taillieu and Boyce (2003) have argued that the linguistic and ritualistic evidence weigh strongly in favor of a strong connection between these cult beverages and *Ephedra* and perhaps the opium poppy in ancient Central Asia, as well as having an important prehistoric association with ancient India and Iran:

> "As for the plant yielding the extract in modern times, the Brahmans regularly used one of the Sarcostemmas (Asclepiads), which are evidently a substitute for ancient *sauma, since they are plants of warm climates. From the late 19th century, it has been known...that the Zoroastrians of Yazd use a variety of *Ephedra* which they call huma, hum and which they supply to their coreligionists in India, where *Ephedra*s do not grow. The plants flourish, however, in Inner Asia, the Indo-Iranian borderlands and Persia. Gradually it was discovered that in a number of living Iranian languages and dialects *Ephedra*s are known as hōm or some similar term, and that in the Indic languages of Gilgit and Kāferestān (Nurestān) they are called som, soma. Together linguistic and ritual evidence seemed decisive" (also see Zhang et al. 2021, Hemphill and Mallory 2004, Taillieu 1998, Chen and Hiebert 1995, Falk 1989).

In addition, an ongoing scrutiny of previously discovered and yet uncovered archaeological and archaeobotanical evidence within the BMAC, along with a more insightful interpretive approach seems needed. We can hope this will shed new light on present accumulation of archaeological information and newly discovered sources within the BMAC; but this will require an explanatory approach at a qualitatively higher level. Such a methodology could produce new insight on the religious and cultural life of the ancient people who inhabited the Central Asian region.

Dannaway (2010) pointed out that *Ephedra* plants have religious, psychoactive and/or medicinal traditional uses, varying from region to region and referred to another Avestan scholar for consideration of a particular *Ephedra* species: "The 'fragrant fuel' of the Avestan texts mentions various aromatics in combination with fragrant *hom* or *homa*, a name for the *Ephedra distachya*, yet another *haoma/soma* candidate" (Falk 1989). Dannaway (2010) also referred to ongoing ritualistic *Ephedra* use: "The burning of magical and psychoactive plants continues with the heirs of these entheogenic traditions, as with the surviving Mandeans, and the Shia of Iran, who burn *Ephedra* and *Peganum harmala* for apotropaic purposes [i.e., to avoid evil influences or misfortune]...The Indo-European complex of holy plants as means of communicating with the gods is found throughout Persian and Indian religious texts that group the plants together in prayers." Some scholars, such as Madhihassan, focus on plants in the genus *Ephedra*.

For example, Madhihassan (1987a) described *Ephedra* as an early source of an "anti-fatigue drink" which later "became a drink of immortality and longevity." As such Madhihassan (1983a) refers to the ritual use of soma as "the first drink of a newly clearly identifying soma of the "Rigveda" with *Ephedra* species as well as its long and continuous use among Zoroastrians.

> "Now the Parsis of Bombay, as Orthodox Zoroastrians, have kept up this custom of administering a few drops of Haoma juice to the new born. Since Haoma, which is *Ephedra*, does not grow in the plains of India the Parsis of Bombay used to import *Ephedra* all the way from Persia where it grows profusely. No mother would tolerate using a substitute of genuine Haoma for that would not assure the longevity of her child".

Thus, Madhihassan (1987a) argues that *Ephedra* evolved culturally from its early use as an anti-fatigue beverage into "a panacea and drink of rejuvenation, finally of longevity, immortality and resurrection":

> "Gods were not born mortals. A drink of immortality made them immortal. This was given as the first drink of a newly born child. This use is mentioned in Rigveda: 3.48.2 and 3.32.9-10. Indra was such a drug made immortal god. West [1901] translates a Zoroastrian Holy scripture which also maintains pouring a few drops of *Ephedra* in the mouth of a new born. To expedite resurrection, it was also given to the dead. This custom has survived up-to-date so that to follow it is to realize Soma = *Ephedra*".

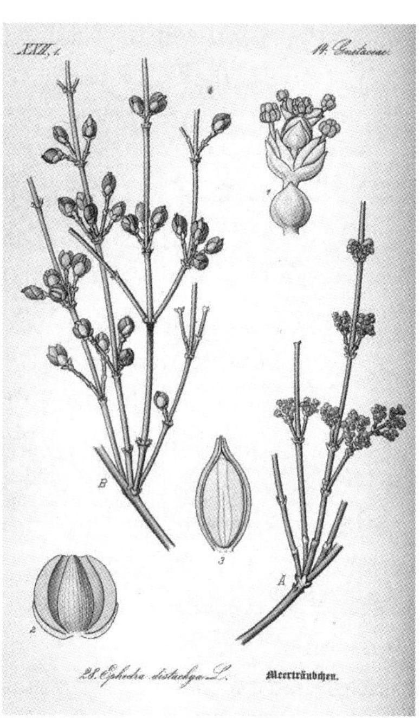

Fig.10 *Ephedra distachya* L. (syn. *E.vulgaris*) is one of a number of *Ephedra* species found in Eurasia. *E, distachya* occurs in some environments from southern Europe to Siberia, and is known to have traditional medicinal use in some areas. *This drawing is flora von Deutschland by Otto Wilhelm Thomé (1885).*

In addition to Madhihassan's many articles as well as other scholarly publications supporting the identification and association of *soma* and *haoma* with one or more species of *Ephedra* notwithstanding, it can be fairly asserted that further investigation in the disciplines of botany, ethnobotany and pharmacology are still needed to better determine the complex nature of the composition of the BMAC "cult beverage," and, more generally, the level of the plant knowledge of Central Asian priests involved with the relevant rituals and their putative botanical and alkaloidal sources of psychoactive inspiration.

In their review of the botanical or fungal identification of the sacred Soma, Ahirrao and colleagues (2022) provided a total of 26 plant species "that have been claimed clearly representing Soma plant, including a fungal and a gymnospermic [*Ephedra*] species," and in conclusion, they suggested that "Vedic Soma plant still remains a botanical enigma."

BRONZE AGE *EPHEDRA* CONSUMED BY HUMANS IN WESTERN EURASIA

"Ancient hair reveals psychoactive drug use" (Jacobs 2023).

A remarkable discovery of ephedrine, along with two psychoactive tropane alkaloids, atropine and scopolamine, was recently found in ancient human hair recovered from Es Càrritx, a Bronze Age cave on Menorca, the second largest of the Balearic Islands in the Western Mediterranean Sea. This finding provides us with rare evidence of the direct use of botanically produced mind-altering substances. (Guerra-Doce et al. 2023).

Menorca, in this Western Mediterranean archipelago has reportedly been inhabited continuously from about the second half of the third millennium BCE. The Menorcan cave of Es Càrritx and its extraordinary contents were discovered intact by speleologists in 1995. The stimulant alkaloid ephedrine found in the ancient human hair found in the Es Càrritx cave is assumed to have been extracted and from *Ephedra fragilis* which occurs on Menorca Island. The ephedrine identified in the ancient hair provides the first specific direct evidence of human consumption of *Ephedra* in Eurasia (Guerra-Doce et al. 2023); furthermore, evidence of the two other psychoactive alkaloids, atropine and scopolamine, also identified in the ancient human hair found in the ritual and funerary cave of Es Càrritx, suggests that the people who lived on Menorca 3,000 years ago or more incorporated mind-altering, medicinally effective plant use in their lives using compounds found in plants that grow on the island; and these plants include not only psychoactive, potentially therapeutic *Ephedra* but also *Datura* (most likely *D. stramonium*). It should be noted here that both *Ephedra* and *Datura* have lengthy histories of use to relieve asthmatic symptoms (e.g., Jackson 2010), and discovery of their alkaloids together in the hair of an ancient person suggest that a therapeutic, psychoactive combination of plant parts were ingested for a common respiratory ailment and/or for ceremonial purposes.

In sum, the examples presented in this essay support the proposition that psychoactive *Ephedra* plants alone or in combination with substances from other species have been used for therapeutic and ritualistic purposes in a great variety of places across the vast continent of Eurasia for a very long time.*

* Recently, a large research team reported the "presence and possible uses of *Ephedra*" approximately 15,000 years ago during the Late Pleistocene; plant identification was based on the analysis of remarkably well-preserved macrofossils found in ancient archaeological deposits in Grotte des Pigeons located in northeastern Morocco across the Mediterranean from Western Eurasia (Morales et al. 2024): "This cave has yielded the earliest carbonized plant macrofossils of *Ephedra*, which were found concentrated in a human burial deposit along with other special finds." The archaological team suggested that the charred cone bracts of *Ephedra* they uncovered probably "represent residues of the processing and consumption of the plant's fleshy cones, which may have been valued for both their nutritional and therapeutic properties." Moreover, the archaological team interpreted "the presence of *Ephedra* and its deposition in the burial area as evidence that this plant played a significant role during the funerary activities."

BIBLIOGRAPHY

Abourashed, E.A, A.T. El-Alfy, I.A. Khan & Walker, L. 2003. *Ephedra* in perspective--a current review. *Phytotherapy Research* 17: 703–712.

Abdullaev, K. 2010. Sacred Plants and the Cultic Beverage Haoma. *Comparative Studies of South Asia, Africa and the Middle East*, Volume 30, Number 3, 2010, pp. 329-340.

Advokat, C.D., Comaty, J.E. & Julien, R.M. 2018. *Julien's Primer of Drug Action: A Comprehensive Guide to the Actions, Uses, and Side Effects of Psychoactive Drugs*, Worth Publishers, UK, 14th edition.

Ahirrao Y.A. & D.A. Patil, D.A. 2022. Identity And Understanding of Soma Plant In Perspective of Indian Bioculture And Medicine *International Journal of Scientific Research in Science and Technology* 9 (2) : 327-337.

Aitchison, J.E.T. 1888. The Botany of the Afghan delimitation commission. *The Transactions of the Linnean Society of London. Second Series, Botany*. Volume III, Part I. 139pp.

Andrews K.M. 1995. *Ephedra*'s role as the precursor in the clandestine manufacture of methamphetamine. *Journal of Forensic Science* 40: 551-560.

Angmo, K., Bhupendra, S.A. & Gopal S.R. 2012. Changing aspects of Traditional Healthcare System in Western Ladakh, India. *Journal of Ethnopharmacology* 143: 621-630.

Bakels, C.C. 2003. Report concerning the contents of a ceramic vessel found in the "white room" of the Gonur Temenos, Merv Oasis, Turkmenistan. *Electronic Journal for Vedic Studies* (EJVS). http://www.ejvs.laurasianacademy.com/ejvs0901/ejvs0901a.txt.

Bennett, C. 2010. *Cannabis and the Soma Solution*. Trine Day, Walterville, Oregon, USA.

Bensky. D. & Gamble. A. 1993. *Chinese Herbal Medicine: Materia Medica*. Seattle, WA.: Eastland Press.

Bergman, F. 1939. *Archaeological Researches in Sinkiang, Especially the Lop Nor Region*. Bokförlags Aktiebolaget Thule, Stockholm, pp. 51-117.

Blumenthal, M. & King, P. 1995. Ma Huang: Ancient herb, modern medicine, regulatory dilemma. *HerbalGram* 34: 22–27, 42–3, 56–7.

Blumenthal, M. 2003. *The ABC Clinical Guide to Herbs*. American Botanical Council, Austin, Texas.

Bowman, R.A. 1970. Aramaic Ritual Texts from Persepolis. Chicago Oriental Institute Publications, Vol. XCI. University of Chicago Press, Chicago.

Boyce, M. 1975. A History of Zoroastrainism, 2 Vols. Brill, Leiden.

Bryant, E. 2001. *The Quest for the Origins of Vedic Culture: The Indo-Aryan Migration Debate*. Oxford University Press, Oxford.

Caveney, S., Charlet, D.A., Freitag, H., Maier-Stolte, M. & Starratt, A.N. 2001. New observations on the secondary chemistry of world *Ephedra* (Ephedraceae). American Journal of Botany 88(7): 1199-208.

Chang, C. 1962. *Chinese History of Fifty Centuries*. Volume 1. Institute for Advanced Chinese Studies, Taipei, pp. 30-31.

Chen, K.K. 1974. Half a Century of *Ephedra*. *American Journal of Chinese Medicine* 2(4): 359-365.

Chen, K. & Hiebert, F. T. 1995. The late prehistory of Xinjiang in relation to its neighbors. *Journal of World Prehistory* 9: 243–300.

Chopra, R.N. 1982. *Ephedra gerardiana* Wall. (Gnetacae) and Allied Species. In: *Chopra's Indigenous Drugs of India: Indigenous Drugs of India: Their Medical and Economic Aspects*. Academic Press, Kolkata, 2nd edition. pp. 144-161.

Chopra, Sir R.N., Chopra, I.C., Handa, K.L. & Kapur, L.D. 1982. *Indigenous Drugs of India: Indigenous Drugs of India: Their Medical and Economic Aspects*. Academic Press, Kolkata, 2nd edition.

Chovanec, Z., S. M. Rafferty, S.M. & Swiny, S. 2012. Opium for the Masses: An Experimental Archaeological Approach in Determining the Antiquity of the OpiumPoppy. *Journal of Ethnoarchaeology* 4(1):5-35.

Chovanec, Z., Bunimovitz, S. & Lederman, Z. 2015. Is There Opium Here? Analysis of Cypriot Base Ring Juglets from Tel Beth-Shemesh, Israel. *Journal of Mediter-ranean Archaeology and Archaeometry* 15(2):175-189.

Clarke, R.C. & Merlin, M.D. 2013. *Cannabis*: Evolution and Ethnobotany. University of California Press, Berkeley and Los Angeles.

Clarke, R.C. & Merlin, M.D. 2016. *Cannabis* Domestication, Breeding History, Present-day Genetic Diversity, and Future Prospects. *Critical Reviews in Plant Science* 35(5-6): 293-327.

Crocq, M.A. 2003. Alcohol, nicotine, caffeine, and mental disorders. *Dialogues in Clinical Neuroscience* 5(2):175-85.

Dannaway, F.R. 2011. Strange Fires, Weird Smokes, and Psychoactive Combustibles: Entheogens and Incense Traditions. *Journal of Psychoactive Drugs* 42(4): 485-497.

Eng, Y. S., Lee, C.H., Lee, W.C., Huang, C.C. & Chang, J.S. 2019. Unraveling the molecular mechanism of traditional Chinese medicine: formulas against acute airway viral infections as examples. *Molecules* 24(19): 3505–3534. Falk, H. 1989. Soma I and II. *Bulletin of the School of Oriental and African Studies* 52/1 (1): 77–90.

Fitzpatrick, S.M. (ed.) 2018 Ancient Psychoactive Substances. University Presses of Florida, 2018.

Flattery, D.S., & Schwartz, M. 1989. *Haoma and harmaline: the botanical identity of the Indo-Iranian sacred hallucinogen "soma" and its legacy in religion, language, and Middle-Eastern folklore*. University of California Press, Berkeley.

Flaws, B., ed. 1998. T*he divine farmer's materia medica: a translation of the Shen Nong Ben Cao Jing*. (translator: Shou-Zhong, Y.). Blue Poppy Press, Boulder, Colorado.

Florin, R. 1933. Über einige neue order wenig bekannte asiatische *Ephedra* Arten der Sect. *Pseudobaccatae* Stapf. *Kungl Svenska Vetenskapsakademiens Handlingar Ser* 3(12): 1–44.

Freitag H. & Maier-Stolte M. 1989. The *Ephedra*-species of P. Forsskal: identity and typification. *Taxon* 38: 545–556.

Freitag H. & Maier-Stolte M. 1993. *Ephedra*. In: Tutin T.G., Burges N.A., Chater A.O., Edmondson, J.R., Heywood, V.H., Moore, D.M., Valentine, D.H., Walters S.M. & Webb D.A. (Eds.), *Flora europaea, 2, 1*. Cambridge University, Cambridge, p. 49

Freitag H. & Maier-Stolte M. 1994. Ephedraceae. In: Browicz K. (Ed.), *Chorology of trees and shrubs in Southwest Asia and adjacent regions 10*. Poznan: Polish Scientific Publishers, pp. 5-16, 39-52.

Fu, L.K., Y.F. Yu & Riedl, H. 1999. Ephedraceae. In: C. Y. Wu and P. Raven (Eds.), *Flora of China, 4, Cycadaceae through Fagaceae*, Science Press, Beijing, China, pp. 97–101.

Guerra-Doce, E., Rihuete-Herrada, C., Micó, R., Risch, R., Lull, V. & Niemeyer, H.M. 2023. Direct evidence of the use of multiple drugs in Bronze Age Menorca (Western Mediterranean) from human hair analysis. *Nature: Scientific Reports* 13(1).

Hardy, K., Buckley, S., Collins, M.J., Estalrrich, A., Brothwell, D., Copeland, L., García-Tabernero, A., García-Vargas, S., de la Rasilla, M., Lalueza-Fox, C., Huguet, R., Bastir, M., Santamaría, D., Madella, M., Wilson, J., Cortés, A.F. & Rosas, A. 2012. Neanderthal medics? Evidence for food, cooking, and medicinal plants entrapped in dental calculus. *Naturwissenschaften* 9(8): 617-26.

Hardy K. 2021. Paleomedicine and the Evolutionary Context of Medicinal Plant Use. *Revista Brasileira de Farmacognosia-Brazilian Journal of Pharmacognosy* 31(1):1-15.

Hedin, S.A. & Bergman, F. 1944. *History of the expedition in Asia, 1927-1935*. Göteborg, Elanders boktryckeri aktiebolag, Stockholm 3: 215.

Houben, J.E.M. 2003. The Soma-Haoma problem: Introductory overview and observations on the discussion. *Electronic Journal for Vedic Studies* (EJVS). http://www.ejvs.laurasianacademy.com/ejvs0901/ejvs0901a.txt.

Hemphill, B.E. & Mallory, J.P. 2004. Horse-mounted invaders from the Russo-Kazakh steppe or agricultural colonists from western Central Asia? A craniometric investigation of the Bronze Age settlement of Xinjiang. *American Journal of Physical Anthropology* 124: 199-222.

Huang, J, & Price, R. 2003. Estimation of the Age of Extant *Ephedra* Using Chloroplast RBCL Sequence Data. *Molecular Biological Evolution* 20(3): 435-440.

Huang, J., Giannasij, D.E., & Price, R.A. 2005. Phylogenetic relationships in *Ephedra* (*Ephedra*ceae) inferred from chloroplast and nuclear DNA sequences. *Molecular Phylogenetics and Evolution* 35: 48–59.

Hummel, K. 1959. Aus welcher Pflanzen stellen die arischen Inder den Somatrank her? *Mitteilungen der Deutschenpharmazeutischen Gesellschaft und der pharmazeutischen Gesellschaft der DDR* 4: 57-61.

Ickert-Bond, S.M., & Renner, S.S.. 2016. The Gnetales: Recent insights on their morphology, reproductive biology, chromosome numbers, biogeography, and divergence times. *Journal of Systematics and Evolution* 54:1–16.

Ickert-Bond, S.M., Skvarla, J.J. & Chissoe, W.F. 2003. Pollen dimorphism in *Ephedra* L. (*Ephedra*ceae). *Review of Palaeobotany and Palynology* 124: 325–.

Jiang, H. E. et al. 2006. A new insight into *Cannabis sativa* (Cannabaceae) utilization from 2500-year-old Yanghai Tombs, Xinjiang, China. *Journal of Ethnopharmacology* 108(3): 414–422.

Jiang, H.E., Li, X., Ferguson, D.K., Wang, Y.F., Liu, C.J. et al. 2007. The discovery of *Capparis spinosa* L. (Capparidaceae) in the Yanghai Tombs (2500 years BP), NW China, and its medicinal implications. *Journal of Ethnopharmacology* 113: 409-420.

Jiang, H.E., Wu, Y., Wang, H.H., Ferguson, D.K. & Li, C.S. 2013. Ancient plant use at the site of Yuergou, Xinjiang, China: implications from desiccated and charred plant remains. *Vegetation History and Archaeobotany* 22: 129-140.

Jiang, H., Wang, L., Merlin, M.D. Clarke, R.C., Pan, Y., Zhang, Y., Xiao, G. & Ding, X. 2016. Ancient *Cannabis* burial shroud in a Central Eurasian Cemetery. *Economic Botany* 70(3): 213–221.

Jackson M. 2010. "Divine stramonium": the rise and fall of smoking for asthma. *Medical History* 54(2):171-94.

Jacobs, A. 2023. Ancient hair reveals psychoactive drug use. New York Times, Science section, April 9.

Jones D. 1999. *Ephedra* (Ma-huang); Today and Yesterday: Traditional and Topical Aspects of its Nutritional and Clinical Applications. Presented at AHPA *Ephedra* International Symposium, Arlington, VA, December 1999.

Kakiuchi N., Mikage M., Ickert-Bond S., Maier-Stolte M. & Freitag H. 2011. A molecular phylogenetic study of the *Ephedra* distachya/E. sinica complex in Eurasia. *Willdenowia* 41: 203-215.

Kashikar, C.G. Antecedents of the vedic Soma. *Hamdard-Medicus*. (1980) 23 (1-2), 62.

Kellen, J. 1995. "Haoma," In: van der Torn, K., Becking, B. & van der Horst, P.W. (Eds.) *Dictionary of Deities and Demons in the Bible.* E.J. Brill, New York, p. 384-385.

Kennedy, D.O. 2014. *Plants and the Human Brain*. Oxford University Press, Oxford.

Kramer, J.C. & Merlin, M.D. 1983. The use of psychoactive drugs in the ancient Old World. In: *Discoveries in Pharmacology*, Volume 1: *Psycho- and Neuro-pharmacology*, M. J. Parnham and J. Bruinvels eds., Elsevier Science Publishers B. V., Amsterdam, The Netherlands, pp. 23-48.

Kritikos, P.G. & Papadaki, S.P. 1967. *The History of the Poppy and of Opium and Their Expansion in Antiquity in the Eastern Mediterranean Area*, translated from Greek by George Michalopoulos. In two parts in *Bulletin of Narcotics* 19(3): 17-38, and 19(4): 5-10.

Kubitzki, K. 1990. Gnetatae. In: *K. U. Kramer & Green, P.S. (Eds.) The Families and Genera of Vascular Plants, vol. 1, Pteridophytes and gymnosperms. Springer-Verlag, Berlin, pp. 378–391.*

Kufterin, V. & Dubova, N. 2013. A Preliminary Analysis of Late Bronze Age Human Skeletal Remains from Gonur-depe, Turkmenistan. *Bioarchaeology of the Near East* 7: 33-46.

La Barre, W. 1970. Old and New World Narcotics: A Statistical Question and an Ethnological Reply. *Economic Botany* 24: 73-80.

Langley, M. C., Clarkson, C. & Ulm, S. 2008. Behavioral complexity in Eurasian Neanderthal populations: A chronological examination of the archaeological evidence. *Cambridge Archaeological Journal* 18: 289-307.

Linares, V., Jakoil, E., Be'eri, R., Lipschits, O., Neuman, R. & Gadot, Y. 2022. Opium trade and use during the Late Bronze Age: Organic residue analysis of ceramic vessels from the burials of Tel Yehud, Israel. *Archaeometry* 1: 1-18 (2022).

Lisitsyna, G. N. & Prishcepenko, L.V. 1977. Paleoethnobotanischeskie. Nakhodki Kavkaza I Blizhnego Vostoka. Nauka, Moscow, pp. 64, 71, 85.

Lee, M.R. 2011. The history of *Ephedra* (ma-huang). *Journal of the Royal College of Physicians, Edinburgh* 41: 78-84.

Leroi-Gourhan, A. 1975. The Flowers Found with Shanidar IV, a Neanderthal Burial in Iraq. *Science.* 190(4214): 562-564.

Leung, A.Y. 1999. Ephedrine, *Ephedra*, Mahuang, Mahuanggen-What are They? Presented at AHPA *Ephedra* International Symposium, Arlington, VA.

Li, J., Abuduresule, I., Hueber, F.M., Li, W., Hu, X., Li, Y. & Li, C. 2013. Buried in Sands: Environmental Analysis at the Archaeological Site of Xiaohe Cemetery, Xinjiang, China. *PLoS ONE* 8(7): e68957. doi:10.1371/journal.pone.0068957.

Lietava, J. 1992. Medicinal plants in a middle Paleolithic grave Shanidar IV? *Journal of Ethnopharmacology* 35(3):263-266.

Long C.F., Kakiuchi N., Takahashi A., Komatsu K., CaiS. Q. & Mikage M. 2004. Phylogenetic Analysis of the DNA Sequence of the Non-Coding Region of Nuclear Ribosomal DNA and Chloroplast of *Ephedra* Plants in China. *Planta Medica* 70(11): 1080-1084.

Long, T., Wagner, M., Demske, D., Leipe, C. & Tarasov, P.E. 2017. Cannabis in Eurasia: Origin of human use and Bronze Age transcontinental connections. *Vegetation, History and Archaeobotany* (26): 245–258.

Lubotsky, A. 2001. The Indo-Iranian Substratum. In: Carpelan, C., Parpola, A. & Koskikallio, P. *Early Contacts between Uralic and Indo-European: Linguistic and Archaeological Considerations*. Suomalais-Ugrilainen Seura, Helsinki, pp. 301-317.

Mahdihassan, S. 1987. *Ephedra*, the oldest medicinal plant with the history of an uninterrupted use. *Ancient Scientific Life* 7(2): 105-109.

Mahdihassan, S. 1963. Identifying *Ephedra* as Soma. *Pakistan Journal of Forestry* 13(4): pages

Madhihassan, S. 1978. The vedic words soma and sura traced to Chinese. *Hamdard-Medicus*. 198(21) 7-12.

Madhihassan, S. 1981. Haoma of Irano Aryans, as the medicinal plant *Ephedra. Hamdard-Medicus* 24(3-4): 3-28.

Madhihassan, S. 1982. Evolution of *Ephedra* as the Soma of Rigveda. *Ancient Science of Life* 2(2): 93–97.

Madhihassan, S. 1983a. Soma juice as administered to a newly born child being mentioned in Rigveda. *American Journal of Chinese Medicine* 11 (1-4): 14-15.

Madhihassan, S. 1983b. Identifying the soma plant as *Ephedra* from Rigveda and Avesta. *Hamdard-Medicus*: 26(3). pages

Madhihassan S. 1984. Soma as Energizer-Cum-Euphoriant, versus Sura, an Intoxicant. *Ancient Science of Life*: 3(3): 161-168.

Madhihassan, S. 1987a. *Ephedra*, the Oldest Medicinal Plant with the history of an uninterrupted use. *Ancient Science of Life* 7(2): 105-109.

Madhihassan, S. 1987b. Soma of the Aryans and Ash of the Romans. *Annals of the Bhandarkar Oriental Research Institute.* 68(1/4): 639-644.

Madhihassan, S. 1987c. *The History and Natural History of Ephedra as Soma.* Pakistan Science Foundation, Islamabad.

Madhihassan, S. 1989. The Seven Theories Identifying the Soma Plant. *Ancient Science of Life.* 9(2): 86-89.

Madhihassan, S. 1990. A brief account of the fractions of soma. *Ancient Science Life* 9(4): 207-208.

Madhihassan, S. & Mehdi, F.S. 1989. Rigveda and an Attempt to Identify It. American Journal of Chinese Medicine 17(1-2):1-8.

Makino, Y., Urano, Y. & Nagano, T. 2005. Investigation of the origin of ephedrine and methamphetamine by stable isotope ratio mass spectrometry: a Japanese experience. *Bulletin of Narcotics* 57(1-2): 63-78.

Manandhar, N.P. 1980. *Medicinal Plants of Nepali Himalaya.* Rama Pustak Bhandar, Kathmandu.

McGovern 2008. *Uncorking the Past: The Quest for Wine, Beer, and Other Alcoholic Beverages.* University of California Press, Berkeley.

Meier-Melikyan, N. R. 1990. Analysis of Plant Remains from Togolok-21 [in Russian, Opredelenie Rastitel'nix Ostatkov iz Togolok-21]. In: V. I. Sarianidi. *Drevnosti Strani Margush*, pp. 203–205 and figs. 55–58. Ilim, Ashkabad. Turkmenistan/Togolok

Merlin, M. 1972. *Man and Marijuana: Some Aspects of their Ancient Relationship.* Fairleigh Dickinson University Press, Rutherford, New Jersey, hardback, (2nd edition 1973); [paperback, Perpetua Books, South Brunswick, New Jersey, 1973].

Merlin, M. 1984. *On the Trail of the Ancient Opium Poppy: Natural and Early Cultural History of Papaver somniferum.* Associated University Presses, East Brunswick, New Jersey, 324 pp.

Merlin, M. 2003. Archaeological Record for Ancient Old World Use of Psychoactive Plants. *Economic Botany* 57(3): 295-323.

Merlin, M. 2013. Some aspects of the traditional use of *Ephedra* species in eastern Eurasia. *Ethnobotany* 25 (1&2): 1-17 [Invited article for Silver Jubilee Volume of Journal].

Merlin, M. 2014. "Medicinal and spiritual use of *Ephedra* species in ancient Xinjiang, China: archaeological and historical evidence." Fifth International Conference on Turfan Silk Road. Turfan, Xinjiang China, October 19-23.

Merlin, M. 2018. Ancient use of *Ephedra* in Eurasia and the Western Hemisphere. In: Fitzpatrick, S. (ed.). *Ancient psychoactive substances.* Gainesville: University Presses of Florida. Chapter 3, 71-111.

Merrillees, R. S. 1962. Opium trade in the Bronze Age Levant. *Antiquity* 36: 287–292.

Merrillees, R. S. 1979. Opium again in antiquity. *Levant* 11: 167–171.

Meyer, S. E. 1995. *Ephedra.* Provo, UT: USDA Forest Service, Rocky Mountain Research Station.

Miller, N. 2003. University of Pennsylvania. Personal Communication.

Monnier, G. 2012. Neanderthal Behavior. *Nature Education Knowledge* 3(10):11.

Morales, J., Carrión Marco, Y., Cooper, J.H. *et al.* 2024. Late pleistocene exploitation of *Ephedra* in a funerary context in Morocco. *Science Reports* 14, 26443 (2024). https://doi.org/10.1038/s41598-024-77785-w.

Motomura, H., Noshiro, S. & Mikage, M. 2007. Variable wood formation and adaptation to the alpine environment of *Ephedra pachyclada* (Gnetales: *Ephedra*ceae) in the Mustang District, western Nepal. *Annals of Botany* 100: 315–324.

Mukerjee, B.L. 1922. The Soma Plant. *Journal of the Royal Asiatic Society*, Calcutta, pp. 241-244.

Parpola, A. 1994. *Deciphering the Indus script.* Cambridge University Press, New York.

Price, R. A. 1996. *Systematics of the Gnetales: a review of morphological and molecular evidence. International Journal of Plant Science* 157 *(Suppl.): 40-49.*

Rätsch, C. 1998. The Encyclopedia of Psychoactive Plants: Ethnopharmacology and Its Applications. Park Street Press, Rochester, Vermont.

Ren, M., Tang, Z., Wu, X., Spengler, R., Jiang, H., Yang, Y. & N. Boivin. 2019. The origins of cannabis smoking:

Chemical residue evidence from the first millennium BCE in the Pamirs. Science Advances 12;5(6): eaaw1391. doi: 10.1126/sciadv.aaw1391.

Ross, I.A. 2001. *World Medicinal Plants of the World*. Humana Press Inc., New Jersey, Vol. 1, pp 131-139.

Rydin, C & Korall, P. 2009. Evolutionary relationships in *Ephedra* (Gnetales), with implications for seed plant phylogeny. *International Journal of Plant Science* 170(8):1031–1043.

Samorini, G. 2003. Personal Communication, March.

Samorini, G. 2019. The oldest archaeological data evidencing the relationship of Homo sapiens with psychoactive plants: A worldwide overview. *Journal of Psychedelic Studies* 3(2): 63-80.

Sarianidi, V. 1994. Temples of Bronze Age Margiana: traditions of ritual architecture. *Antiquity* 68:388–397.

Sarianidi, V. 1998. *Margiana and protozoroastrism*. Kapon, Athens.

Sarianidi, V. 2003. Margiana and Soma-Haoma. *Electronic Journal of Vedic Studies* 9 Issue 1c (May 5) edited by Jan E.M. Houben, Leiden University. http://www.heritageinstitute.com/zoroastrianism/merv/sarianidi.htm.

Schultes, R.E., Hofmann, A. & Rätsch. 2002. *Plants of the Gods: Their Sacred, Healing and Hallucinogenic Powers*. 2nd revised edition, Healing Arts Press, Rochester, Vermont.

Sharma, P., Uniyal, P.L. & Hammer, O. 2010. Two New Species of *Ephedra* (*Ephedra*ceae) from the Western Himalayas. *Systematic Biology* 35:4, 730-735.

Shipley, G.P. & Kindscher K. 2016. Evidence for the Paleoethnobotany of the Neanderthal: A Review of the Literature. *Scientifica* (Cairo). Article ID 8927654, 12 pages. http://dx.doi.org/10.1155/2016/8927654.

Singh, H. 2009. Sir Ram Nath Chopra: A profile. *Journal of Young Pharmacists* 1(3): 192-4. http://www.jyoungpharm.in/text.asp?2009/1/3/192/57062.

Small, E. 2016. *Cannabis: A Complete Guide*. CRC press, Boca Raton, Fl.

Smith, R.K., Stacey, R.J., Bergstrom, E. & Thomas-Oates, J. 2018. Detection of opium alkaloids in a Cypriot base-ring juglet. *Analyst* 143: 5127–5136 (2018).

Solecki, R.S. 1975. Shanidar IV, a Neanderthal Flower Burial in Northern Iraq. *Science* 190 (4217): 880–881.

Sommer, J.D. 1999. The Shanidar IV "flower burial": re-evaluation of neanderthal burial ritual. *Cambridge Archaeological Journal* 9(1):127-137.

Stapf. O. 1889. Die Arten der Gattung *Ephedra*. *Denkschr Math-Naturwiss* Cl K Akad. Wiss. 56. Kaiserlich-Königlichen Hof-und Staatsdruckerei, Wien.

Stein, A. 1931. On the *Ephedra*, the Hum Plant, and the Soma. *Bulletin of the School of Oriental Studies* 4 (1931): 501-514.

Stevenson, D. W. 1993 . *Ephedra*ceae. *In:* Flora of North America Editorial Committee (Eds.) *Flora of North America*. Oxford University Press, New York, pp. 428-434.

Taillieu, D. 1995. Old Iranian haoma: A Note on Its Pharmacology. Acta Orientalia Belgica 9: 187-91.

Taillieu, D. 1998. Haoma Plant. The Circle of Ancient Iranian Studies. http://cais-soas.com/CAIS/Religions/iranian/Zarathushtrian/haoma_plant.htm.

Taillieu, D & Boyce, M. 2002. Haoma. *Encyclopaedia Iranica*. New York: Mazda Pub.

Tang, S.; Ren, J.; Kong, L.; Yan, G.; Liu, C.; Han, Y.; Sun, H. & Wang, X.-J. 2023. Ephedrae Herba: A Review of Its Phytochemistry, Pharmacology, Clinical Application, and Alkaloid Toxicity. *Molecules* 28, 663. https://doi.org/10.3390/molecules28020663.

Tang, W. & Eisenbrand, G. 1992. *Chinese Drugs of Plant Origin*. Springer-Verlag, Berlin, pp. 481-490.

Teuscher, E. 1979. *Pharmakognosie*. Akademie-Verlag, Berlin.

Wang, B. 1983. Agricultural archaeology in Xinjiang. *Nongye Kaogu* (Agricultural Archaeology) 1: 102-121 (in Chinese).

Wang, B.H. 1993. Archaeological excavations at Gumugou Site, Kongque River and a preliminary study on the discoveries. In: B. Wang (Ed.) *Archaeobiological Survey of the ancient Silk Road*. Xinjiang People's Publishing House, Urumchi (in Chinese).

Wang, L., Kakiuchi, N. & Mikage, M. 2010. Studies of *Ephedra* plants in Asia. Part 6: Geographical changes of anatomical features and alkaloids content of *Ephedra sinica*. *Journal of Natural Medicines*. 64(1): 63-69.

Wangchuk, P., Ugyen, S. Thinley, J. & Afaq, S.H. 2008. High Altitude Plants used in Bhutanese traditional Medicine (*gSo-ba-rig-pa*). *Ethnobotany* 20: 54-64.

Wasson, R.G. 1968. *Soma: divine mushroom of immortality*. Harcourt, Brace, Jovanovich, New York.

Wenke, M., ed. 1986. *Farmakologie*. Avicenum, Praha.

Welwitsch, F. 1861. *Journal of the Proceedings of the Linnean Society, Botany* 5: 182-*187*.

West, E. 1901. W. *Pahlavi Texts* SBE 5, p. 222.

Weyrich, L., Duchene, S., Soubrier, J. *et al.* 2017. Neanderthal behaviour, diet, and disease inferred from ancient DNA in dental calculus. *Nature* 544, 357–361 (2017). https://doi.org/10.1038/nature21674

Wikimedia Commons. 2006. *Erbil Governorate Shanidar Cave. Wikimedia Commons.* https://commons.wikimedia.org/wiki/File:Erbil_governorate_shanidar_cave.jpg.

Witzel, M. 2005. Central Asian Roots and Acculturation in South Asia. Linguistic and Archaeological Evidence from Western Central Asia, the Hindukush and Northwestern South Asia for Early Indo-Aryan Language and Religion. In: Osada, T. (Ed.), *Linguistics, Archaeology and the Human Past.* Indus Project, Research Institute for Humanity and Nature, pp. 87-211.

Xia, L. 1997. The ancient Loulan People's adaption to the environment—a cultural interpretation of the funeral *Ephedra* in Lop Nur area. *Social Sciences in China* 3:115–129 (in Chinese).

Xie, M., Yang, Y., Wang, B.& Wang, C. 2013. Interdisciplinary investigation on ancient *Ephedra* twigs from Gumugou Cemetery (3800b.p.) in Xinjiang region, northwest China. *Microscopy Research Technique* 76: 663–672.

Yang, Y. 2010. A Review on Gnetalean Megafossils: Problems and Perspectives. *Taiwania*, 55(4): 346-354.

Yang, Y., Dezhi, F. & Guanghua, Z. 2003. A new species of *Ephedra* (Ephedraceae) from China. *Novon* 13: 153.

Yang, Y., B. Geng, D. L. Dilcher, Z. Chen & Lott, T.A. 2005. Morphology and affinities of an Early Cretaceous *Ephedra* (Ephedraceae) from China. *American Journal of Botany* 92: 231–241.

Yang, Y. 2010. A Review on Gnetalean Megafossils: Problems and Perspectives. *Taiwania*, 55(4): 346-354.

Zhang, F., Ning, C., Scott, A. *et al.* 2021. The genomic origins of the Bronze Age Tarim Basin mummies. *Nature* 599: 256–261.

Zhang, J.S., Tian, Z. & Lou, Z.C. 1989. [Quality evaluation of twelve species of Chinese Ephedra (ma huang)]. Yao Xue Xue Bao 24(11): 865-7. In Chinese. PMID: 2618686.

Zheng, Q., Mu, X., Pan, S., Luan, R. & Zhao, P. 2023. Ephedrae herba: A comprehensive review of its traditional uses, phytochemistry, pharmacology, and toxicology. *J. Ethnopharmacol.* 307, 116153.

Identifying Depictions of *Anadenanthera* in the Iconographic Records of Cupisnique, Paracas, and Nazca Cultures

Colin Domnauer, Doctoral Candidate

Ethnobiologist | Mycologist | University of Utah

> *"The importance of psychoactive plants in many major pre-Columbian Andean cultures is well-documented, with an abundance of convincing evidence for their use in diverse geographical locations and time periods. However, significant gaps remain in the archaeological record, where the current evidence of hallucinogen use in certain cultures is scarce or non-existent. This presentation attempts to address such gaps in our knowledge."*
>
> —COLIN DOMNAUER

This paper explores art history, archaeobotany and psychedelic use amongst ancient cultures of the Andes.

Humans have a long and intimate relationship with hallucinogens, and it is the aim of this work is to examine the distribution, uses, and cultural associations of the most ancient and widely sed hallucinogen in pre-Columbian South America. This is the plant Anadenanthera spp., also referred to as "vilca". Due to the ability of such mind-altering substances to impart an unparalleled profundity upon an individual, hallucinogens serve as powerful agents for shaping the collective cultures that employ their use. In particular they influence iconography. As we will see, this fact is quite clearly evident in many major pre-Columbian Andean cultures as they reflected their relationship with vilca in a range of material objects including cloth, ceramic, and stone. From iconographic analysis, we are offered a unique window into the beliefs, practices, and worldview surrounding the use of vilca in these ancient Andean societies.

The importance of psychoactive plants in many major pre-Columbian Andean cultures is well-documented, with an abundance of convincing evidence for their use found in diverse geographical locations and time periods. With chemical residues analyzed, botanical specimens recovered, paraphernalia unearthed, and iconography deciphered, it is clear that vilca (*Anadenanthera spp.*) was one of the most ancient and widespread plant hallucinogens employed across the pre-Colombian Andes. The earliest archaeological evidence for its use consists of bone pipes found along with vilca seeds in Inca Cueva, Northwest Argentina, with radiocarbon tests dating them back to 2130 BCE. Chemical tests of these smoking pipes revealed the presence of tryptamine alkaloids that are present in *Anadenanthera* (Torres and Repke, 2006, 30). More recent studies have continued to uncover chemical traces of *Anadenanthera* in well-preserved shamanic paraphernalia dated to later pre-Columbian times in other locations of the Andes (Miller et al., 2019; Horta-Tricallotis, 2019).

Archaeological research has identified the presence of vilca in many major Andean cultures including Chavin, Moche, Huari, and Tiwanaku (Sharon, 1972; Furst, 1974; Cordy-Collins, 1977; Burger, 1995; Knobloch, 2000; Torres, 2018a). Within the shamanic tradition which defined pre-Columbian Andean religion, it is believed that vilca was highly regarded and intentionally used for its powerful psychotropic effects. Iconographic studies have yielded insightful and convincing evidence of vilca's use in ceremonial contexts at major religious sites such as the temples of Chavin de Huantar (ca. 900-300 BCE), Huacas de Moche (CA. 100–900 CE), and Tiahuanaco (ca. 100-1000 CE) (Rick, 2004; Burger, 2011; Torres, 2018b).

However, despite this extensive research, significant spatial-temporal gaps remain in the archaeological record where the use of vilca within certain cultures has never been clearly elucidated, despite its probable presence being suspected. This paper seeks to address this knowledge gap by contributing novel iconographic evidence of *Anadenanthera* occurring in three major Andean cultures which had previously exhibited no known evidence of vilca use (Cupisnique) or any hallucinogen use (Nazca and Paracas), thereby contributing to the growing body of evidence demonstrating the significance of psychoactive plant use in the pre-Columbian Andes.

IDENTIFICATION OF VILCA ICONOGRAPHY

Just as our experiences with psychoactive substances are shaped not only by the drug itself, but by social and psychological factors surrounding its use (the so-called set and setting), it is vital that the study of psychoactive plants and fungi includes discourse about the cultural contexts in which they are utilized. Therefore, research into the historical uses of psychoactive substances is valuable because it expands and enriches our appreciation for the variety of ways that humans interact with these substances. This arguably offers just as much insight and perspective as studying the pharmacology itself.

Establishing the historical use of psychoactive plants in ancient cultures may be achieved through a variety of different approaches. Torres (2008, 237) outlines four major categorical strata of what may be considered substantial archaeological evidence: 1. Remains of psychoactive plants themselves, in a relevant context, 2. Implements related to the use of psychoactive materials, 3. Representations of psychoactive plants, and 4. Depictions of the use of psychoactive materials. This study focuses specifically on examining the iconographic representations of psychoactive plants and their associations.

To recognize any plant's depiction in Andean art, the botanical traits characteristic of that plant must be known. In the case of *Anadenanthera*, these features are "the bipinnately compound leaves and the sinuate, irregularly contracted pods with cuspidate apices", spherical flowers, and rounded, dimpled seeds (Torres, 2008, 247) (Figure 1). However, depictions of *Anadenanthera* in the archaeological record are rarely identical to the natural morphology, as much of pre-Colombian art is highly stylized or symbolically illustrated.

In order to identify the more stylized iconographic forms of *Anadenanthera* in pre-Columbian Andean cultures, Patricia Knobloch (who has investigated this intensively) notes the following symbolic attributes of vilca in her analysis of Wari artifacts: "1) circled dots, usually two, at the top of the icon representing the spherical flowers; 2) two, symmetrically positioned ovate or rectangular shapes with interior lines representing the leaves, usually positioned below the circled dots; and, 3) oblong or rectangular shape with interior dots representing the seedpods" (Knobloch, 2000, 391). Also indicative of vilca seed pods is the general motif of "linear clusters of circular elements" (Cordy-Collins, 1982). Many previous researchers have also observed these common motifs of vilca appearing in multiple different Andean cultures across time and space, thus bolstering our confidence in the interpretation of the intended meaning of these symbols (Cordy Collins, 1982; Knobloch, 2000; Burger, 2011; Torres, 2018b; Domnauer, 2020).

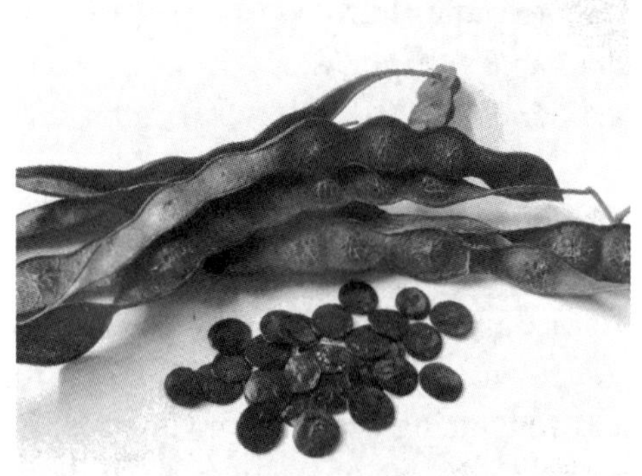

Fig.1 *Anadenanthera* seed pods and seeds.
Courtesy of Cathy L. Costin

In addition to identifying naturalistic and/or stylized depictions of the *Anadenanthera* plant itself, another form of iconographic insight into the ancient use of psychoactive plants is obtained through recognizing imagery associated with shamanism or non-ordinary states of consciousness. Because a culture represents the collective beliefs, emotions, and behaviors of its people, and psychoactive substances directly influence these subjective experiences, the art that comes from this culture is therefore in part reflective of and inspired by encounters with the mind-altering drugs that are used. In other words, the experiences in non-ordinary states of consciousness resulting from the use of psychoactive plants may be expected to appear within that culture's iconography. In fact, it has been argued that some of the earliest artwork produced by humans-cave paintings dating back as early as 45,000 -10,000 years ago- were produced as a result of ecstatic visionary experiences brought about through the ingestion of certain mind-altering plants (Lewis-Williams, 2011). This similarly applies in the pre-Columbian Andes, as Torres and Repke (2006, 198) explains: "Throughout the pre-Hispanic world, psychoactive plants are considered intermediaries between the human and the supernatural realm; they are capable of participating in the interpretation and creation of cultural elements". Anthropologist Christain Rätsch, recounting his personal experience of inhaling vilca snuff and the subsequent realizations it forced upon him, observes this directly, noting the obvious parallel between his subjective experience and the iconographic forms present in pre-Columbian artwork: "A panorama of flowing designs-the exact patterns depicted in the nimbus surrounding the head of the Chavin deity! I marveled for minutes at the interlocking tessellation of these geometric shapes. They possessed a multiple interlocking penetrated arrangement which matched the characteristic style of Tiahuanaco artwork. At that moment I was convinced that the Tiahuanaco artists used this snuff to inspire their work" (Rätsch, 1996, 60-61 in Torres and Repke, 2006, 185).

IDENTIFICATION OF SHAMANIC ICONOGRAPHY

A shaman may be defined as a person who achieves direct contact with the spirit world, fulfilling the function of an intermediary between the physical and mystical realms that, although invisible and inaccessible to ordinary individuals of the culture, is nevertheless believed to be present and capable of influencing the health and well-being of the community (Harner 1973, xi). The spirit world to which the shaman journeys is a place where the shaman achieves unique knowledge, insights, and healing abilities, applied for the benefit and well-being of the community. Central to this faculty of the shaman is transcendence into a non-ordinary state of consciousness. In the Andes, this has been (and still is) most often accomplished through the ingestion of psychoactive plants such as vilca. The iconographic depiction of vilca may be more easily recognized if we are able to consider and discern representations of these common themes of shamanism and the shamanic experience, thus providing a larger context in which frequently observed motifs can be adequately interpreted and their intended meaning properly identified.

The primary shamanic motifs pertinent to the understanding of pre-Columbian Andean iconography are that of 1) separation from the body taking magical flight, 2) transforming into animal form, and 3) gaining access to non-ordinary realms of consciousness where encounters with spirits and deceased ancestors may occur (Harner, 1973, 158; Eliade, 1964, 479). Referring to the first point, leading authority on the study of shamanism Michael Harner notes that "the soul is believed to separate from the physical body and make a trip, often with the sensation of flight" (Harner, 1973, 158). Additionally, general distortions in bodily perception and coordination also occur. This experience of departing from one's physical human body connects to another aforementioned motif, that across all indigenous cultures of the world exists an intimate relationship between shamans and animals, for "it is the shaman who turns himself into an animal…who becomes an animal-spirit, and speaks, sings, or flies like the animals" (Eliade, 1964, 98). Such zoomorphic imagery commonly appears in South American art and shamanism, as "thematic units with a widespread geographical distribution include avian, feline, and ophidian representations" (Torres & Repke, 2006, 197).

Succinctly summarizing all three of these themes, Rebecca Stone describes the journey of the shaman in her book *The Jaguar Within*, writing: "during trances, the corporeal is reported to fall away, and gravity's weight is replaced by a feeling of soaring flight. Plants, animals, and humans merge and exchange identities with one's human self in rapid flashes of transformation, and a shared animation pervades all things, even remaking death itself within a large cosmic flux" (Stone, 2011, 1). This shamanic transformation of identity is a crucial point to consider when attempting to make sense of iconography in the pre-Columbian Andes. The presence of such shamanic imagery by itself does not constitute sufficient evidence for the use of vilca particularly. However when it is considered in context alongside motifs specific to vilca, these two visual categories combined provide supporting and compelling evidence indicative of the use of vilca as a consciousness transforming agent.

Lastly, it is also helpful to note the subjective effects specific to the ingestion of vilca. In concordance with themes of the shamanic experience outlined previously, the experience of receiving the vilca snuff is perceived by the indigenous people as "direct communication with the spirits of animals, plants, deceased relatives and other supernatural's" (Furst, 1976, 131). Moreover, the effects of vilca are characterized by a feeling of being "turned upside down and that men are walking on their feet in the air"; "a twitching of the muscles, slight convulsions, and lack of muscular coordination, followed by nausea, visual hallucinations, and disturbed sleep. Also present are distorted perceptions of objects' size (macropsia), feelings of the world being turned upside down, and when taken as a snuff, a profuse flow of mucus from the nose" (Schultes, 1976, 89). To summarize, in order to track the occurrence of vilca in pre-Columbian artwork, we should be prepared to recognize the symbology associated with the shamanic experience in general as well as the physical symptoms and encounters resulting from the ingestion of the hallucinogenic vilca snuff.

PREVIOUS EVIDENCE OF VILCA IN THE FORMATIVE PERIOD

Before presenting any novel archaeological evidence, it is important to have a basic contextual understanding of the interconnections between the various cultures to be discussed, including those with known evidence for vilca use. These groups are often related spatially or temporally, and establishing a given culture's clear connection and interaction with another society that has already established evidence for vilca use, strengthens the plausibility of any novel arguments for vilca's presence and use in this new culture. It also provides more context where the interpretation of shared motifs and iconography argued to represent vilca can be more wholly understood.

The Formative Period (ca. 1800 BCE–500 BCE) of Andean history represents the emergence of such early influential cultures as Cupisnique (ca. 1000–200 BCE) located on the North Coast of Peru, Chavin (ca. 900-300 BCE) located in the central highlands of Peru, and Paracas on the South Coast of Peru (ca. 800-100 BCE). Previous research investigating psychoactive plants portrayed in Formative Period artwork has mostly focused on the San Pedro cactus (*Trichocereus* spp); the evidence for its presence and use in both Chavin and Cupisnique societies has been extensively discussed and is now considered to be well-accepted (Cordy Collins, 1977, 1982; Sharon, 1978, 2000; Sharon and Donnan, 1977). However, unlike the well-accepted use of San Pedro throughout Formative Period cultures, the case for vilca is much less substantial. Evidence for vilca's presence in Cupisnique and Paracas has remained entirely absent, while examples of vilca imagery have only recently emerged in the study of Chavin.

Chavin is well-known for its religious ceremonial temple of Chavin de Huantar, which is extensively decorated with depictions of shamanic transformation and hallucinogenic plants. Elaborately engineered at the confluence of two rivers, this temple features a system of underground stone labyrinths leading to a stone obelisk/deity carved with surreal imagery. Recent tests have shown these narrow tunnels to be acoustically resonant, so the sound of rushing water (which was diverted from the nearby rivers) would have been amplified, both by the architectural engineering as well as from the ingestion of powerful mind-altering plants. It has long been well established that the religious rituals performed at Chavin de Huantar were shamanistic in nature and based upon the consumption of hallucinogenic plants (Burger, 1995; Cordy Collins, 1977, 1980; Sharon, 1972).

This hallucinogen hypothesis was based entirely on depictions of San Pedro cactus, while the evidence for *Anadenanthera* specifically at Chavin de Huantar has only recently emerged. A stone carving was found to contain naturalistic depictions of plant parts matching that of *Anadenanthera* leaves and seed pods, all of which adorned a figure transforming from human into animal form (Figure 2a) (Burger, 2011). This led to the initial proposal that *Anadenanthera* was another hallucinogenic plant in Chavin's pharmacopeia employed by their religion. Other compelling indications that vilca was consumed at Chavin de Huantar come not from images of the plant itself, but rather scenes of the effects following vilca's ingestion. Specifically, there are a number of examples of nasal discharge emerging from the nostrils of anthropomorphic heads carved in stone. The best explanation for this is offered by the fact that vilca is traditionally taken as a snuff through the nostrils, and consequently, produces a copious flow of mucous (Torres, 2008, 243). The shaman would apparently then experience being transformed into an animal form as the effects of vilca took hold, a theme we also see depicted in a series of stone tenon heads decorating the temple walls at Chavin de Huantar which illustrate the progressive stages of transformation from human to feline form (Figure 2b).

Another potential source of evidence for vilca use in Chavin culture comes from the so-called "Shamanism Textile", recovered from an Early Horizon Ica valley site but which likely originated from Chavin. Appearing in this textile is "a linear cluster of circular elements", which has been argued to represent the similarly shaped vilca seed pods (Cordy-Collins, 1982, 147). What is particularly noteworthy in this case is the context in which the vilca motif appears. Alongside it is depictions of San Pedro cactus (another hallucinogenic plant), animals associated with shamanism (e.g. jaguar, hummingbird), and a deity figure (Cordy-Collins, 1982). Moreover, imagery of mucus flow is also observed, which as previously discussed likely indicate insufflation of vilca

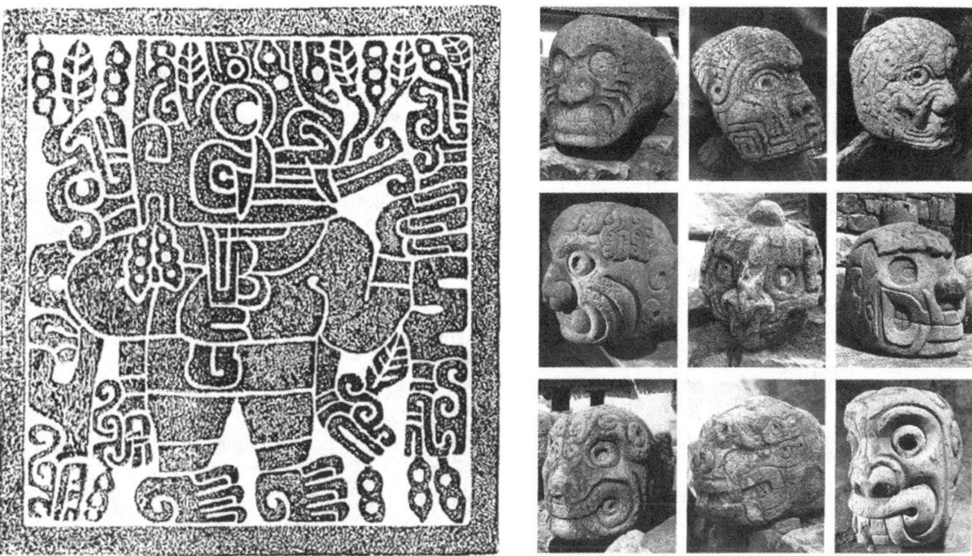

Fig.2 a) Stone carving at Chavin de Huantar, depicting *Anadenanthera* leaves and seed pods alongside a shaman in the act of transformation into animal form (Burger, 2011) b) Stone heads portraying the progressive stages of metamorphosis from human into feline form (Burger, 1995).

snuff (Cordy Collins, 1982, 148). All such images appearing within a single textile, of a clearly shamanic theme reinforces the interpretation of this symbol as a stylized representation of hallucinogenic vilca seeds.

In total, this abundance of iconographic evidence strongly suggests vilca was consumed as a snuff at Chavin de Huantar. Moreover, this argument is supported by noting the precedence of the snuffing practice; the oldest evidence for snuffing comes from the Peruvian coast at Huaca Prieta in the Chicama Valley, where snuff trays and bird bone tubes were dated to 1200 BCE, thus preceding the time of Chavin de Huantar (Bird, 1948, 27). To conclude, iconographic studies have formed a compelling case that in addition to the consumption of San Pedro cactus, vilca was also utilized in the religious rituals performed at Chavin de Huantar (Cordy-Collins, 1980). This thus establishes a reasonable context for vilca to possibly appear in related Andean cultures.

CUPISNIQUE

Based on similarities in religious artifacts, architecture, and iconography, previous research has pointed out the widespread influence of the Chavin tradition on the contemporaneous cultures in other areas of the Andes, particularly the Paracas on the south coast and the Cupisnique on the north coast of Peru (Cordy-Collins, 1979; Nesbitt, 2012). In fact, the societies of Chavin and Cupisnique share such similar artistic styles in their iconography that for a long time they were believed to be of the same origin, with scholars commonly referring to Cupisnique as coastal Chavin. Thus, this relatedness between Cupisnique and a contemporaneous Andean culture known to have utilized vilca (as well as other psychoactive plants) in a shamanic context not only indicates a sharing of artistic styles, but likely of religious traditions and practices as well, thereby providing plausible historical context for the use of vilca amongst the Cupisnique.

Also suggesting the possible presence of *Anadenanthera* in Cupisnique, is the shared traditions and iconography with another related (although later period) Andean culture known to have used vilca: the Moche. The evidence for vilca in Moche culture is well-established and has been written about extensively and so will not be discussed here (Torres and Repke, 2006; Torres, 2018a). Suffice to say numerous Moche artifacts (mostly ceramic drinking vessels) have been recovered which clearly display *Anadenanthera* in naturalistic form (Figure 3).

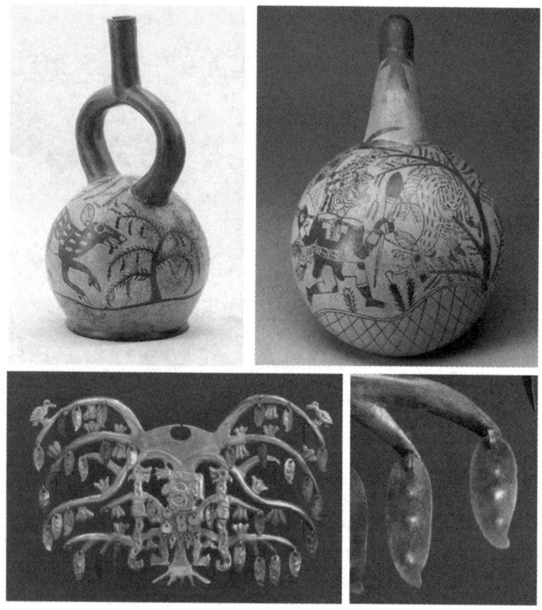

Fig.3 Moche artifacts depicting *Anadenanthera* in naturalistic form. Two ceramic drinking vessels and one elaborate nose piercing. *Fowler Museum X73.237; AIC 1955.2277; MFA Houston 2010.543.*

Also occupying the North Coast of Peru in later times, the Moche share many iconographic motifs and themes with their predecessors, the Cupisnique, thus indicating that the Moche were inheritors of cultural elements and traditions established by the Cupisnique (Cordy-Collins 1992). In fact, in her analysis of Northern Coast symbolism, Alana Cordy-Collins concludes that certain major supernatural iconographic themes present in both Cupisnique and Moche are so similar that they must be seen to indicate "a direct transference [from Cupisnique to Moche] of religious belief..." (Cordy-Collins, 1992, 217). Likewise, Izumi Shimada writes "the early phases of the mochica culture were clearly built upon the widespread antecedent and contemporary North Coast cultures known as the Cupisnique, Salinar, and Gallinzao" (Shimada, 1994, 61). Thus, despite distinct differences in artistic style, the Moche and Cupisnique clearly share many overlapping religious motifs, which suggests the possibility of a continuity of certain religious beliefs and/or practices which would have originated in earlier (Cupisnique) times. From this fact, combined with the evidence for vilca in the contemporaneous Chavin culture, there exists a reasonable plausibility that vilca was used in Cupisnique as well. Nonetheless, the study of Cupisnique iconography has yet to uncover any clear evidence for such a claim. However, I will present new evidence from Cupisnique ceramics which I believe to be clear depictions of both vilca and the subjective effects upon its consumption, which can be interpreted as referencing the use of vilca as a consciousness transforming agent by the Cupisnique people.

VILCA IN CUPISNIQUE CERAMICS

Cupisnique ceramics have long been known to contain a rich and abundant display of shamanic themes, including images of bodily transformation and the hallucinogenic San Pedro cactus. In fact, Cupisnique art consists almost entirely of surreal and supernatural imagery, and of those natural objects which are occasionally present, they nearly always appear within a religious context (Cordy-Collins, 1992, 207). For these reasons, Cupisnique society is seen as one strongly rooted in and absorbed by religion. Moreover, as previously mentioned, the use of San Pedro cactus amongst the Cupisnique is already well-accepted. Thus, for these reasons and the historical contextual reasons discussed, the occurrence of another plant hallucinogen (vilca) within the shamanic pharmacopeia and iconography of the Cupisnique culture logically fits within our understandings of their religious practices and traditions.

Various botanical components of *Anadenanthera* are seen the Cupisnique ceramics shown in Figure 4. The stirrup-spout vessel is covered in fine surface etchings of a comb-like, chevron shaped lines in exactly the same pattern which has been identified by previous scholars to represent the bipinnate

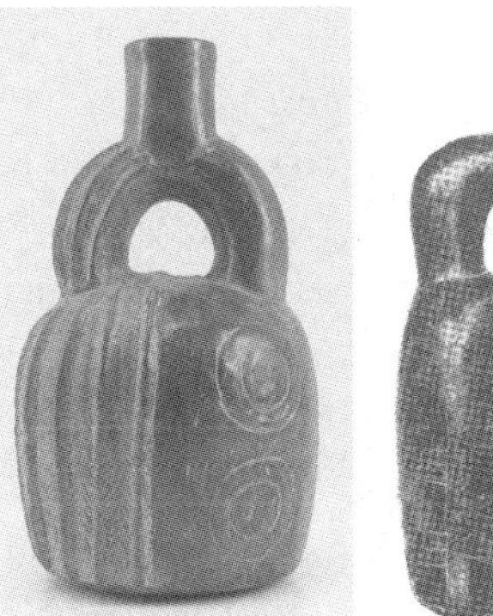
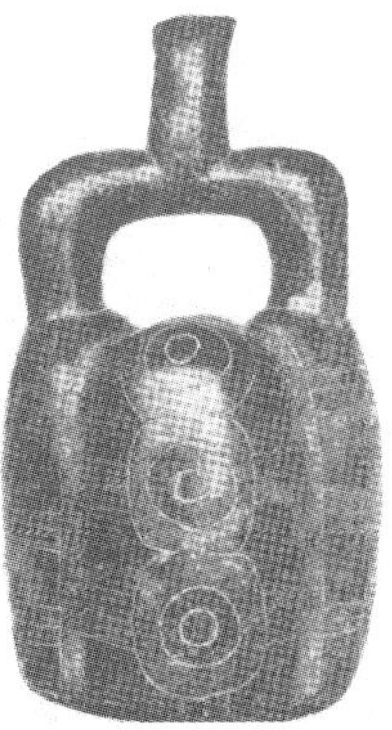
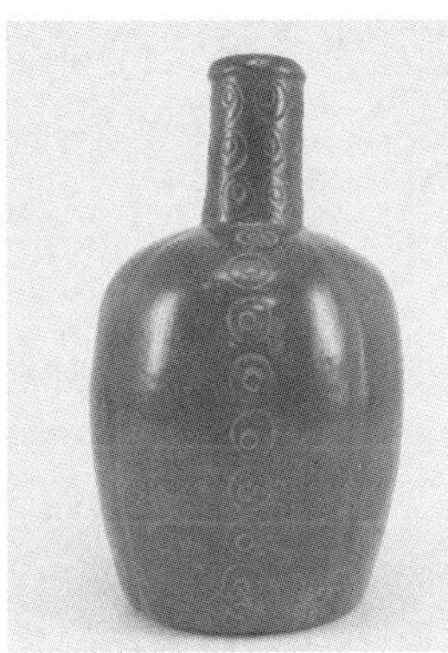

Fig.4 Cupisnique ceramic vessel with etchings of linear columns of inscribed circles. *Museo Larco ML15102; Alva 1986: Fig 22B*

opposite leaf shape of *Anadenanthera*. Additionally, there are two large circles with central dots which resemble known representations of the flowers or seeds.

Perhaps the most intriguing evidence for vilca is seen in a Cupisnique stirrup-spout ceramic vessel shown in Figure 5. Indeed, one could hardly imagine a clearer depiction of pre-Columbian Andean shamanism contained within a single artifact. Here we see the shamanic animal familiars of the jaguar and the serpent, the San Pedro cactus, and as I will argue here, vilca seeds. As such, this vessel may be attempting to portray multiple features of Cupisnique shamanism and psychoactive plant use combined into a single image, a context into which vilca would have logically belonged, and thus could be expected to be visually depicted.

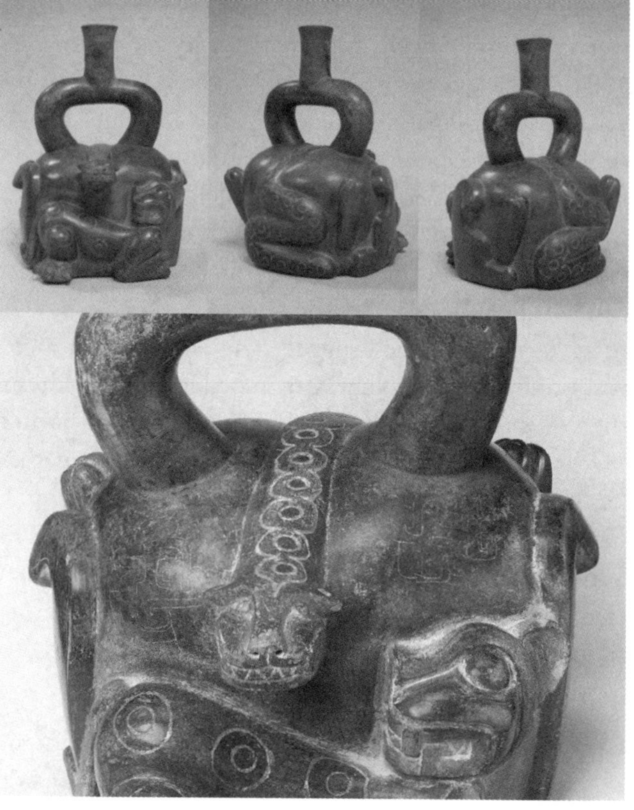

Fig.5 Cupisnique ceramic vessel depicting the legume pod motif in serpent, alongside shamanic familiar of the jaguar dotted with the same circle symbol, as well as another psychoactive plant, the San Pedro cactus. *Metropolitan Museum of Art 67.239.17*

The linear column of connected inter-constricted circles seen along the serpent's body is a well-known motif of vilca seed pods, the so-called "legume pod-motif". It is a naturalistically accurate representation of *Anadenanthera spp.* seed pods and almost always appears in combination with other shamanic imagery, most commonly a serpent as it does here.

The legume pod motif is seen in several other Cupisnique artifacts as well. In Figure 6, the vilca legume pod motif is once again present inside the body of the serpent and occurs near what appears to be two curved cacti (likely San Pedro cactus). While this vertical column of connected circles morphologically resembles vilca seed pods, it is the simultaneous co-occurrence of this motif with a serpent and another hallucinogenic plant that further strengthens the interpretation that the intended meaning of this symbol is to the represent vilca.

As will be discussed later, this legume pod motif has also been identified as depicting vilca in an analysis of Paracas and Nazca art, where the vilca image (as in Figure 5) similarly appears within the body of serpents, thus highlighting this common motif's portrayal across Andean cultures over time (Domnauer, 2020). In other words, this symbol is not only virtually identical in style to its occurrence in other Andean cultures, but it also appears within a similar symbolic context, further strengthening the interpretation that this motif is representing the shamanic use of vilca in Cupisnique pottery. This linear column of connected circles being interpreted as a legume pod representing vilca is supported by its 1) morphological resemblance to *Anadenanthera* seed pod, 2) occurrence in the iconography of other Andean cultures within a similar context (noted by previous scholars), 3) logical appearance alongside shamanic imagery and another hallucinogenic plant (San Pedro cactus), and 4) reasonable plausibility given the overlapping religious practices and iconography between the Chavin- who are known to have utilized vilca- and the Cupisnique.

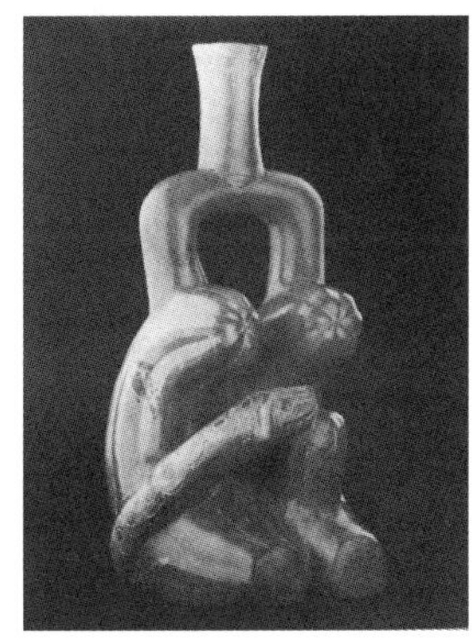

Fig.6 Cupisnique ceramic vessel depicting the legume pod motif in serpent's body, alongside the psychoactive San Pedro cactus. *Bonavia 1994: Figure 17*

Focusing now on the body of the jaguar, we see the exact same shape of individual circles inscribed with smaller interior circles, closely resembling the legume pod motif seen on the serpent, only in this instance the dots are disconnected. Of course, this could simply be portraying the jaguars' naturally dotted fur as previous scholars have suggested, but this motif may also be considered multivalent in its meaning, serving a dual symbolic purpose of also representing vilca seeds (Domnauer & Costin, 2022). For one, these dots are drastically oversized if the artist was simply intending to replicate the naturalistic morphology of jaguar spots. As previously discussed, the ingestion of hallucinogenic plants was often experienced as a transformation from human into animal form. As Burger (1995, 157) describes: "One important feature of Chavin ideology was the belief that its priests could transform themselves into jaguars in order to contact and affect the behavior of supernatural forces. Hallucinogenic snuffs and beverages apparently catalyzed these changes". In fact, this association between vilca and felines traces back to the earliest evidence for *Anadenanthera* use (2100 BCE), as vilca seeds and tryptamine residues were found with pipes made of puma bone. Moreover, there are many examples of closely related Andean cultures making similar stylistic choices to depict a zoomorphically transformed shaman blended with the psychoactive plants they utilized as their vehicle for transformation, as previously shown in Figure 2. Additionally, in an animistic worldview, it is normal to perceive parallels or equivalences in meaning between isomorphic forms, such as the irregularly rounded spots of a jaguar and the similarly irregularly rounded vilca seeds. Similarities are seen to be meaningful rather than random, indicative of an underlying connection between seemingly "separate" phenomena. Therefore, given the strong associations among jaguars and plant-induced trances in South American shamanic rituals, it is likely that these circular spot motifs are multivalent in their meaning, referencing not only shamanic avatars but also the means by which the shaman connected with (or in fact transformed into) them. In other words, whereas the connected column of circles (legume pod motif) represents the entire vilca seed pod, the same circles, when individually separated, could represent individual vilca seeds.

A clear example of this potential is outlined in Figure 7, where we see two remarkably similar Cupisnique vessels, with one notable difference. In one case is a column of connected circles on the interior of a serprent's body (i.e. the legume pod motif), while in the other vessel, this same form is separated into individual circles. That this individual circle motif appears in a nearly identical situation on a vessel which clearly depicts the legume pod motif suggests that it is in fact

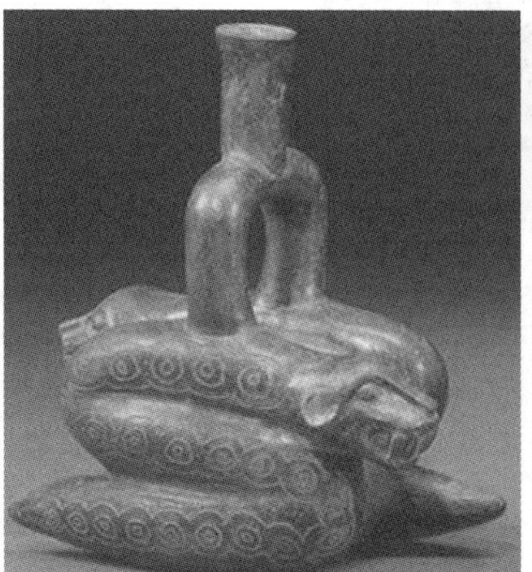
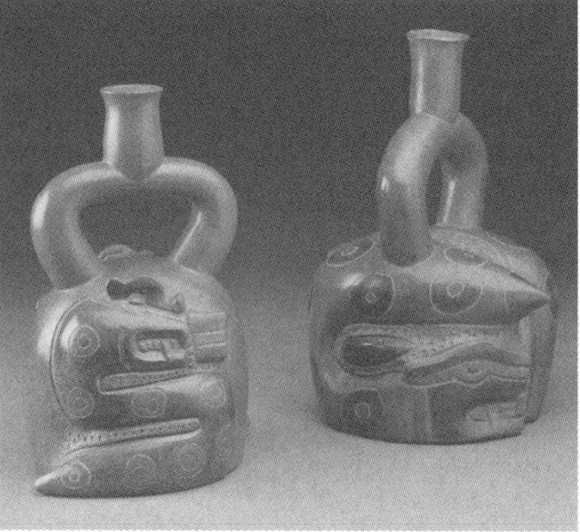

Fig.7 Two Cupisnique vessels show similar seed motif inside the body of a serpent. In one case they are connected as a single column while in the other they are disconnected, potentially representing the entire vilca seed pod and individual seeds, respectively. *Metropolotin Museum of Art 67.239.17; Museo Larco 10481,10501*

an attempt to represent the vilca seeds. Additional support for this interpretation comes from the fact that this same seed motif has been seen in artifacts across many major Andean cultures including Paracas, Chavin, Nazca, and Tiwanaku, where it is similarly found associated with shamanic images. For example, this exact same circular shape motif also appears at Tiwanaku on monoliths which have been identified to be holding vilca snuffing trays, and at Chavin on a stone carving of a jaguar (Torres, 2018b) (Figure 8). Therefore, in both of these cases, this circular seed image is associated with an aspect of vilca ingestion: snuffing paraphenelia and animal transformation, respectively. It is thus reasonable to assume that this motif carries a meaning associated with vilca, which I believe to be a symbol of vilca seeds. For all these reasons discussed, I believe this circle-shaped motif cannot be simply dismissed as random "spots" on an animal, but has a more plausible interpretation of carrying a deeper meaning associated with *Anadenanthera*, specifically being images of vilca seeds.

Less direct evidence for vilca in Cupisnique (but still worth noting) comes from a multitude of artifacts depicting subjective experiences of non-ordinary states of consciousness which would have been brought about by the ingestion of such powerful plants as vilca (Costin 2018, 2019a, 2019b). In Figure 9 we see a Cupisnique stirrup-spout vessel in the fascinating shape of a contorted human figure with an arched back and the head upside down contacting the ground. This contortion of bodily perception is strikingly similar to the subjective feelings experienced upon the ingestion of vilca: effects are characterized by a feeling of "...the world being turned upside down…and that men are walking on their feet in the air" (Schultes, 1976, 89). Other signs of bodily distortion from vilca include "a twitching of the muscles, slight convulsions, and lack of muscular coordination" (Schultes, 1976, 89). The feeling of "walking on their feet in the air" is clearly illustrated in the vessels shown in Figure 9.

Held in each of the hands of Figure 9 is what appears to be a rattle or musical device. The use of rhythmic instruments is a well-known aspect of shamanism, both ancient and modern, thus

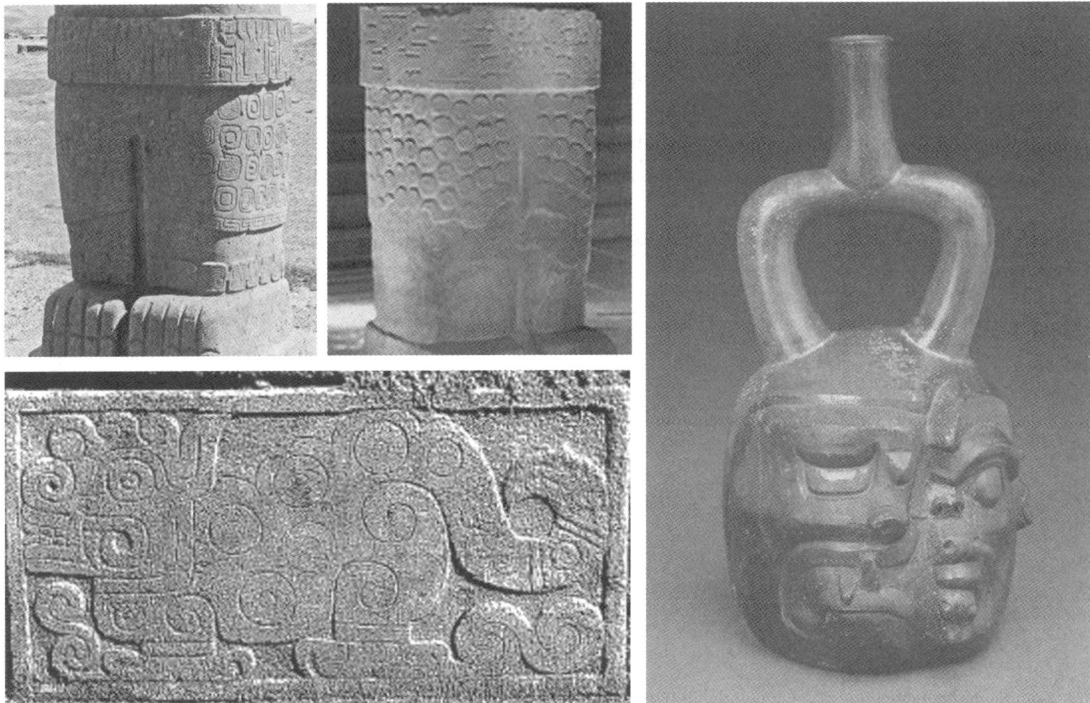

Fig.8 Additional examples of the vilca seed motif appearing on monoliths holding vilca snuffing trays at Tiwanaku , a stone jaguar carving at Chavin, and a Cupisnique ceramic depicting shamnic transformation. *Museo Larco ML040218*

supporting the interpretation of the vilca seed pod motif appearing in a shamanic context (Costin 2019a, 2019b). Lastly, on the figure's kneecap we see the etching of the previously encountered vilca seed motif. There are many other examples of Cupisnique ceramics also portraying similar bodily distortion (Figure 10). Particularly noteworthy in these cases are the serpents adorned to the person's head, which as previously discussed is another common image associated with vilca. Lastly, Figure 11 shows a ceramic drinking vessel covered with esoteric etchings in a style similar to Chavin, shaped in the form of a crouched human pouring a liquid into a small bowl, perhaps suggesting that vilca was consumed orally in liquid form (Costin 2018). Here again, the vilca seed motif appears on the figure's shoulder and knee. Also relevant is how the eyes are upturned, apparently rolled to the back of the head. This rolled eye trait is also seen in the famous Chavin stone carving of the anthropomorphic shaman holding San Pedro cactus. Showing the eyes unturned in this way is likely an intentional detail attempting to convey a state of trance of transcendence.

While any single example presented here may not be convincing evidence of vilca, when observed across multiple artifacts depicting common motifs and themes related to the use of vilca the evidence becomes substantial. This includes symbols of the *Anadenanthera* plant itself within a shamanic context, to illustrations of the subjective effects following its ingestion to the evidence for vilca being portrayed in Cupisnique iconography.

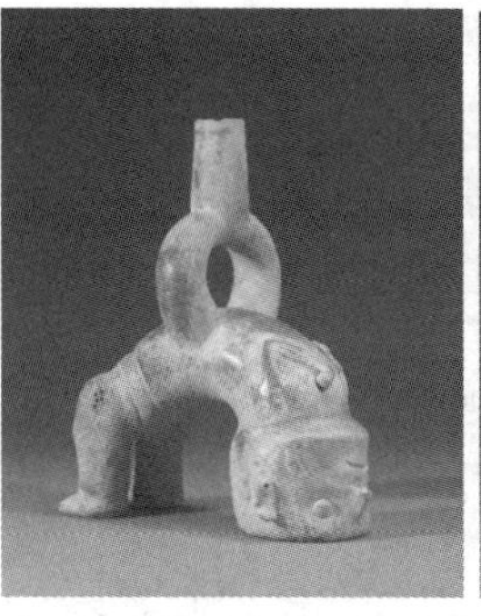
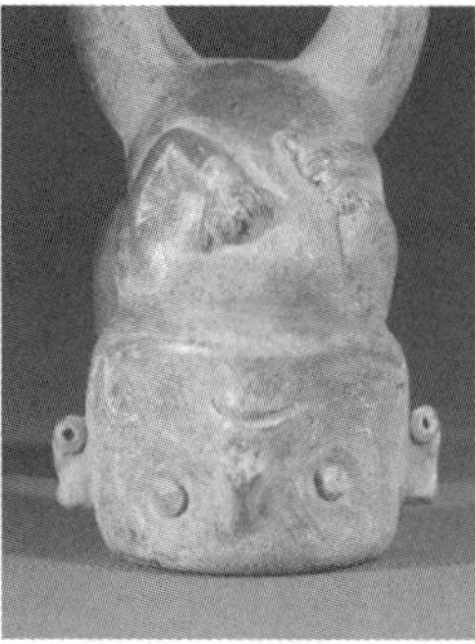
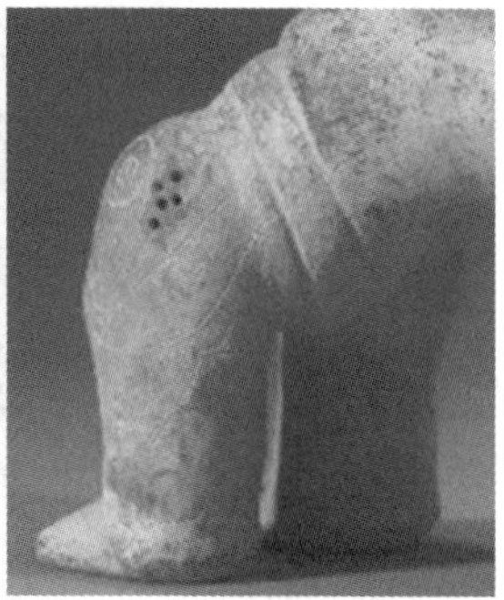

Fig.9 Cupisnique vessel portraying bodily and sensory contortion. Note the rattle held in the shaman's hand and vilca seed motif on knee. *Walters Art Museum 2009.12.11*

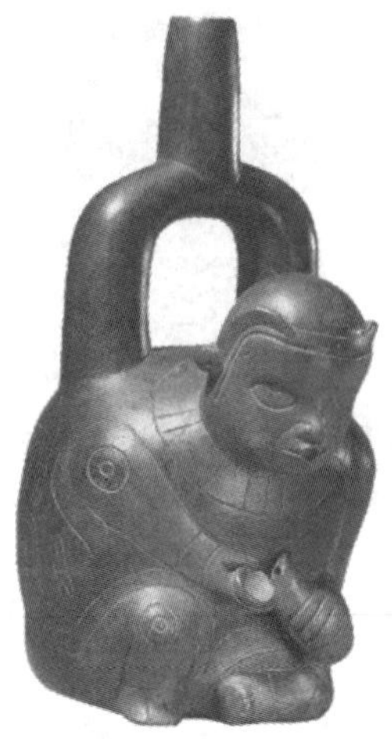

Fig.11 Cupisnique ceramic showing a crouched figure, their back covered in surreal/esoteric etchings, pouring liquid into smaller bowl, eyes rolled to the back of the head indicating a trance state, with the vilca seed motif on their shoulder and knee. *American Museum of Natural History 41.2/7768*

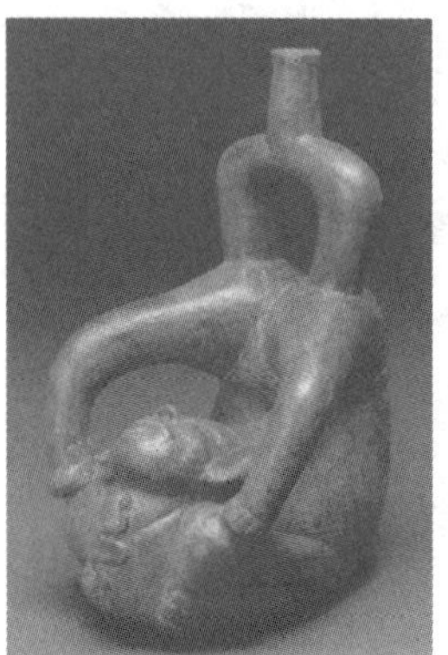
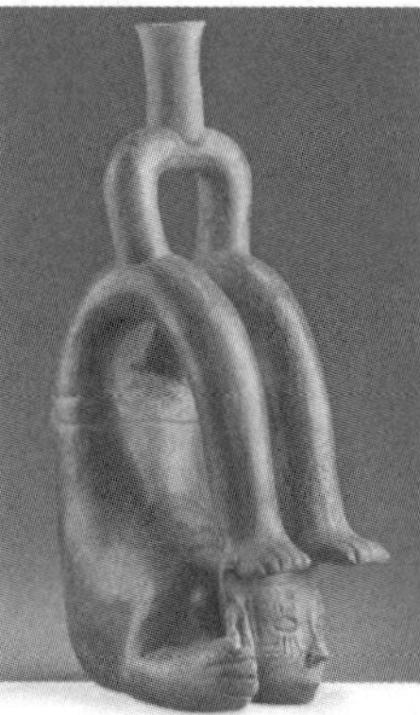
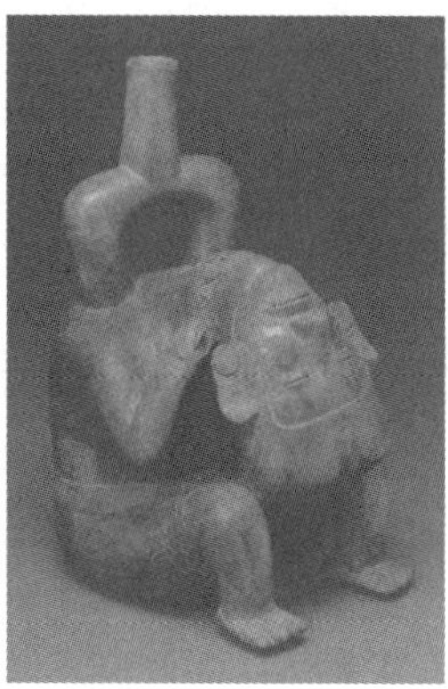

Fig.10 Cupisnique vessels portraying intense bodily contortion, a common subjective feeling following the consumption of vilca. *MNAAHP C-63693; MALI 2007.16.10; Museo Nacional de Colombia 10914*

PARACAS

The Paracas culture occupied the south coastal desert of Peru from roughly 800-100 BCE, also during the Formative phase contemporaneous with (though geographically separated from) Chavin and Cupisnique. Less concerned with ceramics, the Paracas are renowned for their incredible textile creations. These embroideries were prominently featured in Paracas culture, from intricate ritual attire worn by the elite as a visual expression of power, to mummy burials wrapped in finely decorated bundles of cloth. One of the most ubiquitous iconographic depictions seen in Paracas textiles are highly decorated, mythical, supernatural, or anthropomorphic figures. The most commonly recognized form is the so called "Occulate Being", aptly named for its characteristically large eyes with a surreal body (Menzel et al., 1964, 199). While the nature of what this figure represents has been the subject of debate, one argument is that such characters represent shamans in the process of transformation in order to commune with supernatural realms, achieved through the ingestion of certain visionary plants (Burger, 1992). However, the lack of any clearly identifiable hallucinogenic substances in the archaeological record of Paracas has limited the strength of this argument for Paracas. Here I present iconographic evidence for the depiction of *Anadenanthera* in Paracas textiles. Furthermore, *Anadenanthera* is represented alongside such mythical, anthropomorphic figures which inspires the conclusion that we are in fact observing visual illustrations of shamanic metamorphosis induced through the use of vilca in Paracas culture.

Like all pre-Columbian Andean cultures, the Paracas lived with an animistic worldview, where everything was imbued with a living quality or essence seen to be capable of exercising power and agency in the affairs of the living. In line with this perception, death was not conceived as an absolute cessation of activity, but just a transformation. Consequently, deceased members of the Paracas culture were ritually buried below ground wrapped in enormous, multilayered bundle wrappings of elaborately woven textiles, where they were believed to remain active participants of the world (Bolin 2010; Paul 2000: 79). The significance of this belief was reflected in these weavings covering the dead, as they were so meticulously constructed that artisans would have had to spent much of their lives creating these mantles. The iconographic details found on these burial wrappings gives insight into the underlying beliefs and practices of Paracas culture.

The realms of experience visited by shamans were possibly equated to the realms considered to be inhabited by the deceased members of the community, while shamanic techniques (such as the ingestion of hallucinogenic plants) operated as the vehicle to travel between the world of the living and the dead. As Michael Harner points out, "there can be little doubt that the use of the more powerful hallucinogens tends to strongly reinforce a belief in the reality of the supernatural world and in the existence of a disembodied soul or souls" (Harner 1973: XLV). In such a case, images related to the practice of Paracas shamanism may be expected to appear in a materialized form within mummy bundle textile iconography.

In Figure 12 we see a number of anthropomorphic figures exhibiting notable experiential qualities of vilca ingestion such as weightlessness (i.e. "magical flight") depicted as flying through the air, and the head being turned upside down. This figure possessing these traits is such a recurring image in Paracas art that it has been identified and dubbed as the "Ecstatic Shaman" motif. It has been observed in over 40 Paracas weavings across 18 different Paracas bundles, representing a comparatively larger fraction of occurrence than most other iconographic themes, which on average have only four appearances in the archaeological record (Paul and Turpin, 1986, 23). Obviously, therefore, this motif was of great significance to the Paracas people. Curiously, however, despite all the known depictions of shamanic themes, the presence of any hallucinogenic plants has never previously been recognized in Paracas iconography.

In the examples shown in Figure 12, we see several Paracas textiles which contain the legume pod motif of *Anadenanthera*, and once again appear within the body of a serpent. The textiles also contain images of snuffing tubes and symbols of the star-shaped San Pedro cactus slices, providing an obvious context of hallucinogenic plant ingestion. The snuffing tubes would indicate the use of vilca, not San Pedro cactus. Thus, vilca would logically be depicted here, which strengthens the interpretation of this more stylized symbol of the legume pod motif. The beings in these textiles appear to be flying through the air, with large eyes and tilted heads, likely conveying a sense of weightlessness, pupil dilation, and distorted bodily perception. All these features

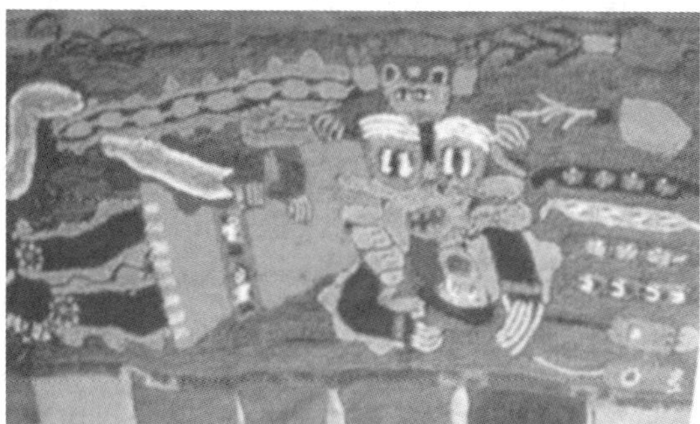

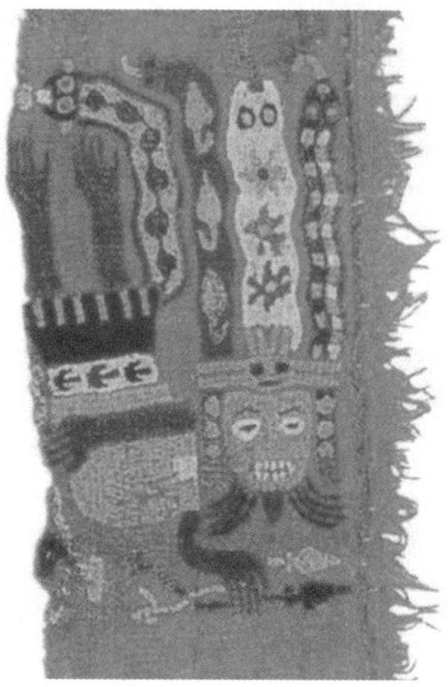

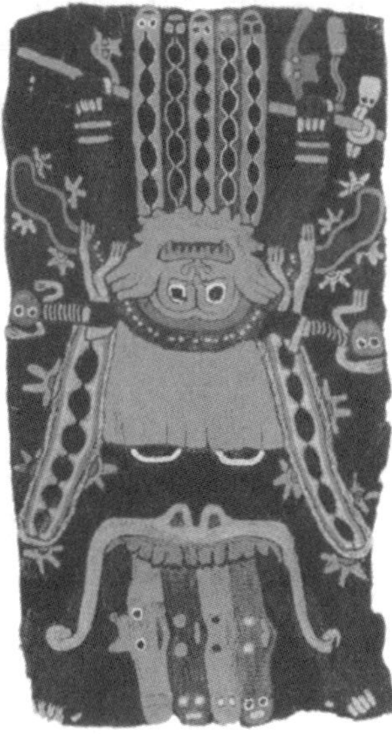

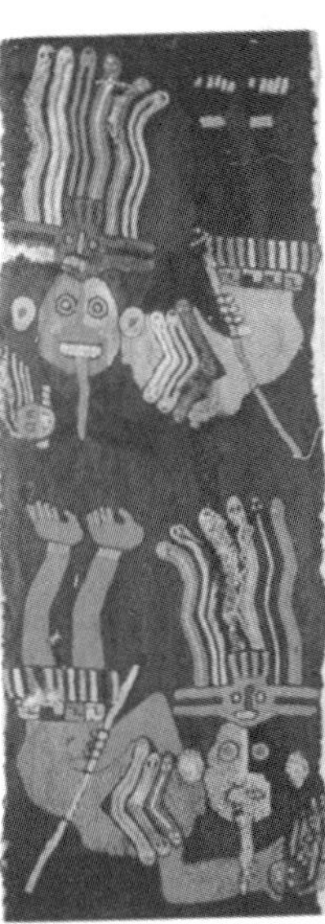

Fig.12 Paracas textiles showing an abundance of shamanic imagery, including snuffing tubes, symbols of hallucinogenic plants, and magical flight. *Campora (1990, 56); Yale University Art Gallery Collection No. 2018.22.23; Yale University Art Gallery Collection No. 2017.40.20; Paul and Turpin (1986, 25)*

are known to be associated with the non-ordinary state of consciousness that would have been evoked following the ingestion vilca. In total, these Paracas embroideries are clear illustrations of the shamanic use of vilca.

Interestingly, this imagery of shamans and hallucinogenic plants appear to have been closely associated to traditions surrounding death as these cloths were ultimately used to bury the deceased. Upon recognizing the association between these figures and the subjective effects of the shamanic experience, it can be seen that many of these supernatural beings can most accurately be recognized as shamans in the process of transformation, induced by the use of hallucinogenic plants with specific evidence for the vilca snuff. In some case's the figures appear concurrently with naturalistic and stylized depictions of hallucinogenic plants and snuffing paraphernalia. From all of this we can conclude that these shamanic figures and related rituals played an important and central role in the lives and worldview of the Paracas people, being associated with traditions surrounding both life and death, the worlds seen and unseen.

NAZCA

The Nazca people occupied the arid south coast of Peru from roughly 100-800 CE, temporally following the Paracas culture in the same geographic region. As the Nazca culture directly descended from the Paracas people, it is not surprising to expect an overlap of similar artistic symbolism and iconography. Moreover, if the Paracas culture did indeed possess knowledge of the hallucinogenic properties of vilca and utilized this plant in a ritual context, it follows that the Nazca descendants would have likely maintained such a tradition in some capacity as well.

Indeed, several Nazca period artifacts have been discovered to contain depictions of the legume pod motif (Figure 13). In these Nazca ceramics we find the legume pod motif as a linear column of connected circles concurrent with imagery of serpents, jaguar, and San Pedro cactus, matching this motif's context in Cupisnique and Paracas iconography. Strengthening the previous argument that the vilca seed motif indeed represents vilca seeds and not simply the naturalistic spots of an animal, in this piece we see that the circles with a central dot covering the surface of the jaguar are connected by a joining line, a detail which the artists would not have included if they were solely trying to replicate the spots of a jaguar. To conclude, there are a number of Nazca artifacts containing symbolic representations of *Anadenanthera* appearing in an appropriate context of shamanic imagery, similar to the examples of vilca iconography in the Paracas and Cupisnique cultures.

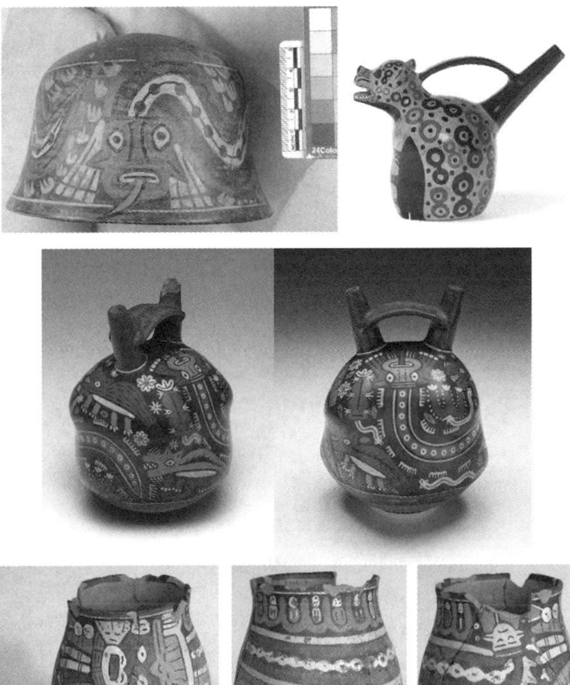

Fig.13 Nazca ceramics showcasing the legume pod motif. *Phoebe A. Hearst Museum University of California, Berkeley Collection No. 4-8803; Metropolitan Museum of Art 33.149.23; Art Institute Chicago 1955.2137; Phoebe A. Hearst Museum, University of California, Berkeley, Collection #4-8629*

ANIMISM AND *ANADENANTHERA*

A regular feature of vilca's representation in the iconographic record across Andean cultures appears to be its depiction with animals such as the serpent and jaguar. For example, the vilca seed pod ("legume pod motif") is virtually always depicted concurrently with a serpent such that these two images (the serpent and the seed pod) may be treated as a singular motif. In making these two forms inseparable, perhaps the Andean artists were attempting to convey the perceived animistic quality of vilca. Appending eyes or a face to an otherwise "inanimate" object is a practice often seen in pre-Columbian iconography with the intent to attribute a living quality to an object. The vilca seed motif has also been seen appearing on the coat of feline imagery. While other scholars have suggested these are simply the spots of a jaguar, I argue that the intended meaning was more complex, representing both jaguar spots and the similarly shaped vilca seeds. From an animistic perception, parallels between common morphologies are not viewed as random coincidences, but rather as expressions of an underlying commonality. This is still seen in some modern Amazonian societies who associate the twisting, crawling vine of *Banisteriopsis caapi* with serpent imagery. This parallelism is of course due to the common morphology, but it is also further reinforced through their direct encounters with serpent imagery in the visions induced following the consumption of this plant. Perhaps we are seeing a similar expression of animistic parallelism between a shamanic plant and animal in these ancient Andean artifacts featuring *Anadenanthera*, with vilca seed pods resembling the serpent and the individual vilca seeds corresponding to the spots on a jaguar.

CONCLUSIONS

Specific symbolic depictions believed to represent vilca have been identified and traced through the artistic record of multiple important Andean cultures that exhibited no previous evidence for the use of vilca: Cupisnique (ca. 1000–200 BCE), Paracas (ca. 800-100 BCE), and Nazca (100–800 CE). Supporting the interpretation that such stylized symbols indeed represent vilca, the occurrence of these motifs virtually always appear in combination with themes associated with shamanism and non-ordinary states of consciousness.

Although no previous evidence had been found for the use of *Anadenanthera* in Cupisnique culture, it was long known that they shared many similarities with the contemporaneous culture of Chavin and the later culture of Moche, both of which had well-established evidence for the ceremonial use of vilca. Through iconographic analysis of Cupisnique ceramic vessels, several artifacts with representation of *Anadenanthera* were identified. The ubiquitous appearance of vilca iconography on drinking vessels, in combination with the lack of any snuffing paraphernalia on the North Coast, suggests that vilca was consumed orally by the Cupisnique. This remains to be confirmed through chemical analysis of ceramic artifacts. Moreover, these motifs frequently appeared in combination with various shamanic themes, as well as other well-known hallucinogenic plants, thus providing a logical context for the depiction of vilca which supports the interpretation of these stylized motifs to indeed be symbols of vilca. On the south coast, there had been no previous evidence for the use of any hallucinogens within Paracas and Nazca culture. However, through examination of textile and ceramic artifacts, numerous examples of vilca iconography were identified. Again, these vilca motifs occurred in a logical visual context, appearing alongside shamanic imagery indicating their familiarization with the subjective effects of vilca ingestion. The iconographic evidence suggests that in these societies, *Anadenanthera* was utilized in a shamanic context and indicates that it was culturally important enough for artists to devote a substantial amount of time and resources to reflect these themes of vilca and shamanism in the material record through the creation of detailed ceramics, intricate textiles, or elaborate stonework. This new visual evidence therefore acts to further expand and reinforce our understanding of the prevalence and significance of vilca in the pre-Columbian Andes.

As new evidence continues to be uncovered of *Anadenanthera*'s widespread use and significance in various Andean cultures across space and time, we expand our appreciation for the prevalence and importance of this plant in the pre-Columbian Andes. The iconographic analysis of Cupisnique, Paracas, and Nazca artifacts discussed here helps to fill in gaps of evidence for vilca use in the archaeological record where no previous evidence had been identified. In conclusion, throughout these pre-Columbian Andean cultures spanning thousands of years, we have discovered iconographic representations of *Anadenanthera* in contexts that make clear not only its presence, but its intentional use, as well as the culturally significant role it played in the lives and worldviews of pre-Columbian Andean people.

ACKNOWLEDGEMENTS

I would like to acknowledge Dr. Cathy Costin for her collaboration and support, as much of the analysis of Cupisnique ceramics was built upon her previous work and large collection of images which she so generously provided.

BIBLIOGRAPHY

Bird, Junius B. 1945. "Preceramic Cultures in Chicama and Virú." *Memoirs of the Society for American Archaeology* 4 (January): 21–28. https://doi.org/10.1017/s0081130000000320.

Bolin, Inge.1999. "Rituals of Respect: The Secret of Survival in the High Peruvian Andes." *Choice Reviews Online* 36 (09): 36–5153. https://doi.org/10.5860/choice.36-5153.

Bonavia, Duccio, and Luis Enrique Tord. 1994. "The Origins of Andean Civilization."

Art and History of Ancient Peru: Enrico Poli Bianchi Collection . South Bank, *London: Thames and Hudson*.

Burger, Richard L. 2011. "What Kind of Hallucinogenic Snuff Was Used at Chavín de Huántar? An Iconographic Identification." *ÑAwpa Pacha* 31 (2): 123–40. https://doi.org/10.1179/naw.2011.31.2.123.

Campora, Pierantoni.1990. "The Paracas Culture: Thirty Centuries of Textile Art."

Cordy-Collins, Alana.1977. "Chavín art: its shamanic/hallucinogenic origins." *Pre-Columbian Art History, Selected Readings*: 353-362.

Cordy-Collins, Alana. 1979. "Cotton and the Staff God: analysis of an ancient Chavin textile." In *The Junius B. Bird Pre-Columbian Textile Conference*, pp. 51-60. Washington, DC: The Textile Museum and Dumbarton Oaks.

Cordy-Collins, Alana. 1980. "An artistic record of the Chavin hallucinatory experience." *The Masterkey for Indian Lore and History* 54, no. 3: 84-93.

Cordy-Collins, Alana. 1992. "Archaism or tradition?: The decapitation theme in cupisnique and moche iconography." *Latin American Antiquity* 3, no. 3: 206-220.

Costin, Cathy L. 2019a. Seeing Shamanic Practices in Ancient Peruvian Pottery. Invited Lecture presented in conjunction with the exhibit "Pleasure, Poison, Prescription, Prayer: The Worlds of Mind-Altering Substances" at the Phoebe A. Hearst Museum of Anthropology, University of California, Berkeley. October.

Costin, Cathy L. 2019b. Revisiting North Coast Formative Period Ceramic Iconography: the Case for Foundational Ritual Power. Institute for Andean Studies Annual Meeting. Berkeley, CA. January

Cathy, Costin L. 2018. Didactic Imagery, Transmission of Esoteric Knowledge, and the Rise of Complexity on the North Coast of Peru. Paper Presented in the Session "Political Matters in Prehistory: Papers in Honor of Antonio Gilman Guillén." 24th Annual Meeting European Association of Archaeologists. Barcelona. September.

Domnauer, Colin. 2020. "The Legume Pod Motif as a Symbolic Representation of the Shamanic Hallucinogen, Vilca (Anadenanthera spp.), in Pre-Columbian Andean Cultures." Ñawpa Pacha 40, no. 2: 163-173.

Domnauer, Colin and Cathy L. Costin. 2022. Iconographic Evidence for the Use of Vilca (Anadenanthera spp.) During the Formative Period on the North Coast of Peru. Paper presented in the Symposium Altered States of Consciousness: Recent Research on Mind-Altering Substances and Practices in the Ancient Americas. 87th Annual Meeting of the Society for American Archaeology.

Eliade, Mircea. 1964. "Shamanism: Archaic Techniques of Ecstasy, trans." *WR Trask, Princeton.*

Furst, Peter T.1974. *Hallucinogens in Precolumbian art.* Texas Tech Press.

Harner, Michael J. 1973. *Hallucinogens and shamanism.* Oxford U. Press.

Horta-Tricallotis, Helena, Javier Echeverría, Verónica Lema, Alethia Quirgas, and Alejandra Vidal.2019. "Enema syringes in South Andean hallucinogenic paraphernalia: evidence of their use in funerary contexts of the Atacama and neighboring zones (ca. AD 500–1500)." *Archaeological and Anthropological Sciences* 11, no. 11: 6197-6219.

Knobloch, Patricia J. 2000. "Wari ritual power at Conchopata: An interpretation of *Anadenanthera colubrina* iconography." *Latin American Antiquity* 11, no. 4: 387-402.

Lewis-Williams, David. 2011. *The mind in the cave: Consciousness and the origins of art.* Thames & Hudson.

Menzel, Dorothy, John Howland Rowe, and Lawrence E. Dawson. 1964. *The Paracas pottery of Ica: a study in style and time.* Vol. 50. Berkeley: University of California Press.

Miller, Melanie J., Juan Albarracin-Jordan, Christine Moore, and José M. Capriles. 2019. "Chemical evidence for the use of multiple psychotropic plants in a 1,000-year-old ritual bundle from South America." *Proceedings of the National Academy of Sciences* 116, no. 23: 11207-11212.

Nesbitt, Jason. 2012. "Excavations at Caballo Muerto: an investigation into the origins of the Cupisnique Culture." PhD diss., Yale University.

Paul, Anne, and Solveig A. Turpin. 1986. "The ecstatic shaman theme of Paracas textiles." *Archaeology* 39, no. 5: 20-27.

Paul, Anne. 2000. "Bodiless human heads in Paracas Necrópolis textile iconography." *Andean Past* 6, no. 1: 7.

Rick, John W. 2004."The evolution of authority and power at Chavín de Huántar, Peru." *Archaeological Papers of the American Anthropological Association* 14, no. 1: 71-89.

Schultes, Richard Evans, and Elmer W. Smith. 1976. *Hallucinogenic plants.* Vol. 35. New York: Golden Press.

Shimada, Izumi. 1994. *Pampa Grande and the Mochica culture.* University of Texas Press.

Stone, Rebecca R. 2012. *The jaguar within: Shamanic trance in ancient Central and South American art.* University of Texas Press.

Torres, Constantino M., and David B. Repke. 2014. *Anadenanthera: visionary plant of ancient South America.* Routledge.

Torres, Constantino Manuel.2008. "Chavin's psychoactive pharmacopoeia: the iconographic evidence." *Chavín: Art, Architecture, and Culture*: 239-260.

Torres, Constantino Manuel. 2018a. From Beer to Tobacco: a Probable Prehistory of Ayahuasca. Ethnopharmacologic Search for Psychoactive Drugs. Vol. II. *Synergetic Press.*

Torres, Constantino Manuel, William H. Isbell, Mauricio I. Uribe, A. Tiballi, and Edward P. Zegarra. 2018b. "Visionary plants and SAIS iconography in San Pedro de Atacama and Tiahuanaco." *Images in action: the southern Andean iconographic series*: 287-326.

Tiwanaku and Wari. Visionary Plants and Politics in the Central Andes, ca. 300–1000: Superficial Similarities and Profound Divergences

Constantino Manuel Torres, PhD

Professor of Art History at Florida International University in Miami | Author

"Plants and fungi have been shared across cultures for millennia, and so have customs and beliefs. This paper shares the history and biocultural links between ancient Andean societies and the psychoactive plants they used, and how these plants influenced their respective polities." —Constantino Manuel Torres

INTRODUCTION

The presence of objects associated with the Tiwanaku (Tiahuanaco), and Wari (Huari) cultures define the Middle Horizon (*ca.* 300-900 AD) period of Andean Pre-Columbian history (Table 1). These two pre-Inca cultures of the Central Andes (Fig. 1) shared an iconographic system, and the use of diverse psychoactive plants, *Anadenanthera* (*vilca*, *yopo*, *cebil*), tobacco, and coca. The enactment of their respective politics, however, differs greatly. Wari expansion was one of colonialist control. In the Wari sphere of influence there is clear evidence of colonial outposts with the presence of emissaries whose burials mostly consisted of Wari implements, including elaborately decorated textiles, ceramics, and metal objects. Tiwanaku expansion was of a different nature. There is no evidence of colonial envoys, or military enforcement of ideologies. In the oasis of San Pedro de Atacama, Chile, Tiwanaku integrates with local expressions, as well as with objects from NW Argentina and southern Bolivia, revealing anarchic forms of organization. In comparison, the Tiwanaku periphery is less hierarchical and less prone to central control than Wari organization.

The differences and similarities between these two cultures provide the opportunity to observe the impact of psychoactive agents in their respective political contexts. Both use the seeds of *Anadenanthera colubrina*, rich in bufotenine, as part of their visionary preparations. The Tiwanaku favored snuffing and smoking, while the Wari favored drinking *chicha* (beer) de *molle* (*Schinus molle*) sometimes with the addition of *Anadenanthera* seeds (Biwer et al., 2022: 1-2; Sayre *et al.*, 2014). The Wari conducted large feasts with heavy drinking during which hundreds

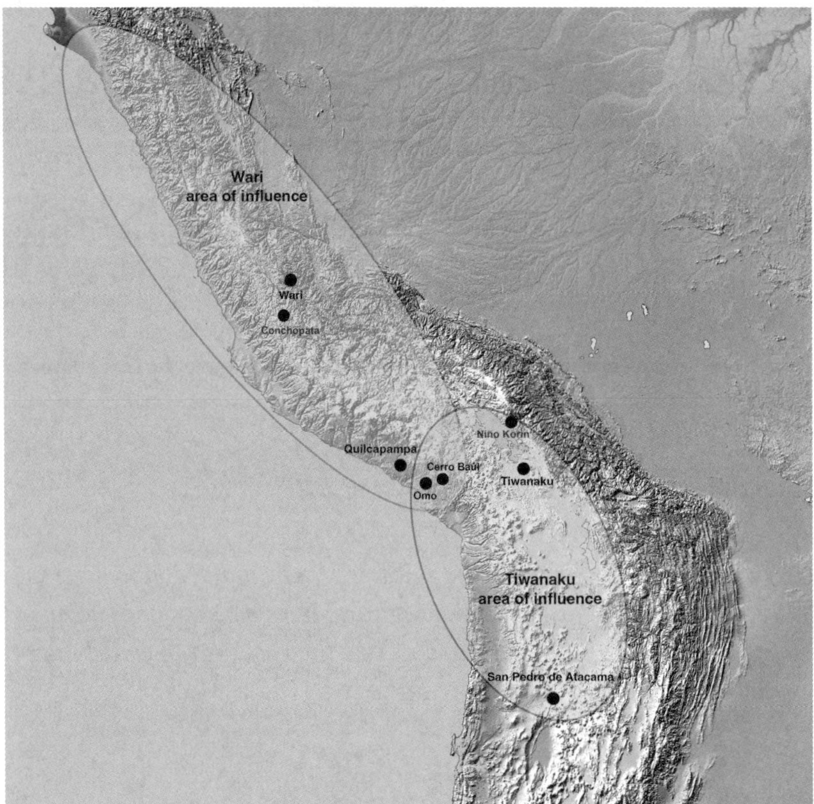

Fig. 1 Map of the Central Andes indicating the extent of Tiwanaku and Wari territories.

of liters of chicha with admixture plants including *vilca* were consumed* (Biwer et al. 2022; Moseley et al. 2005: 17267; Nash, 2012). The Wari demonstrate scant evidence for smoking or snuffing. In the Tiwanaku area of the South-Central Andes there is a preference for snuffing and smoking, and this is supported by extensive archaeological evidence (Horta, 2014; Torres. 2006; Wassén, 1967). In the Andes, snuffing paraphernalia is portable and intimate, and so not likely to be used in large collective activities. The question is how does the practice of drinking and snuffing determine societal configurations? Could the narrative structure of the visionary event correspond to cultural and individual organizational patterns?

TIWANAKU AND WARI-PRIMARY COMPARISONS

This paper investigates the Wari (500-1000 AD) and Tiwanaku (300-1000 AD) cultures of the Central Andes (Bergh, 2012; Isbell et al., 2018; Schreiber, 1992: Vranich and Stanish. 2013; Young-Sánchez, 2004). The question of whether Wari and Tiwanaku could be classified as empires has been debated for decades. That is a discussion beyond the scope of this investigation.

* To learn more about vilca and Anadenanthera spp., see our paper "Identifying Depictions of Anadenanthera in the Iconographic Records of Cupisnique, Paracas, and Nazca Cultures" by Colin Domnauer.

TIMETABLE—CENTRAL ANDES								
Period	**North Coast**	**Central Coast**	**South Coast**	**North High-lands**	**Central High-lands**	**South High-lands**	**Titicaca Region**	**Atacama Desert**
Formative 3500-900 bC	Cerro Sechín Huaca Prieta							Chinchorro Alto Ramirez
Early Horizon 900-100 bC	Cupisnique	Moche	Paracas	Chavín				Pisagua
Early Intermediate 100 bC-400 CE	Moche		Nasca	Recuay			Pukara	San Pedro de Atacama
Middle Horizon 400-1100 CE	Moche	Wari	Wari	Wari	Wari	Wari Tiwanaku	Tiwanaku	San Pedro de Atacama
Late Intermediate 1100-1430 CE	Chimú	Chancay						San Pedro de Atacama
Late Horizon 1430-1535 CE	Inka	Inka	Inka	Inka	Inka	Inka	Inka	Inka

Table 1 Timetable of Pre-Columbian cultures of the central Andes.

Wari fits the concept of empire with a central control that oversees a vast and diverse territory. Schreiber (1992; 2001) labeled such a diverse empire as an "imperial mosaic". Tiwanaku is not so easily classified as their expansion strategies differ greatly. The Wari exhibited traits that could be equated to central colonial control, and clearly established outposts in areas remote from the city of Wari in Ayacucho. Tiwanaku expansion does not include colonial emissaries with foreign individuals going to expand the sprawling state. Its expansion was more likely guided by ideologies generated by the snuffing and smoking of bufotenine (5-Hydroxy-dimethyltryptamine) rich powders. This paper delves into the nature of these modes of control, and compares Wari (a more domineering and hierarchical institution), to Tiwanaku's anarchic form of organization and expansion. Anarchic forms of organization are characterized by voluntary collaboration, no obedience to central control, they are functional relative to a given situation, and are generally temporary, shifting to some mode of centralized control according to the needs of the circumstances. This permits seasonal variations to social organization. Mink'a, voluntary collective labor, is a tradition that survives in the Andes. It ranges from community projects to helping a family in harvest time, creating a web of reciprocity that contributes to define the identify of individuals and communities. Regarding issues of seasonal variation, Lévi-Strauss documents how the Nambikwara of the Matto Grosso during the rainy season occupied villages on higher ground with appointed chiefs to lead them. In the dry season they dispersed into small groups of foraging bands, living effectively in two societies, (Graeber and Wengrow, 2021: 98-99).

To allow for more detailed and specific comparison this discussion concentrates on Wari affiliated Nasca sites on the south Peruvian coast, and San Pedro de Atacama (300-1000 AD), the southernmost presence of Tiwanaku. One significant difference lies in the Wari preference for chicha de molle (*Schinus molle*), and Tiwanaku for chicha de *jora*, a corn-based beer with multiple plant additives and variations, and the emphasis on snuffs in Tiwanaku. Specifically, this work concentrates on the impact these substances might have had in their respective politics of expansion.

During the Andean Middle Horizon (300-1000 AD) Wari was located in the Huamanga Basin, near the present-day city of Ayacucho, Perú. This civilization covered large expanses of the Central Andes and adjacent coast including Nasca territory, and archaeological sites such as Conchopata, and Pikillacta (Bergh, 2012). Wari was one of the largest cities in the Andes. The central core was densely occupied, and it was composed of large rectangular, multi-storied enclosures with few entrances and no windows (Schreiber, 2001: 81, 92).

As previously mentioned, Tiwanaku cannot be easily classified as an empire. Tiwanaku emerged *ca.* 300-400 AD. It soon controlled the southern Lake Titicaca Basin and influenced the Moquegua Valley. To the south, Tiwanaku objects are found in Cochabamba, Bolivia and San Pedro de Atacama, Chile. The Omo settlement represents the only location outside the altiplano with Tiwanaku religious monumental architecture (Williams et al., 2020: 206). The city of Tiwanaku was designed as a performance space, with monumental stairways (Fig. 3), gateways, and plazas with sculptures of finely cut stone (Fig. 2), that could accommodate large crowds, suggesting routes with the arrangement of plazas, mounds, and built compounds. In contrast, Wari architecture limits public gatherings and ritual movement, and there were no large plazas (Browman, 2002; Isbell and Vranich, 2004:174–175, 181). Wari could be described as a centralized expansive state, while Tiwanaku could be seen as a less intrusive expansion. In San Pedro de Atacama, approximately 1000 kms away from the Tiwanaku core, there are no Tiwanaku settlements or architecture, no plazas, or significant mounds.

Mortuary practices in San Pedro de Atacama are homogenous. Tiwanaku objects, such as snuffing equipment, textiles and pottery mixed in the burials with local and regional artifacts, mostly from NW Argentina. It should be noted that besides its obvious presence in San Pedro de Atacama, Tiwanaku objects have never been found in the Argentine northwest. Wari presence in Nasca differs in the creation of colonial outposts, the introduction of burial methods, and imported Wari ceramics. At least 40 Wari affiliated sites have been located in the Nasca area. One has two D-shape plazas, a characteristic of Wari architecture, absent in Tiwanaku (Conlee et al., 2021: 1529).

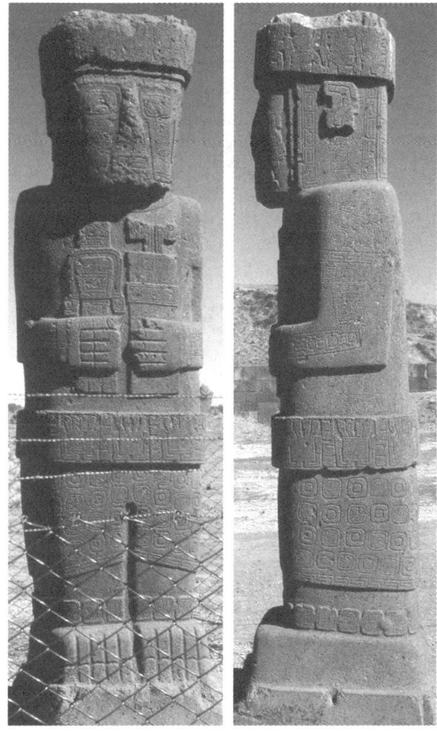

Ponce Stela, 3.05 mt Tiwanaku, Bolivia

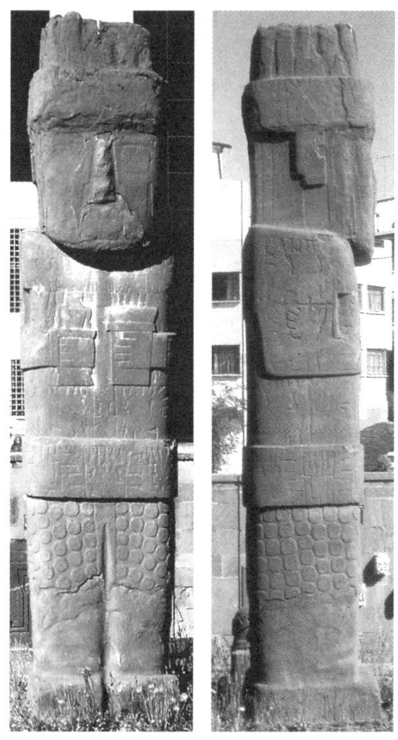

Bennett Stela, 5.5 mt, Tiiwanaku, Bolivia

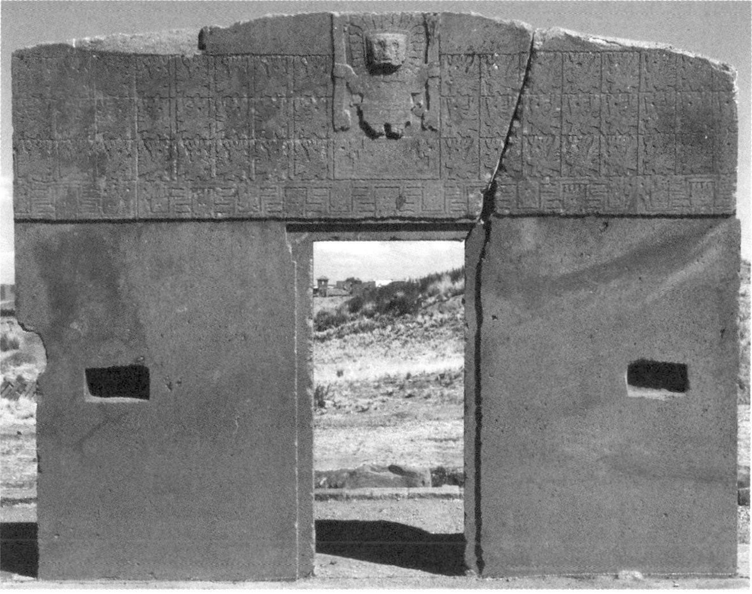

Gateway of the Sun
Tiwanaku, Bolivia

Fig. 2 Three monolithic sculptures from Tiwanaku, Bolivia. *Photos C. M. Torres*

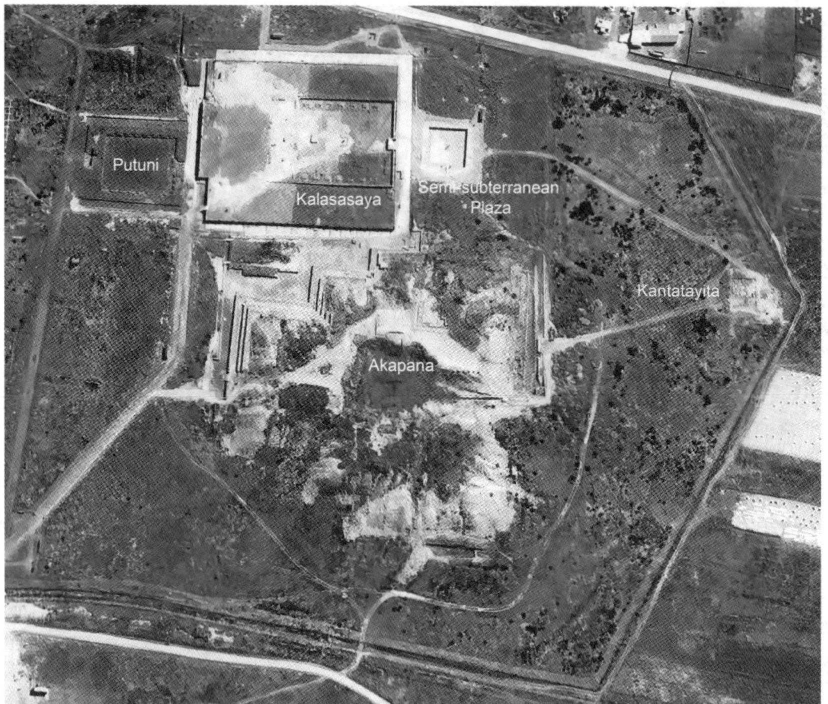

Fig. 3 Aerial view of the core of the city of Tiwanaku. *Google Earth*

Tiwanaku and Wari shared a similar iconographic system, basically a frontal staff-bearing personage and a profile staff-bearing entity frequently depicting avian and feline attributes (Fig. 4). The basic configurations differ in component elements. This becomes evident, for example, when staffs, face details, and crowns are compared. The repertoire of motifs that compose these images is more varied in Tiwanaku than in Wari iconography (Torres, 2018). Numerous Wari chicha-drinking vessels depict elements of Wari ideologies (Fig. 5). Wari style tends to be more geometric than Tiwanaku. The shape of Wari icons is determined by framing devices. Most of the extant iconographic corpus of Wari consists mostly of textiles and painted pottery. These textiles (Fig. 6) geometric and colorful style appealed to the modernist taste of mid-twentieth century collectors, provoking a demand for such textiles and consequent looting. Wari textiles consisted of tapestry-woven tunics (*unku*), mantles, and four-pointed hats (Bergh, 2012: Pls. 146, 147). Numerous textiles survive, found in the arid Peruvian south coast. The imagery on these textiles is limited and icons are repeated over the tunic's surface in complex arrangements (Fig. 6). Wari tunics consist of two woven rectangles stitched together to form a seam that falls in the center on the front and back of the garment. The warp frequently consisted of alpaca thread, and the weft of cotton. Tiwanaku textiles in contrast, had warp and weft of camelid fiber and were made from one large rectangular piece that was not stitched at the center. These structural characteristics were probably meaningful. The iconography depicted on the few extant Tiwanaku textiles consist of one thematic unit (Fig. 7), mostly the profile staff bearing personage, repeated

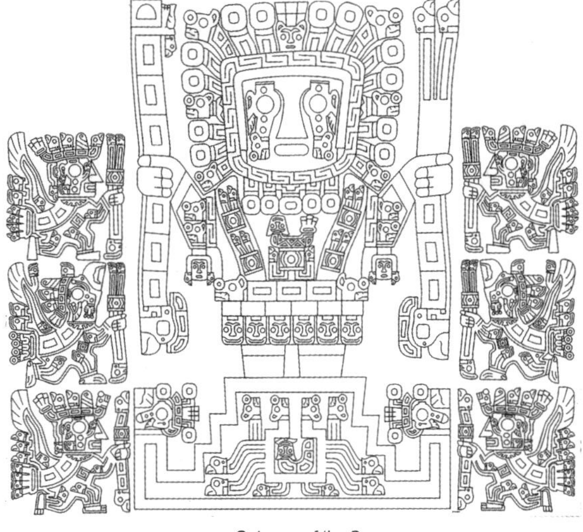

Gateway of the Sun

Painted ceramic vessel, Wari

Fig. 4 Tiwanaku and Wari icons of widespread distribution (after Bergh 2012: Fig. 76b).

but with color permutations of its component elements. In the central Andes, textiles, partly due to portability, were carriers of information and markers of compromises and alliances.

The Wari placed a strong emphasis on feasting and drinking chicha. The production and consumption of alcohol created an interactive web of reciprocity. The structure of the feast, including which goods are provided and how they are served, consolidated social positions (Jennings and Bowser, 2008: 5). These were large feasts with numerous participants, requiring complex technology that provided the setting for creating alliances, and modifying identity by colonial dominant pressures on the host culture (for example, Wari presence on the Nasca populations on the south Peruvian coast). Chicha brewing goes through several standard production steps: selection and removal of the grain; soaking and germination (to increase sugar content); drying, grinding and

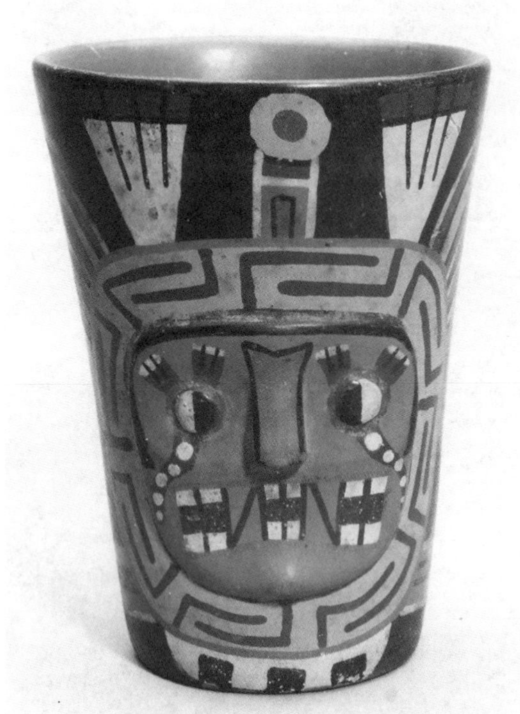

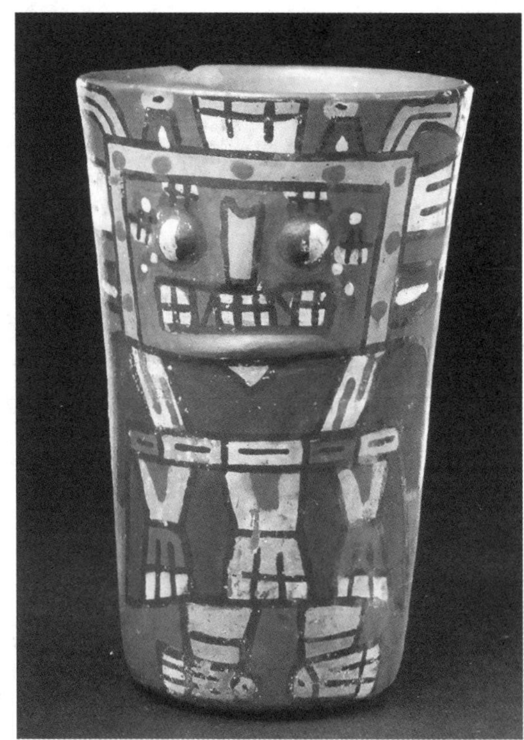

Fig. 5 Wari drinking cups (after Bergh 2012: Figs. 122, 243)

cooking; followed by straining and fermentation (Moore, 1989: 686). Vegetable sources for chicha additives are varied. Chicha de *jora* (germinated corn chicha), is common today but chicha is also produced from a variety of plant sources and additives. Chicha de molle (*Schinus molle*) brewed from the bright red drupe of the molle tree is preferred by the Wari (Sayre, 2012: 233). *Aloja*, or *algarrobo* (*Prosopis* species) chicha is brewed throughout the Atacama Desert. The addition of *vilca* (*Anadenanthera colubrina*) seeds has been documented since the early colonial period (Cobo, 1964, 1: 272; Ondegardo 1916, 3: 29-30). A recent study (Quiroga, 2019) on the representation of *vilca* (*Anadenanthera colubrina*) seeds on Tiwanaku stone sculpture, incorporates among the authors three Traditional Specialists (Especialistas Tradicionales) from the Tiwanaku community to aid in iconographic interpretation. These specialists reported to Quiroga (2019: 52, 61) that they added vilca snuff powder to chicha. Excavations at the Wari outpost of Quilcapampa in southern Peru (Biwer *et al.*, 2022), recovered *vilca* seeds in association with molle (*Schinus molle*) drupes, presumably for making chicha. Wari serving vessels sometimes represent *vilca* (Knobloch, 2000: Fig. 2).

The following quote by Garcilaso de la Vega (1970: 499, published 1609) clearly mentions the addition of other plants to the chicha during the brewing process:

"Some Indians, more passionate about inebriation than the rest of the community, steep the corn (*sara*) until it begins to sprout. They then grind it and boil it in the same water as other

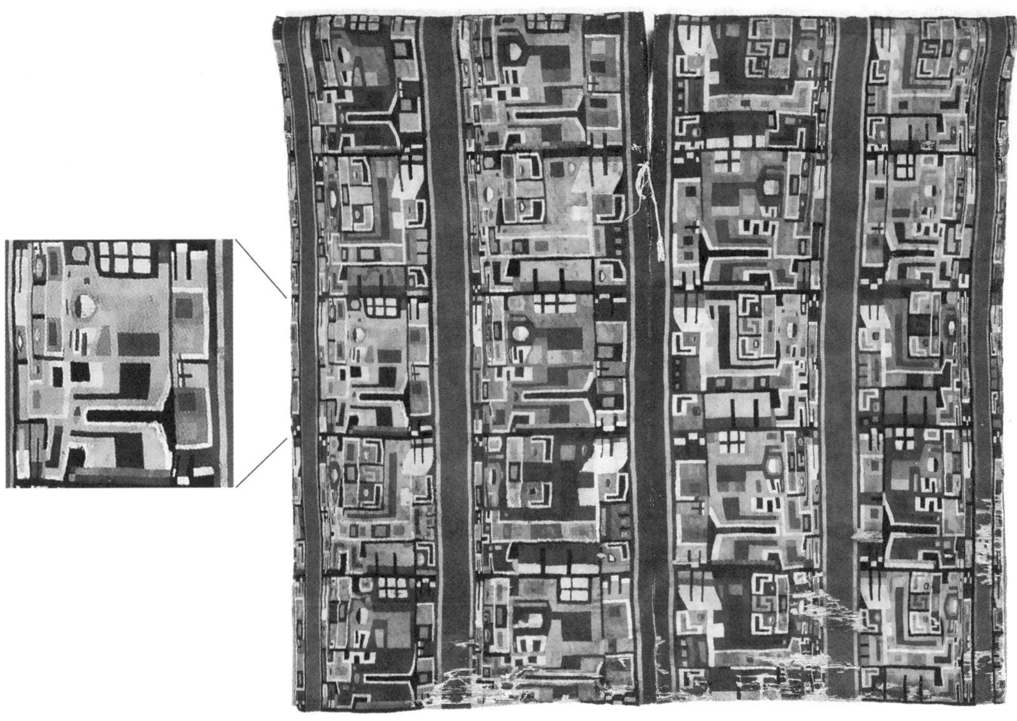

Fig. 6 Wari tunic, camelid fiber and cotton, with representation of upward-looking genuflect profile figure (after Bergh 2012: Fig. 153).

things. Once this is strained it is kept until it ferments. A very strong drink, which intoxicates immediately, is thus produced…"

The Guahibo, from the plains (llanos) of eastern Colombia, prepared a fermented drink called yaraque, obtained from yuca (*Manihot esculenta*) which included yopo powder (*Anadenanthera peregrina var. peregrina* seeds) (Fabo, 1919-1920: 31; von Reis Altschul, 1972: 31). Mario Califano (1976: 16-18, 46), in his study of shamanism among the Wichi (Mataco) of the Gran Chaco, mentioned the drinking of vino de *cebil*, a fermented *Anadenanthera*-based potion, in relation to shamanic initiation.

Wari and Tiwanaku greatly differ on issues of psychoactive substances, the Wari preferred drinking chicha de molle (Jennings, 2008; Sayre 2012), while the evidence clearly suggests that Tiwanaku preferred snuffing (Berenguer, 2001; Quiroga, 2019; Torres, 2018). Evidence for snuffing is scarce within the Wari sphere of influence. A discussion of mechanisms of drug action must include characteristics of the modes of production, such as infrastructure (buildings and areas for production, transport, and storage), production of manufacturing implements such as ceramic cooking and serving ware, moving technicians from production site to production site, and trade requirements. Ritual requirements probably needed specialists deployed within the sphere of influence. Perhaps collective use within the context of feasting or intimate use with only a few individuals participating in the event? Drinking seems more conducive to collective

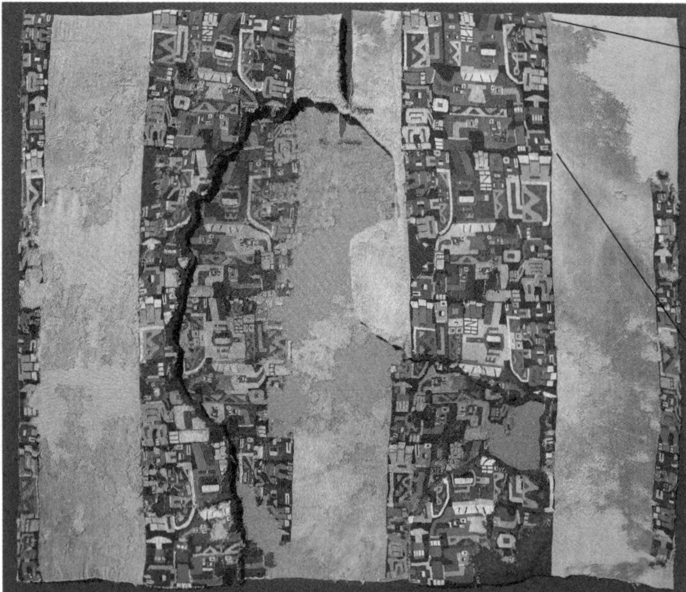
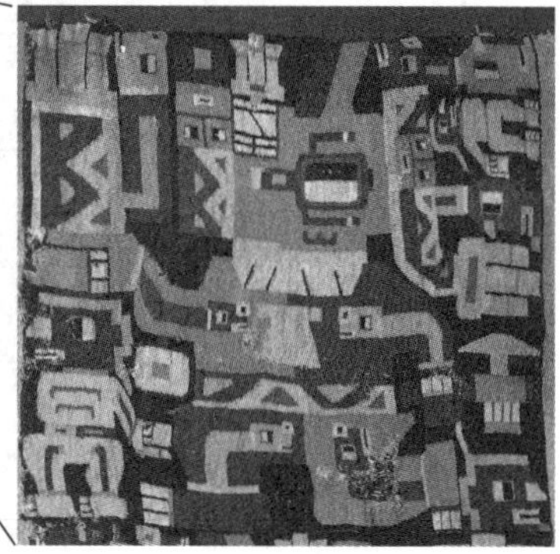

Fig. 7 Tiwanaku tunic, Pulacayo, Bolivia. *Photo courtesy Fernando Maldonado*

events, while snuffing was perhaps a more intimate affair. The frequency of snuffing implements in San Pedro de Atacama suggests individual use. For example, in the Quitor 6 cemetery on the western side of the oasis one of every three burials contained a snuffing kit. The typical snuffing kit was kept inside a woolen bag containing a rectangular wooden snuff tray, a snuffing tube generally made of wood or bird bone, a spoon or spatula generally made of bone, and one or two leather pouches with the snuff powder (Fig. 8). Manufacturing of snuff powder begins with the importation of the *A. colubrina* seeds from the eastern slopes of the Andes, as *Anadenanthera* is not present in the arid western slopes. The seeds were dried and roasted to facilitate grinding into a very fine powder. Tobacco and sometimes an alkaline mixture were added. The alkaline component was usually obtained from calcined shells or ashes from a vegetable source.

Wari brewery construction required a large outlay of labor. The monumental brewery atop Cerro Baúl, on the Moquegua River basin, included a trapezoidal structure with separate compartments for milling, boiling and fermentation. The fermentation room contained twelve large vats where the liquid fermented for 3-5 days depending on taste and desired alcohol content. Each vat had a capacity of approximately 150 liters of beer. This is one of the largest breweries in the Andes, capable of producing 1800 liters per batch (Moseley *et al.*, 2005: 17267). Construction of such a large brewery with complex architecture required the moving of supplies from the valley to the mesa top, the making of pottery vessels for cooking and fermenting, and a variety of serving ware with painted Wari iconography, including the labor of builders, farmers, potters, artists, and brewers. This complex series of activities likely required the transportation of technicians and materials affiliated with the Wari center in Ayacucho, approximately 400 kms away. This extraterritorial presence is evident in Nasca with the incidence of colonial outposts and emissaries, changes in settlement patterns and the introduction of mortuary practices

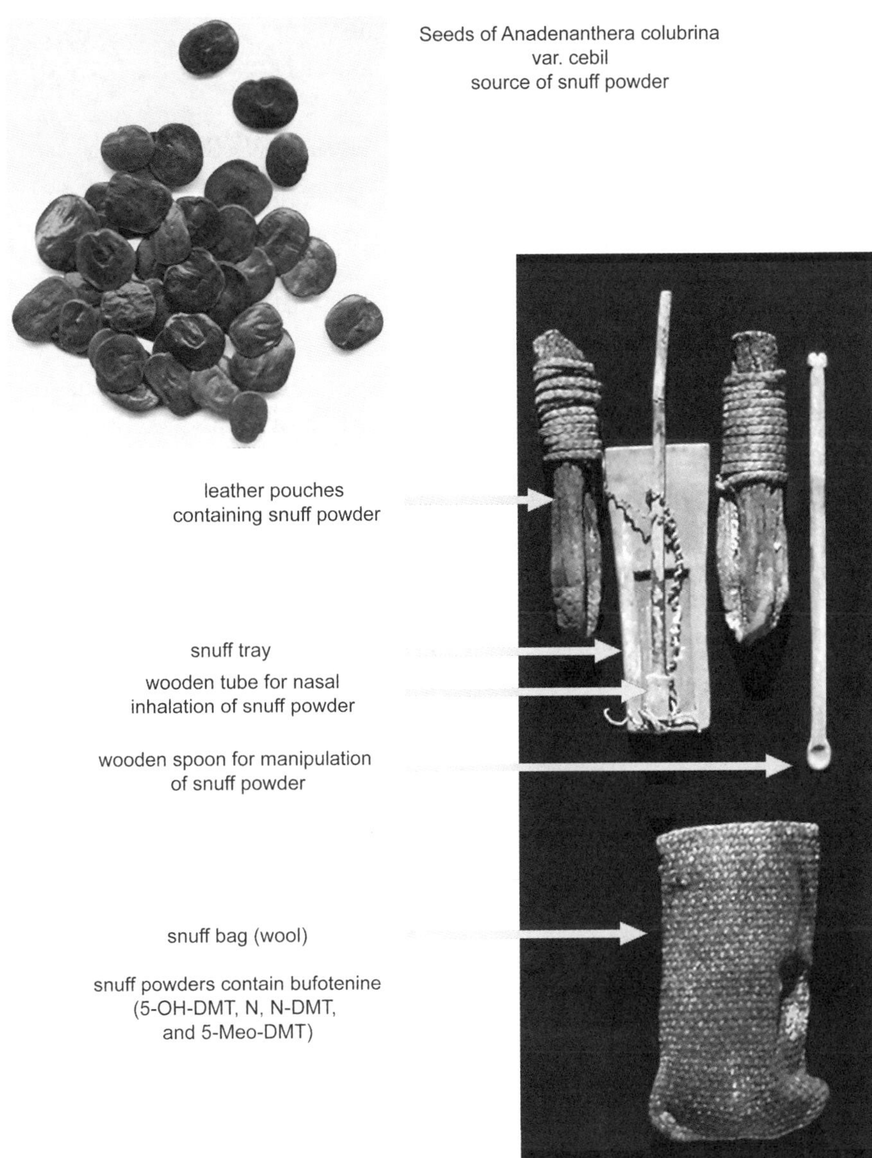

Fig. 8 Components of a snuffing kit.

(Conlee *et al.*, 2021: 1529). Feasting and drinking chicha fostered conversation and discussion bringing people together and creating reciprocal obligations and agreements. As Jennings and Bower state "the production and consumption of alcohol are central to the creation of identity, the construction and maintenance of power, the functioning of social networks, and the practice of religions" (Jennings and Bower, 2008: 3-5).

Objects bearing Tiwanaku iconography are distributed over a vast area in the southern Andes. San Pedro de Atacama is the southernmost archaeological zone with a significant Tiwanaku presence. The Moquegua Valley, including Cerro Baúl, lies at the northern extremes of Tiwanaku influence. It is in this area that Tiwanaku and Wari interface.

SUPERFICIAL SIMILARITIES AND PROFOUND DIVERGENCES

Comparing the Tiwanaku monumental city with Wari in the Ayacucho Valley illuminates clear differences. Tiahuanaco is arranged as a series of performance spaces with plazas at different levels that include large stone sculptures which clear references to visionary plant use. This display of psychoactive drug use in public monumental sculpture (Figs. 9, 10) suggests some degree of government sponsorship. The buildings are composed of finely cut stone, unlike Wari, where the stone is not so finely dressed. Wari sites limit public gatherings; there are no large plazas.

The site of Tiwanaku is composed of a series of plazas and mounds (Fig. 3), with entrances and monumental sculptures, including the Ponce, and Bennett monoliths, and the Gateway of the Sun (Fig. 2). Most of the icons represented in monumental sculpture are also represented in textiles and snuffing paraphernalia. These are portable objects distributed throughout the Tiwanaku sphere of influence. In localities such as San Pedro de Atacama and Niño Korin, Bolivia (Torres 2018: 11.15) snuffing paraphernalia is carved with complex and varied manifestations of Tiwanaku iconography (Fig. 11). The Ponce stela (Figs. 9, 10) was excavated in 1957 by Carlos Ponce Sanginés (1999: 230), in the central plaza of the area known as Kalasasaya (Isbell, 2018: 15.9; Fig. 2). The sculpture represents a standing anthropomorphic individual, with

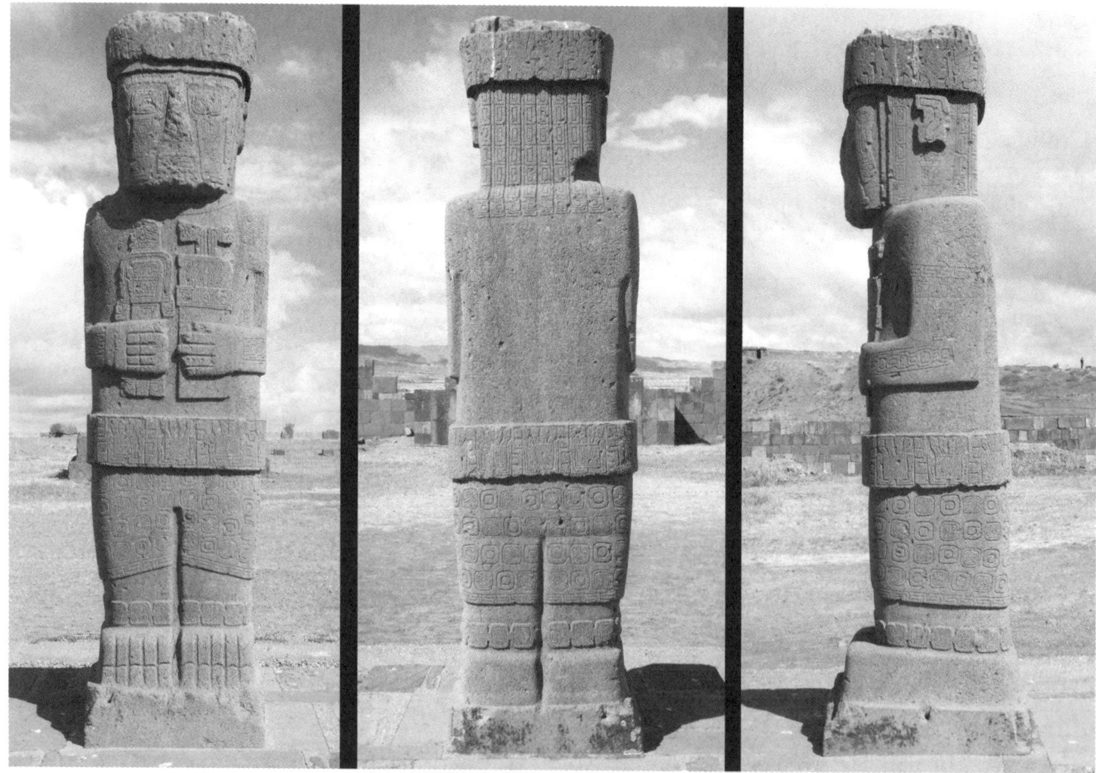

Fig. 9 Ponce stela, 3.05 mt, central courtyard of the Kalasasaya, Tiwanaku. *Photos C. M. Torres*

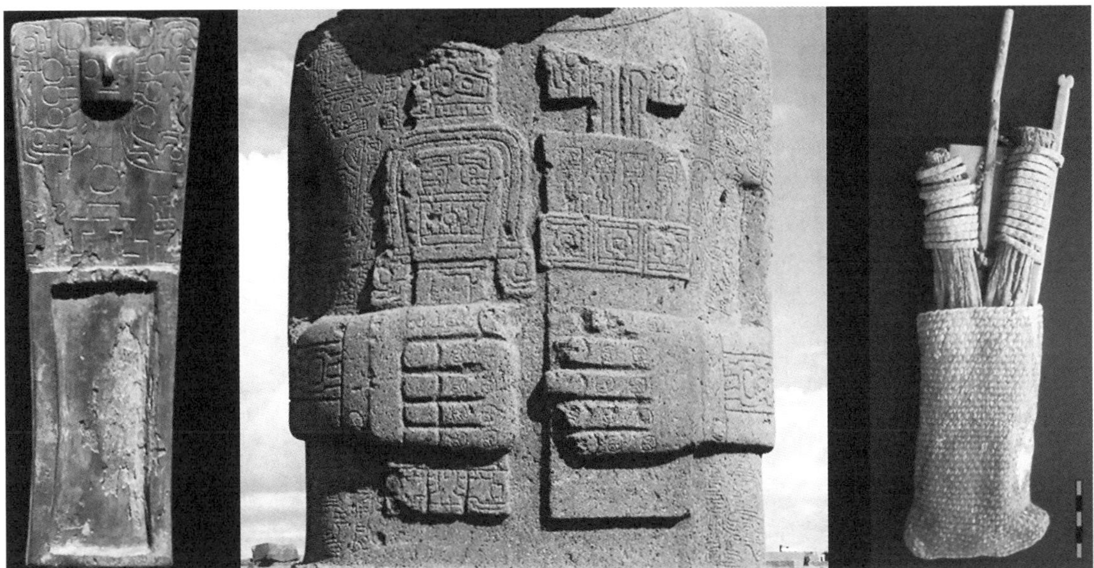

Fig. 10 Ponce stela, held objects detail, snuff tray and bag. *Photos C. M. Torres*

an elaborate crown and attire, carrying two objects in front of his torso (Fig. 10). The two held objects have been identified as a snuff tray and a woolen bag containing snuffing paraphernalia or perhaps a kero (Berenguer, 2001: 67; Torres and Torres, 2014: 64). This figure serves as a scene for the representation of a series of processions made up of a great variety of characters. In contrast Wari stone sculpture is smaller, and not so detailed as Tiwanaku.

Tiwanaku strategies of expansion have not been properly elucidated. In San Pedro de Atacama there are a few foreign individuals, but these are not affiliated with Tiwanaku artefacts (Torres-Rouff *et al.*, 2015: 593). Burials in San Pedro de Atacama consist of a cylindrical pit with a corpse seated with knees flexed against the chest, wrapped in several layers of textiles, surrounded by bags, ceramics, and baskets (Fig. 12). Males most frequently carried a snuffing kit and bow and arrows. Tiwanaku objects are scattered among the graves. There are no complete Tiwanaku burials in San Pedro. Occasional artefacts, mixed with local objects and other foreign finds, are mostly from NW Argentina and southern Bolivia. Tiwanaku textiles and ceramics in San Pedro de Atacama are scarce. San Pedro de Atacama is the archaeological culture in South America with the highest evidence for psychoactive use. Chemical analysis of a snuff sample from a snuffing kit excavated at the site of Solcor 3, tomb 112 (Fig. 12), yielded 5-hydroxy-DMT (bufotenine), and in lesser amounts N,N-DMT (*dimeltryptamine*) and 5-Meo-DMT (Torres *et al.*, 1991). A bag containing snuffing equipment was found at the archaeological site known as Cueva del Chileno (*ca.* 1000 AD), on the Lipez plateau, in SW Bolivia. Analysis of the contents of this bag revealed the presence of bufotenine (5-OH-DMT), N,N-DMT (*dimeltryptamine*), nicotine, and *harmine* (Miller *et al.*, 2019). The presence of bufotenine in these samples suggest *Anadenanthera colubrina* var. *cebil* as its source. This tree is abundant in NW Argentina, on the eastern side of the Andes, opposite San Pedro de Atacama. The occurrence of harmine in this sample suggests the presence of plants containing harmala alkaloids in southern Bolivia and NW Argentina.

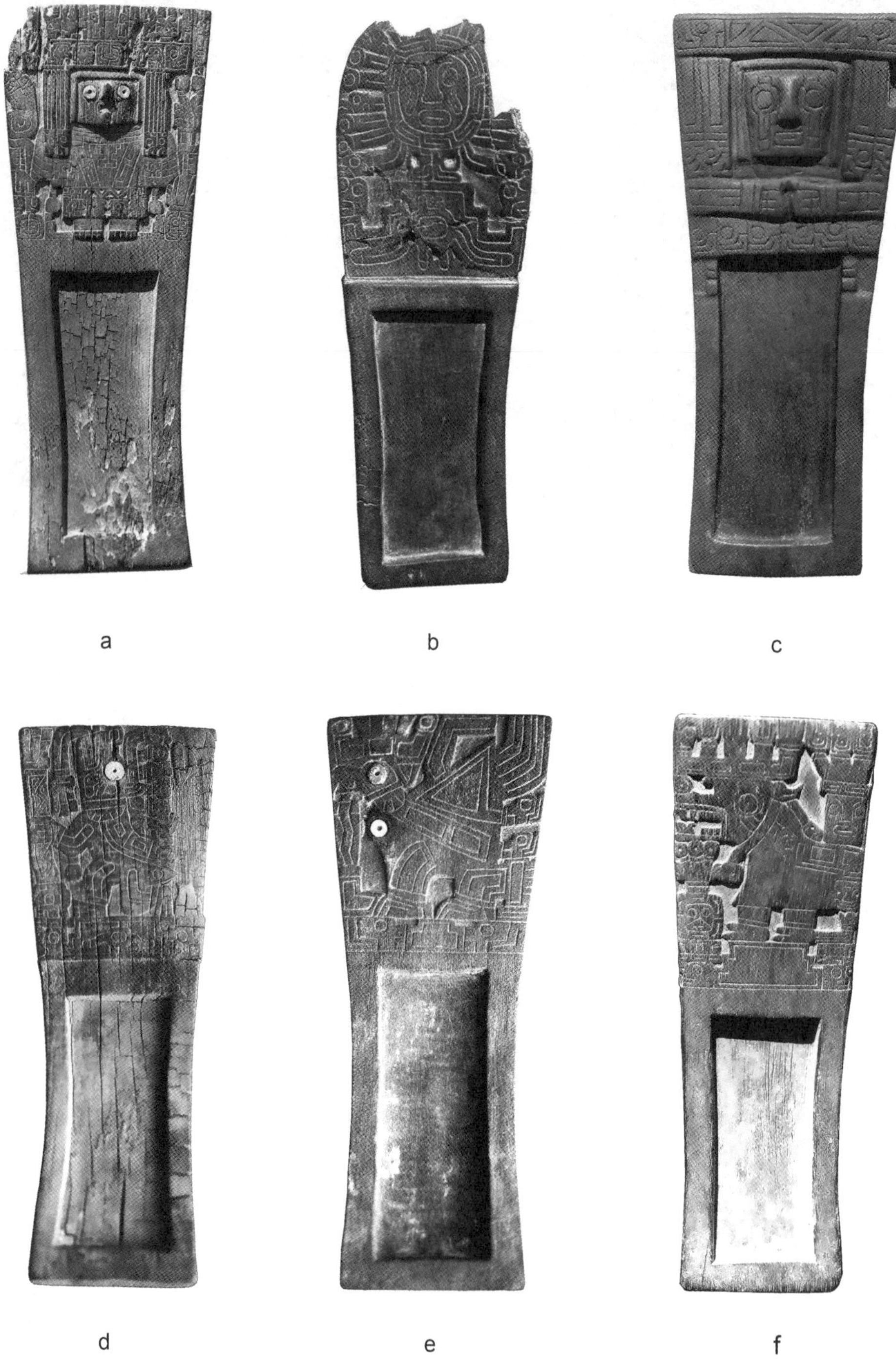

Fig. 11 Six Tiwanaku snuff trays from San Pedro de Atacama. a. Frontal staff bearing entity; b. Disembodied rayed head; c. Frontal entity with arms over chest; d. Profile genuflect entity holding staff; e. Bird-headed entity; f. Camelid bearing cargo (Photos C. M. Torres).

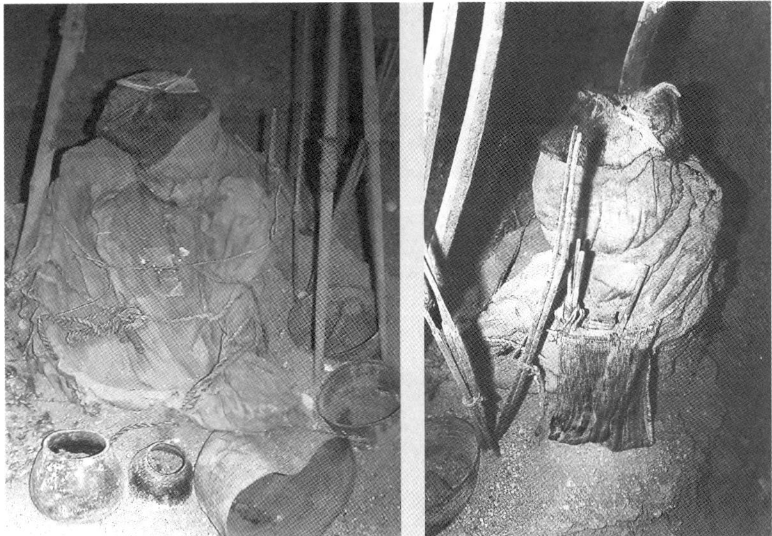

Fig. 12 Tomb 112 (in situ), Solcor 3, San Pedro de Atacama, ca. 780±60 CE (Beta-12447). Right photo showing one of two snuffing kits.

It should be emphasized that there is no evidence of Tiahuanaco emissaries or colonial outposts in this area. Only a handful of foreign individuals have been identified in San Pedro de Atacama, individuals that, as previously mentioned, were not associated with Tiwanaku objects. Approximately 700 snuff trays have been found there. Of these, sixty-four exhibit Tiwanaku iconography. The earliest date associated with a snuff tray bearing this type of iconography is *ca.* 190 AD, and the latest date is 920 AD* (Torres, 2018: Pls. 11.4-11.10).

It should be noted that the presence of a snuff tray from San Pedro de Atacama (Fig. 13) engraved with a representation of a profile genuflect personage early in the development of Tiwanaku iconography raises questions concerning center-periphery relationships and suggests trade patterns that might have included knowledge and ideologies. This tray could predate the development of this iconography at Tiwanaku itself.

Several of these thematic units survived through the centuries and are shared with Wari and other south central Andean cultures. Prominent among these themes (Torres, 2018: Pls. 11.31-35) because of wide geographical and temporal distribution are:

a. Frontal staff bearing entity (Fig. 11a)
b. Disembodied rayed head (Fig. 11b)
c. Frontal entity with arms over chest (Fig. 11c)
d. Profile entity holding staff (Fig. 11d)
e. Bird-headed entity (Fig. 11e)
f. Camelid bearing cargo (Fig. 11f)

* For high resolution images please visit: https://dig.ucla.edu/sais/images-in-action-visual-database?field_chapter_target_id=360).

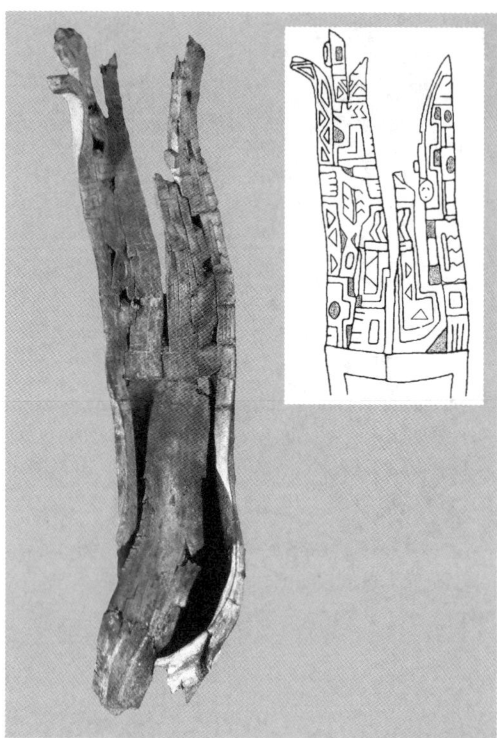

Fig. 13 Snuff tray from Toconao, ca. 190±140 CE San Pedro de Atacama. *Photo C. M. Torres, line drawing Donna Torres*

This shared iconography could conceal deep ideological differences. This is readily observable in Christian iconography and rituals where icons are shared, basically of a crucified and wounded human being. A Christian ritual performed in Rome notably differs from a Christian event in the south of the USA, although both emphasize a sacrificed human being. These differences range from the social to the domestic environment, with radical differences in the performance of politics. Notable divergence in political strategies between Tiwanaku and Wari, raise questions as to what caused these variances. Inebriating substances, the different modifications of consciousness produced, issues of manufacturing and distribution influenced the behavior of the political entity. In addition, the structure of the visionary event contributed to the definition of societal configurations, interacted, and modified cultural and individual organizational patterns.

Snuffing the seeds of vilca (*Anadenanthera colubrina* var. *cebil*) was the preferred mode of administration in Tiwanaku. The manufacture of snuff powders differs greatly from chicha production as was previously described for Wari. Vilca does not grow on the western slopes of the Andes. It is abundant on the eastern slopes down to sea level. It prefers open savannas and does not favor forested areas. Given the importance of snuffing in San Pedro de Atacama, it can be assumed that they had established a secure supply of seeds. The seeds probably moved through well-established llama caravan routes across the Andes. A question that arises is whether psychoactive substances and related ritual paraphernalia journeyed via regular transport caravans or had a separate way of traveling, perhaps an exclusive pattern dependent on ritual specialists and manufacturers. The style and iconography of the Tiwanaku snuff trays suggest a movement across the southern altiplano and the Atacama Desert. Detailed analysis of the 64 Tiwanaku snuff trays from San Pedro de Atacama has not revealed engravers or carvers with an idiosyncratic style. Side by side stylistic comparisons of San Pedro de Atacama Tiwanaku snuff trays denote that they are different enough to indicate that these elaborate objects were each made by a different artist. Consequently, it has not been possible to identify two or more trays created by the same hand. The criteria used in this work to define style refers to a constant series of design elements that remain relatively unchanged when observed within the transformation process of a coherent series of objects or themes (Gell, 1998: 167; Kübler, 1981: 129-130), The absence of individual artists in this sample suggest that snuffing paraphernalia circulated over this vast territory. The seeds traveled from the east across the Andes. Does the snuff move ready-made or do the seeds travel in their pods and get made into a snuff powder to meet local demands, with variations in plant admixtures including beta carboline-containing plants (as, for example, in the previously mentioned Cueva del Chileno, Miller *et al.*, 2019), and as documented among the Piaroa (Rodd, 2002: 276)? It is not possible to know with the evidence available so far if the seeds or the prepared snuff traveled from its source to San Pedro de Atacama. Snuff enthusiasts of the Atacama probably preferred to prepare their own powder. One argument regarding this factor is that prepared snuff, a very finely ground powder would lose potency faster than stored seeds. Preparation of the snuff itself was a simple procedure, not necessitating complex infrastructure and foreign specialists to accomplish the task of snuff production.

The production of the snuffing paraphernalia, particularly those which implement motifs from Tiwanaku iconography, were probably manufactured elsewhere, and traveled across the Andes. The high quality of craftmanship of the Tiwanaku snuff trays implies a sustained tradition to allow well trained artists to emerge. To effectively carve the stories engraved in these implements the artist would have to be well informed about mytho-historical events. San Pedro de Atacama is the only archaeological site with such a high presence of snuffing equipment. In addition, considering the absence of identifiable individual artists in San Pedro suggests that medical technology, ideological, and artistic knowledge circulated over the South-central Andes. Surely, future investigations will reveal archaeological sites with the same high percentage of visionary preparations as San Pedro de Atacama.

Society was not, at least with the evidence provided by the mortuary evidence, highly stratified. Few differences are discerned in the graves of San Pedro de Atacama; they are all a cylindrical pit with the body of the deceased seated with knees flexed, facing East toward the high peaks of the Andes (Fig. 12). Some burials included foreign objects such as snuff trays and tubes, foreign pottery including a few Tiwanaku ceramic vessels, and textiles. Most likely, these individuals were associated in some way with long range caravan routes, and not necessarily members of hierarchical elites with some sort of central control over the communities occupying the oasis. Differences in wealth do not necessarily imply the capacity to give orders and be obeyed.

The San Pedro oasis is located 15 kms north of the Tropic of Capricorn, at an elevation of 2447 mts (8028 feet). Agriculture is limited by low rainfall and mineralized water high in Boron in amounts well above the limit for irrigation. The water is of poor quality with much dissolved mineral matter. The limited and poor quality of the water coupled with the hyper-arid climate of the area restrict crops to a few species (Dingman, 1967: 2). This is not an area of intense corn cultivation, hence the manufacturing of chicha from *algarrobo* and not corn or molle. This limited agriculture is a factor that suggests a reliance on trade and caravan routes. Trans-Andean llama caravans circulated through a vast area beyond the Atacama salt flats all the way to the Pacific coast. Evidence for this circulation has been found in caravan circuits and waystations with rock art. The inventory of objects included, according to Gallardo *et al.* (2022: 71):

"… the quality of the foreign craftsmanship in circulation is quite remarkable. Among the known inventory of objects there is modeled, decorated, and polished pottery; stone sculptures, cups, and pipes with delicate finishes; hallucinogenic seeds of *Anadenanthera colubrina*; beads and red pigment containers made with land snails (*Strophocheilus oblongus*)."

The entity that is currently called San Pedro de Atacama did not exist during the Middle Horizon; the oasis was divided into separate communities today referred to as *ayllus*. During certain times of the year the requirements of ayllu organization most likely shifted. *Ayllus* had well delineated territories and consisted mainly of extended families or kin groups. In San Pedro de Atacama there is no evidence for central domination of the *ayllu* groups or command of a specific *ayllu*, although centralized control could have intermittently existed in the ebb and flow of caravan movement and climate. Communities may have lapsed to a hierarchical and a more authoritarian way of life during preparations for caravan arrivals and departures, where more of a cohesive force was needed. Then, they may have returned to less domineering forms of organization, akin to foragers with limited agriculture. This desert culture demonstrates a high degree of adaptability to shifting cultural needs (see the work of Graeber and Wengrow, 2021: 98-102, for a discussion of shifting political strategies).

To summarize, the production of chicha involved more infrastructure needs, and therefore required the movement of people. They were not only involved with chicha production but also it contributed to the nature of political interaction. Snuff production was a far simpler affair compared with the brewing of chicha. At this point in our discussion, it would be advisable to consider the nature of the effects of alcohol with admixture of *Anadenanthera* seeds, (likely a proto-ayahuasca potion), or just plain chicha, and the effects of snuffed *Anadenanthera* seeds with admixture of tobacco and harmine containing plants. The tryptamine alkaloids contained in the snuff powder produce a dynamic visionary experience. While chicha, with its low alcohol content might produce a somewhat lethargic state conducive to conversation. However, the definition of modified states of consciousness is impossible to confirm when diverse factors such as issues concerning time, place, and people are considered.

Careful stylistic analysis of the 64 Tiwanaku snuff trays in San Pedro de Atacama demonstrate, as previously mentioned, that they were all carved by different hands. This suggests that the snuff trays and the other components of the snuffing paraphernalia circulated in a vast area. Stops along the way provided additional objects, plants, stories, technologies, thus enriching and contributing variations to Tiwanaku iconography. Tiwanaku snuffing paraphernalia and seeds would travel, and in more intimate encounters in the path compromises and obligations were created. Tiwanaku snuff trays are engraved with stories that most likely were part of oral traditions. Through the journey the story goes and grows, variations are added that define social connections and create ideologies. In this way regional communities could define their social identity autonomous from direct control from Tiwanaku itself. This argument is strengthened by the absence of foreign individuals in San Pedro de Atacama (Torres-Rouff *et al.*, 2015: 593) that could have been emissaries of Tiwanaku and the southern Lake Titicaca Basin. No human agents or central control necessary, the visionary plants were the agents. One cannot help but wonder what the San Pedro de Atacama oasis could have contributed to trade with neighboring peoples. There is little evidence suggesting export of any commodities. Exchange of ideas and pharmaceutical technologies were likely part of exchange. The San Pedro *ayllus*, located in a crossroad between the Andes and the Pacific Ocean, perhaps provided knowledge, rituals, stories, songs, and dances. Surely, complex information was being exchanged through the caravan routes.

BIBLIOGRAPHY

Berenguer, José, 2001. Evidence for snuffing and shamanism in Prehispanic Tiwanaku stone sculpture. *Eleusis* 5: 61-83, Telesterion and Museo Civico di Rovereto, Trento, Italy.

Bergh, Susan, 2012. *Wari: Lords of the Ancient Andes*. Thames & Hudson.

Biwer, Matthew E., Willy Yépez Álvarez, Stefanie L. Bautista, and Justin Jennings, 2022. Hallucinogens, alcohol and shifting leadership strategies in the ancient Peruvian Andes. *Antiquity* 96 (385): 142-158, Cambridge University Press.

Browman, David L., 2002. Thoughts on the theater aspects of Tiwanaku. Paper presented at the 51st International Congress of Americanists (courtesy of the author), July 2003, Santiago, Chile.

Califano, Mario, 1976. El chamanismo Mataco. *Scripta Ethnologica* 3, 3, part 2: 7-60, Centro de Estudios de Etnología Americana, Buenos Aires.

Cobo, Bernabé, 1964. *Historia del Nuevo Mundo*, 2 vols.. Biblioteca de Autores Españoles, vols. 91, 92, Ediciones Atlas, Madrid.

Conlee, Christina A., Corina M. Kellner, Chester P. Walker, Aldo Noriega, 2021. Early imperialism in the Andes: Wari colonization of Nasca. *Antiquity* 2021 Vol. 95 (384): 1527-1546.

Dingman, Robert J., 1967. Geology and ground-water resources of the northern part of the Salar Atacama, Antofagasta Province, Chile. *Geological Survey Bulletin* 1219, Washington, DC.

Fabo, P. 1919-1920. Etnografía y lingüística de Casanare (Colombia, América meridional. *Anthropos* 14-15: 21-32, Vienna, Austria.

Gallardo, Francisco, Benjamín Ballester, Gloria Cabello, Carole Sinclaire, Itací Correa, Gonzalo Pimentel, and Estefanía Vidal. 2022. From northwestern Argentina to the Atacama Desert. Circulation, goods, and value (900 BC–AD 400). *Caravans in Global Perspective. Contexts and Boundaries*. Persis B. Clarkson and Calogero M. Santoro, editors. Routledge.

Gell, Alfred, 1998. *Art and agency. An anthropological theory*. Oxford University Press.

Graeber, David, David Wengrow, 2021. *The dawn of everything: A new history of humanity*, Farrar, Straus and Giroux, NY.

Horta Tricallotis, H. (2014). Lo propio y lo ajeno. Definición del estilo San Pedro en la parafernalia alucinógena de los oasis del salar de Atacama. *Chungará*, 46(4), 559-583.

Isbell, William, Mauricio I. Uribe, Anne Tiballi, and Edward P. Zegarra,. *Images in Action. The southern andean iconographic series*, 2018. Cotsen Institute of Archaeology Press, University of California Press, Los Angeles.

Isbell, William H., and Alexei Vranich, 2004. Experiencing the Cities of Wari and Tiwanaku. in *Andean Archaeology*, edited by Helaine Silverman, pp. 167-182. Blackwell Studies in Global Archaeology. Blackwell, Oxford.

Jennings, Justin and Brenda J. Bowser, 2008. *Drink, Power, and Society in the Andes*. University Press of Florida.

Knobloch, Patricia J., 2000. Wari ritual power at Conchopata: An interpretation of *Anadenanthera colubrina* iconography. *Latin American Antiquity* 11 (4):387-402. Society for American Archaeology, Washington, D.C.

Kubler, George, 1981. Period, style and meaning in ancient american art. In *Ancient Mesoamerica*, J. Graham, ed., pp. 11-23. Palo Alto: A Peek Publication.

Miller, Melanie J., Juan Albarracin-Jordan, Christine Moore, and José M. Capriles, 2019. Chemical evidence for the use of multiple psychotropic plants in a 1,000-year-old ritual bundle from South America. *Proceedings of the National Academy of Sciences*, May 6, 2019.

Moore, Jerry, 1989. Pre-Hispanic Beer in Coastal Peru: Technology and Social Context of Prehistoric Production. *American Anthropologist* 91(3): 682–695.

Moseley, Michael E., Donna J. Nash, Patrick Ryan Williams, Susan D. deFrance, Ana Miranda, Mario Ruales, 2005. Burning down the brewery: Establishing and evacuating an ancient imperial colony at Cerro Baúl, Peru. *Proceedings of the National Academy of Sciences of the United States* 102 (48): 17264–17271.

Nash, Donna, 2012. The Art of Feasting: Building an Empire with Food and Drink. In *Wari: Lords of the ancient Andes*, edited by Susan Bergh, pp. 82-101. Thames and Hudson.

Ondegardo, Polo de, 1916. Informaciones acerca de la religión y gobierno de los Incas. En *Colección de libros y documentos referentes a la historia del Perú*, vols. 3 and 4. Sanmartí y Ca., Lima.

Ponce Sanginés, Carlos, 1999. *Tiwanaku: 200 años de investigaciones arqueológicas*. Centro de Investigaciones Antropológicas Tiwanaku and Producciones CIMA, La Paz.

Quiroga, Juan Carlos, Dennis Ricaldi, Arturo Argueta , Jose Tata, Dionisio Tata, N.N., 2019. Iconografía de Villca en estelas líticas del sitio arqueológico de Tiwanaku. *Revista Ciencia, Tecnología e Innovación* 2019, 17-20: 51-64. Bolivia.

Reis Altschul, Siri von, 1972. *The Genus Anadenanthera in Amerindian Cultures*. Botanical Museum, Harvard University, Cambridge, Massachusetts.

Rodd, Robin, 2002. Snuff synergy: preparation, use and pharmacology of *yopo* and *Banisteriopsis caapi* among the Piaroa of southern Venezuela. *Journal of Psychoactive Drugs*, 34 (3): 273-9, San Francisco.

Sayre, Matthew, David Goldstein, William Whitehead, Patrick Ryan Williams, 2012. A marked preference. Chicha de molle and Huari state consumption practices. *Ñawpa Pacha, Journal of Andean Archaeology*, 32, (2): 231–282. Institute of Andean Studies, Berkeley, California.

Schreiber, Katharina J., 1992. Wari Imperialism in Middle Horizon Peru, *Anthropological Papers Series* Book 87, Museum of Anthropology University of Michigan.

Schreiber, Katharina J., 2001. The Wari empire of Middle Horizon Peru. The epistemological challenge of documenting an empire without documentary evidence. In *Empires: Perspectives from Archaeology and History*, edited by Susan E. Alcock, Terence N. D'Altroy, Kathleen D. Morrison, Carla M. Sinopoli, pp. 70-92. Cambridge University Press.

Torres, Constantino Manuel, 2018. Visionary Plants and SAIS Iconography in San Pedro de Atacama and Tiahuanaco. In editors Isbell, William H.; Mauricio Uribe;, Anne Tiballi; Edward P. Zegarra. *Images in Action. The southern andean iconographic series*, Chapter 11: 287-326 Cotsen Institute of Archaeology Press, University of California Press, Los Angeles. https://dig.ucla.edu/sais/

Torres, Constantino Manuel, and David B. Repke, 2006 *Anadenanthera, Visionary Plant of Ancient South America*. Haworth Press, Binghamton, New York.

Torres, Constantino Manuel, Donna Torres, 2014. Un analisis iconografico de la estela Ponce, Tiwanaku, Bolivia. *Art & Sensorium—Revista Interdisciplinar Internacional de Artes Visuais da UNESPAR/EMBAP*, 1 (01): 49-74. Universidade Estadual do Paraná—Campus de Curitiba, Brasil.

Torres, Constantino M., David Repke, Kelvin Chan, Dennis McKenna, Agustín Llagostera, and Richard Evans Schultes, 1991. "Snuff powders from Pre-Hispanic San Pedro de Atacama: Chemical and contextual analysis." *Current Anthropology* 32, 5: 640-649.

Torres-Rouff, Christina, Kelly J. Knudson, William J. Pestle, Emily M. Stovel, 2015. Tiwanaku Influence and Social Inequality: A Bioarchaeological, Biogeochemical, and Contextual, Analysis of the Larache Cemetery, San Pedro de Atacama, Northern Chile. *American Journal of Physical Anthropology* 158: 592–606

Vega, Garcilaso de La 1970 (orig ed. Lisbon, 1609). *Royal Commentaries of the Incas, and General History of Peru: Part One*. University of Texas Press, Austin.

Vranich, Alexei, Charles Stanish, 2013. *Visons of Tiwanaku*. Monograph 78, Cotsen Institue of Archaeology Press. University of California Press, Los Angeles.

Wassén, S. Henry 1967. Anthropological survey of the use of South American snuffs." In *Ethnopharmacologic Search for Psychoactive Drugs*, edited by Daniel H. Efron *et al.*, 233-289, Public Health Service Publication 1645, U.S. Department of Health, Education, and Welfare, Washington, D.C. Reprinted in *Ethnopharmacologic Search for Psychoactive Drugs: 50 years of research* (Vols. 1 & 2, Synergetic Press, Santa Fe, New Mexico, 2018.

Williams, Patrick Ryan, Donna Nash, Patricia Chacaltana, 2020. Wari and Tiwanaku. Early Imperial Repertoires in Andean South America. In *Archaeologies of Empire. Local participants and imperial trajectories*, Chapter 8: 199-227. Edited by Anna L. Boozer, Bleda S. Düring, and Bradley J. Parker. School for Advanced Research, University of New Mexico Press, Albuquerque.

Young-Sánchez, Margaret, 2004. *Tiwanaku: Ancestors of the Inca*. University of Nebraska Press

Ethnosphere

Contemporary Cultures of Psychoactive Plant Use

Coca: The Divine Leaf of Immortality

Wade Davis, PhD

Professor of Anthropology | BC Leadership Chair in Cultures and Ecosystems at Risk at the University of British Columbia | Ethnobotanist | Author | Filmmaker

> *"A legal market in coca will generate for Colombia tax revenues that will allow a long-suffering nation to pay the price of peace, having drained its treasury for 50 years to cover the costs of a war only made possible by the sordid profits of prohibition."* —WADE DAVIS

This paper shares an interdisciplinary perspective on the potential and power of the coca plant, as well as the devastating impact tht its vilification has caused.

COCA: LEAF OF THE GODS

As darkness fell over the Colombian Amazon, the shaman lit a torch dripping in resin, and a red glow illuminated the circle of low stools where the Barasana had gathered, as they do every night. From the other end of the *maloca*, the community longhouse, came the rustle of women and children making ready to sleep. A young man played an instrument made from the head of a deer; another blew softly over a large shell, a sound intended to stir the spirits. To one side, a boy kindled a fire beneath a large clay griddle, upon which he placed the leaves we had harvested earlier in the day. He tossed the coca with a steady rhythm, chanting and singing. His brother swept clean the dirt floor before setting fire to a large pile of dried leaves from the *yarumo* tree; the flames flared well over his head, and quickly died back, leaving a mound of white ash. Tobacco was passed, a powerful snuff that caused the head to spin and beads of sweat to soak the fingertips.

When the coca was ready, the leaves lightly toasted and brittle, the brothers placed several handfuls into the mouth of a large wooden mortar, and began to pound them with a long pestle, taking turns. It was hard steady work, and sweat soon fell from their brows. Once the coca had been reduced to a bright green powder, they poured the contents of the mortar into a large calabash and mixed in some ash, roughly a handful for every two handfuls of coca. The color turned a rich gray-green. The next step involved wrapping the powder in palm fibre, securing the bundle to a stick, and shaking the contents vigorously inside a covered vessel. As small clouds of green dust filled the air, one of the men asked if I had ever tried *mambe*. At the time, I was only familiar with the coca of the highlands, where the leaves are taken whole, with alkali added to the quid. My new friend cringed at the thought. "*Qué bárbaro*," he said, "How barbaric."

He handed me the calabash. I followed his instructions and placed a large spoonful of the powder gently on my tongue. Within seconds, I coughed and great puffs of green smoke blew out of my mouth and nostrils. The Barasana roared with laughter. Never talk, I was told, just wait and let the *mambe* come together. I tried again, and soon could feel the coca trickling down my throat. The flavour was smoky and delicious. Within a few minutes the inside of my cheek was numb and a sensation of well-being had spread throughout my body. It was a subtle feeling that lasted long into the night, even as the men spoke of the primordial journey of the *Ayawa*, the Thunders, the four culture heroes who brought order and harmony to the world, along with the gifts of the Anaconda, the sacred plants; tobacco, Yagé, and coca.

The next morning we left for the forest early. Fortified by a huge wad of *mambe*, I moved effortlessly over rough terrain and, for the first time, felt truly oblivious to the tropical heat. The renowned botanical explorer Richard Evans Schultes, my professor at Harvard, used coca every day during his 12 years in the Amazon, beginning in 1941. It was no wonder. I smiled to recall how, like a sommelier recommending a favourite vintage, he had urged me to seek out the *mambe* of the Tanimukas, a delicious recipe, he claimed, infused with aromatic resin of a rare forest tree. Schultes once pulled out a can of *mambe* at a society party in Bogotá. In measured tones, he explained to anyone who would listen that the preferred ash came from the large palmate leaves of *Cecropria sciadophila*, not the decidedly inferior foliage of *Cecropia peltata*. He naturally had the good stuff.

GREEN COCAINE

On October 31 2020, WPVI Action News, an ABC affiliate in Philadelphia, led its evening report with a sensational account of a rare drug bust at Philadelphia International Airport. US Customs and Border Protection (CBP) officers had seized more than 12 pounds of what was described as green cocaine, along with a mysterious "brown tar-like substance" which had tested positive for nicotine. The powder had tested positive for cocaine. According to authorities, the green hue was a way of camouflaging the drug, which through a chemical process using gasoline, ammonia and other chemicals, could be turned white, the implication being that, ounce for ounce, it was just your ordinary blow, tinged with another colour. "This seizure," reported Casey Durst, head of CBP's Baltimore Field Office, "perfectly illustrates how Customs and Border Protection officers use keen instinct and professional scientific analysis to intercept dangerous drugs being smuggled into our communities." In Cincinnati, Port Director Richard Gillespie heralded those singularly responsible for having "kept this dangerous green powder out of our neighbourhoods."

Beneath the righteous pose, however, was a farce worthy of Moliere. The source of nicotine reported in the bust I knew well. It was *ambil*, a native paste with very high concentrations of tobacco, an addictive and potentially lethal drug that, when smoked, is responsible for the death of 480,000 Americans each year. Tobacco being legal, this substance was of no concern to the customs agents. The green powder in question was *mambe*. As early as 1957, Schultes had reported its use as a mild stimulant and essential component of the nutritional regime of the peoples of the Northwest Amazon; daily consumption more than satisfied the Recommended Dietary Allowance for calcium, iron, phosphorous, vitamin A and riboflavin. Prepared from an

Amazonian variety of coca with notably low concentrations of the alkaloid, less than 0.5 percent dry weight, *mambe* is food as much as stimulant, as innocuous as a cup of black tea or coffee, and far better for the health.

The news reports from WPVI noted that the "green cocaine" had been sent to labs in Savannah and Newark for analysis. Not reported were the actual results of the assays, trivial amounts of cocaine equivalent to the concentrations of caffeine in a coffee bean. Had anyone tried to snort the powder, they would have simply plugged their nostrils most unpleasantly with a substance the consistency of talcum powder; *mambe* is always consumed orally. To suggest that smugglers might import *mambe* to extract cocaine, even assuming it could be done given the large quantities of ash in the preparation, makes about as much sense as suggesting that someone would import Dom Perignon to secure by chemical processing pure extracts of ethyl alcohol. Like champagne, *mambe* is a specialized item, made by trained individuals on a small scale, a labour-intensive process that yields a highly valued and unique natural product. Drug cartels that have successfully shipped cocaine by the ton into the United States for nearly fifty years are not about to waste their time with it.

What transpired at the airport in Philadelphia was a drug bust on par with Elliot Ness mistaking a truckload of potatoes for vodka and seizing the entire works as a violation of the Volstead Act. It's one thing to note with regret that after 50 years of a "war on drugs", there are more people in more places using worse drugs in worse ways than ever before. It's quite another to acknowledge that having spent billions of dollars a year on this misguided crusade, $1 trillion altogether, our front line defenders still do not know the difference between a pure alkaloid first isolated and extracted as a drug in 1859, and coca, a benign and highly nutritious plant, revered today by millions of indigenous people, and long celebrated by the ancient civilizations of South America as the divine leaf of immortality.

SOCIALLY DISRUPTIVE PLANTS

New drugs have a way of upsetting the social order. The French Revolution was caused, at least in part, by caffeine. For generations, it had been impossible to drink the water in any European city for fear of succumbing to disease, cholera and dysentery in particular. People slaked their thirst with alcohol—gin and rum, whiskey, wine, ale and mead. The entire continent was mildly besotted, which was fine as long as the main economic activities remained farming and handcrafted manufacturing.

Then, over the course of several decades, three botanical treasures appeared, all central nervous system stimulants: tea from India and China, chocolate from Guatemala, and coffee from Abyssinia by way of Brazil and the tropical lands of the New World. All had to be prepared with boiled water, which killed the pathogens, rendering them safe to drink. As each was a highly valued commodity, especially in the early years of the trade, their sale was concentrated in shops that, in time, became centers of intellectual and political intrigue, attracting the likes of Voltaire and Rousseau, Isaac Newton and Christopher Wren.

Rather than hanging out in the local tavern with their brows in their beer, those who patronized these new establishments became wired on caffeine and they couldn't shut up. The writings of Alexander Pope, Samuel Pepys and Jonathan Swift are positively infused with the drug. The coffee houses of London and Oxford became known as penny universities, a reference to the cost of admission and the presence of the finest minds of the era engaged in open discourse and debate. Those of Paris served as fountains of revolution as equally talkative men took note that Louis XIV's chateau at Versailles was a bit bigger than their digs. The call to arms that led to the storming of the Bastille originated at the Café de Foy, Voltaire's favourite coffee house. From there the mob gathered and marched.

Not surprisingly, those in charge, royalty across Europe and beyond, tried their best to curtail the use of the drug. In 1633, having imposed the death penalty for coffee drinkers throughout the Ottoman Empire, Sultan Murad IV stalked the streets of Istanbul in disguise, ready to decapitate anyone caught with the brew. Charles II infiltrated the coffee houses of London with spies; in 1675, he ordered them all to close. As late as 1777, Frederick the Great of Germany attempted to outlaw coffee that his people might return to beer, which yielded a more docile and manageable citizenry.

A dull and passive work force was, in fact, the last thing the emerging industrial economy needed. One could harvest a field after a few tumblers of beer, but hardly operate an unforgiving machine tool. Along with steam and coal, coffee and tea fueled the Industrial Revolution, two stimulants that kept workers alert, while providing rare moments of relief and satisfaction. A cup of tea became the salve for any crisis, even as the coffee break was institutionalized in every corporate office, union hall, school, hospital, fire station and church priory, a brief but inviolable suspension of work allowing employees to imbibe with predictable regularity another dose of the drug.

Coffee, initially employed exclusively as a medicine, and only later serving as a spark of sedition, had by the 19th century been tamed and domesticated, in good measure because it allowed men and women to work, and industrial production to soar. Its pharmacology, the raw potential for good or ill, had not changed. Rats fed large doses of caffeine become aggressive and violent; a caffeine crazed rat may even attack itself, ripping apart its own flesh. The drug's undoubted potential for harm, however, did not ultimately result in its prohibition; caffeine was needed and thus its chemical essence was reconfigured and culturally redefined.

As a consequence, there is today no black market with extortionate prices that would bankrupt coffee drinkers and drive the most desperate among them to lives of crime, while delivering enormous profits to those in control of the dark trade. Instead, coffee is sold at prices that reflect a healthy and dynamic free market, generating both legitimate employment and significant tax revenues for countries and governments throughout the world. What's more, the ready availability of the natural product—coffee beans and tea leaves in scores of flavours and blends—has effectively precluded the emergence of a significant market for chemical extracts of caffeine, which is fortunate. It is an axiom of pharmacology that the purer the drug, the greater the potential for abuse.

THE HISTORY OF COCAINE IN THE WEST

The first drug distilled in pure form from a plant was morphine. Cocaine was the second, isolated in 1859 by Albert Nieman, a German chemist. The drug came into its own in 1884 when Carl

Koller, a close friend of Sigmund Freud, recognized its anesthetic properties, which led to the first application of local anesthesia in surgery. To this day, cocaine remains our most powerful topical anesthetic, notably for nose throat and ear surgery, a perfect illustration of the adage that there are no good and bad drugs, only good and bad ways of using them.

The Corsican chemist Angelo Mariani came down on the good side in 1863 when he patented *Vin Tonique Mariani*, a combination of red bordeaux wine, coca leaf extract, and a sprinkling of pure cocaine. Needless to say, it was a hit. Mariani was responsible for two U.S. presidents, four kings, two popes, three princes, one Russian tsar, a shah and the Grand Rabbi of France turning on to coca and cocaine. Pope Leo XIII carried a flask of the wine on his hip. In the United States, an ailing Ulysses S. Grant managed to complete his memoirs with the aid of a teaspoon a day for the last five months of his life. Louis Bleriot sipped Vin Mariani as he became the first to fly the English Channel in 1909. Among those who provided Mariani with testimonials were Thomas Edison, H.G. Wells, Jules Verne, Auguste Rodin, Henrik Ibsen, Sarah Bernhardt and the Prince of Wales.

As the most popular prescribed medicine in the world, Vin Mariani inspired a host of imitators. In 1885, John Pemberton, pharmacist in Atlanta, registered the trademark for a preparation called *French Wine of Coca: Ideal Nerve and Tonic Stimulant.* A year later, he removed the wine and added the kola nut of Africa, rich in caffeine, as well as citrus oils for flavouring. Two years after that, he replaced the water with soda water, because of its association with mineral springs and good health, and began to market the product as an "intellectual beverage and temperance drink." In 1891, Pemberton sold his patent to Asa Griggs Candler, another pharmacist from Atlanta, and a year after that the Coca-Cola Company was launched. Sold as a treatment for headache, a "sovereign remedy" for hangovers, Coca-Cola soon found its way into every drugstore in the land. The soda fountain, a kind of poor man's health spa, became an institution, and all over the country men and women were strolling into their pharmacies and ordering their favourite drink by asking for "a shot in the arm".

Although Coca-Cola removed cocaine from its formula in 1903, to this day it relies on the source plant as a flavouring agent. The Stepan Company in Maywood, New Jersey, imports tons of leaves every year, removing the cocaine to sell on the pharmaceutical market, before shipping the residue containing the essential oils and flavonoids to Atlanta. The company doesn't advertise its position as the only legal importer of coca in the country, but the leaves are the reason Coca-Cola can legitimately lay claim to be, as its advertising slogan has long professed, the real thing. That the company earns $3 billion a year selling cocaine, mostly to Mallinckrodt, the country's largest manufacturer of opioids, is just a bonus.

By the 1880s, cocaine was being marketed and sold in scores of products—sweets, cigarettes, ointments, sprays, throat gargles, over-the-counter injections and cocktails. Articles in leading medical journals recommended cocaine for the treatment of a host of afflictions ranging from seasickness to stomach pain, hay fever, depression, and even that scourge of the 19th century, female masturbation, for which one physician recommended a "topical dose to the clitoris for prevention." The wave of popularity peaked in 1884, the year Sigmund Freud published his misguided paper, *On Coca*, in which he celebrated cocaine as a panacea, recommending it in particular for alcoholism and opium addiction.

It soon became apparent, however, that the cure could be worse than the disease. By 1890, the medical literature contained more than 400 cases of acute toxicity brought on by the drug, psychotic episodes in which patients experienced horrific tactile hallucinations, haunting illusions of insects crawling beneath their skin. The reversal of fortunes was immediate and dramatic. Within a few years, cocaine went from being promoted as the most beneficial stimulant known to man, the tonic of choice of presidents and popes, to being perceived as a modern curse.

As laws increasingly circumscribed its use and availability, cocaine was condemned as a narcotic, which it is not, and culturally marginalized as a symbol of decadence, employed only by artists and assorted degenerates, most of them conveniently black. As both physicians and politicians came to consider cocaine and morphine as equally dangerous, coca became associated with opium, and the public was led to believe that the ruinous effects of habitual opium use would inevitably befall those who regularly chewed coca leaves. Thus, a mild stimulant that had been used for at least 5,000 years before Europeans discovered cocaine came to be viewed as an addictive drug.

But coca is not cocaine, and to equate the leaf with the raw alkaloid is as misguided as suggesting that the delicious flesh of a peach is equivalent to the hydrogen cyanide found in every peach pit. Yet, for nearly a century, this has been precisely the legal and political position of nations and international organizations throughout the world.

AN ETHNOBOTANICAL PERSPECTIVE

The US government, in particular, has long demonized the plant. In Peru, programs to eliminate the traditional fields, supported by the United States, began 50 years before a black-market trade in the drug existed. The real issue was not cocaine but, rather, the cultural identity and survival of those who traditionally revered coca. The call for eradication came from officials and physicians, Peruvian and American, whose concern for the well-being of the Andean peoples was matched in its intensity only by their ignorance of Andean life.

In the 1920s, as physicians from Lima looked up into the Andes, they saw only abject poverty, illiteracy, poor health and nutrition, and high rates of infant mortality. With the blindness of good intentions, they searched for a cause. Since political issues of land, economic disparity and raw exploitation struck too close to home, forcing them to examine the structure of their own world, they settled on coca. Every possible ill, every source of embarrassment to their bourgeois sensibilities, was blamed on the plant.

Carlos A. Rickets, who first presented a plan for coca eradication in 1929, described coca users as feeble, mentally deficient, lazy, submissive, and depressed. Referring in 1936 to Peru's "legions of drug addicts," Carlos Enrique Paz Soldán, a doctor and university professor, raised the battle cry: "If we await with folded arms a divine miracle to free our indigenous population from the deteriorating action of coca, we shall be renouncing our position as men who love civilization."

In the 1940s the push for eradication was led by Carlos Gutiérrez-Noriega, chief of pharmacology at the Institute of Hygiene in Lima. Considering coca "the greatest obstacle to the improvement of Indians' health and social condition," Gutiérrez-Noriega established his reputation with a series of dubious scientific studies, conducted exclusively in prisons and asylums, which concluded that coca users tended to be alienated, antisocial, inferior in intelligence and initiative, prone to "acute and chronic mental alterations," as well as other reputed behavioral disorders such as "absence of ambition." The ideological thrust of his science was blatant. In a report published in 1947 by the Peruvian Ministry of Public Education, he wrote, "The use of coca, illiteracy and a negative attitude towards the superior culture are all closely related."

It was largely as a result of Gutiérrez-Noriega's lobbying that the United Nations dispatched a team of experts in the fall of 1949 to look into the coca problem. Not surprisingly, their findings, published as the 1950 Report on the Commission of Enquiry on the Coca Leaf, condemned the plant and recommended a 15-year phasing out of its cultivation. Such a conclusion was never in doubt. Eleven years later both Peru and Bolivia signed the Single Convention on Narcotic Drugs, an international treaty that called for the complete abolition of coca chewing and the end of coca cultivation within 25 years.

Incredibly, in the midst of this hysterical effort to purge the nation of coca, none of the Peruvian public health officials did the obvious: analyze the leaves to find out exactly what they contained. It was, after all, a plant consumed every day by millions of their countrymen and women. Had they done so, their rhetoric might have softened.

In 1973, the Botanical Museum at Harvard, under the direction of Professor Schultes, secured support from the US Department of Agriculture (USDA) to conduct the first comprehensive and modern scientific study of the botany, ethnobotany, and nutritional value of all cultivated species and varieties of coca. At the time, despite growing concerns about the illicit use of cocaine, surprisingly little was known about the source plant. The botanical origin of the domesticated species, the chemistry of the leaf, the pharmacology of coca chewing, the geographical range of the cultivated species and the relationship between the wild and cultivated species all remained mysteries. No concerted effort had been made to document the role of coca in the religion and culture of Andean and Amazonian peoples since W Golden Mortimer's classic book, *History of Coca,* published in 1901.

Leading the research effort was the botanical explorer Timothy Plowman, whose mandate from the US government, made deliberately vague by Schultes, was to travel the length of the Andean Cordillera and locate, among other things, the place of origin of the sacred plant. It was the dream academic assignment of the 1970s, and it was my good fortune to serve as Plowman's field assistant for two years. Also on the trail of coca at the time was another Schultes protégé, Andrew Weil, then in the midst of a multi-year odyssey studying altered states of consciousness around the world. A graduate of Harvard Medical School with a profound knowledge of medicinal botany, Weil was fascinated by the healing properties of coca and the plant's role in nutrition and well-being.*

With coca purchased in a public market in Bolivia, Plowman and Weil, in collaboration with Jim Duke of the USDA, examined 15 nutrients found in the leaves, comparing their concentrations with the levels of the same nutrients in 50 common Latin American foods; coca

* Professor Andrew Weil has written a paper for this ESPD55 publication called "The therapeutic potential of coca".

was higher than the average in calories, protein, carbohydrates and several minerals. The study also revealed that coca leaves contain a host of vitamins, more calcium than any other cultivated plant—especially useful for Andean communities that traditionally lacked dairy products—and enzymes that enhance the body's ability to digest carbohydrates at high altitude, an ideal complement for a potato-based diet. To the disappointment and horror of some of our backers in the US government, the results confirmed that coca, as consumed by Indigenous Peoples, serves as a mild and benign stimulant that is beneficial to the health and highly nutritious, with no evidence of toxicity or addiction.

As a physician, Weil went on to report that coca facilitates well-being, eases digestion, and demonstrably relieves the symptoms of altitude sickness, or *soroche.* His studies indicated that coca can be helpful in the treatment of rheumatism, dysentery, stomach ulcers and nausea, with the leaves having a positive influence on respiration and a capacity to cleanse the blood of toxic metabolites, notably uric acid. Daily use of the leaves clears the mind, elevates mood and tones and strengthens the digestive tract, enhancing the assimilation of foods, even while promoting longevity. Citing a popular Andean legend, Weil concluded that coca was indeed a gift from the heavens, a sacred leaf intended only to better the lives of all people dwelling in all places on the earth.

TRADITIONAL USE AND BOTANY

None of this will come as a surprise to students of South American history. For the Inca, coca figured prominently in every aspect of ritual and daily life. Before a journey, priests tossed leaves into the air to propitiate the gods. Unable to cultivate the plant at the heights of Cusco, they replicated it in gold and silver, in sacred gardens enclosed by temple walls. At the *Coricancha*, the Temple of the Sun, sacrifices were made to the plant, and supplicants could approach the altars only if they had coca in their mouths. Soothsayers read the future in the venation of the leaves and in the flow of green saliva on fingers, skills of divination acquired only by those who had survived a lightning strike. At initiation young Inca nobles competed in arduous foot races, while maidens offered coca and chicha, a fermented drink. At the end of the ordeal each runner was presented with a *chuspa,* a woven bag filled with the finest leaves as a symbol of his new manhood.

Long caravans carrying as many as 3,000 large baskets of leaves regularly moved between the lowland plantations and the valleys leading to Cusco. Without coca, armies could not be maintained or marched across the vast expanse of the empire. Coca allowed the imperial runners, or *chasquis*, to relay messages across 4,000 miles in a week. When the *yaravecs* (court orators) were called on to recite the history of the Inca at ceremonial functions, they were aided only by a system of knotted strings, called *quipus*, and coca to stimulate the memory. In the fields, priests and farmers scattered leaves to bless the harvest. A suitor presented leaves to the family of the bride. Official travelers lay spent quids of leaves on rock cairns dedicated to *Pachamama* and placed at intervals along the paths of the empire. The sick and dying kept leaves at hand, for if coca was the last taste in a person's mouth before death, the path to paradise was assured.

Just as the Inca venerated the plant, so, too, did the other peoples of the Andes. Archaeological evidence suggests that coca was used as early as 3000 BCE at Valdivia on the Santa Elena Peninsula in western Ecuador; on the coast of Peru, it was commonly grown by 2500 BCE. Lime pots and ceramic figurines depicting humans chewing coca have been found at virtually every major site from every era of pre-Columbian civilization on the coast, Nazca, Paracas, Moche, Chimu. The very word coca is derived not from Quechua but from Aymara, the language spoken by the descendants of the Tiwanaku, the empire that predated the Inca on the altiplano and in the basin of Titicaca by 500 years. The root word is *khoka*, a simple term meaning bush or tree, implying that the source of the sacred leaves is the plant of all plants. An active trade was established in the Bolivian highlands as early as 400CE, a thousand years before the dramatic expansion of the Inca.

The plant itself is a beautiful if delicate shrub, with small white flowers and fruits the size and colour of rubies. The texture and shape of the leaves varies, for there are two cultivated species, each with two distinct varieties. *Erythroxylum coca* var. *coca* is the classic leaf of the southern Andes, grown in the upper reaches of the tropical valleys that fall away to the Amazon, the harvest making its way to the markets of Cusco and La Paz.

Colombian coca, *Erythroxylum novogranatense var. novogranatense*, is distinct. Adapted to hot, seasonally dry habitats and highly resistant to drought, it produces small narrow leaves of a bright yellowish green hue. Named in 1895 after the colonial name for the country, Nueva Granada, this was the coca of the 13th-century Muisca and Quimbaya goldsmiths, the stimulant of the unknown peoples who carved the monolithic statues of San Agustín, the plant that Amerigo Vespucci encountered on the Paria Peninsula in 1499, when he recorded the first European description of coca chewing. Once extensively grown along the Caribbean coast of South America, in adjacent parts of Central America, and in the interior of Colombia, it is now found in traditional context only in the rugged mountains of Cauca and Huila and in the Sierra Nevada de Santa Marta. Throughout Colombia it is known as *hayo*. Curiously, the coca of the north-west Amazon, *Erythroxylum coca var. ipadu*, the source of *mambe*, is derived not from *hayo*, but rather from cuttings or seeds carried downriver from southern Peru or Bolivia in pre-Columbian times. Finally, there is *Erythroxylum novogranatense* var. *truxillense*, now grown in the coastal desert valleys of northern Peru. With just a hint of wintergreen oil, this was the preferred coca of the Inca, not to mention the key ingredient in the secret formula of Coca-Cola.

Significantly, DNA analysis suggests that the progenitor of both domesticated species and all four varieties is *Erythroxylum gracilipes*, a wild species found the length of the Andes in the lowland forests of the western Amazon. Such botanical sleuthing may seem arcane, but to have two highly valued cultigens derived independently from a common ancestor, separate processes of artificial selection occurring thousands of miles apart, is an astonishing story of parallel invention, made all the more wondrous when the plants in question are revered throughout the entire range of the cultivated species as the very essence of the sacred.

COLONIALIZATION AND COCA

In the wake of the conquest, the Spaniards shattered every shrine, violated every temple, laid waste to an empire the scale and achievements of which they could not begin to fathom. All that was most precious to the Inca invoked the wrath of the conquerors, including coca, which was demonized as "the work of idolatry and sorcery", a plant serving only to strengthen "the wicked in their delusions, and asserted by every competent judge to possess no true virtues; but on the contrary, to cause the death of innumerable Indians, while it ruins the health of the few who survive."

That none of this was true ultimately proved convenient for the Spanish crown, especially as it became clear that natives would not toil in the mines without access to the leaves. In 1573, with his eye on gold and silver, Francisco de Toledo, Viceroy of Peru, revoked earlier laws prohibiting coca, and, by decree, removed all obstacles to its cultivation. Even as he forcibly relocated much of the population to new settlements, condemning thousands to death—at Potosí alone an average of 75 would die each day for 300 years—Toledo made sure the workers had coca.

Secularized and commercialized on a scale unknown to the Inca, coca became the foundation of the colonial economy, with taxes on its cultivation and exchange providing the church with its largest source of revenue. Christ's mission in Peru for three centuries was made possible by a plant the clergy had initially condemned as the "weed of the devil".

Many of the early chroniclers, scholars who sincerely sought to understand these new found lands, wrote glowingly about the coca plant. In his *Royal Commentaries,* Garcilaso de la Vega stated that the magical leaf "satisfies the hungry, gives new strength to the weary and exhausted, and makes the unhappy forget their sorrows." Pedro Cieza de Léon, who traveled throughout the Americas between 1532 and 1550, noted: "When I asked some of these Indians why they carried these leaves in their mouths . . . they replied that it prevents them from feeling hungry, and gives them great vigor and strength. I believe that it has some such effect."

Throughout the colonial era and well into the 19th century, praise for coca was effusive, often taking a tone of reverence and devotion, even adulation. José Hipólito Unánue, the most famous Peruvian physician of the 18th century, heralded the leaves as a panacea, the most powerful herb in a healer's repertoire. The Swiss naturalist and explorer Johann Jakob von Tsudi, who spent five years in the Andes, was impressed by the longevity of those who, over the course of their lives, by his estimate, "have consumed no less than 2700 pounds of leaves, yet nevertheless enjoy perfect health." Writing in 1846, he concluded: "I am clearly of the opinion that moderate use of coca is not merely innocuous, but even very conducive to health."

In Scotland, Sir Robert Christison, President of the Royal Society of Edinburgh (1868-73) and President of the British Medical Association (1875), decided to put the leaves to the test as he and ten students set out to walk thirty miles over hilly countryside, including an ascent of Ben Vorlich, which rises 3232 feet above Lock Earn. "On arrival home before dinner," he reported, "I felt neither hunger nor thirst, after complete abstinence from food and drink of every kind for nine hours, but upon dinner appearing in half an hour, ample justices was done to it." At the time of his experiment, Christison was 78.

Such qualities, of course, had long been reported by scientifically minded travelers in South America. J.T. Lloyd, who published *A Treatise on Coca* in 1913, wrote of the native porters of Popayán in southern Colombia: "After eating a simple breakfast, they would start with their heavy packs, weighing 75 to more than a hundred pounds, strapped to their backs. All day long they traveled at a rapid gait over steep mountain spurs at an altitude that to us, without any load whatever, was most exhausting. On these trips the Indians neither rested anywhere nor ate at noon but sucked their wads of coca throughout the entire day. These Indians we found very pleasant, always cheerful, happy and good natured, in spite of the fact that their daily toil subjected them to the severest of hardships and the most frugal fare." Lloyd concluded that coca was surely the key to their good health and good spirits. "Not only is it not harmful, it is said to provide nourishment for the body and to be useful in the treatment of many kinds of illnesses."

Perhaps the most fulsome praise came from the surgeon W. Golden Mortimer, author of *History of Coca* (1901). Among his more amusing testimonials is an account of the Toronto La Crosse Club which, in 1877, while hosting the world championships, decided to use coca in all their matches. As Mortimer reported: "The Toronto Club was composed of men accustomed to sedentary work, while some of the opposing players were sturdy men accustomed to out of door exercise. The games were all very severely contested, and some were played in the hottest weather of one summer; on one occasion the thermometer registered 110F in the sun. The more stalwart appearing men were so far used up before the match was completed that they could hardly be encouraged to finish the concluding game, while the coca chewers were as elastic and apparently free from fatigue as at the commencement of play."

Mortimer acknowledged coca as a panacea, noting its virtues as a medicine, tonic, and food. But what truly fascinated him was the subtlety of its mode of action. It was a stimulant to be sure and yet, at the same time, its subjective effect on the body was unlike that of any other stimulant known to science. As the physician W.S. Searle wrote in 1881, "It is not a little remarkable that while no other known substance can rival coca in its sustaining power, no other has so little apparent effect. To one pursuing the even tenor of his usual routine, the chewing of coca gives no especial sensation, in fact the only result seems to be a negative one, an absence of the customary desire for food and sleep. It is only when some unusual demand is made upon mind or body that its influence is felt... Those expecting some internal commotion or sensation are disappointed."

Andrew Weil captured this quality of the coca experience beautifully in his description of his first exposure to *mambe* whilst visiting the Cubeo in the Colombian Amazon in 1973. The effect of coca, he reported, was so subtle that it could not be compared to any other natural product similarly employed; it had to be learned to be appreciated, with set and setting playing a significant role. His first taste of *mambe* occurred at night, leaving him with a good feeling "that lasted for some time after I had nothing more in my mouth; in fact, it never really ended but simply trailed off imperceptibly." It was only in the morning, as he huddled with the men as they exchanged a calabash full of the delicate green powder, that he came to understand what all the fuss was about. "I found myself marching along in the column of Cubeos, swinging my machete, humming a tune, and feeling increasingly happy. The coca seemed stronger at this hour of the morning. Its warm glow spread from my stomach throughout my body. I felt a subtle vibrational energy in my muscles. My step became light, and there was nothing I wanted to do more than just what I was doing."

SOCIAL AND SPIRITUAL USES OF COCA

The difference between coca and cocaine, anthropologist Enrique Mayer once quipped, is the difference between traveling by donkey and jet plane. A clever line, but one that misses an essential point. The actions of coca and cocaine are not comparable. Each gives a sense of well- being, but while cocaine assaults the central nervous system, the effect of coca is modified by any number of naturally occurring compounds found in the leaves and not present in cocaine. Indigenous people who have traditionally used and celebrated coca show no preference for leaves with high levels of the alkaloid. The preferred leaves are always those rich in aromatic compounds and essential oils and low in cocaine. *Mambe* is made from leaves that have the lowest concentrations of cocaine of any of the cultivated varieties.

What's more, the cultures of coca and cocaine consumption could not be more distinct. What draws people to cocaine is the exotic decadence, the mystique of a rich man's drug, the ritual of a handful of the select few slipping into the shadows of a party to snort a few grains of a mysterious crystal that these days could be just about anything. Inclusion in the clandestine circle in the corner of the room, the stall in the bathroom, a private office at work, declares that one has arrived. Everyone at the party knows what is happening, which again is intentional. One of the privileges of membership in a secret society, as anthropologists have long reported, is the right to periodically flaunt the secrecy in public. Otherwise, what's the point of belonging? A lingering legacy of the cocaine culture of the 1980s is a small epidemic of hepatitis C, contracted by those who in their youth found it glamourous to stick up their noses a $100 note, damp with the snot of a stranger.

Coca, by contrast, is less a high than a meditation. Consumed in the Colombian Amazon as *mambe*, the plant is more commonly taken as whole leaves, which are held in the mouth as a quid for about 40 minutes, and then removed and placed on the ground in a respectful and deliberate gesture. To chew coca, or at least to absorb efficiently the small amount of the alkaloid in the leaves, one must modify human saliva by the addition of alkali. Any basic compound— baking soda, ash, limestone— will do. The Barasana and Makuna fire yarumo leaves to secure the ash. The Kogi and Arhuaco of the Sierra Nevada de Santa Marta, mountains that soar to 20,000 feet above the Caribbean coastal plain of Colombia, prefer seashells, which they acquire by trade or gather as part of elaborate pilgrimages to the ocean.

For the *Mamos*, the sun priests of the Kogi and Arhuaco, the chewing of *hayo* represents the most profound expression of culture. Their spiritual ideal would be to refrain from sex, eating and sleeping while staying up all night, chewing the leaves and chanting the names of the ancestors. As the guardians of the world, they believe that their rituals and prayers maintain the cosmic and ecological harmony of nature. At night, before they rest, they taste the leaves, deep in contemplation of the day that has passed; and in the morning *hayo* welcomes a new dawn. Every adult man consumes roughly a pound of leaves each day, beginning at marriage and continuing until his final breath.

In the mountains of the southern Andes, distance is measured not in miles but in *cocadas*, the length of time that a traveler is sustained by a single chew of leaves. When men and women meet on a trail, they pause and exchange *k'intus* of coca, three perfect leaves arranged to form a cross. They then turn to face the nearest of the *Apus*, the protective mountain deities that hover over every community and direct the destinies of all those born in their shadows. With eyes lifted toward the summits, they bring the leaves to their mouths and blow softly, a ritual invocation that sends the essence of the plant back to the earth, the community, the sacred places, and the souls of the ancestors. The exchange of leaves is a social gesture, a way of acknowledging a human connection. But the blowing of the *phukuy*, as it is called, is an act of spiritual reciprocity, for in giving selflessly to the earth, the individual ensures that in time the energy of the coca will return full circle, as surely as rain falling on a field will inevitably be reborn as a cloud. This subtlety of gesture is, in its own way, a prayer for the well-being of the entire world.

The etiquette of *hallpay*, the totality of the act of using coca—the exchange and salutations, the way one places the leaves in the mouth, the attitude of reverence and respect—in a very real sense defines what it means to be *Runakuna*, a child of Pachamama. Throughout the entire Andean world, as anthropologist Catherine Allen writes: "One cannot function as a social being unless you partake in the ritual, and you must do it properly." Nothing causes more offence than tourists and travelers who stuff their mouths with leaves, like horses eating hay.

Whether the leaves are taken in the presence of a friend or a stranger, alone or together with all the community, to chew coca, to *hallpay*, is to transcend self and become part of the social, moral and spiritual nexus that in the Andes gives meaning to life. Coca alone makes possible direct communication with the divine, with some saying today that the first to taste the leaves was Santísima María, mother of Christ, who according to legend lost her holy child, and chewed on the leaves to allay her grief. Thus, for the people of the Andes to be without coca is a form of social and spiritual death, an excommunication from existence itself. Efforts to deny the *Runakuna* access to the leaves, to eradicate the traditional fields, are not analogous to outlawing, for example, beer in Germany, coffee in the Middle East, or betel chewing in India. They are the policies of cultural genocide.

THE DESECRATION OF COCA

The war on drugs began in 1971 when Richard Nixon took hold of fear and turned it into a political movement. Caring little about drug use, as John Ehrlichman, his closest domestic advisor later acknowledged, Nixon concocted the crisis strictly as a political ploy to galvanize his base ahead of his re-election campaign in 1972. At the time, most Americans had never heard of cocaine. The illicit trade, such as it was, remained in the hands of the independent drifter; young travelers who rotated through Colombia from El Salvador and Peru, drawn to a good life, which they financed by smuggling into the US small packets of coke, hidden in their luggage or crammed uncomfortably into various body orifices.

Today, 50 years on, more cocaine is being produced and trafficked than ever before. Thanks to prohibition, the US is the only developed country to have more citizens with criminal records than university degrees. In Colombia, an actual war, funded almost exclusively by the profits of the drug trade, left 400,000 dead, and seven million internally displaced; in the past five decades, millions more have abandoned the country, some by choice, others desperate to escape.

Cocaine has been Colombia's curse, but the engine driving the trade has always been consumption. The cartels rose out of the barrios and country clubs of Medellín and Cali, but the ultimate responsibility for Colombia's agonies lies in good measure with every person who has ever bought street cocaine and every foreign nation that has made possible the illicit market by prohibiting the drug without curbing its use in any serious way.

Even were the complete removal of the plant to be desirable, it's highly unlikely that countries like Colombia and Peru could ever eliminate the cultivation of coca. The financial incentives for small family farmers are too great, and the potential growing areas too vast and inaccessible, especially in the ecological and altitudinal zones where cultivated coca thrives.

Crop substitution programs are delusional. Coca produces three harvests a year, generating returns that dwarf those of any other crop. Aerial eradication is doomed to failure, even as it compromises pristine forests and taints the soil and waterways with toxins. Juan Manuel Santos, Nobel Laureate for Peace in 2016, served as minister of defense under Álvaro Uribe and subsequently two terms as Colombia's president. No one in the world, as he suggested in a recent podcast, has been responsible for eliminating more coca plants than him and his government, policies that proved, in his own words, to have been a total failure. Santos now advocates the only rational solution, the cleansing stroke of legalization, without which the corrosive influence of cocaine will never subside.

The war on drugs has not only been a grotesque failure, it has blackened the name and robbed us of the promise of one of the most beneficial plants known to botanical science. When, in the 1970s, Weil and Plowman attempted to develop coca-based products that had the potential to wean Americans from their addictions to coffee and tobacco, they were shut down by a government hellbent on the pursuit of egregious policies that have only made a bad situation worse with each passing year. In her classic book, *The March of Folly*, the historian Barbara Tuchman defined folly as the acts of political leaders who, though in full possession of the facts, nevertheless pursue policies contrary to the best interests of their people and nations. By any objective measure, the war on drugs has been the most misguided crusade in the history of public policy, save perhaps for the actual Crusades, and we all know how they ended. Yet, the drug war goes on, month after month, decade after decade, with no one held accountable for its failures, and no end in sight.

We remain stuck for a simple reason, something I came to understand many years ago, soon after I returned from South America, in 1975. There was a position advertised at the USDA that Tim Plowman wanted me to apply for, though he warned that if I took the job, he'd kill me. Intrigued, I went out to the USDA campus in Beltsville, Maryland, and found my way to the office of a corpulent bureaucrat who clearly was no agricultural agent. He was DEA (Drug Enforcement Administration), head to toe.

The first thing I noticed was that he was an addict; I could hardly see across the room for the cigarette smoke. The shelves of his bookcases were cluttered with drug paraphernalia. It was like going into the office of anti-pornographer and finding the walls papered with pornography. The man was wearing a bright orange jacket over a shirt with a wide butterfly collar that showed off a hairy chest. The hair was red. Around his neck were gold chains; his wristwatch had small nuggets of gold on the band. It was soon clear that all he had gleaned from our research was that Tim and I were good at finding coca fields. The job description called for me to return to Peru to collect any organism—insect, fungus, mold—that attacked and caused damage to coca plants. I was to bring them back to the lab so they could be genetically manipulated and then reintroduced, presumably with more lethal capabilities. When I suggested that this might be a somewhat hazardous assignment, he stuck his hand under his shirt and brought out a gold dog tag, inscribed with the names of field agents he had lost.

As the interview came to an end, I realized that, although we had never met before, I knew him well. In the early 1970s, I crossed paths in Medellín with many who later made their names in the drug business, and if the future of the trade remained unclear at the time, the dark essence of these men and women was more than evident.

As I left the office at Beltsville, I understood in a heartbeat that the man asking me to manipulate nature in order to destroy coca was cut from exactly the same cloth as those making fortunes smuggling cocaine. Energetically, they were one and the same, two sides of the same coin, the DEA and the anti-drug crusaders, and the cartels and all of their *sicarios*. Neither had the slightest interest in ending the war on drugs. The drug traffickers would see their empires implode, with profits plummeting. Interest in cocaine, truth be told a shitty drug, might well fade to nothing once the scent of money was removed from the scene. As for those in the DEA, a victorious end to their obsessive war would find them all out on the streets, looking for work. As long as they can maintain the folly, with enemies to pursue, their appropriation is the safest in the US federal budget, garnering support from every branch of the bureaucracy because virtually every agency has a piece of that $50bn pie. For this reason alone, the war on drugs will never be won, for ending it is not in the interests of either side.

Needless to say, I didn't take that job, but apparently someone did. Twenty-five years after Tim Plowman, working for the USDA, revealed coca to be a mild and benign stimulant, essential to the diet, culture and spiritual life of Andean and Amazonian peoples, the US approved the use of a novel fungus, *Fusarium oxysporum*, developed by scientists at the USDA with the specific goal of wiping out coca wherever the plant was found. They also experimented with a moth, *Eloria noyesi*, known throughout the Amazon as the "gringo" because of its insatiable appetite for coca. In the end, much to the disappointment of the DEA, the scheme was cancelled by Bill Clinton, who was concerned that the unilateral use of biological agents would be perceived diplomatically, especially in Latin America, to be a form of biological warfare, which, of course, it was.

Frustrated on one front, those dead set on eradicating coca turned to defoliants. Beginning in 1990, and continuing for more than two decades, U.S. contractors in Colombia sprayed glyphosate, commonly known as Round Up, over 4.4 million acres. The herbicide kills plant life indiscriminately, leaving the forests, in the words of Colombian botanist Alberto Gómez, "burnt to ashes."

Gómez worked seven years on the eradication campaign, but came away disillusioned, convinced that little was accomplished by aerial fumigation save the destruction of the wild, and the violation of local people who, faced with hunger in the ruin of their gardens, readily turned against the state. If sprayed, he reported, coca fields were immediately harvested and the crop salvaged. In time, all such lands could be replanted, and most were. The impact on cocaine production was negligible. The acreage dedicated to coca in Colombia grew steadily each year through 2007, and then, even as eradication efforts began to be felt in some regions, overall production declines were offset by increases in productivity in the healthy fields.

In 2015, the then president, Juan Manuel Santos, suspended the program out of concern for the health of the nation's children; it was reported that in some indigenous communities, 80 percent of children exposed to aerial spraying had fallen sick with skin rashes, fever, diarrhoea, and eye infections. Every acre of coca destroyed, if not replanted, only forced growers deeper into the pristine forests of the Amazon, resulting in soaring rates of deforestation.

In 2019, cocaine production in Colombia reached an all-time high, only to increase again in 2020. Even as the country struggled with the biggest humanitarian crisis in the history of the hemisphere, offering food, housing, medical care, schooling and the right to work to two million Venezuelan refugees, the US government threatened to revoke more than half a billion dollars in foreign aid if the Colombian government did not resume aerial spraying with glyphosphate, despite a 2014 WHO report suggesting that the defoliant may be carcinogenic. President Iván Duque agreed to do so, making Colombia the only Latin American nation willing to tolerate the presence of American contractors fully intent on saturating the air and soils of the nation with chemicals designed to kill everything green that grows. "The drug war has tried in vain to keep cocaine out of people's noses," remarked Sanho Tree, director of the Drug Policy Project at the Institute for Policy Studies, "but could result instead in scorching the lungs of the earth."

A GIFT FOR THE WORLD

Surely, it is time to find another way. Rather than yielding to American pressure to expand the aerial use of herbicides, it's not unreasonable to ask why any of Colombia's biodiversity, perhaps its greatest national asset, not to mention the health and well-being of its children, should be put at risk to satisfy the misguided policies of a foreign country. Having endured the consequences of the illicit trade for so many years, perhaps now is the time for Colombia to reclaim a stolen legacy by celebrating coca for what it really is, what the Inca saw it to be.

Marketed as a tea, perhaps as a chewing gum for those not keen on dried or powdered leaves, the sacred plant could be Colombia's greatest gift to the world- dwarfing the commercial success of coffee, in good measure because coca is simply a better product. Who would not want to experience a sense of enhanced energy and mental clarity, a mild suppression of hunger, a gentle feeling of creative confidence, a lightness to one's step lasting throughout the day, knowing that the source of your slight elevation of mood was a benign and highly nutritious leaf that has been revered by the peoples and ancient civilizations of South America for five thousand years?

In a digital economy in which work for so many implies long hours staring at screens, what could be more welcome or promising than a natural product that facilitates focus and concentration, even while inducing a subtle sense of contentment and well-being? Truth be told, coca is the ideal companion for any creative endeavour, be it the writing of poetry or code, composing music or simply basking in the silence of the stars.

Those who experience coca invariably come away astonished by its subtle yet pleasant effects, and its practical use. Coca works, and it works for everyone, in idiosyncratic ways. In my case, a writer happily cursed with a frenetic travel schedule, coca allows me take a seat on an aeroplane after a busy day, and return immediately to the task at hand, picking up right where I left off in a text, watching as the words flow from my fingers, oblivious to all distractions.

At the moment, coca is listed in Schedule II of the US federal Controlled Substance Act, a category reserved for drugs with acknowledged therapeutic use, but also a high potential for abuse. Technically, physicians can prescribe coca, as Andrew Weil has written, but in practice they can't, for there is no legal source and the therapeutic indications have not formally been specified. Marijuana, by contrast, along with ecstasy, mescaline, and LSD, have long been listed in Schedule I, classified as drugs with serious abuse potential but no recognized medical applications; drugs in this category are deemed to be the most dangerous, the greatest threats to society.

And yet today, even as Canada and 40 other nations have legalized the use of cannabis, and hallucinogens are being heralded as the therapeutic instruments of a psychedelic renaissance that will transform the treatment of mental health, coca, despite its long history as a healing plant, remains off limits, simply because of its association with the cocaine trade.

This has to change. Some weeks ago, I called Andy Weil. We hadn't been in touch for some time, and yet it felt as if we had never been apart. Our thoughts turned, as they often have over the years, to memories of our long-departed friend, Tim Plowman, who died in 1989. Tim devoted his professional life to the study of coca—the plant had no greater champion—only to have his research, the results of years of botanical exploration in the most difficult and remote reaches of a continent, denied and betrayed by the very government that had sponsored his work. Andy and I decided to once again take up the cause of this sacred plant, if only to expose the folly of those who have kept Tim's dreams from being realized, even while promoting policies that have only brought violence, corruption and pain to the world.

Our mission is to stimulate research that will document coca's medical and therapeutic benefits, with the goal of making available for all people a plant that promises to improve their well-being and ease the day-to-day challenges of their lives. A wide array of coca-based products will bring delight to consumers, even while supporting the 130,000 Colombian families who grow the plant for a living, allowing them to sever their ties to the cartels. The liberation of the leaves will undermine the black-market trade, and reduce deforestation by opening up for cultivation lands long ago cleared and abandoned. Through taxation, it will generate for Colombia the revenues that will allow a long-suffering nation to pay the price of peace, having drained its treasury for 50 years to cover the costs of a war only made possible by the sordid profits of prohibition.

We are not alone in this quest. Colombia is on side with the plant, as are the people of Peru, and those of Bolivia who are sick and tired of their patrimony being denied, their gift to the world insulted and refused. Throughout Andean South America there are scores of new enterprises, all focused on the beneficial potential of the leaves as food, medicine, stimulant and sacrament.

A new generation of political leadership in Latin America has found the courage to defy American pressure, setting their nations on new paths that will bring an end to policies that have only served the interests of criminals, profiteers and state institutions with a vested interest in prosecuting their war on drugs indefinitely, no matter the consequences.

Within weeks of his inauguration, Gustavo Petro, newly elected president of Colombia, made good on his campaign promise to end the forced eradication of coca. He is on record as supporting legislation that will decriminalize and regulate cocaine sales. The president has taken such a stand not because he endorses the use of the drug, but because he knows that only by destroying the illicit trade, and the profits that fuel it, will it be possible to secure peace, stability and prosperity for the Colombian people.

Should President Petro succeed, undercutting the black market with the cleansing stroke of legalization, even while bringing the gift of coca to the world, he will both inspire his supporters and give pause to his opponents, those who view his young presidency across a chasm of uncertainty and trepidation. What better way to signal a new beginning for all of Colombia, a nation divided, but a people long united in hope, resilience and faith. An end at last to the war on drugs.

A stolen legacy returned to its rightful status. A sacred plant, long defiled, heralded, as in the time of the Inca and all the ancient civilizations of the Andes, as a gift of the gods, coca, the divine leaf of immortality.

BIBLIOGRAPHY

Acosta, José de. Historia natural y moral de las Indias. Madrid, Ramón Anglés. 1894. (Original: Seville. 1588).

Allen, C.J. 1988. *The Hold Life Has: Coca and Cultural Identity in an Andean Community*, Smithsonian Institution Press, Washington, DC.

Allen, C.J. 1981 "To Be Quechua: The Symbolism of Coca Chewing in Highland Peru", American Ethnologist, Vol 8, No.1 (Feb.,1981), pp.157-171

Bohm, B, F. Ganders, and T. Plowman, 1982 "Biosystematics and Evolution of Cultivated Coca (Erythroxylaceae), *Systematic Botany* 7(2):121-33.

Burchard, R.E.,1974. "Coca Chewing: A New Perspective", in Rubin, V. (ed.) Cannabis and Culture, Mouton, The Hague, pp. 463-84.

Cieza de Leon. 1959. The Incas of Pedro de Cieza de Leon, (trans. Harriet de Onis, edit, von Hagen), University of Oklahoma Press.

Cobo, El P. Barnabé.1890. Historia del Nuevo Mundo. I and IV, Sevilla, Imp. de E. Rasco, Bustos Tavera.

Conzelman, C. and D. White. 2016. "The Botanical Science and Cultural Value of Coca Leaf in South America", in *Roadmaps to Regulation: Coca, Cocaine and Derivatives*, The Beckley Foundation.

Davis, W. 1996. *One River: Explorations and Discoveries in the Amazon Rainforest*, Simon & Schuster, New York.

Dillehay, T.D., J. Rosen, D. Ugent, A. Karathanasis , V. Vásquez and P. Netherly, 2010. "Early Holocene Coca Chewing in Northern Peru", Antiquity 84: 939-953

Duke, J.A., D.Aulik, and T. Plowman. 1975. "Nutritional Value of Coca", Botanical Museum Leaflets 24(6):113-19, 1975

Forsberg, A. 2011. *The Wonders of the Coca Leaf*, Academia.

Gade, D.W. 1979. "Inca and Colonial Settlement, Coca Cultivation and Endemic Disease in the Tropical Forest", *Journal of Historical Geography*, 5,3 263-279

Garcilaso de la Vega. 1966. Royal commentaries of the Incas and general history of Peru, I and II, (trans. Livermore). Austin, University of Texas Press.

Gutierrez-Noreiga, C. and V. W. von Hagen. 1951. Coca—the mainstay of an arduous life in the Andes. Economic Botany, V, 145–152.

Gutiérrez-Noriega, C. and V. Zapata Ortiz. 1947. "Estudios sobre coca y la cocaína en el Perú", Ministerio de Educación Pública, Lima.

Henman, A. 2008. *Mama Coca*, Biblioteca del Gran Cauca, Cali.

Leon, Luis A. 1952. "Historia y extincion del cocaísmo en el Ecuador", *America Indígena*, XII, 7–32, Mexico.

Lloyd, J. T. 1913. *A Treatise on Coca*. Drug Treatise XXVII. Cincinatti, Lloyd Brothers.

Mariani, A. 1890. *Coca and its Therapeutic Application*. J. N. Jaros, New York.

Markham, C. R. 1892. *A History of Peru*. Charles Sergei and Co. Chicago.

Martin, R.T. 1970. "The Role of Coca in the History, Religion and Medicine of South American Indians," *Economic Botany* 24(4):422-38.

Metaal, P., M. Jelsma, M. Argandoña, R. Soberón, A. Henman and X. Echeverría. 2006. "Coca Yes, Cocaine, No?:Legal Options for the Coca Leaf", *Drugs & Conflict Debate Papers* No.13, Transnational Institute, Amsterdam.

Monge Medrano, C. 1952. "La necesidad de estudiar el problema de la masticacion de las hojas de la coca", *Peru Indígena*, III, 131–135, Lima.

Mortimer, W.G. 1901. *History of Coca: The Divine Plant of the Incas*, J. H. Vail & Co., New York.

Moser, B. and D. Tayler, 1965. *The Cocaine Eaters*, Longmans, Green and Co., London.

Pacheco, K. (ed.) 2022. *Historias, memorias y recorridos de la hoja de coca: Antología, siglos XVI-XXI*, Ceques Editores, Cusco.

Pacini, D. and C. Franquemont (eds), 1985. *Coca and Cocaine*, Cultural Survival Report 23, Cambridge.

Plowman, T.1979. "The Identity of Amazonian and Trujillo Coca", *Botanical Museum Leaflets* 27:45-68.

Plowman, T. 1979. "Botanical Perspectives on Coca", Journal of Psychedelic Drugs, 11(1-2): 103-117, Jan-Jun.

Plowman, T.1981. "Amazonian Coca", *Journal of Ethnopharmacology* 3:195-225.

Plowman, T.1984."The Ethnobotany of Coca", *Advances in Economic Botany* 1:62-111.

Plowman, T.1984. "The Origin, Evolution and Diffusion of Coca, Erythroxylum spp., in South and Central America", in Stone, D. (ed), *Pre-Columbian Plant Migration*, papers of the Peabody Museum of Archaeology and Ethnology, vol.76:125-63.

Puga I. and A. Mario, 1951."El indio y la coca", *Cuadernos Americanos*, X, 39–51, Mexico.

Ricketts, C.A. 1952. "El Cocaísmo en el Perú" América Indígena, XII, pp. 309-322, Mexico.

Ricketts, C.A. 1954. "La masticacion de las hojas de coca en el Peru". América Indígena, XIV, pp.113–126, Mexico.

Schultes, R.E.,1980. "Coca in the Northwest Amazon", *Botanical Museum Leaflets* 28(1):47-59.

Schultes, R.E., 1957. "A New Method of Coca Preparation in the Colombian Amazon", *Botanical Museum Leaflets* 17(90):241-246.

Stolberg, V.B., 2011. "The Use of Coca: Prehistory, History and Ethnography", *Journal of Ethnicity in Substance Abuse*, 10:126-146.

Tschudi, J.J. von., 1847. *Travels in Peru during the years 1838–1842.* David Bogue, London.

Unanue, Hipólito.1794. "Disertacion sobre el aspecto, cultivo, commercio, y virtudes de la famosa planta del Peru nombrada coca", *Mercurio Peruano XI*, 205–250, Lima.

Valdez, L.M.,2015. "Ancient Use of Coca Leaves in the Peruvian Central Highlands", Journal of Anthropological Research, vol.71, pp. 231-258.

Weil, A.T.,1981. "The Therapeutic Value of Coca in Contemporary Medicine", *Journal of Ethnopharmacology*, 3:367-76.

Weil, A.T.,1980. "The Green and the White: Coca and Cocaine", in The Marriage of the Sun and the Moon, pp.139-165, Houghton-Mifflin, Boston.

White, D., J. Huang, O. Adolfo Jara-Muñoz, S. Madriñán, R. Ree and R. Mason-Gamer, 2021"Origins of Coca: Museum Genomics Reveals Multiple Independent Domestications from Progenitor *Erythroxylum gracilepes*", *Systematic Biology* 70(1):1-13.

WPVI Action News, 2020. "'Green' cocaine confiscated by CBP officers at Philadelphia International Airport" October 31, 2020 https://6abc.com/green-cocaine-philadelphia-international-airport-customs-and-border-protection/7514258/

The Therapeutic Potential of Coca

Andrew Weil, MD

Medical Doctor | Founder and Director of Arizona Center for Integrative Medicine | Author | Editorial Director of DrWeil.com

> *"Educating health professionals about potential uses of coca in contemporary medicine and about the great difference between whole coca and isolated cocaine is a priority."*
>
> —Andrew Weil

A transcribed speech edited by Andrew Weil, on the medicinal and historical uses of the coca plant.

I think I am the only person here who was at that original conference in 1967. The other person there was my mentor Richard Evans Schultes, the long-time director of the Harvard Botanical Museum. Two years prior to that conference, in 1965, he sent me to South America with one of his graduate students. I had just finished my first year of medical school, and we were tasked with collecting for a US pharmaceutical company a large quantity of leaves of a tree from the forest around Leticia, Colombia. After a stay in Colombia, we traveled to Peru and Bolivia. Just before I left, Dick Schultes told me, "Be sure to chew coca when you're in Peru and Bolivia and get to know that plant.", so I did.

That summer I spent time in the Andes and tried coca for the first time. I wanted to learn as much as I could about it, especially it's uses in indigenous medicine in the region. What I found out got me thinking about how coca might be used in Western medicine. I began writing about this in the 1970s and 1980s and put a lot of effort into trying to educate people in both North and South America about the differences between coca and cocaine, about the therapeutic potential of coca, and about the possibility of making it more widely available. It was slow going. Now, more than forty years later, I'm extremely gratified to see real momentum developing for rehabilitating coca—freeing it from years of persecution and denigration and rejection by the medical profession.

So, I want to tell you some of what I've learned about coca, especially how it can contribute to modern medicine. Coca has a low concentration of cocaine and contains other alkaloids (Jenkins, 1996). The intensity of the effects of stimulant drugs, their toxicity and potential for dependence are more related to the rate of increase of concentration of the substance in the blood than to the dose administered. That means that a smaller dose of a drug given directly to the bloodstream will be more powerful and more dangerous than a larger dose given by a slower route of administration.

When coca leaves are chewed, a low dose of cocaine absorbed through the oral mucosa leads to a slow rise of cocaine in the blood. When people snort cocaine, smoke it, or inject it, there is a rapid rise in blood concentration, a much greater stimulant effect, and a much greater potential for trouble. The route of administration is critical. Additionally, with coca, the pharmacological activity of cocaine is modified by the other alkaloids present (Novak, 1984).

In traditional Andean medicine coca is the major remedy for all gastrointestinal conditions: Curiously, indigenous users say that coca treats both diarrhea and constipation. That makes very little sense from the point of view of Western pharmacology, but it is an interesting claim that deserves attention; I'll discuss it in a moment. Coca is also used to treat acute motion sickness and acute altitude sickness, as a remedy for fatigue, and as an aid to doing physical work (Biondich, 2016). Of course, this is all in addition to its important role as a social lubricant and mild stimulant. The stimulating effect of coca is qualitatively different from that of coffee. Cocaine is rapidly metabolized and eliminated from the body, giving it a shorter duration of action than amphetamine and related drugs (Cone, 1998).

These uses of coca in indigenous medicine attracted very little attention from physicians in both North and South America for a remarkably long time. It was really not until 1860 that there was any interest from the medical profession in coca. What sparked it was a widely circulated and translated essay by an Italian neurologist about the effects of the leaf. Soon after, a variety of coca products flooded European and North American markets, promoted as tonics and energizers. Unfortunately, at the same time, a German chemist isolated cocaine from coca. It was released to the world and promoted by pharmacologists as the sole component of importance in coca, the one responsible for all of its beneficial effects. Physicians recommended cocaine enthusiastically, with the result that many patients became dependent on it and suffered adverse effects. A wave of reaction eventually turned medical opinion against cocaine and the plant from which it came (Ashley, 1975; Grinspoon & Bakalar, 1974). That was the end of scientific interest in coca; thereafter, research focused only on isolated cocaine.

I find it remarkable and astonishing that so little research has been done on a plant of such great cultural, economic and medical significance. That must be remedied. The effects and reported benefits of coca demand investigation. Much of the literature on coca is motivated by a desire of governments and non-Indigenous people to demonize the plant and the habit of chewing the leaves and ascribe to them negative effects on health and behavior. For instance, coca is cited as a cause of malnutrition in the Andean population, even of interference with intellectual function and normal growth and development. While heavy use of coca has been associated with people who are living in not great conditions and of course health may be poor, this is in great contrast to what you see in the Amazon basin.

After I observed coca use in the Andes, I spent time in the Amazon basin, with the Cubeos in the Vaupés territory of Colombia. Amazonian natives live in much more favorable climatic conditions and are more well-nourished than their Andean counterparts. And even though they use coca heavily (as *mambe,* the powdered form), they do not suffer from the health problems associated with coca chewers in the mountains. I conclude that most of the ill effects ascribed to coca result from environmental conditions, not from coca chewing. I have never seen toxic reactions to the leaf in the Cubeo groups I studied, nor any dependence. Cubeo men who go for work to regions where coca is not available say they miss it because they like its effects, but they don't experience withdrawal syndromes. I think it would be very worthwhile paying more attention to coca use among Amazonian tribes.

I have recommended coca to some patients, teaching them how to use it in the indigenous manner: that is, to chew leaves with some form of alkali and slowly swallow the liquid that accumulates while retaining the solid material. Some people have difficulty learning how to do it, but this way of administration is much more effective than drinking a hot water infusion of leaves. Coca tea is commonly served at high altitude, especially to tourists arriving in Cusco from Lima. The tea is pleasant and has a warming and soothing effect on the stomach but lacks the additional actions obtained from using the leaves in the traditional manner.

Some of these patients reported rapid and often permanent relief of a wide variety of gastrointestinal ailments, both of the stomach and of the lower gastrointestinal tract. I know people who have used coca successfully to wean themselves off coffee. For many, coffee is a stomach irritant and strong stimulant of the lower GI tract. Coca is soothing to the GI tract. I find the stimulation of coffee to be harsher—more "jangling"—than that of coca, due possibly both to pharmacological differences between cocaine and caffeine and to the modifying effects of the other alkaloids in coca. There is a wide range of sensitivity to caffeine; for people who are very caffeine sensitive, coffee can be a very strong, irritating drug. If coca were legally available, I would recommend it as a substitute.

Coca can also be used as an aid to weight loss. It is an appetite suppressant, gives you something to do with your mouth, and provides a pleasurable taste experience. Also, its energizing effect on muscles encourages physical activity.

Perhaps the most interesting therapeutic potential of coca is its normalizing effect on metabolism, especially of carbohydrates. Some research suggests that coca may protect Indigenous Peoples of the Andes from developing type-2 diabetes, even though they have a genetic propensity for the condition. If they adhere to their traditional diets, are physically active, and chew coca, they are less likely to become diabetic, but risk increases in those who move to lower altitudes, as they generally eat more fat and more high glycemic-load carbohydrate (especially more sugar), and stop chewing coca. We also have some evidence from both mice and humans that chewing coca normalizes blood sugar, whether it's too high or too low (Burchard, 1980; Vitti, 1979). If we can confirm these findings with larger studies, coca would be indicated as a useful component in the prevention and management of type-2 diabetes through lifestyle modification and dietary adjustment.

I mentioned above the curious claim of indigenous coca users that the leaf treats both diarrhea and constipation. As I said, it makes no sense in terms of Western pharmacology. Like other drugs that stimulate the sympathetic nervous system, cocaine increases gut motility, making it a rapid (if overly intense) remedy for constipation, but it can only worsen diarrhea. That is the action of isolated cocaine. In coca, that action is modified by the other alkaloids present. They have never been studied, but I find them very interesting, because their molecular structure puts them (along with cocaine) in the tropane series of alkaloids, which are abundant in solanaceous (nightshade family) plants. Well-known tropanes are atropine and scopolamine. Many stimulate the parasympathetic nervous system and act as gut paralytics. Some have been used in medicine of the past to treat diarrhea. So, looking at the structure of the coca alkaloids, one would think they would be gut paralytic, yet cocaine is a gut stimulant.

This is a pattern I see in the composition of many medicinal plants. Nature produces complexes of related molecules, and often in these complexes there are both agonists and antagonists: that is, compounds that push and compounds that pull against mammalian physiology. How does the body respond to a mixture of compounds with this kind of ambivalent action? I believe it "chooses" how it does so—by means of which receptors are available for binding. This is a very different way of treating the organism than giving a single compound that pharmacologically pushes it in one direction. Most of the medications in use today are isolated compounds with single actions that give the body no choice in how to respond. Whole-plant remedies with ambivalent potential allow the body to participate in the therapeutic equation.

A number of botanical remedies valued as tonics in traditional medical systems have normalizing actions on body functions. For example, the traditional Chinese pharmacopeia includes herbs that are said to both raise low blood pressure and lower high blood pressure. I believe coca is such a tonic. Cocaine is certainly a key component, responsible for the leaf's local anesthetic properties and much of its stimulant and energizing effect. But I think coca's effects on the GI system and on metabolism result from the complex mixture of related compounds. Here is a fascinating area of study. The molecular structure of the coca alkaloids suggests one action, yet isolated cocaine has an opposite action.

I have put a lot of effort into trying to educate people about the unique properties and benefits of coca and informing medical colleagues about its uses. Coca happens to be in Schedule 2 of the US Controlled Substances Act, defined as substances with high abuse potential but accepted therapeutic use (it's there only because cocaine was put there; cocaine is used in dentistry and in ophthalmology). Physicians can obtain, dispense, and prescribe Schedule 2 drugs. That makes it much easier to change attitudes and policy about coca than about Schedule 1 drugs like cannabis and psychedelics, which are defined as substances with high potential for abuse and no therapeutic potential. The obstacle in North America to making coca available for medical use is that despite the scheduling there is no legal source of it. Also, the US Food and Drug Administration does not recognize any indications for the medical use of coca.

It's probably not realistic to expect patients to chew a mouthful of dried leaves with an alkaline substance. I have suggested using coca in the form of a lozenge or chewing gum containing a whole extract of the leaf combined with an alkali. A chewing gum would closely approximate the way that native peoples use coca, allowing slow absorption of alkaloids through the oral mucosa. It would provide a pleasant oral experience as well as require some muscular effort through mastication.

I'm very gratified at the moment to see momentum building after all these years for rehabilitation of the sacred leaf, including exploration of ways to export it legally from producing countries, to open markets for it throughout the world, to make it legally available to physicians, and, most importantly, to educate people about the great differences between coca in whole leaf form and isolated cocaine.

Obviously, there are many challenges to making coca available as a therapeutic agent. The greatest one, in my opinion, remains confusion of coca with cocaine. Also, the idea that single compounds act differently from complex natural mixtures is not yet widely accepted in contemporary medicine.

I am delighted to see coca addressed in this Conference. And I'm grateful to Cody Swift and the River Styx Foundation for supporting the effort to change coca policy in both North and South America.

BIBLIOGRAPHY

Jenkins, A. J., Llosa, T., Montoya, I. D., & Cone, E. J. (1996). Identification and quantitation of alkaloids in coca tea. *Forensic Science International*, *77*(3), 179–189. https://doi.org/10.1016/0379-0738(95)01860-3

Novák, M., Salemink, C. A., & Khan, I. A. (1984). Biological activity of the alkaloids of Erythroxylum coca and Erythroxylum novogranatense. *Journal of Ethnopharmacology*, *10*(3), 261–274. https://doi.org/10.1016/0378-8741(84)90015-1

Biondich, A. S., & Joslin, J. (2016). Coca: The History and Medical Significance of an Ancient Andean Tradition. *Emergency Medicine International*, *2016*, 1–5. https://doi.org/10.1155/2016/4048764

Cone, E. J., Tsadik, A., Oyler, J. M., & Darwin, W. D. (1998). Cocaine Metabolism and Urinary Excretion After Different Routes of Administration. *Therapeutic Drug Monitoring*, *20*(5), 556–560. https://doi.org/10.1097/00007691-199810000-00019

Ashley, R. (1975). *Cocaine. Its History, Uses and Effects.* St Martin's Press. https://doi.org/10.7326/0003-4819-84-2-237_6

Grinspoon, L., & Bakalar, J. B. (1974). Cocaine: A Drug and Its Social Evolution. *Contemporary Sociology*, *8*(4), 600. https://doi.org/10.2307/2065189

Granier-Doyeux, M. (1962, January 1). *Some sociological aspects of the problem of cocaism.* United Nations : Office on Drugs and Crime. https://www.unodc.org/unodc/en/data-and-analysis/bulletin/bulletin_1962-01-01_4_page002.html

Burchard, RE., (1975) Coca chewing: a new perspective. *Cannabis and Culture,* Mouton, The Hague, 463-84

Vitti, TG, (1979) "Recent biochemical research on coca alkaloids: metabolic implications". Paper presented at Congress of Americanists, Vancouver.

Ethnopharmacology of Psychoactive Substances in Chinese Culture

Jonathan Lu

Co-founder VCENNA Inc.

> *"Why is China, which is home to a celebrated ancestral tradition of plant-based medicine (Traditional Chinese Medicine aka TCM), the world's oldest continuous civilization, and history's earliest documented pharmacopeia left out from the ethnobotanical study of psychoactive plants?"* —JONATHAN LU

This deeply rich interdisciplinary paper shares historical, social and cultural perspectives on the use of mind-altering substances throughout Chinese history.

ABSTRACT

The history of mind-altering substances in Chinese culture is as complex as the nation itself. While there are many similarities between how psychoactive plants and fungi were used in China and Western countries, unique aspects of Chinese culture have led to profound differences in public perception and acceptance. This paper analyzes how Chinese culture developed with a Confucian-inspired shame orientation, as well as a value for social unity and order, that continues to influence the prevailing negative view of mind-altering substances in Modern China.

INTRODUCTION

The use of psychoactive plants and fungi holds a storied tradition in 4 of the world's 5 oldest civilizations: Mesopotamia, Indus Valley, Ancient Egypt, and Mayan. Why is China, which is home to a celebrated ancestral tradition of plant-based medicine (Traditional Chinese Medicine aka TCM), the world's oldest continuous civilization, and history's earliest documented pharmacopeia left out from the ethnobotanical study of mind-altering substances?

For the past century, the majority of research on the historic shamanistic use of psychoactive plants and fungi has centered on Western civilizations (Clottes 1998), and the predominant image of a shaman in modern society is that of the Amazonian or Indo-European medicine man, not the Daoist sage. Even the renowned Harvard biologist Richard Schultes, considered the father of modern ethnobotany, states in his magnum opus, *Plants of the Gods,* that:

"Notwithstanding the greater age of cultures and the widespread use of hallucinogens in the Eastern Hemisphere, the number of species so used is far greater in the Western Hemisphere (Schultes 1979, 28-29)."

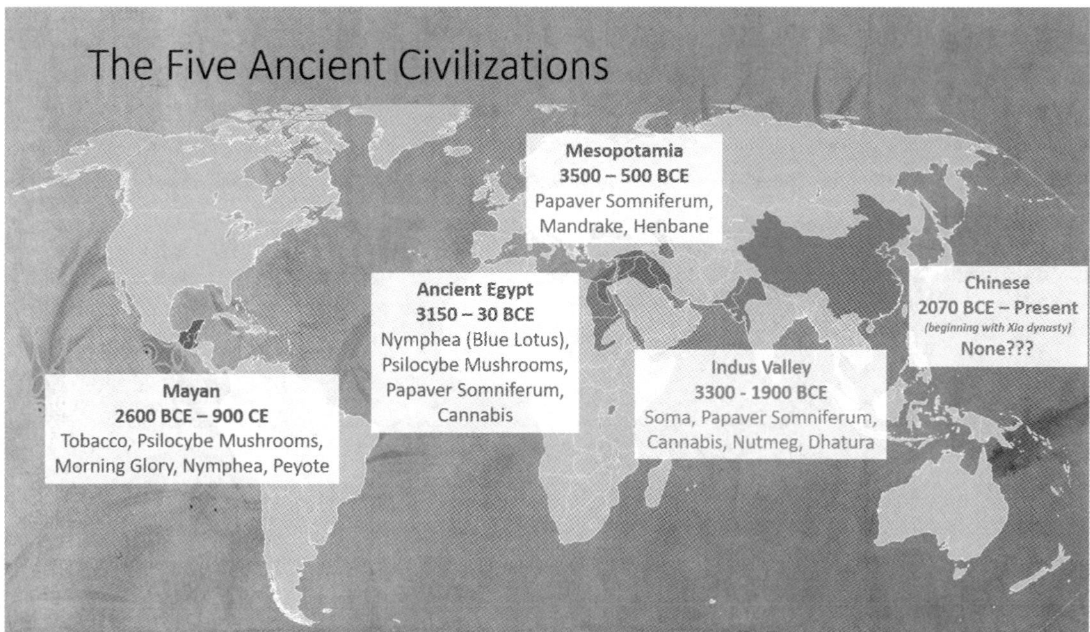

Fig.1 World map with the five oldest civilizations highlighted, including their popularly known use of psychoactive substances.

Schultes supports this statement with a map of the native use of major hallucinogens, that demonstrates a rich history of psychoactive use by early populations across fertile lands of the Americas, Africa (minus the Saharan desert), Europe, and South Asia. Overlaying his map onto a map of global population density by country (Balakhadze n.d.), the exclusion of populous countries in East Asia such as China, Japan, Korea, and Indonesia becomes conspicuous.

Schultes acknowledges that there is no significant difference between the geographical preponderance of hallucinogenic plants between the Eastern and Western Hemispheres, and attributes the disparity in usage to "cultural reasons." Noted scholars such as Terence McKenna (McKenna 1992, 153-159) and Mark Merlin (Clarke 2016, 211) have postulated the central role that psychoactive plants have played in the anthropological development of human civilizations. Are we to believe that Chinese and East Asian cultures developed differently, in the absence of psychoactive plants and fungi? Or as Wang Jichao, researcher of Ancient Chinese Cultural History at the Hubei Provincial Museum, questioned:

"Is it because the Chinese are so rational that we don't use hallucinogens in religious activities, or there are no similar intoxicating plants in China? I am not so certain." (Wang 2005)

In this paper we will review the historical context of how psychoactive plants and fungi played an important role in China's cultural and medicinal development over the past 4,000 years, in ways that were "the same but different" as compared to the West. We will unpack how Chinese culture became dominated by the shame-oriented pragmatic Confucian school of thought that values social order, and how this continues to influence the prevailing negative view

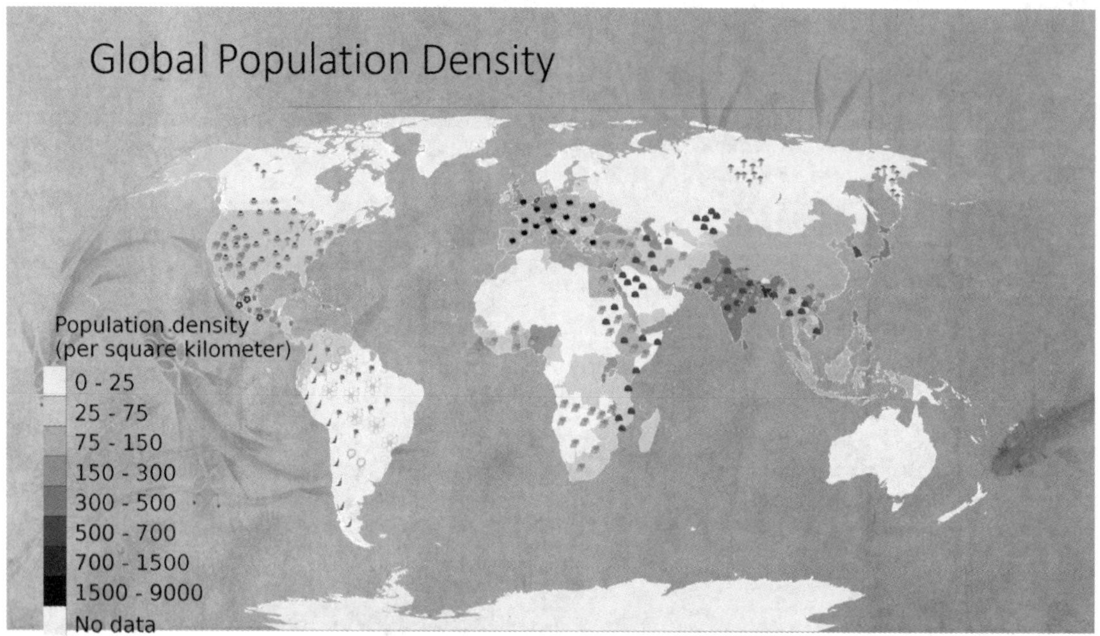

Fig.2 World map of population density (2018) by country, overlaid with Richard Schultes's map of native use of 13 major psychoactive substances. *Template from Balakhadze (2020)*

of psychoactive substances in Modern China, as well as what it means for the future of psychedelic science and research in the world's second largest economy (as of 2022).

PSYCHEDELIC SCIENCE AND LEXICOGRAPHY

Since the 1950's, psychologists and psychiatrists have pursued medical research into the therapeutic applications of mind-altering compounds for treatment of mental disorders such as depression, anxiety, and post-traumatic stress disorder. Long before Albert Hoffman kicked off the psychedelic science revolution by synthesizing LSD in 1938, as far back as 5,000 BCE indigenous tribes around the world used naturally occurring mind-altering substances ritually in pursuit of healing, spiritual insight, and social cohesion (Akers 2011). To label these shamanistic practices as religious is incomplete, as religion, astrology, alchemy, and medicine were closely intertwined; healers followed an amalgam of beliefs and practiced a myriad of techniques together with the objective of holistic healing.

Thanks to scientific advancements in neuroscience, psychology, and pharmacology, we have a better understanding today of the medicinal practices that our ancestors discovered long ago. These scientific advancements have spurred a recent renaissance in psychedelic medical research, following the hiatus that began in the 1970's as a government response to the anti-war, anti-authoritarian, and counterculture movement that embraced the use of psychedelics such as LSD for mind expansion. The regulatory policy enacted back then was accompanied by promotion of misinformation, politicization, and irrational fear in an effort to garner public support for banning clinical research with mind-altering compounds (Belouin 2018).

While the US government's objective for intervention in psychedelic research is beyond the scope of this paper, it is of relevance how their choice of words in spreading anti-psychedelic propaganda was effective at painting mind-altering compounds in a negative light; and how the popular choice of lexicography serves as an indicator for public perception and acceptance of mind-altering substances as dangerous vs. therapeutic. Words matter. Our choice of words impacts the way we see the world, ourselves, and our own belief structures (Boroditsky 2001). Just as how the selection of different words to describe colors affects how our brain's visual cortex processes the sight of color (Whorf 1964), the words we choose to describe mind-altering compounds also have a profound effect on our individual biases and collective opinion.

The English word first used to describe this class of mind-altering compounds in the early 1950's was "psychotomimetic" (imitating a psychotic state), as American and European scientists believed that these substances made people temporarily insane. In 1957 the British-Canadian psychiatrist Humphrey Osmond introduced the term "psychedelic," with its roots in the Greek words "psyche" (mind) and "delic" (manifesting). While the term "psychedelic" has come to be viewed with skepticism and alarm as a result of the ideological war of the past, Osmond meant for it to bring a more expansive and favorable connotation than "psychotomimetic". Today, the term "psychedelic" is popularly used by supporters to describe compounds that develop the potential of the human mind, and scientifically by researchers to describe compounds that induce an altered state of consciousness characterized by agonism of serotonin 2A neuroreceptors. "Hallucinogenic" is another term that is often used synonymously with "psychedelic" but carries a more recreational rather than therapeutic connotation. Other English words with less baggage include the more neutral "psychotropic" (mind changing) and "psychoactive" (mind affecting) whose broader definitions can encompass even commonly used compounds such as caffeine, alcohol, and sugar (Weill 2004, 9).

Three important Chinese words used in the context of early medicinal practice are wū (巫), dú (毒), and gǔ (蛊 simplified, 蠱 traditional), each with its own profound meaning and context. The earliest applications of medical alchemy in China are wū (巫), which almost always referred to a concoction of different plants rather than a single substance. Wū (巫) is translated as shamanism, but can also mean witchcraft, magic, or sorcery, and is a combination of the characters for work (工) and person (人). Wū (巫) can be interpreted pictorially as "people dancing around a pillar" in reflection of social shamanistic practices, and carries a romantic implication of unreal mysticism.

Gǔ (蛊) is translated as venom, but can also mean putrefaction or infestation, and is a combination of the characters for insect (虫) and container (皿). Gǔ (蛊) can be interpreted pictorially as "poisonous insects in a container," in reflection of the dark magic practice of concocting a strong venom by putting a poisonous snake, centipede, scorpion, toad, and spider in a jar such that the surviving creature will be imbued with the most complex toxins. While not related to plants and fungi, gǔ (蛊) is an example of medical lexicon with a clearly negative implication that is related to parasites and improper sorcery.

Dú (毒), the most important Chinese word in the context of medicine, originally meant a plant that was poisonous or harmful, but came to take on a more nuanced definition over time akin to potency. Originally written as a combination of the characters for grass (屮) and immoral person (毐), by the time of early Han Dynasty (3rd century BCE), dú (毒) was written together as a 2-character word with the word for medicine yào (药), referring to drugs in general (Liu 2021, 21-24). Dú (毒) came to be seen as a potent class of poison that could be used curatively, similar to the use of chemotherapy in modern medicine today. The dualistic nature of dú (毒) is reflected in two Chinese idioms: "every medicine is part poison" (shì yào sān fēn dú 是药三分毒), and "fight poison with poison" (yǐ dú gong dú 以毒攻毒); Eastern versions of "the dose makes the poison," from 1,500 years before Paracelsus.

Just as the use of English words such as "psychedelic" and "hallucinogenic" carry cultural biases, so do the contextual use of Chinese words such as wū (巫) and dú (毒). In the next section, we will discuss how the use of these words has evolved China's history of medicinal practice with psychoactive plants.

HISTORY OF PSYCHOACTIVE COMPOUNDS IN CHINA

Starting with the Neolithic period of Ancient China, early cultures from as far back as 6,000 BCE, such as the Majiabang and Hemudu people (in present day Zhejiang and Jiangsu provinces), are believed to have engaged in shamanistic practices with wū (巫) (L. a. Liu, The Archaeology of China: From the Late Paleolithic to the Early Bronze Age 2012, 194-196). Many of these early Chinese cultures were nomadic, in search of food, shelter, and safety during a period of warring tribal chiefdoms and frequent famine.

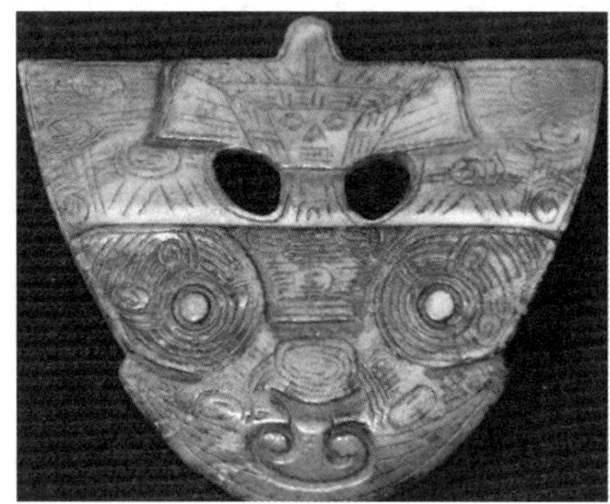

Fig.3 Jade Cong featuring a Sun deity (3300–2300 BCE), from the Liangzhu Culture Museum in Hangzhou, China.

Artifacts from this era depict the polytheistic tribal worship of spirits imbued with the power of the sun, fertility, and the sky and heavens. Similar to the practices of early Western cultures, religion, alchemy, and medicine were also inseparable in Neolithic Chinese cultures, and served complementarily for ritual healing and hope. While Western cultures often view shamanism positively in a romantic and idealistic light, the school of intellectual thought that has come to dominate Chinese culture over the past millennia does not. Use of the word shaman (sàmǎn 萨满) was not even adopted until 12th century Song dynasty, when it was first coined to derogatorily describe an elder sorceress of the minority Jurchen tribe (Guo Mar 2006).

Pre-Historic Era (3000–2070 BCE): Multipurpose use of Cannabis

It is unclear whether early cultures of China engaged in ritualistic consumption of psychedelic substances, but one mind-altering plant in particular is known to have played an important role in pre-historic societies: cannabis (dàmá 大麻) (Chang 1968). Archaeological discoveries in China have dated the cultivation of cannabis as far back as 4,000 BCE (Geng 1985) (Li 1973); its strong fibers were used in textile, rope, and paper making; its seeds and oils were a food source;

and importantly its leaves and roots were used medicinally (Merlin 1973, 48-49) (Abel 1980, 4-7).

Similar to the early history of Christianity, study of the early history of shamanic practices in China is limited by the dearth of textual material (Kleeman 2016). Evidence as to the ritual use of cannabis in pre-historic China is supported by phytochemical studies and archaeological discoveries. A 2021 genome sequencing study of 82 different *Cannabis sativa* strains concluded that cannabis was first domesticated in China, and was used historically as a multipurpose crop until bred for increased fiber or drug production beginning in 2000 BCE (Ren 2021). Archaeological finds that lend support to the shamanic use of cannabis in early Chinese history include the discovery of cannabis burned on hot stones within wooden braziers at the Jirzankal burial site (800–400 BCE) (M. e. Ren 2019), and a large quantity of 789g of cannabis stored in the leather basket of a traveling shamanic healer buried at the Yanghai tombs (700 BCE) (Russo 2008).

Zhou Dynasty (1046–256 BCE): Advances in Medical Science and TCM

The pre-historic era came to an end with the unification of warring tribes that led to the earliest Chinese dynasties, notably the Zhou Dynasty that ruled for nearly 800 years beginning in 1046 BCE (X. Li 2002). It was during this era that the basis of Traditional Chinese Medicine (TCM) emerged from the early shamanic use of medicinal plants, evolving to wǔxíng (五行), a form of cosmology based on the interaction of five elements: wood, fire, earth, metal, and water.

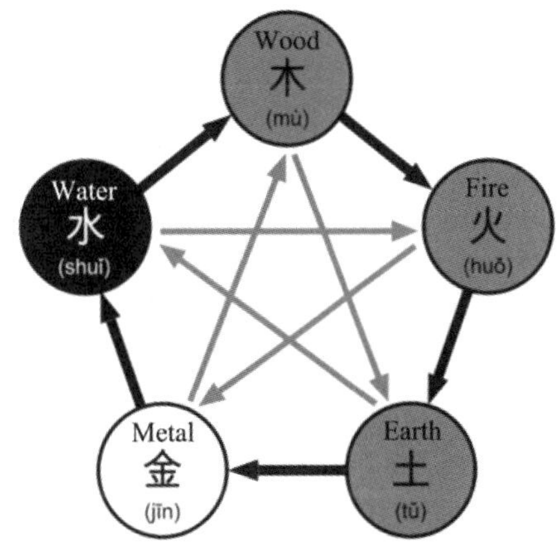

Fig.4 Diagram of the interactions between the wǔxíng (五行). *Catic et al. 2018*

It was the advent of wǔxíng (五行) from which alchemy and medicine began to emerge as unique sciences distinct from religion and ritual ceremony. Religion had begun to evolve from ancestral worship to a moral view of destiny (Strickmann 2002, 322). Towards the end of this era in late 4th century BCE, during the Warring States period, we find the first written record of the medicinal use of aconite in the eponymous Daoist text of Zhuāngzi (莊子) (DaoBudMed6D n.d.). Classified today as a deliriant, *Aconitum carmichaelii* (fùzǐ 附子 or wūtóu 烏頭) was one of many species of aconite used medicinally, and referred to as the "lord of the hundred drugs" (Obringer 1997).

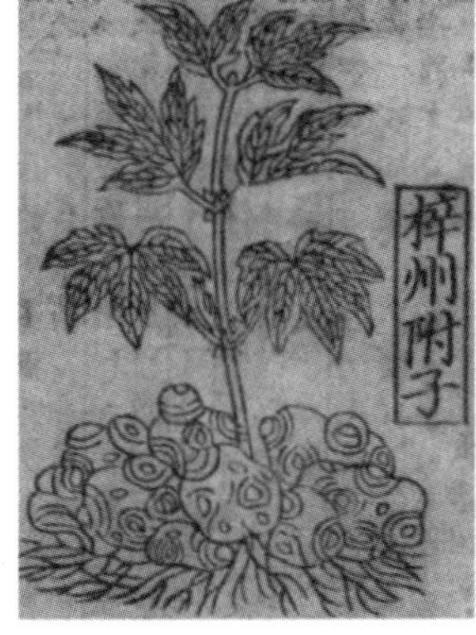

Fig.5 Botanical illustration of *Aconitum carmichaelii* (fùzǐ 附子). *Liu 2021, 48*

Aconite was known to be fatal at high doses, but it was used for its anesthetic properties, suggesting an early understanding of the dual nature of dú (毒) as both poison and medicine. "For all things under heaven, nothing is more vicious than the poison of aconite. Yet a good doctor packs and stores it, because it is useful"—Wisdom of the Huainan Masters (2nd century BCE).

Importantly, during the Warring States, both Lao Tze, the father of Daoism, and Confucius were born; although their cultural impacts would not become profound until the succeeding centuries.

Qin Dynasty (221–207 BCE): History's 1st military dictatorship

The fall of the Zhou dynasty, and end of Ancient China, came during a time known as the Warring States Period, a de facto civil war between seven states. The beginning of Imperial China came at the hands of Emperor Qín Shǐ Huáng (秦始皇), whose short-lived but impactful reign unified these warring states for the 1st time between 256–221 BCE. The Qin dynasty was a militaristic and totalitarian regime that brought order to the nation after years of internal conflict, and not only completed military construction of the Great Wall but instituted a standard for weights and measures that would become critical to future scientific and medical progress (Needham 1964).

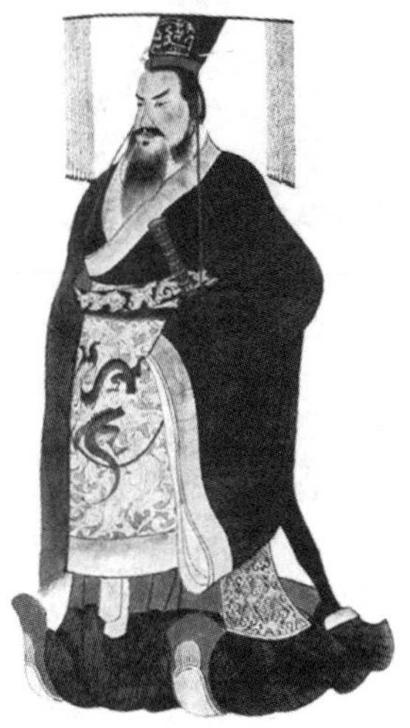

Fig.6 Portrait of Emperor Qín Shǐ Huáng (秦始皇). *Katz 2017*

Emperor Qin ruled with an iron fist, suppressing intellectual discourse in promotion of unity of thought. Although written language had been developed 1,000 years earlier, much historical knowledge has been lost due to the "burning of books and burying of scholars" (fénshū kēngrú 焚書坑儒) of this era. It was during the Qin dynasty that we find early written evidence of alchemical practice for more than just treating ailments, but the pursuit of eternal life. Emperor Qin was obsessed with immortality and later in life would regularly consume toxic cinnabar (mercury sulfide), with the belief that its blood-red color could help him live forever. He commissioned an expedition to the Eastern Sea in search of an immortality elixir, and constructed the Terracotta Warriors, where he is believed to be buried in an unopened tomb encircled by mercury (Afshari 2019).

Han Dynasty (207 BCE–220 AD): Era of Progress and the Spread of Confucianism

Following the death of Qín Shǐ Huáng (秦始皇), as is common following a totalitarian regime, China entered a thriving 400-year period of economic success, state progress, and social advancement with the emergence of the Han Dynasty. It was during this time period that scholar-officials coopted Confucianism both as a symbol of national pride, and as an organizing principle of political bureaucracy to manage a growing nation of 65 million people (more than 1/3 of global population at the time). Advancements in paper-making technology meant that much of history, which had been passed down through oral traditions, was finally recorded.

Three texts of medical importance were written during this period: *The Divine Farmer's Materia Medica* (Shénnóng Běncǎo Jīng 神农本草经), the world's earliest pharmacopeia as categorized by Shénnóng (神农) the Chinese father of medicine and agriculture who is believed to have been born in 2737 BCE; *The Yellow Emperor's Classic of Internal Medicine* (Huángdì Nèijīng

黄帝内经), the writings of the legendary Emperor Huángdì (黄帝) who was believed to have ruled during pre-historic times and promotes a rational view of health over shamanistic beliefs; and *The Biography of the Transcendents* (Lièxiān Chuán 列仙传), an early Daoist text with alchemical recipes for psychoactive medicines. These texts are notable as the earliest Chinese literature that unambiguously describe the use of mind-altering substances (Chen 2021).

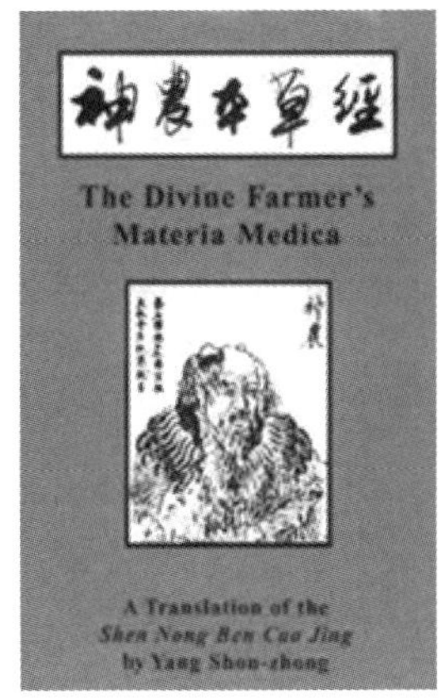

Fig.7 *The Divine Farmer's Materia Medica. Shou-Zong 1998*

Also notable during the Han Dynasty was the emergence of the Southern Silk Road, beginning trade between China and the Indian subcontinent. This resulted in the introduction of Buddhism to China from India, that led to a competition with Daoist religions for prestige and influence (Mollier 2008, 144). Daoism had fallen out of favor and with the ruling political classes and found greater popularity in the poorer rural parts of the country (Schipper 1993, 9-14).

The Silk Road also introduced two plants of importance from India: henbane or *Hyoscyamus niger* (làngdàng 莨菪), and *Datura stramonium* (màntuóluó 曼陀罗). These tropane-containing plants, similar to aconite, are also classified today as deliriants and were similarly used in pain relief and anesthesia (Xiao 1983)—suggesting a persisting perception of the dual nature of dú (毒) as both poison and medicine.

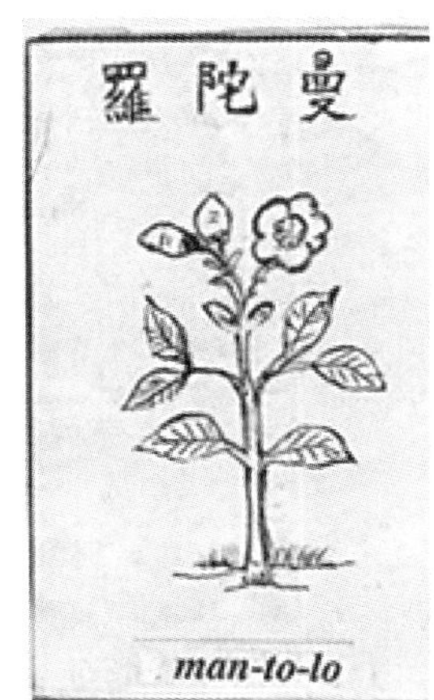

Fig.8 Botanical illustration of *Datura stramonium* (Màntuóluó 曼陀罗). *Fu 2009*

Aconite served more than just a medical purpose, as Daoists used it in the alchemical pursuit of transcendence. One character is described in *The Biography of the Transcendents* (Lièxiān Chuán 列仙传) as having achieved transcendence from a practice of consuming melon seeds, cinnamon, and aconite (Stanley-Baker, Liu and Chang 2018), and the Daoist sect known as the Celestial Masters (Tiān shī dào 天师道) were believed to have engaged in communal ceremonies of ingesting herbs with mind-altering properties (Kleeman, Celestial Masters: History and Ritual in Early Daoist Communities 2016, 197). The psychoactive properties of these plants were known, as it was even written about henbane (làngdàng 莨菪) in *The Divine Farmer's Materia Medica* that:

> "It may make one walk briskly and behold ghosts. Taking too much of it may make one run frenetically. Protracted taking will make the body light, enabling one to run as fast as a galloping horse, fortify the will, boost the physical force, and enable one to communicate with spirits." (Shou-Zong 1998, 76)

Post-Han Era (220–420 AD): Evolution of Daoism

The social inequalities faced by Daoist religions during the Han Dynasty led to the rise in influence of marginalized sects such as the Way of Supreme Peace (Tàipíng Dào太平道) and the Celestial Masters (Tiān shī dào 天师道) whose rebellion ultimately led to the fall of the

Han Dynasty (Lo 2013, 63). From the 3 Kingdoms Era (220–280 AD) to the Jin Dynasty (260–420 AD), the philosophy of Daoism evolved as part of an intellectual renewal that led to its adoption by many from the educated aristocratic classes (Zürcher 2007, 46) which began to merge Confucian and Daoist principles (Chan 2019).

Many Daoist texts were published by prominent alchemists, such as Gé Hóng's (葛洪) *Master Who Embraces Simplicity* (Bàopǔzi抱朴子) that taught the attainment of immortality through

Shénnóng (神农), The Divine Farmer

In Chinese legacy, the three sovereigns are deified heroic figures who made priceless contributions to human knowledge and societal development. Shénnóng (神农) is one of the three sovereigns who is celebrated for introducing agricultural techniques such as the use of the plow, employ of beasts of burden, and introduction of 5 staple crops (rice, wheat, sorghum, millet, and beans) that helped combat a repeated history of famine. Known as the "Divine Farmer" he also discovered tea and is known as the father of medicine, reflecting an ingrained cultural belief about food as both nutrition and medicine. It's unknown exactly when he lived since the compendium of his life's work The Divine Farmer's Materia Medica (Shénnóng Běncǎo Jīng 神农本草经) was not written until the Han Dynasty, but the folk belief is that he lived from 2737–2697 BCE. As a legendary figure whose knowledge was passed down orally across generations, it's likely that he was not one person, but a composite of multiple people including women.

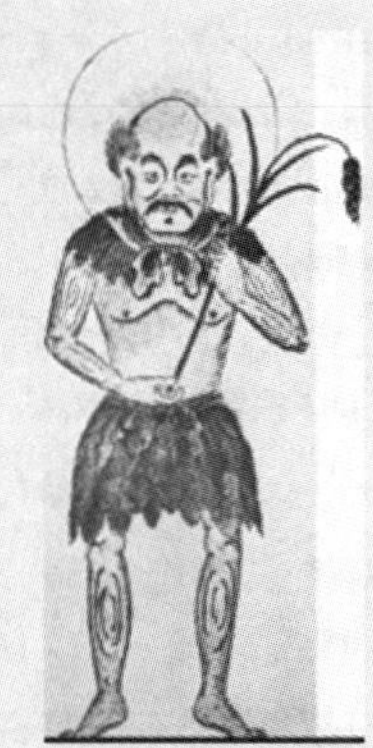

Fig.9 Portrait of Shénnóng (神农). *Schultes 1979, 92*

Shénnóng (神农) is said to have possessed a transparent stomach which allowed him to observe the absorption, distribution, and metabolism of the substances that he ingested and documented through self-experimentation. The 365 drugs in his pharmacopeia are organized hierarchically with the presence of dú (毒) as the defining criteria for each category: of the 125 lowest-level drugs, most possess dú (毒) and are meant for treating illnesses; next are 120 middle-level drugs of which some dú (毒) and are meant for replenishing a weak body; and 120 highest-level drugs of which few possess dú (毒) and serve a preventative nature towards the achievement of immortality (considering death as a sickness). In this respect, the class structure of *The Divine Farmer's Materia Medica* is reflective of both the bureaucratic nature of the Han Dynasty in which it was written, as well as the Daoist legacy of transcendence. From this book a core tenet of TCM is derived: the use of small remedies rather than chronic treatment, and treatment of the whole body rather than a single symptom (Y.-C. Cheng 2003). Per the Chinese idiom: "the sage only treats people who are not yet sick, not people who are already sick."

ritual movement and alchemy with mind-altering elixirs (Robinet 1997, 78-113) (Poo 2005, 123-139); and The Book of the Five Talismans of Lingbao (太上靈寶五符序) that provides transcendent recipes for divine wine (神酒) including the use of cannabis and aconite (Stanley-Baker, Shen and Chang, Markus encoded 太上靈寶五符序, DR-NTU (Data), V1 2018).

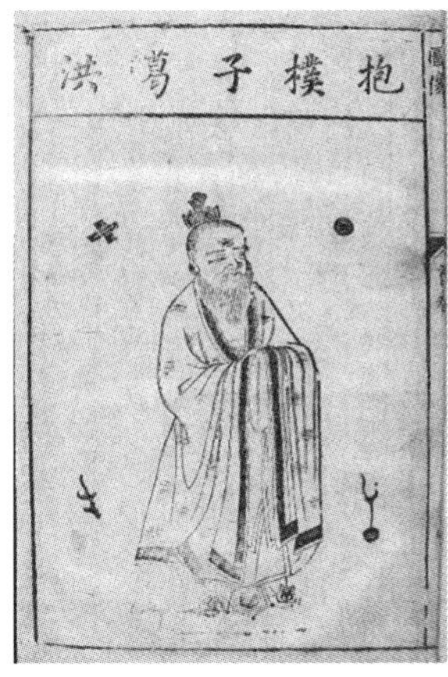

Fig.10 *Master Who Embraces Simplicity* (Bàopǔzi抱朴子) by Gé Hóng (葛洪).

While thought of today as more a philosophy than religion (largely due to the influence of Jesuit missionaries in the 1500's who saw the opportunity for religious backwards-compatibility), the many forms of Daoism as practiced prior to the 10th century were indeed esoteric religions focused on healing and personal transcendence (Irwin 2004). As the duality of yin and yang as an indivisible whole is central to Daoism, so is the dualistic interpretation of dú (毒) as both a poison and a medicine (Cheng 2003). The legacy of early Daoist religions on medicinal practice in China is well summarized by Yan Liu in his 2021 book *Healing with Poisons: Potent Medicines in Medieval China*:

"The central idea underlying the poison-medicine paradox in China is transformation: no fixed distinctions exist; all things are subject to perpetual change. To harness poisons, therefore, one must grasp the techniques of judiciously transforming them into therapeutic agents." (Liu 2021, 38)

"Tellingly, there is no concept of side effects in classical Chinese medicine. A clear distinction between the two opposing effects—an intended effect as distinguished from unintended effects—does not hold in many traditional healing cultures, because the outcome of therapy is often interpreted as dynamic, systemic, and processual." (Liu 2021, 145)

The problematic use of mind-altering substances also began during this period, notably 5-stone powder (wǔ shí sàn 五石散), that had been used for hundreds of years as an invigorating tonic but developed a recreational use as a psychoactive nootropic with both depressant and deliriant properties (Yeung 2008).

Tang Dynasty (618–907 AD): Medical Safety and Regulation

By the time of the Tang Dynasty, medicine had become a social currency of the elite and 5-stone powder, a toxic combination of chalcanthite, cinnabar (mercury sulfide), realgar, arsenolite, and magnetite, had become a drug of the wealthy. In the 5-stone powder formulation, arsenolite, a toxic source of arsenic, was considered to be the source of dú (毒).

Many are believed to have died from ingesting 5-stone powder, including five emperors, beginning the shift in perception of dú (毒) towards a singular definition as poison. The Tang Dynasty commissioned a series of protective medical regulations in response (Liu 2021, 131-133). With 80 million people (1/3 of global population), and often referred to as the "Golden Age of China," the Tang published the 1st government sponsored medical text, *The Newly Revised Canon of Materia Medica (Xīn xiū běncǎo* 新修本草*),* and oversaw the creation of three civil ser-

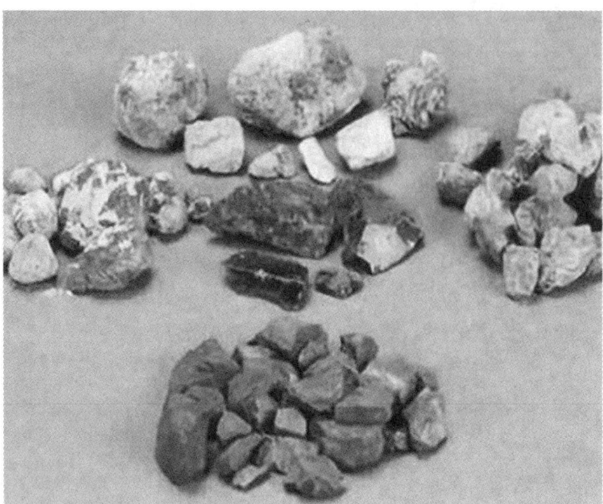

Fig.11 Minerals used in 5-stone powder (Wǔ shí sàn 五石散).

vice departments: the Imperial Medical Office, which served as the health ministry; the Palace Drug Service, which served as the drug enforcement agency; and the Pharmaceutical Bureau, which was responsible for drug production.

These bureaucracies implemented such strict rules for pharmaceutical production and transport to prevent drug diversion, even stipulating the weight of harvested plants that a donkey could carry. In response, an underground countercultural movement began led by the intelligentsia, who continued to consume 5-stone powder as an escape from what they considered as oppressive regulation, which in turn led to an even more stringent crackdown by the Tang's regulatory bodies (H.-L. Li, The Origin and Use of Cannabis in Eastern Asia: Linguistic-Cultural Implications 1974).

Song Dynasty (979–1279 AD): The Rise of Neo-Confucianism

By the end of the Tang Dynasty, both the ritual and recreational use of mind-altering substances had declined substantially. Part of this can be attributed to the impact of the government regulatory agencies, and part to the fatalities from elixir poisoning. Daoists had evolved from teaching "outer alchemy" to "inner alchemy" meditative practices to reach transcendence endogenously rather than through the use of mind-altering substances (Pregadio 2020, 464-497). Even still, Daoist practitioners and their pursuit of personal transcendence were viewed as antisocial by the Neo-Confucianists (B. Wang 2022).

900 years after the rise of Confucianism during the Han Dynasty, the Song Dynasty introduced a revival of neo-Confucianism, emphasizing its social, political and cultural promotion of communal values. These values were based on the teachings of Confucius (Csikszentmihalyi 2004, 5-11), as savvy officials again learned to coopt the brand of "Confucianism" for political value in pushing their agenda of intellectualism, elitism, and technocracy (Hinrichs 2022). Core aspects

of modern Chinese culture, such as the prioritization of logic over emotion, the well-being of the state over the individual, and preservation of propriety (e.g. "saving face") were particularly strengthened during this period (C.-Y. Cheng 1996). When it came to the use of medicine, in comparison with prior Daoist practice that had focused on longevity and the individualistic attainment of transcendence, the co-evolution of Confucianism, Buddhism, and Doaism resulted in a shift towards health as public welfare for the preservation of social stability (M. D. Stanley-Baker 2013).

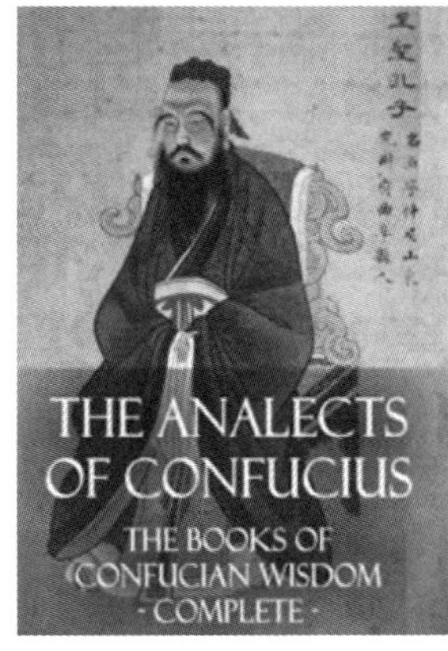

Fig.12 The Analects of Confucius (Lúnyǔ 論語) (Confucius 2018).

Governmentally, the Bureau of Medical Texts, a new bureaucratic department with responsibilities similar to the US FDA, was created and shamanism (萨满) and wū (巫) were banned by imperial edict as seen in conflict with Neo-Confucian values. The Chinese population had surpassed 100 million, and Daoism, Buddhism, and Confucianism had come to coexist peacefully and even begin to "borrow" traditions from each other. By the end of the Song Dynasty in 1279 AD, the ritual and recreational use of mind-alter-

Confucius (Kǒng Fūzǐ 孔夫子)

Confucius (551–479 BCE) is the pre-eminent Chinese philosopher whose master work The Analects (Lúnyǔ 論語) continues to be one of the most studied books for the last 2,000 years. Similar to Aristotle, John Locke, and the prophet Zoroaster, Confucius promoted the concept of a universal natural law based on personal morality, humanism, and the aversion of impropriety, particularly for the benefit of collective society (Csikszentmihalyi 2004). He was deeply concerned with sincerity, and saw external appearances as equally important as internal thoughts such that good actions match good intentions.

The core tenets of Confucianism are the moral ideal of five virtues: benevolence, righteousness, ritual propriety, wisdom, and trustworthiness. While early belief structures from Ancient China centered on social hierarchies for those blessed with a spiritual mandate from the heavens, Confucianism taught that value is for those who benefit society (i.e. meritocracy) and righteousness comes from personal morality. It is from this school of thought that Chinese cultural values originate: technocracy, ignoring emotions, and pride (i.e. "saving face") (C.-Y. Cheng 1996). Ironically, while Confucius taught the rejection of traditional hierarchy based upon wealth and position, the adoption of Neo-Confucianism as a political tool led to the creation of new hierarchies implicit in social and economic inequalities, such that Confucianism came to be rejected with the rise of the Communist Party in the 1940's.

ing drugs had become nearly non-existent (Lo, Professor of History, University College London 2022).

Ming and Qing Dynasties (1368–1912 AD): End of Imperial China

By the time of the 17th century Ming Dynasty, the view of dú (毒) had shifted almost exclusively to that of a dangerous poison; an extensive portion of the great medical text Běncǎo gāngmù (本草綱目) written in 1596 by Lǐ Shízhēn (李時珍) is even dedicated to the removal of dú (毒) in medical preparation (Y. Liu, Professor of History, SUNY Albany 2022).

Any discussion about the role of mind-altering substances in Chinese history must eventually confront the elephant in room: the Opium War. While viewed by the Chinese as vile for the past century, and even labeled by British missionaries to China "as an evil which is devastating to the East" (Matheson 1857, 24), opium was originally seen as a panacea, with medical use dating back to the 8th century for pain, sleep, diarrhea, and virility among others. With the arrival of the Jesuits to China in the mid-15th Century came a period of trade expansion as China became more economically prosperous and its population began to approach 200 million. To address a widening trade imbalance due to an increasing appetite by its citizens for tea and spices, the British instituted a commercial policy to get Chinese citizens addicted to opium (Pollan 2021, 110-111).

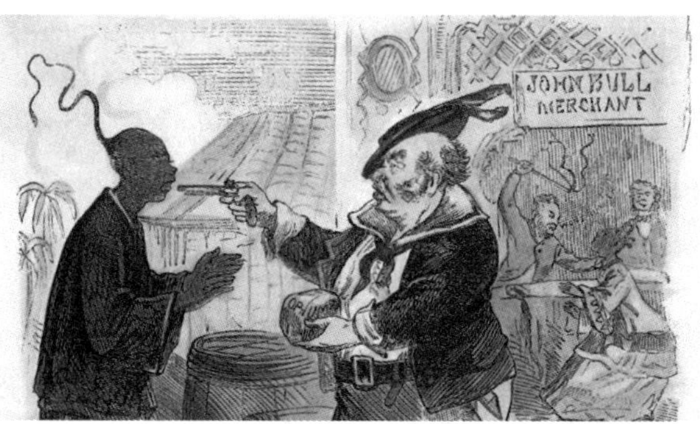

Fig. 13 'To the Weak Relation.' Cartoon from an American newspaper showing John Bull (England) forcing China to accept opium. Cartoon, 1864. *Sarin Images 1864*

The ensuing war led to the "Century of Humiliation" and end of Imperial China, a source of shame that continues to be the source of distrust and enmity towards the West today (Lovell 2011). China's attempt to modernize in an effort to catch up with the technological advancements of the West resulted in a movement to ban TCM, resulting in the destruction of even more historical works of materia medica, of which the remaining medical and pharmacology texts today are thought to comprise less than 10% of historical record (J. (. Li 2000).

With the rise of the Peoples' Republic of China following World War II, China's population had grown to almost 700 million (1/4 of global population) by the time of the disastrous Great Leap Forward and famine that claimed over 30 million lives (W. a. Li 2005). More than starvation, many died from consuming poisonous plants, as the folk knowledge of plants (Métailié 2007) had been lost to time as a victim of modernization and rapid population growth (Sheng-Ji 2001).

MODERN DAY CHINESE CULTURE

While famines were not new to China, nor the rest of the world—as Thomas Malthus claimed in 1798 "Famine seems to be the last, the most dreadful resource of nature" [to combat population growth]"—the Great Chinese Famine of 1959 was unique for its size. Across world history, famine deaths have typically accounted for 2–3% of a country's population, which makes this tragedy proportionate but magnanimous given the size of the Chinese population at the time (Devereux 2000). The Great Famine left an indelible mark on Chinese Culture, not least of all its culture of food.

A common Chinese greeting of endearment, akin to "how are you?" is "have you eaten? (chīle ma? 吃了吗?). The origin of this greeting dates back to the institution of the Confucian values of ritual propriety during the Song Dynasty, as published in an etiquette manual by the government meant for rural populations:

"Whoever you visit, you should ask them if they have eaten or not……if they are about to eat, don't enter the house until after they finish the meal. Otherwise, you would be intruding."—Lu's Township Covenant (吕氏乡约), 1076 AD (Yang 2005)

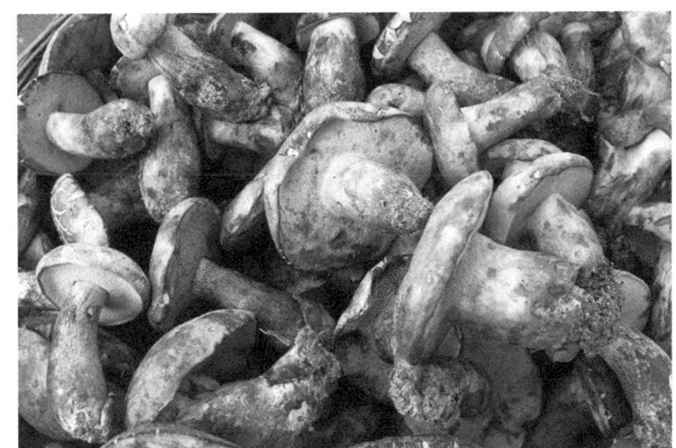

Fig.14 Jiàn shǒu qīng (见手青) mushrooms.

Following the Great Famine, the greeting "have you eaten?" (chīle ma? 吃了吗?) assumed a more profound meaning, implying a concern for well-being.

Across the world, food is central to culture. A legacy that remains in Chinese food culture is that vegetables are almost never consumed raw. Out of concern for poisoning, in Chinese cuisine, vegetables are almost always cooked or pickled. This applies to mushrooms as well, as evidenced by the curious case of jiàn shǒu qīng (见手青), the "*Boletus speciosus*"* or Xiaomei Boletus mushrooms indigenous to Yunnan province. Sometimes referred to as xiǎo rén rén (小人人), "little people" as they have been purported to cause "Lilliputian hallucinations," these mushrooms are considered a delicacy and always prepared by boiling for 30–45 minutes so as to remove the mind-altering components through cooking (Arora 2008).†

From my own experience consuming these mushrooms at a restaurant in 2014 in Yunnan province, I was instructed to boil them for at least 30 minutes so as to remove dú (毒). The waiter's instructions were notably indicative of 1) the modern cultural perspective that dú (毒) is poison; and 2) the common view of mind-altering substances as poisonous. This is also reflected in a 2006 report from the Chinese Institute of Microbiology about mushrooms and their toxins. This paper, that describes 110 species of hallucinogenic mushrooms indigenous to China, reveals detailed historical records maintained by the Chinese government regarding poisoning and fatal-

* There is some controversy about the species identification of *Boletus speciosus* as it is yet to be properly elucidated.

† Read our paper "Reports of Psychoactive Boletes" by Colin Domnauer and Professor Bryn Dentinger for more information on this fungi species.

ities, and even groups the neuropsychiatric effect of psychedelic compounds such as muscimol and psilocybin as a type of poisoning (similar to respiratory or hepatic failure) (Mao 2006).

While very strict drug enforcement laws exist in China today, and substance abuse is less problematic than other parts of the world (0.2% in China vs. 0.6% globally of adult population) (Zhang 2015) (Hurst 2019), the public view of mind-altering substances in China today is predominantly one of bemusement and avoidance. From 1,200 years ago, the popular view of psychoactive substances had fully transitioned away from ritual value to dangerous poison.

PHARMACOLOGY OF PSYCHOACTIVE PLANTS AND FUNGI IN CHINA

The use of mind-altering substances in Chinese history holds many similarities to Western cultures. Originally used in shamanistic rituals of spiritual healing and social cohesion, psychoactive plants and fungi came to play a significant role in medicine. Just as the dominant powers of the Catholic Church and centralized governments in Europe and the Americas regulated and suppressed the use of mind-altering substances out of concern for public health and threats to social order, so too did Chinese governments. With the backdrop of 1) a significantly larger population and population density; 2) a history of internal rather than external conflict due to geopolitical isolation; 3) the highly centralized communal control of Chinese governance; 4) the devastating memory of the Opium War; and 5) the legacy of Confucianism: ritual propriety, portraying benevolence / "saving face," and rejection of emotions in favor of pragmatism (Stephens 2009); the perception of mind-altering compounds carries a different nuance in China as compared to Western countries. This historical context, or what Richard Schultes referred to as "cultural reasons," is made revealing by an analysis of the compounds commonly used in Chinese medicinal history.

Figure 15 shows the relative selectivity of mind-altering substances used throughout Chinese history to neurotransmitter receptors that are implicated in altered states of consciousness, using

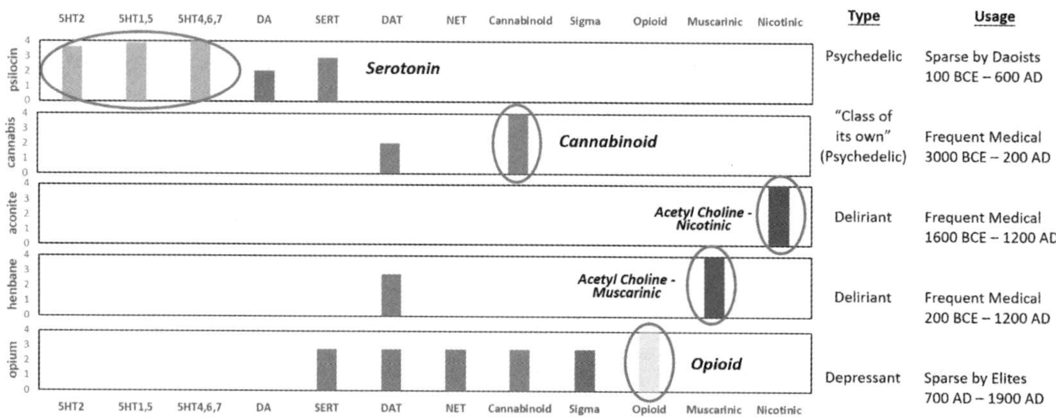

Fig.15 Relative selectivity of mind-altering substances used throughout Chinese history by neurotransmitter receptor family.

published inhibitory constant values from the University of North Carolina's Psychoactive Drug Screening Program Ki database (Roth n.d.). For each substance profiled, selectivity for each neuroreceptor is shown relative to the highest binding affinity neuroreceptor, listed on a logarithmic scale (i.e. a value of 4 is 10x higher than 3, and 100x higher than 2), and provided only for those within 100-fold of the highest binding affinity neuroreceptor (below which binding affinity is not expected to be sufficient, i.e. no relative values below 2 are listed) (Ray 2010).

On this chart, selectivity cannot be compared in absolute terms between substances; a value of 4 does not mean that cannabis is as selective for the cannabinoid neuroreceptor family as opium is for the opioid neuroreceptor family, it means that cannabis has the strongest affinity for the cannabinoid neuroreceptor family and opium has the strongest affinity for the opioid neuroreceptor family. This chart is meant to be interpreted in relative binding affinity terms per substance, so as to demonstrate which neuroreceptor families are targeted by each substance.

The earliest psychoactive plants and fungi, used primarily by Daoists in pursuit of transcendence, were psilocybin-containing mushrooms (primarily of the Panaeolus genus) (Ishida 2000) and cannabis. Psilocin, the pro-drug of psilocybin, is a strong serotonin (5HT) agonist and considered along with LSD to be the classic psychedelics. While Western cultures do not consider cannabis to be psychedelic, the Chinese do—consistent with Dr. Andrew Weill's classification of cannabis as a drug "in a class of its own" (Weill 2004, 114). For nearly 1,500 years, the use of psychedelics has been nearly non-existent in China.

The most commonly used psychoactive plants and fungi in China for nearly 3 millennia were aconite (e.g. *Aconitum carmichaelii*, fùzǐ 附子), henbane (*Hyoscyamus niger*, làngdàng 莨菪), and datura (*Datura stramonium*, màntuóluó 曼陀罗). These plants are classified today as deliriants, given their selectivity for the nicotinic and muscarinic acetyl choline receptors (nAChR and mAChR). Not listed on this chart is 5-stone powder, which produced depressant and deliriant effects due to behavioral and motor function deficits from the neurotoxic effects of mercury and arsenic poisoning. And finally, opium, whose use became recreational and problematic towards the end of Imperial China, that is classified as a depressant given its selectivity for opioid receptors.

Why is it that the use of psychedelics was discontinued long ago, and more prevalent throughout history was the use of deliriants and depressants? What are the "cultural reasons," as referred to by Richard Schultes, why this might be the case?

Going back thousands of years, Chinese culture has rewarded bureaucratically, familiarly, educationally, and professionally a portrayal of personal morality and adherence to social norms. The Confucian virtues of righteousness and ritual propriety, portrayal of benevolence (i.e. "saving face"), means that China has developed to become a shame-oriented society as compared to the guilt-oriented culture of the West.

"The conformity of an individual in Chinese society is regulated by a culturally instilled sense of shame. The Confucian personality is a shame-oriented personality. The Western personality tends to be more guilt-oriented."—Wolfram Eberhard, Former Professor of Sociology at the University of California at Berkeley (Eberhard 1967)

"The opium user was more likely to remain pacific and sedated, and thus not challenge social norms. Cannabis, with its stimulation of erratic effects, was likely to induce acts that might bring shame upon the user or his family."—Li Hui-Lin (王纪潮), Former Chairman of the Department of Botany at the University of Pennsylvania (H.-L. Li, The Origin and Use of Cannabis in Eastern Asia: Linguistic-Cultural Implications 1974)

Psychedelics that develop the potential of the human mind and induce an altered state of consciousness (including cannabis) promote individualism, as was their intended use by Daoists that sought personal transcendence. They are often consumed in a social or group ritual, and present a greater risk of standing out and bringing public shame. Whereas deliriants and depressants are more often consumed alone, and while the effects may not always be pacific, they are less likely to be externally visible.

The combination of 1) the strong top-down centralized authority of the Chinese government; 2) an equally strong bottom-up social view of psychedelics as bemusing and to be avoided; and 3) a shame-oriented culture preoccupied with maintaining appearances results in a society with low knowledge and interest in psychedelics. The shame associated with mind-altering drugs persists strongly today, as the Chinese, with a strong sense of nationalism, are quick to point out (falsely and wishfully) that drugs did not originate in the country but were brought in externally (Hinrichs 2022), reflecting a personal drive to avoid admitting mistakes as well as a pervasive view of drugs as mistakes.

FUTURE OF PSYCHOACTIVE SUBSTANCES IN CHINESE CULTURE

Without passing moral judgement, a shame-oriented culture is useful for mass alignment and coordination in the economic and technological development of a growing nation. Such a culture also presents challenging social trade-offs. Also impartially, the powerhouse that China has grown to become over the past 40 years is nothing short of an economic marvel in lifting 800 million people out of poverty (Jakovljevic 2019). This also means that 800 million people no longer worry about their physical needs of survival but now struggle with fulfilling their eudemonic needs of purpose and self-fulfillment.

In a pragmatic society that celebrates individual sacrifice for group well-being, it is not surprising that economic progress in China has led to the adoption of 9-9-6 culture: a 72-hour standard workweek comprising of 9am to 9pm workdays 6 days per week, that is reflective of a pervasive drive for accomplishment. Combined with the surveillance-state history that accompanied the rise of the Communist Party in the not-so-distant past and encouraged neighbors to spy on neighbors and families to spy on families, and the psychological effects of extended isolation as a result of China's extreme measures to combat COVID-19 (Dong 2020), China today faces a significant mental health crisis that a culture of "saving face" makes difficult to even acknowledge. As Chinese-American entrepreneur/philanthropist Bo Shao, who is working with the Multidisciplinary Association for Psychedelic Studies to bring MDMA-assisted therapy to China (Gillespie 2020), stated:

"We all have so much hurt inside of us and everywhere [...] so many of us develop certain views of oneself that we somehow think that there's something wrong with us, that we are not worthwhile, that we have no value other than the things we do."

"It's just breathtaking how much suffering there is [...] China went through some very tough periods after World War II [...] that really traumatized an entire generation of people." (Shao 2022)

What does this mean for the future of mind-altering substances and psychedelic medicine in China? As Mark Twain famously said, "History doesn't repeat itself, but it often rhymes." Figure 16 showcases a historical timeline of notable events in the use of psychoactive substances dating back to 5,000 BCE across geographic cultures.

Common patterns emerge across cultures and geographies, such as 1) The early shamanic use of psychedelics for healing, social cohesion, ancestral reverence, knowledge transfer, and pursuit of purpose in early civilizations, where "early" can be roughly quantified by population density < 25 per square mile; 2) The growing concern of exogenous threats to social order and cultural/political influence as civilizations progress, roughly quantified by when population density reaches 30–35 per square mile; and 3) The eventual regulation or suppression of psychoactive use by the dominant power upon reaching a stage of civil maturity, roughly quantified by when population density surpasses > 50 per square mile.

Today, cultures across the world are characterized by a lack of social cohesion, nostalgia for days past, shortfall of knowledge combined with an overload of data, a crisis of purpose, and need for healing. Rather than an exogenous threat to social order, nations face common endogenous threats to social order that are similar to the reasons why mind-altering substances came to be used in early shamanic rituals of healing. Life has become more complex than ever as population densities have skyrocketed: 87 per square mile across the US, 62 per square mile across Latin America, 110 per square mile across Europe, and 459 per square mile across China (as of 2022), while technology-enabled isolation has also become prevalent.

Given its massive manufacturing scale and ability to control economic development through

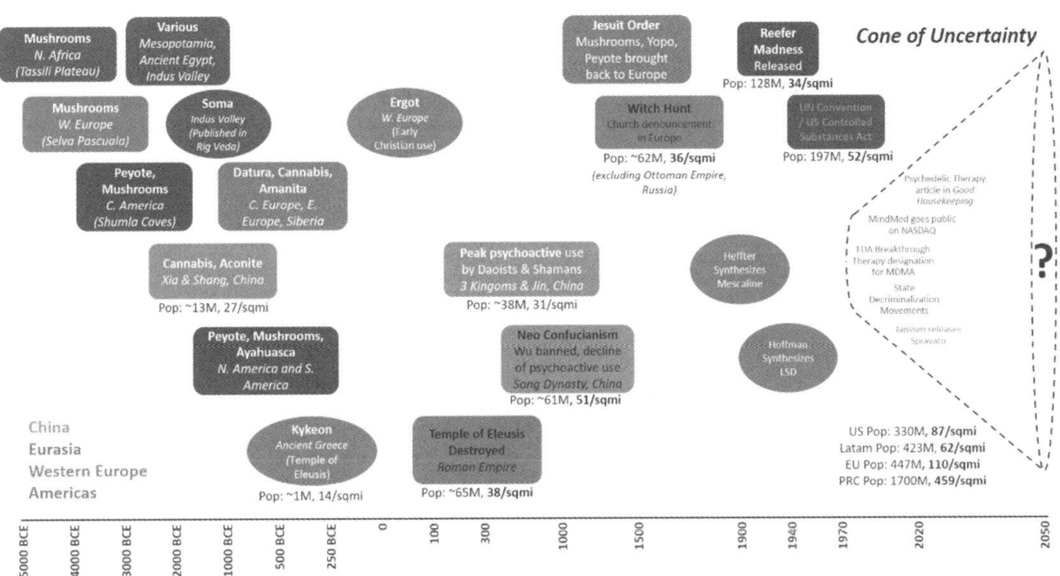

Fig.16 Back-cast of notable events in the use of mind-altering substances across global history.

a unique system of public-private partnerships, China is home to the world's pharmaceutical supply chain. Following the natural cycle of economic advancement (Kenessey 1987), Chinese companies have begun to play a more prominent role upstream in pharmaceutical development which is beginning to extend to psychedelic medicine as well. There are nearly as many post-graduate programs in pharmacology at Chinese universities as in the US and Europe combined (140 vs. 170 as of 2022 (Quacquarelli Symonds Limited n.d.)), and in 2019, M2 Biosciences, the publicly traded South African affiliate of the Chinese public/private conglomerate Wuhan General Group, announced that they would be entering the psychedelic medicine market (Wuhan General Group (China), Inc., 2019).

How will psychedelic medicine progress in China as compared to Western countries? An indication of how history may rhyme is revealed by the January 2022 publication in *Science*, from the laboratory of Professor Wang Sheng of the Chinese Academy of Sciences: "Structure-based discovery of non-hallucinogenic psychedelic analogs" (Cao 2022). In the West, even for a native English speaker, the ambiguous lexicographical distinction between "hallucinogen" and "psychedelic" makes this paper's title challenging to define. But the nuance of intentional word selection is informative. Whether we label mind-altering substances as psychedelic ("mind manifesting") or psychoactive ("mind affecting"), in China a hallucinogen (causes apparent perception of something not present) that may be used recreationally is bad. In an interview with NetEase (the Chinese internet and media technology company, similar to Yahoo! in the US), Professor Wang goes on to state that:

> "To engineer hallucinogens, we must find their hallucinogenic mechanism to solve their addiction problem (如果要改造其他致幻剂，不仅需要找到它们的致幻机制，还要解决其成瘾问题)." (文汇报 2022)

It is unclear if this statement represents Professor Wang's personal scientific belief. Having completed his post-doctoral studies in the prominent laboratory of Professor Bryan Roth at the University of North Carolina School of Medicine, Professor Wang is a leading scientific authority in neuropsychopharmacology research, and also holds a public responsibility as a representative of China's most prestigious state sponsored research institute. This quote does indicate, consistent with historical and cultural context, that psychedelic research in China will likely focus on developing sub-perceptive compositions.

CONCLUSION

China possesses a deeply rich psychedelic history, but has been left out from the ethnobotanical study of mind-altering substances for both external and internal "cultural reasons." Evaluation by Western scholars is challenging since so much of historic medical literature has been lost to time or destroyed intentionally, few texts have been translated into English, and in the absence of cultural or botanical knowledge the illustrative use of language in Daoist texts makes it challenging to discern which historical plants possess mind-altering properties—e.g. the Jin dynasty text from the Lingbao school of Daoism (靈寶無量度人上品妙經) states that consumption of língzhī (靈芝) or reishi mushrooms will provide "a rejuvenating feeling that makes your bones feel light and body float into the heavens", poetic descriptors of deep meditation without psychoactivity (Stanley-Baker and Chang, Markus encoded 靈寶無量度人上品妙經", DR-NTU (Data), V1 2018).*

Internally, the use of mind-altering substances had come to be seen negatively as irrational, antisocial, and shameful, in a pragmatic society that prioritizes achievement and shies away from admitting fault, especially in consideration of the devastating Opium War and legacy of opium addiction. In the context of China's growth to massive population scale with geopolitical isolation and Confucian-inspired values, China's nearly 8,000-year history of psychoactive plant and fungi has evolved from early use of psychoactive plants for personal spiritual development, to a view of mind-altering substances as socially harmful and poisonous.

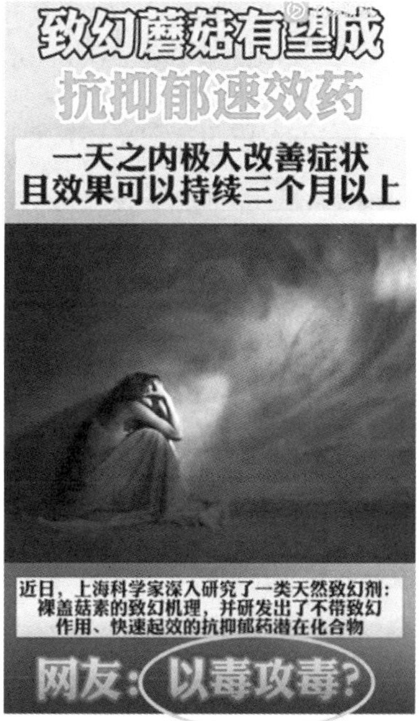

Fig.17 Promotion for NetEase article covering the publication of Professor Wang Sheng's laboratory's paper in *Science*, with slug-line highlighted (文汇报 2022).

In light of the burgeoning mental health crisis, and increasing research in psychedelic science, might there be room for a return to a more progressive view of psychoactive medicine and nuanced understanding of dú (毒)? In a culture of achievement, where scientists are celebrated in a manner similar to athletes in the West, the social media promotion for the NetEase article covering the publication of Professor Wang Sheng's laboratory's paper in *Science* offers a ray of hope as to where public perception may evolve:

While the article uses the Chinese term for hallucinogen (huànjué 幻覺) to describe mind-altering substances, it also highlights the idiom以毒攻毒 (yǐ dú gong dú): "fight poison with poison"—a hint from state-run public media towards the dualistic definition of dú (毒).

Throughout this paper, the simplified Chinese writing (used in Mainland China) has been displayed (毒), but the traditional Chinese writing (used in Hong Kong, Taiwan, and Macau) of the word is closer to its historical glyphic form 毒 (grass 屮 + immoral person 毐). The traditional writing of 毒 as compared to the simplified writing of 毒 differ in the radical used in the bottom half of the character 毋 vs. 母. These two radicals have different meanings, and the simplification of 毒 to 毒 almost certainly had nothing to do with an intended change in the meaning of the word. But, an alternative interpretation of the simplified Chinese construct 毒 could be 生 (plant or life) + 母 (mother).

* To learn about medicinal herbs and fungi, TCM and herbalism see educational charity www.herbalreality.com for monographs and articles about these topics. To learn about reishi see this reishi monograph www.herbalreality.com/herb/reishi/

Words matter. Maybe, just maybe, we may begin to see a subtle shift in Chinese belief structures about the curative value of mind-altering substances.

ACKNOWELEDGEMENTS

First and foremost, I sincerely thank Dennis McKenna for his ongoing guidance, support, and amiability in inviting me to present at the Ethnopharmacological Search for Psychoactive Drugs Conference 55; Annette Badenhorst for her tireless efforts, together with the other organizers of the ESPD55 Conference; and Dinah and Nick Ashley-Cooper for their warm hospitality in hosting this transformative event. I am grateful to Ban Wang, Yung-Chi Cheng, Fan Pen Li Chen, T.J. Hinrichs, Vivienne Lo, Yan Liu, Michael Stanley-Baker, Mark Csikszentmihalyi, and Snu Voogelbreinder for their graciousness in offering time, knowledge, and feedback.

And most of all, I would not be here today if not for my friend and business partner Shauheen Etminan, my life partner Michelle Paulin, and my reasons for being: Daniela Avicenna Lu, Maya Angel Lu, and Valeria Ada Lu.

BIBLIOGRAPHY

Abel, Ernest. 1980. *Marihuana: The First Twelve Thousand Years*. New York: Spring Science.

Afshari, Reza. 2019. "Mercury Poisoning, Emperor Qin Shi Huang and his Terracotta Army." *BC Toxicology News*, vol. 4, Jan 2019, pp. 407-430.

Akers, B.P., et al. 2016. "A Prehistoric Mural in Spain Depicting Neurotropic Psilocybe Mushrooms?" *Economic Botany*, vol. 65, no. 1, pp. 121–128, 2011. DOI: 10.1007/s12231-011-9152-5

Clarke, Robert, and Mark Merlin. *Cannabis: Evolution and Ethnobotany*. Berkeley: University of California Press.

Arora, David.2008. "Xiao Ren Ren: The 'Little People' of Yunnan." *Economic Botany*, vol. 62, no. 3, Nov 2008, pp. 540-544. DOI:10.1007/s12231-008-9049-0

Balakhadze, Giorgi. 2020. *Population Density of Countries 2018 World Map, People per Sq Km. Svg—Wikimedia Commons. Commons. Wikimedia. Org.* https://commons.wikimedia.org/wiki/File:Population_density_of_countries_2018_world_map,_people_per_sq_km.svg.

Belouin, Sean J., and Jack E. Henningfield. 2018. "Psychedelics: Where we are now, why we got here, what we must do." *Neuropharmacology*, vol. 142, no. 1, pp. 7-19, Nov 2018. DOI: 10.1016/j.neuropharm.2018.02.018

Boroditsky, Lera. 2001. "Does language shape thought? Mandarin and English speakers' conceptions of time." *Cognitive Psychology*, vol. 43, no. 1, pp. 1–22, 2001. DOI: 10.1006/cogp.2001.0748

Cao, Dongmei, et al. 2022. "Structure-based discovery of nonhallucinogenic psychedelic analogs." *Science*, vol. 375, no. 6579, Jan 2022, pp. 403-411. DOI: 10.1126/science.abl8615

Catic, Tarik, Ivana Oborovic, Edina Redzic, Aziz Sukalo, Armin Skrbo, and Izet Masic. 2018. "Traditional Chinese Medicine—an Overview." *International Journal on Biomedicine and Healthcare* 6 (1): 35. https://doi.org/10.5455/ijbh.2018.6.35-50.

Chan, Alan. 2019. "Neo-Daoism." *The Stanford Encyclopedia of Philosophy* (Summer 2019 Edition), Edward N. Zalta (ed.), URL = https://plato.stanford.edu/archives/sum2019/entries/neo-daoism/

Chang, Kwang-Chih. 1968. *The Archeology of Ancient China*. New Haven: Yale University Press, 1968.

Chen, Fan Pen Li. 2021. "Hallucinogen Use in China." *Sino-Platonic Papers*, vol. 318, Oct 2021.

Cheng, Chung-Ying. 1986. "The Concept of Face and Its Confucian Roots." *Journal of Chinese Philosophy*, vol. 13, no. 3, Sep 1986, pp. 329-348. DOI: 10.1111/j.1540-6253.1986.tb00102.x

Cheng, Yung-Chi. 2003. A Comprehensive Guide to Chinese Medicine. Singapore: World Scientific Publishing Company.

Clottes, Jean, and David Lewis-Williams.1998. *The Shamans of Prehistory*. New York: Harry N. Abrams Inc.

Confucius, and James Legge. 2018. *The Analects of Confucius: The Books of Confucian Wisdom—Complete*. Adansonia Press, 2018.

Csikszentmihalyi, Mark. 2004. *Material Virtue: Ethics and the Body in Early China*. Leiden: Brill, 2004.

Devereux, Stephen. 2000. *Famine in the Twentieth Century*. Institute of Development Studies, vol. 105, Jan 2000.

Dong, Lu, and Jennifer Bouey.2020. "Public mental health crisis during COVID-19 pandemic, China." *Emerging Infectious Diseases*, vol. 26, no. 7, Jul 2020, pp. 1616-1618. DOI: 10.3201/eid2607.200407

Eberhard, Wolfram.1967. "Guilt and Sin in Traditional China." *The Journal of Asian Studies*, vol. 27, no. 3, 1967, pp. 618-619. DOI: 10.2307/2051167

Ferriss, Tim (host). 1999. "Bo Shao — His Path from Food Rations to Managing Billions, the Blessings and Burdens of Chasing Perfection, Building the eBay of China in 1999, Pillars of Parenting, and Pursuing the Unpopular." *The Tim Ferriss Show, episode 584*, 6 Apr. 2022. https://tim.blog/2022/04/06/bo-shao/

Fu, Louis. 2009. "Surgical history of ancient China: part 1." *ANZ Journal of Surgery*, vol. 79, no. 12, Dec 2009, pp. 879-885. DOI: 10.1111/j.1445-2197.2009.05138.x

Geng, Jianting (耿鉴庭), and Liang Liu (刘亮). 1985. "Plants unearthed from the Shang Dynasty site in Taixi, Gaocheng (藁城台西商代遗址中出土的植物)." *Cultural Relics Publishing House (文物出版社)*, vol. 3, 1985, pp. 193-196.

Gillespie, Nick. 2020. "People Should Have the Fundamental Right To Change Their Consciousness." *Reason*, Jul 2020.

Guo, Shuyun (郭淑云). 2006. "Hallucinogenic Drugs and Shamanic Experience (致幻药物与萨满通神体验)." *Western Regions Studies (西域研究)*, vol. 71, no. 7, Mar 2006.

Hinrichs, T.J. 2022. (Professor of History, Cornell University). Interview. Conducted by Jonathan Lu, 28 Apr 2022.

Hurst, Terri. 2019. "World Drug Report." *The encyclopedia of women and crime*, Aug 2019. DOI: 10.1002/9781118929803.ewac0543

Irwin, Lee. 2004. "Daoist Alchemy in the West: The Esoteric Paradigms." *Esoterica*, vol. 6, 2004, pp. 31-51.

Ishida, Hidemi. 2000. (石田秀實). "Spirit drugs (見鬼藥考)." *Journal of Eastern Religions (東方宗教)*, vol. 96, Oct 2000, pp. 38-57.

Jakovljevic, Mihajlo, et al.2019. "The impact of health expenditures in BRICS nations." *Journal of Sport and Health Science*, vol. 8, no. 6, Nov 2019, pp. 516-519. DOI: 10.1016/j.jshs.2019.09.002

Katz, Brigit. 2017. "2,000-Year-Old Texts Reveal the First Emperor of China's Quest for Eternal Life." *Smithsonian Magazine*, Dec 2017.

Kenessey, Zoltan. 1987. "The Primary, Secondary, Tertiary, and Quaternary Sectors of the Economy." *The Review of Income and Wealth*, vol. 33, no. 4, Dec 1987, pp. 359-385. DOI: doi.org/10.1111/j.1475-4991.1987.tb00680.x

Kleeman, Terry. 2016. Celestial Masters: History and Ritual in Early Daoist Communities. Cambridge: Harvard University Press, 2016.

Kleeman, Terry.2016. "Reconstructing Taoism's Transformation in China." Interview by Ian Johnson. New York Times, 8 August 2016.

Li, Hui-Lin. 1973. "An Archaeological and Historical Account of Cannabis in China." *Economic Botany*, vol. 28, no. 4, Oct 1973, pp. 437-448. DOI: 10.1007/BF02862859Li, Hui-Lin. 1974. "The Origin and Use of Cannabis in Eastern Asia: Linguistic-Cultural Implications." *Economic Botany*, vol. 28, no. 3, Jul 1974, pp. 293-301. DOI: 10.1007/BF02861426

Li, Jianmin (李建民).2000. *The Territory Between Life and Death (死生之域)*. Taipei: Academia Sinica, 2000.

Li, Wei, and Dennis Tao Yang.2005. "The Great Leap Forward: Anatomy of a Central Planning Disaster." *Journal of Political Economy,* vol. 113, no. 4, Aug 2005. DOI: 10.1086/430804

Li, Xueqin.2002. "The Xia-Shang-Zhou Chronology Project: Methodology and Results." *Journal of East Asian Archaeology*, vol. 4, Jan 2002, pp. 321–333. DOI:10.1163/156852302322454585

Liu, Li, and Xingcan Chen. 2012. *The Archaeology of China: From the Late Paleolithic to the Early Bronze Age*. New York: Cambridge University Press, 2012.

Liu, Yan. 2021. *Healing with Poisons: Potent Medicines in Medieval China*. Seattle: University of Washington Press, 2021.

Liu, Yan (Professor of History, SUNY Albany). 2022. Interview. Conducted by Jonathan Lu, 12 May 2022.

Lovell, Julia. 2011. *The Opium War: Drugs, Dreams, and the Making of Modern China.* New York: Overlook Press, 2011.

Lo, Vivienne. 2013. "The Han Period" in T.J. Hinrichs & Linda Barnes (Eds). *Chinese Medicine and Healing.* Cambridge: Harvard University Press, 2013.

Lo, Vivienne (Professor of History, University College London). Interview. Conducted by Jonathan Lu, 3 May 2022.

Pei Sheng-Ji. 2001. "Ethnobotanical Approaches of Traditional Medicine Studies: Some Experiences From Asia." *Pharmaceutical Biology*, vol. 39, no. S1, 2001, pp. 74-79, DOI: 10.1076/phbi.39.s1.74.0005

Giorgi Balakhadze.2018. *File:Population Density of Countries 2018 World Map, People per Sq Km.Svg Wikimedia Commons*. 2020. https://commons.wikimedia.org/wiki/File:Population_density_of_countries_2018_world_map,_people_per_sq_km.svg. licensed under CC BY-SA 4.0.

Pregadio, Fabrizio, and Lowell Skar.2020. "Inner Alchemy (Neidan)" in Livia Kohn (Eds). *Daoism Handbook*. Leiden: Brill, 2020.

Mao, Xiaolan (卯晓岚). 2006. "Species diversity and toxins of toadstools in China (中国毒菌物种多样性及其毒素)." *Journal of Mycology (菌物学报)*, vol. 25, no. 3, 2006. DOI: 10.3969/j.issn.1672-6472.2006.03.004

Matheson, Donald. 1857. *What is the Opium Trade?* Edinburgh: Thomas Constable and Co.

McKenna, Terence.1992. *The Archaic Revival*. San Francisco: Harper Collins.

Merlin, Mark.1973. *Man and Marijuana*. Cranbury: A.S. Barnes and Company Inc.

Métailié, George.2007. "Some Reflections on the History of Botanical Knowledge in China." *Circumscribere: International Journal for the History of Science*, vol. 3, 2007, pp. 66-84.

Mollier, Christine. 2008.*Buddhism and Taoism Face to Face: Scripture, Ritual, and Iconographic Exchange in Medieval China*. Honolulu: University of Hawaii Press.

Needham, Joseph.1964. *Science and Civilisation in China. Volume 1: Introductory Orientations*. London: Cambridge University Press.

Obringer, Frédéric.1997.*Aconite and Orpiment: Drugs and Poisons in Ancient and Medieval China (L'Aconit et l'orpiment: Drogues et poisons en Chine ancienne et médiévale)*. Paris: Fayard.

Pollan, Michael.2021. *This Is Your Mind on Plants*. New York: Penguin Press.

Poo, Mu-Chou. 2005. "A Taste of Happiness: Contextualizing Elixirs in Baopuzi" in in Roel Sterckx (Eds). *Of Tripod and Palate: Food, Politics, and Religion in Traditional China*. New York, Palgrave Macmillan.

Ray, Thomas S.2010. "Psychedelics and the Human Receptorome." *PLoS One*, vol. 5, no. 2, Feb 2010. DOI: 10.1371/journal.pone.0009019

Ren, Guanpeng, et al. 2021."Large-scale whole-genome resequencing unravels the domestication history of *Cannabis sativa*." *Science Advances*, vol. 7, no. 29, Jul 2021. DOI: 10.1126/sciadv.abg2286

Ren, Meng, et al. 2019. "The origins of cannabis smoking: Chemical residue evidence from the first millennium BCE in the Pamirs." *Science Advances*, vol. 5, no. 6, Jun 2019. DOI: 10.1126/sciadv.aaw1391

Robinet, Isabelle. 1997.*Taoism: Growth of a Religion*. Stanford: Stanford University Press.

Russo, Ethan B., et al. 2008. "Phytochemical and genetic analyses of ancient cannabis from Central Asia." *Journal of Experimental Botany*, vol. 59, no. 15, 2008, pp. 4171-4182. DOI: 10.1093/jxb/ern260

Schipper, Kristofer.1993. *The Taoist Body*. Berkeley: University of California Press.

Schultes, Richard Evans, and Albert Hoffman. 1979. *Plants of the Gods: Their Sacred, Healing, and Hallucinogenic Powers*. New York: McGraw-Hill.

Shou-Zong, Yang. 1998. *The Divine Farmer's Materia Medica: A Translation of the Shen Nong Ben Cao Jing*. Portland: Blue Poppy Press.

Stanley-Baker, Michael; Chang, Chao-jan. 2018, "Markus encoded 靈寶無量度人上品妙經", https://doi.org/10.21979/N9/BPD1UW, DR-NTU (Data), V1

Stanley-Baker, Michael. 2013. *Daoists and Doctors: The Role of Medicine in Six Dynasties Shangqing Daoism*." London: University College.

Stanley-Baker, Michael; Liu, Wei-ting; Chang, Chao-jan. 2018. "Markus encoded 列仙傳", https://doi.org/10.21979/N9/UQK3RS, DR-NTU (Data), V1

Stephens, Daniel J.2009. "Confucianism, Pragmatism, and Socially Beneficial Philosophy." *Journal of Chinese Philosophy*, vol. 36, no. 1, Mar 2009, pp. 53-67. DOI: 10.1111/j.1540-6253.2008.01504.x

Strickmann, Michael. 2002. *Chinese Magical Medicine: Asian Religions and Cultures*. Stanford: Stanford University Press.

Wang, Ban 2022. (Professor of Chinese Studies, Stanford University). Interview. Conducted by Jonathan Lu, 26 Mar 2022.

Wang, Jichao (王纪潮).2005. "Concerning the Hallucinogens for Shamanic Ecstasy in Ancient China (中國古代薩滿昏迷中的藥物問題)." *Studies in the History of Natural Sciences (自然科学史研究)*, vol. 24, no. 1, pp. 13-28.

Weill, Andrew T., and Winifred Rosen.2004. *From Chocolate to Morphine: Everything You Need to Know About Mind-Altering Drugs*. Boston: Houghton Mifflin Co.

Whorf, Benjamin Lee. 1964. *Language, Thought, and Reality*. Boston: The MIT Press.

Wuhan General Group (China), Inc. 2019. "Wuhan Enters Mushroom Psychedelic Medicine Market." *GlobeNewswire News Room*, April 5, 2019. https://www.globenewswire.com/news-release/2019/04/05/1797796/0/en/Wuhan-Enters-Mushroom-Psychedelic-Medicine-Market.html.

Xiao, Peigen, and Liyi He.1983. "Ethnopharmacologic investigation on tropane-containing drugs in Chinese solanaceous plants." *Journal of Ethnopharmacology*, vol. 8, no. 1, Jul 1983, pp. 1-18. DOI: 10.1016/0378-8741(83)90086-7

Yang, Jianhong (杨建宏). 2005. "Lu's Township Covenant: Civil Society Control in Song Dynasty (吕氏乡约》与宋代民间社会控制)." *Journal of Social Sciences of Hunan Normal University (湖南师范大学社会科学学报)*, vol. 5.

Yeung, Wai-Song. 2008. "Abuse of Wushi powder in Old China." *Journal of Chinese Medicine*, vol 87, Jun 2008, pp. 19-21.

Zhang, Sheldon X., and Ko-lin Chin. 2015. "A People's War: China's Struggle to Contain its Illicit Drug Problem." *Brookings Institution*, vol. 1.

Zürcher, Erik. 2007. The *Buddhist Conquest of China*. Leiden: Brill Publishing.

文汇报. 2022. "科学》重磅：改善抑郁症一天起效？'致幻蘑菇'有望变身抗抑郁速效药." www.163.Com. January 28, 2022. Accessed May 1, 2022. https://www.163.com/dy/article/GUQE8BFC05506BEH.html.

The Ark: Bio-Cultural Sustainability for the San Pedro Cactus

Laurel Anne Sugden, Doctoral Candidate, and Josip Orlovac Del Río

PhD candidate in interdisciplinary Studies at the University of British Columbia | Ethnobotanist | Co-founder Huachuma Collective

Maestro Huachumero | Co-founder Huachuma Collective

> *"Huachuma, or San Pedro, is a psychedelic cactus in the genus Echinopsis native to the mid-elevation Andes. Shamanic practitioners across huachuma's wide range have prepared the plants as a visionary drink for at least 3,000 years."* —JOSIP ORLOVAC DEL RÍO

> *"This presentation supports anecdotal evidence from traditional San Pedro use in Peru, which suggests that Indigenous communities and practitioners distinguish types of San Pedro which science cannot tell apart."* —LAUREL SUGDEN

Authors' note:

Our first care when publishing this essay on San Pedro's sustainability has been to protect the wild plants and their locations. Illegal extraction of endemic San Pedro in Peru is ongoing, and we are unwilling to publicly provide any information which could further endanger their populations. For this reason, general and well-known place names have been included, while specific place names have been omitted throughout the piece. All translations between Spanish and English are by the authors.

The cactus Huachuma was the sun and stars that illuminated thousands of years of cultural evolution on the coast of what is now called Peru. When the Spanish conquistadors sailed onto that coast and planted a flag, those who carried the knowledge of the plant were violently persecuted, and their practices were driven underground. But Huachuma shone on, the Southern Cross to their ship in the night.

Halfway through the drafting of this essay, the knowledge and traditional uses of the San Pedro cactus were declared "Intangible Cultural Heritage of the Nation" by the Peruvian government. The declaration recognized "the expression of a systemic and integral vision of a cultural universe" that people and plants have created together since the dawn of civilization in the Andes (Guerrero 2022). It was the biggest legal leap for the cactus and its allies in 500 years.

"At last!" was the overwhelming response from the community of surviving elders in North Peru who still carry San Pedro's tradition.

And yet, as I read the declaration, pacing our office with freshly printed pages warm in my hands and Josip on the phone tucked between ear and neck, I couldn't shake a growing feeling of unease.

The ancestral cultures of Peru unleashed the power of the plant over 3,000 years ago during the rise of Andean civilization—civilization which coalesced around a psychedelic sacrament in a way that no other developed culture on Earth has matched. The cacti themselves were associated with flowers, the cosmos, and the regenerative cycle of water as it moves through the earth, holding a mediating role in a world where unpredictable weather was the limiting factor for human survival (Glass-Coffin 2010). Beginning with the unprecedented rise of Chavín, the "mother culture" of the Andes, in the first millennium B.C., a succession of cultures integrated the plant into the deepest levels of government, politics, health, and artistic expression (Sharon and Donnan 1977). Much later, as the Catholic Fathers did their best to annihilate Andean religion, the descendants of those cultures were accused of witchcraft and communion with the devil for the crime of taking the same sacrament. "This is a plant with which the devil had deceived the Indians of Peru... which they used for their lies and superstitions," wrote Father Cobo in 1631. "Transported by this drink, the Indians dreamed a thousand follies and believed them as if they were true" (Cobo and Mateos 1956).

As the remaining San Pedro practitioners—called *maestros* (masters) or *curanderos* (healers) in North Peru—emerge from this long night of persecution, standing with pride in the sunrise of governmental recognition, the ruins are plain to see. The renowned healing cults of the plant survive in urban centers throughout North Peru's coastal areas, where all-night rituals of San Pedro consumption called *mesadas* are still practiced on Tuesday and Friday nights. These rituals retain their Indigenous roots, but their practice also incorporates Catholic symbolism (Sharon 2015). Nearly all of the practitioners in the traditional world of San Pedro are over 60 years old, and many of the greats have already passed on. Their children are the first generation in 3,000 years of uninterrupted cultural relationship with San Pedro who are no longer learning to work with the plants. Many live in extreme poverty.

To add insult to injury, hundreds of miles to the south, in an idyllic valley far from the native habitat of the plants, people who are not from the Andes are making millions selling San Pedro to an exploding global community of spiritual tourists.

But the unease that Josip and I felt, our words tumbling over each other on the phone as we considered the implications of the announcement, did not come from what the Ministry of Culture's report included. It came from what was missing. There was an obvious hole in the resolution: a threat on the near horizon which puts at risk, more than any other single factor, the integrity of the ship on which traditional healers have sailed through the catastrophe of conquest only to emerge in the equally damaging dawn of the modern world.

The document does not say a word about the fact that the San Pedro cactus itself is endangered and disappearing in the wild.

Experts have known about the cactus's conservation issues for fifteen years. All species of San Pedro are considered "endangered in the wild" or "threatened" within Peru (Informe de la

Autoridad Científica CITES Perú 2013). And yet, it appears that reports of endangered cactus populations have had little impact outside government offices, and even less impact outside Peru. Illegal harvest and exportation of the plants has continued to increase exponentially. Even today, the myth persists within Peru and internationally that Peruvian San Pedro is a sustainable source of psychedelic medicine.

The language that the Ministry of Culture uses in their recent declaration leaves no doubt that the direct consumption of the plant is "indispensable" to preserving at-risk cultural knowledge. The document recognizes that "the San Pedro cactus is understood as a vehicle for the knowledge of the spiritual forces that preside over [the Andean] conception of health" and "a medium which allows knowledge of the spiritual world," and "a guide to achieve a vision of sickness and its diagnosis." The plant is the center of the "cultural universe" they aim to protect, but the plant itself is poorly protected (Guerrero 2022).

I conducted my PhD research in Peru's wild San Pedro habitats, surveying their populations and diversity in broad strokes through a swath of the Andes the size of California. When I began, I had no idea of the sustainability crisis that San Pedro was facing. Five field seasons later, I was intimately familiar with the devastation of the plants in so many of these habitats. The story of wild San Pedro is a simple, universal story: that there is always enough of everything until there is not. Less simple are the many factors that have led to the decline of plant populations over the last fifty years.

My husband Josip was guide, co-researcher, and—occasionally—bodyguard during our sustainability surveys, and he was the reason I understood even half of what I was observing in the field. He also happens to know San Pedro better than anyone I've encountered in a decade of immersion in the world of the plant.

Josip was born near Lima, but he lived and studied in North Peru as a teenager. Like most San Pedro *maestros*, he is *mestizo,* mixed-race. His name comes from his Croatian father, who was a World War II refugee to Peru. His maternal grandfather was an Andean man from Arequipa, and through his influence, Josip grew up connected with San Pedro. Josip's lifelong relationship with the plants started when he was a child.

As Josip tells the story:

> "When I was five, with curiosity and innocence, I ate my first raw San Pedro salad with honey in my family garden. I loved honey, so I ate a lot of that salad. I remember when my grandfather, Don Nicolás Del Río, said to my uncle and sisters: 'Stop taking San Pedro, it is not a drug!' He meant that it is a sacred medicine that needs to be taken with respect, with guidance, and with a higher purpose.
>
> I never took a pill in my life until he died. When I was sick, he always came with plant medicine from our garden. Officially Don Nicolás was a marine and a politician, but traditionally he was a *curandero naturista*. Until the 70's, San Pedro was not used very much outside of North Peru, except as a drug for young people. Even though San Pedro grew near where we lived in the mountains of Lima, all the traditional use of the plant was in North Peru.

A few years later I moved with my family to Chimbote in North Peru, and I was fascinated by the legacy of the ancient cultures that worked with San Pedro there: Chavín, Cupisnique, Moche, Sicán. I was understanding how important San Pedro was for them, and how alive the use of the plant was today, in modern society.

There I met Maestro Felipe Pereda. He became my elder brother and from him I learned much about the art of *curanderismo* and the traditional use of San Pedro ceremonially. I worked as the assistant of Felipe for several years, and then I made the decision to follow my own path with San Pedro. At the age of eighteen I was overwhelmed by the amount of commitment and responsibility needed to carry the wisdom of the plant for other people."

As Josip followed his chosen path with San Pedro as a young man, he traveled through many of the plant's habitats in the 1990's, before San Pedro became popular outside its traditional world. Perpetually hitchhiking through Lima, Ancash, La Libertad, Cajamarca, Lambayeque, and Piura, he had lots of time to observe the plants. At that time, before paved roads opened access to the interior, crossing the 13,000-ft passes from the dry Pacific coast to the verdant eastern slopes of the Andes took two long days of travel on bumpy, precipitous dirt roads. On clear days, Josip would stretch out on top of the cab of a cargo truck on the way to a cultural festival in Cajamarca or Huánuco and watch the desert give way to rocky landscapes of San Pedro, sprouting like serpents from every crevice in the cliffs. *Comuneros* call it "San Pedro de peña," San Pedro of the rocks: wild plants which have grown slowly, with little water, and are therefore extremely potent. They are prized above cultivated plants for ceremonial use because their spiritual power is more concentrated.

Wild *Echinopsis pachanoi*, the Northern species of San Pedro, forms great clumps of cacti of up to five meters in height, the columns of which bear modest spines of 1-3 cm that their cultivated counterparts do not. The number of ribs per stalk varies from five to ten, but most bear seven: an auspicious number for *curanderos* (Sharon 2015). When swollen with rainwater, the limbs break and fall of their own accord, only to re-root in the soil beside their mother plants and sprout new cacti from their bodies, using the old tissue as compost. Often hundreds of years old, these self-propagating clumps of cactus can expand interminably. As Josip recalls, many zones in the north, tucked in the valleys and folds of the land far from paved roads, were at one time forests of San Pedro.

A decade before Josip's travels, wild San Pedro was already declining in populated areas. Wade Davis observed the plants in his trip to North Peru at that time, writing "At one time San Pedro grew commonly throughout the valley [of Huancabamba]. By 1981 it was relatively rare, and found almost exclusively in association with house sites, the property of individual families. With the popularity of the healing cult increasing, demand for the plant ran high" (Davis 1998, 169-202).

1981 signaled the beginning of a decade of bloody terrorism which devastated Peru, as guerrilla soldiers in the rural Andes waged war against the Peruvian government. The Shining Path was a violent terrorist group whose philosophy was based in Marxist communism. Its leader, Abimael Guzmán, incited his followers to take up arms against what he called Peru's "bourgeois democracy," declaring that "there will be a great rupture and we will be the makers of a definitive dawn. We will convert the black fire into red and the red into light!" (Gorriti 2000). Even as many Indigenous Andean people were coerced to join or oppose the rebellion, its bloody wake left 70,000 people dead. No one in rural Peru was untouched by violence and hunger. It was impossible to travel safely in the Andes, and for a decade, only guerrillas and Peruvian soldiers traversed the *sierra*.

The 80's displaced hundreds of thousands of rural Andean people and sent them fleeing to the urban centers of Lima, Chimbote, Trujillo, Chiclayo, and Piura (Gorriti 2000). Urban populations exploded, and so did San Pedro shamanism in cities.

Though San Pedro had been present in urban areas for decades already, new population growth exacerbated a widening split between people and plants. San Pedro *maestros* usually worked full time day jobs in addition to their healing practices, and they no longer had time or resources to travel to wild sources to harvest their own plants. Instead, they cooked and served cut lengths of San Pedro purchased from the markets (Sharon 2015).

The Ministry of Culture declaration describes the importance of the relationship between *maestro* and the living, growing plants:

> "The collection of this plant follows a series of ritual procedures, directed by the *curandero*, which are aimed at preventing its qualities from being disturbed. Since it is conceived as the residence of a spirit with which it is necessary to interact in a relationship of respect, this interaction begins at the moment in which the stems and branches of the plant are collected. Before making this collection, the *curanderos* must greet it and pay homage with prayers, songs, ablutions with flower-water and tobacco smoke around the plant that will be cut, even blessing the knife used for this purpose.... By these means it is achieved that the cactus allows itself to be used and that it maintains its qualities. It is important that whoever makes the collection follows a correct life according to traditional parameters. This is also the reason why said person is usually the *maestro curandero* himself.... it is also considered necessary that the person who prepares [the medicinal drink] be the same specialist, or assistant, who collected the plant in order to allow its powers to come to 'life' and to assume its therapeutic functions (Guerrero 2022)."

The bifurcation caused by the lack of access to San Pedro in urban areas had immediate cultural ramifications for the *maestros*, for they no longer related to the spirit of the plant as a living, rooted being. The consequences of the split became more and more evident in the wild plant populations as the years progressed.

On his 1981 trip, Davis observed, "In coastal markets a one-foot section of about eight inches in girth sold for as much as a dollar. A [large cactus] could feed a family for a month" (Davis 1998, 169-202). The cuttings that he describes are twice as thick as the San Pedro found in northern markets today and could only have come from successive cutting of the old-growth plants that still populated rural areas of North Peru at that time. The people cutting the plants for urban markets were, as Davis suggests, making extra money selling the existing wild plants on or near their land, but they did not know how to harvest it in ways that promote regeneration. Market vendors became the middlemen between harvesters and *curanderos,* and those who used the plants no longer communicated with those who cut the plants. As a result, most urban San Pedro *maestros* even today have little idea of the extent of the destruction of San Pedro's wild populations.

Extensive road construction projects under the administrations of Fujimori, Toledo, and Alan García around the turn of the century cut indiscriminately through the habitats of the plants, opening the Andes to easier travel and allowing paved access to new San Pedro harvest zones. There was a mining boom post-terrorism, and new prosperity meant that urban populations were exploding. More people were drinking more San Pedro than at any point since the Spanish conquest.

THE CONSERVATION STATUS OF *ECHINOPSIS PERUVIANA* IN NORTH PERU

"Take the old man a horse, and you can fill a truck with as much San Pedro as it will hold," Oscar Cortéz pleaded. "Do him this favor, Josip. He can't get far enough out to do his rounds anymore, so they're taking all the San Pedro anyway. Any horse, any good horse will do. It's a fine trade" (Oscar Cortéz, personal communication, 2004). It was 2004, and Oscar was bartering the last of the roadside San Pedro from the Laquipampa Wildlife Refuge in North Peru. Josip declined the offer. He preferred his plants from Arequipa and Lima, the lands of his grandfather and father, and more importantly, what Oscar was proposing—plant extraction from a protected area—was illegal. The plants that grow in Laquipampa make up one of the last remaining populations of the most renowned variety of San Pedro of all, the famed Chiclayo plants.

In 2015, a master's student named Lenin Joel Vera completed a survey of San Pedro in Laquipampa, the same zone where Josip had been offered a truckload of San Pedro eleven years earlier. He noted that populations outside of the protected area had already been devastated to such an extent that Laquipampa was the only place he could find to do his survey. In the 687-hectare protected reserve of prime San Pedro habitat, Vera counted a total of just 2,578 individual San Pedro cacti, most of which were growing in areas inaccessible to harvest (Vera Chilcon 2016).

Vera notes that in Laquipampa, "The human pressures to which the populations of San Pedro are subjected are diverse… the deterioration of habitat due to modification of vegetation by cattle entering the area; likewise, areas of extraction of the resource for commercialization were evident…." He clarifies that San Pedro is "…suffering pressures from a part of the [human population who]… enter the area to take pieces of these individuals (stems) to commercialize them and thus generate their income, with the risk that this species could be considerably reduced in number in this protected area due to extraction…. they are cut both at the top and bottom of a distance from twenty to twenty-five centimeters long, which in many cases does not ensure regeneration" (Vera Chilcon 2016).

Vera's conclusions were similar to what we found in our own investigations. Our windshield surveys of San Pedro populations in North Peru were carried out from 2020-2022. We assessed the number and density of plants visually from the roadside and supplemented those observations with walking surveys in areas that were inaccessible by road.

The first task was to distinguish endemic plants from cultivated ones. Anyone who has seen cultivated San Pedro growing in Peru can attest to the plants' prolific nature, and we suspected that the visible presence of cultivated plants near roadsides contributed to the widespread illusion of sustainability. San Pedro is ubiquitously planted by the front doors of houses in Peru. Popular knowledge says that the plants whistle to alert the owners of the house when thieves or delinquents appear. Since guardian plants in front of the house are seen as protectors which repel or neutralize negative energy, these plants are rarely cooked or used as medicine.

Grandma's plant in the back garden does not have the same restrictions. Planted behind homes with the intention of attracting good fortune rather than repelling negativity, these older cultivated plants are often harvested for market. However, the people who have watched their plants grow through the years know their value. It costs more for harvesters to buy cultivated plants than to cut them from the wild. Most had chosen the second option for as long as there were still wild plants to cut.

Decades of this practice had made wild San Pedro scarce. As we searched valley after valley of the rural North in vain, our disbelief grew. The aspect, the elevation, the vegetation… everything about these habitats was perfect. Locals confirmed that even thirty years ago, San Pedro was everywhere in these mountains. Today, the only remaining endemic San Pedro plants were growing in the middle of cliffs, reachable only by binoculars. Here and there we found an old, gnarled San Pedro which was obviously wild, but which had been preserved by its enclosure in a garden or a field. Even these, though, showed evidence of successive harvest over a period of many years, and they were dramatically reduced in size.

There was one account which spoke to the true scarcity of endemic San Pedro in North Peru more than any other. In the rural outskirts of Cajamarca, housewives reported that Chiclayo-based harvesters were, in recent years, making the seven-hour trip across the spine of the Andes to buy the remaining wild San Pedro from their agricultural lands. These notoriously "soft" plants would only be used by Chiclayo shamans as a last resort, once they had already exhausted their local stocks. This detail was the nail in the coffin for endemic *Echinopsis pachanoi.*

By the time we arrived in the North for our surveys, we were a decade too late. The demise of the bulk of the wild plants was complete. As we would soon learn, it didn't take long for the pattern to repeat further south.

THE CONSERVATION STATUS OF *ECHINOPSIS PERUVIANA* IN CENTRAL PERU

In the early 2000's, a new threat to the wild cacti of Peru's central coast emerged. The San Pedro in this area is known to botanists as *Echinopsis peruviana,* and the English-speaking world calls it the Peruvian Torch Cactus. A foot in diameter, loaded with mescaline, and covered in finger-length spines, the plants are impressive. Their traditional cultural uses by people in the area were lost due to colonial and religious forces, and the plants were still fairly abundant here because of a lack of local use.

Though the wild plants have been disturbed in many places, Andean people often integrate San Pedro into cattle grazing and agricultural landscapes in this part of Peru. Fast-growing and spiny, the plants form effective fences that both cattle and cattle thieves are loath to cross. These living fences of San Pedro grow quickly and are pruned back whenever they become too big. The cuttings from the pruning of the mature plants are propagated to create new sections of fence. In the areas where this cultural practice still exists, the damage caused to the plants by the presence of cattle is mitigated.

Perhaps there is something—conscious or subconscious—about the plants' energy of protection that these communities are tapping into, in the same way that Northern Peruvians plant San Pedro by their front doors as guardians. Maybe it was this protective quality which kept their populations intact longer than any other wild San Pedro in Peru. Once discovered, though, it didn't take long for these powerful plants to become the medicine of choice for the budding "spiritual tourism" industry of Cusco.

Josip remembers:

> "I started to live part time in Pisac [near Cusco] in the early 90's. There was no exotic retreat center in Cusco or the Sacred Valley then. No yoga, no ayahuasca. There was Coca. Coca is the most important element of ancestral Andean spirituality. It is the vehicle of social and cultural cohesion in the Andes. Cusco is the center of the world of Coca, and without Coca, nothing exists.
>
> But tourists were just starting to ask about San Pedro in the 90's. I would always answer, 'do you want to have a real San Pedro experience? Go to North Peru.' But people came looking for the superficial charm of psychedelics, not for real rituals.
>
> By the year 2000, more and more tourists were visiting Cusco and the interest in having a psychedelic experience to connect with Andean spirituality became trendy. The only two stalls in the Cusco market that sold San Pedro for local use suddenly received a high demand for cactus.
>
> Within three or four years, the cultivated, mature plants that were coming from Arequipa in South Peru were used up. Then the market was filled with leftover baby sprouts from Arequipa. The strength of the medicine from these babies was lower. New practitioners were disconnected from the traditional way to use these plants, and their answer was to use more and more cactus for dosage.
>
> By 2005, the demand for high-mescaline plants opened the doors for wild plants from Lima and Ancash to come to the market. Hundreds of wild plants started to be shipped to the Cusco market and retreat centers. I knew these new plants. They were endemic to the place where I grew up, near the land of my father, where I had some of my first experiences at age twelve and thirteen, drinking San Pedro in the mountains with my friends. These were old mother-plants, which is why they give people such powerful experiences.
>
> And so, I realized in 2005 that what was happening was going to create a problem with the sustainability of the plant.

Josip's intuition about the sustainability situation in Lima proved apt. The plants began to be harvested *en masse* from community lands in Lima, where living fences of San Pedro suddenly became a hot commodity, and they were transported south 24 hours by truck to Cusco. A stroll through Cusco's San Pedro Market today will reveal an abundance of these plants, recognizable by their 8-12" girth, shiny green and leathery skin, and holes where their long spines have been pulled off with pliers.

In 2006, Dr. Carlos Ostolaza, the top cactus expert in Peru, recommended that *Echinopsis peruviana*—the very plants that were being harvested for shipment to Cusco—be considered "endangered" (Ostolaza et al. 2006, Ostolaza et al. 2007). Unfortunately, ceremonial use in Cusco was not the only new threat to the plants of Lima. The Peruvian Ministry of the Environment (MINAM) published a report in 2013 called *'El San Pedro' or 'Achuma': The genus Echinopsis, Taxonomy, Distribution and Commerce* (Informe de la Autoridad Científica CITES Perú 2013). The report was the first to definitively list both *Echinopsis peruviana* and *Echinopsis pachanoi* as "endangered in the wild." MINAM had noticed an increase in the export of desiccated San Pedro out of Peru, and they surveyed Lima markets to learn where it was coming from. They found that there was a steady supply of packaged "San Pedro powder" available in Lima which was made from wild *E. peruviana*.

MINAM reports that from the years 2009-2013, over 40 tons of San Pedro cacti were harvested, dried, and exported legally with permission from CITES, the international authority on endangered species (Informe de la Autoridad Científica CITES Perú 2013). Of course, they were unable to put a number on how much illegal export was happening under their radar. Though it is impossible to track the harvest that happens illegally, there have been more and more seizures in recent years of unregistered shipments of San Pedro to and from the mountains of Lima. SERFOR, the Peruvian Forestry Service, has road checkpoints in ecologically sensitive areas which manage to stop at least a tiny fraction of the illegal export of wild San Pedro. The recovered shipments are often sent to a cactus nursery in Cieneguilla (Zuzana Knize, personal communication, 2022).

More and more, companies are getting around the problem of transporting large shipments of cactus by having the San Pedro processed and dried on-site in the communities where it is harvested. The resulting product is more compact and easier to transport. Indigenous community members who are employed by these companies to harvest and dry San Pedro tell us that the going rate for a kilo of dried San Pedro there is 10 soles, or the equivalent of about $3 US dollars (Juan Francisco Pérez, personal communication, 2019). According to the MINAM report, each kilo of San Pedro powder takes 46.5 kilos of fresh cactus to make (Informe de la Autoridad Científica CITES Perú 2013). Add to that the work of processing—pulling off the spines and the skin, slicing the outer green layer from the inner white pith, and sun-drying the tissue into "chips," and the resources and work that goes into each bag becomes monumental. The companies who buy dry cactus for $3 per kilo package the product and sell it for $60-120 US Dollars a kilo in Peru (2019 prices observed by the authors in markets of Lima, Cuzco, and Iquitos), and even more internationally. As was the case in North Peru, we observed that declining numbers of mature plants in high-harvest zones of Lima means that the remaining plants are being cut down to their roots, harming their ability to regenerate.

These exploitative practices are only possible because the Indigenous Andean communities who process and sell the plants have lost their cultural connection to the plants after 500 years of colonial and religious onslaught. In one village at the heart of *E. peruviana*'s habitat, a decoction of the plants is used today to "lower fevers in cows… and children" (Ana María Santos, personal communication, 2019). San Pedro no longer holds a spiritual value above that of aspirin, and so the plants are sold for a pittance with little care for how or whether they will regenerate. More than any other factor, it is the loss of culture which allows the blatant destruction of the plants to happen.

Today, Josip and I live 45 minutes from Lima's most active harvest zone. During one of our trips to visit the communities and survey recent harvests, we were gifted a large head of blue-green San Pedro to plant in our garden. It was crowned with a stunning flower in full bloom and several newly sprouting buds. We shimmied the plant into a tote bag to carry it home, getting only slightly bloody from the 4" spines, and the tip with its delicate flower peeked out the top of the bag. We boarded a nearly empty bus, the last of the evening. Dusk was falling quickly in the Andes. An older woman sat alone in the first seat of the bus. She sat up straighter when she saw us.

"Huachuma."

Josip paused. "Not many people call the plant Huachuma around here, *Señora. Espino*, we call it. Where are you from?"

"Of course." She chuckled a little, crossing her arms. "Only *gringos* call it that. We Peruvians call it San Pedro. I am from here, too. Used to live up there by the orange bridge."

"Rosa Saavedra," she introduced herself. "*La Reina del San Pedro*" (Rosa Saavedra, personal communication, 2020).

An involuntary shiver crawled up my spine. The Queen of San Pedro, she had called herself. "I sell more San Pedro than anyone," she boasted. "Sell it to all the *gringos* in Cusco. I used to only take it down to the markets in Lima once a month or so. All my life. Then, one day, maybe fifteen years ago, I get there, and there's this man, a French man. He has been waiting three days to meet me. He wants me to send my plants directly to Cusco. Now I send 200 big heads every month to that foreign woman, you know the one. Have for years and years. It's my sons and I who supply a lot of the retreat centers."

She and Josip conversed in quiet tones as we descended from the Andes. Night had fallen black and moonless outside the windows of the bus when Josip asked at last, "Do you drink the plant, *Señora* Rosa?"

"No, I've never drunk it, it's a drug. They say it makes you see devils. My mother told me, 'Don't you smell that white flower, because it has a worm in it that will enter through your nose and eat your brain.'" Rosa paused, then finished in a voice so low it was almost a prayer. "God forgive me for the business I do." She crossed herself, suddenly self-conscious.

Josip gave her his number when we parted ways. "*Señora* Rosa, the day that you would like to meet the spirit of the plant and listen to the voice of the plant, you know where to find me."

As we stepped off the bus, it occurred to me that Rosa had expressed the same disconnection that had been evident in North Peru. The harvesters did not drink San Pedro, which made it easy to cut hundreds of plants as though they were bucking firewood. The users in Cusco and around the world did not grow or harvest their own plants, cutting them off from the reality of San Pedro as a living being.

Josip, like the most traditional of Northern *maestros,* believes that in that lost connection lies the true medicine of San Pedro. He says:

> "The importance of growing your own plants comes with the teachings that no human *maestro,* facilitator, or shaman can give you. Only San Pedro's spirit, who is the Great Master, can teach you the most important things.
>
> I had been drinking San Pedro with different *maestros* for twenty years. On the night of the full moon in January 2012, I was drinking in my garden in Pisac, with a plant from Arequipa there on the mountainside that was blooming. She was one of the first I ever planted, from 1999.
>
> When the flower opened her mouth and spoke, it was the voice of an old lady that came out. I said, "Why did you never speak to me before?"
>
> The Old Lady said, "I have been speaking all along. Why did you never listen to me before?"
>
> The Old Lady told me many, many, many things that night. She showed me every way that I had caused harm to others in my life. She showed me the ways I was still hurting the people that I loved. At last, I asked her, "If I am so terrible, what hope is there for me?"
>
> "Well, you're the only one who takes care of *me.*" The flower showed me every San Pedro I had planted in my life. How happy they were. How much medicine they held for the people. And then she reached into me and touched the deepest place in my heart and healed what still hurt there. It was the last time the plant ever made me vomit. And the air I breathed in was like springtime.
>
> After the Old Lady spoke to me, I started to serve medicine to other people. It was only at that time that I felt ready to make the commitment to the plant and I understood how to not kill her spirit when I cook her.
>
> Cooking is the traditional way to prepare San Pedro medicine. When we cook medicine with care, we use the four elements: Water in the pot; Fire under the pot; Wind in the words of our prayers, and in the steam that evaporates; and Earth, which is the body of the plant. The four elements become one when you add the fifth element, Love.
>
> These elements are the way to keep the spirit of the plant alive in the medicine. When people use San Pedro powder they lose this alchemy and connection of growing-harvesting-cooking. The powder does not have the whole organic material of the cactus, so its use does not represent the maximum power of the plant. It is not full spectrum the way that traditional cooking is. San Pedro powder kills the spirit of the plant.
>
> When people treat the plant like only a way to make money, without respect, without prayers, without music, without dancing, without strong connection, the

plants don't like to show their full power. It doesn't matter how much you take; the plant will not show her face to you."

Like North Peru's "cultural universe" on a different scale, San Pedro tourism in Cusco has generated its own small world over the last twenty years. It is a world fed entirely by the bodies of the last endemic old-growth San Pedro on Earth. For every kilogram of San Pedro powder that someone buys in Peru or online, a poacher cuts down a cactus that weighs as much as a human being and has been alive much longer. Meanwhile, the plant's rising international popularity is fed by the myth that San Pedro is a sustainable medicine.

Not long after we met Rosa on the bus, I happened to see the social media post of a young foreign woman living in the Sacred Valley of Cusco. She posed with legs twisted into the full lotus position, holding an impressive trunk of old-growth cactus that was scarred along its length where the spines had been torn off. *Dear friends*, the caption read, *I have been blessed to humbly serve 108 cups of Grandfather Huachuma this year. I would like to plant 108 Huachuma seeds in the wild, in reciprocity to the spirit of the medicine. Does anyone have seeds to gift me for this pilgrimage of love?* (Spirit Events Sacred Valley 2021). Though her intentions were good, she expressed in a concise way that she had never seen a San Pedro seed, never germinated one or cared for a seedling as it grew, never come into contact with a San Pedro fruit. If she had, she would have known that cactus seeds only germinate and mature in the wild under specific and rare circumstances, and that even if by some miracle one of her seeds managed to survive, it would take fifty years at the very least—that is, twice as long as she'd been alive—to grow as large and potent as the wild plant whose arm she cradled in her photo.

The post was an example of the sincere love coupled with total lack of connection that is common among people newly discovering the plant. The cultural universe that San Pedro and the ancestors of the North created together was developed over thousands of years of reciprocal relationship in which the plants were cared for by the people, and the people by the plants. Ignorance of that ancient world is widespread, and it is not harmless.

Foreigners in Cusco make millions donning ponchos and serving San Pedro with a side of appropriated Andean spirituality. Meanwhile, the children of the Northern *maestros*, for the first time in 3,000 uninterrupted years, are not learning to work with the plant. Andean communities in the Lima highlands are economically and environmentally exploited for San Pedro, while their own cultural traditions have been ruptured by violent colonialism.

The Ministry of Culture's recognition of the traditional knowledge and uses of San Pedro as Immaterial Cultural Heritage is a vitally important first step in safeguarding the plant's cultural world for the future. The second step is protecting the wild populations of San Pedro on which the survival of that cultural world depends.

For *maestros,* the natural diversity of endemic San Pedro and the land in which it grows is key to the medicine's spiritual power. In the art of ancient cultures spanning thousands of years, Huachuma is depicted rooted in its natural environments, surrounded by the other members of its ecosystem: serpents, pumas, birds, and sacred mountains (Sharon and Donnan 1977). This relationship of the plant's spirit to place still lies at the heart of contemporary practices. The renowned *curanderos* of Huancabamba never import San Pedro for their rituals; they work only with their local varieties, which carry and channel the powers of the nearby highland lakes. In Cajamarca the "soft" San Pedro is prized for the high mineral content of the soil in which it grows, and it is used to induce purging for the purpose of curing physical ailments of the stomach and organs. In Chiclayo, the San Pedro from in and around Laquipampa puts practitioners in contact with the *gentiles* and *encantos*, the spirits of waterfalls and springs that have animated their mountains for a hundred generations. Further south, one population of San Pedro is used specifically for its connection with the generous spirit of the Virgin Mary. The Lima plants may be undervalued by locals today, but they once inspired the magnificent nature-based artwork of cultures such as Nazca and Wari.

How much cultural memory would be lost if even one of these populations became extinct in the wild? How many have already been lost? Josip sums up what is at stake when he says:

> "The Great Spirit of San Pedro is made up of all the plants, in their endemic habitats, over time. This Great Spirit lives in the wild, in the places the plants grow that humans never touch.
>
> All the individual San Pedro cacti on earth are like scales on an enormous winged dragon. The wild populations of San Pedro are its vital life force, and the diversity and spiritual power of all the individual plants is fed and protected by this great dragon.
>
> If wild San Pedro is extinguished, the Great Spirit of San Pedro will be extinguished."

There is a narrow band of effective habitat for wild San Pedro in the Andes. The plants grow in very specific zones which meet their precise elevation, temperature, and water needs. Many of those habitats have already been compromised by agricultural encroachment and road construction. In the majority of active harvest zones, the plants are being harvested at a faster rate than they are able to regenerate, and where old-growth plants still exist, they are being harvested disproportionately.

From our preliminary windshield and walking surveys, we estimate that among all San Pedro's endemic habitats in Peru, less than a quarter are still well-stocked. At this rate, Cultural Heritage declaration or not, Peru is perhaps a decade away from losing the very roots which sustain its living culture: the wild source of Huachuma that built the ancient empires and watched them fall.

CULTIVATING HOPE FOR HUACHUMA

"I thought you were dead!" shouted the old lady. A wrinkled face appeared at the window of the whitewashed house, then disappeared just as quickly (Hermilda Hernandez, personal communication, 2019).

From somewhere in the back came the sound of latches and bolts sliding. A door creaked open, and a cane carried by someone in a hurry rang through the yard.

"*Mi querida* Doña Hermilda," Josip called from the garden gate, his hands folded politely behind his back, "I am a young man yet. If one of us were going to die since we last saw each other, it would have been you."

"Well, I'll drop dead here and now if you didn't bring me toasting corn from Cusco. All the corn here in the Arequipa market is tough."

A tiny woman limped around the corner, wrapped in a colorful knitted sweater that reached her knees. She must have been in her nineties. She flung open the gate, scattering magenta husks of bougainvillea on all three of us. Josip bent nearly double to wrap her in a hug, and she planted two kisses on each of his cheeks.

"Of course, I have the corn, and the coca, and the cacao too, Doña Hermilda." He patted the bag slung over his shoulder. "Everything you like."

Doña Hermilda sat us down at her kitchen table and served chamomile tea in cracked floral china, along with her infamous toasted corn *canchitas.* Josip emptied his bag and she opened her gifts one by one: three colors of quinoa; two pounds of coca leaves from Qosñipata; knitted alpaca gloves, hat, and scarf for the frigid Arequipa winter; maca;* a kilo of cacao; three fat wheels of *queso Andino* to eat with the corn; and bulging sacks of two kinds of toasting corn, *chullpi* and *blanco.*

"And the coffee?" she asked sweetly.

"Ahhhh, no, the coffee! In four years my memory must have failed. Maybe I am getting old, as you say. My deepest apologies, Doña Hermilda. Next time I will bring your coffee, you have my word."

Josip reached into the left breastpocket of his jacket and produced one more packet, smaller than the rest. In it were the creamy white dried petals of San Pedro flowers, with their profuse tentacle-like anthers.

"Maybe this can make up for the coffee. These are the flowers from the plants that we harvested together from your garden in 2007. Today, those plants in Chaclacayo are twice my height, and they make flowers every year. They are your plants, but now they grow in Lima soil. Please, take these to use for your tea when your flowers are not in season."

Doña Hermilda accepted the bag, inhaled the delicate dried scent of the petals, and then pressed the packet to her heart with both spotted hands as she exhaled deeply.

"The plant has bloomed more than ever this year. I use the flowers like you showed me, seven petals in my tea each night. Oh, how they calm me! How they enchant me! I feel sadness, you see, so much sadness about my son. But the flowers help me."

She stood, stowed the dry flowers in a once-transparent plastic Tupperware, and patted me roughly on the back.

"Now it's time to see the plant. *Vamos.*"

Out back of the kitchen, between a pair of feathery *huarango* trees, towered a sleek, blue-green San Pedro plant with no spines at all. It had obviously been pruned and shaped over the years, and looked like a stately tree, shining with health. The thick trunk that formed the base of the plant belied its age: sixty years old at the very least, perhaps eighty. Josip approached it as though greeting an old friend.

---

* To learn more about the medicinal properties of this plant see www.herbalreality.com/herb/maca/

"How beautifully she has grown these last four years!"

"That's what love does," said Doña Hermilda. "The plant protects the house. But you know, an arm fell this summer. My grandchildren play here, and it's getting too tall. It's dangerous. Please take quite a lot this time. Start with that arm there. And this one!"

Josip produced more coca along with a bag of fresh rose petals, and together he and Doña Hermilda showered the plant with them—"...for good luck, for prosperity, for health, for protection, for flowers, for love, for strength, for happiness...."

The offerings joined a pile of dried garden flowers and grains already scattered at the base of the plant, quiet evidence of regular offerings.

Then Doña Hermilda rested in her lawn chair and directed the pruning with vigorous gestures of her cane. Josip carefully separated each arm she pointed to by hand, refusing to use a knife or machete on the living plant. We packed the arms into newspapers, then sacks, then cardboard boxes, and loaded them into the waiting car outside. The work took all morning, and by the time we finished, the high-altitude sun was straight overhead and blistering. The old plant looked lighter but no less impressive, and I guessed that in another four years it would be bigger than ever.

"Are you sure you won't come out to lunch, Doña Hermilda? For a bit of guinea pig *chactado*?"

"No, my son is bringing the children this afternoon, and I don't want to miss them. God bless you. May He light your path and protect you from harm during your travels." She slipped a plastic bag of her toasted corn into Josip's now-empty tote. "For the road home."

The gate swung shut behind us before I heard her shout.

"Don't forget my coffee next time!"

Josip had been growing San Pedro in Pisac since 1999. But in 2007, he took what he had learned on a small scale and began to plant in earnest. He purchased what remained of his father's land in Chaclacayo, east of Lima, and began to fill it with San Pedro. He started with 133 of his most beloved plants, those which came from Doña Hermilda in Arequipa, the birthplace of his grandfather Don Nicolás. Over the years, more San Pedro joined the first group of plants, and today there are thousands of heads comprising at least forty varieties from around Peru.

From the beginning, Josip has held the vision for this land as a place of protection for the plants. It has been a safe space for San Pedro to grow up and grow old, relaxing into its natural diversity and abundance, connected with the sacred mountains of Santa Inés, the rumble of the Río Rimac, and the sea air rushing inland from the coast each morning. The plants have received space and care, sunlight and moonlight, and they bloom flowers each summer. Over the years they have given thousands of cups of medicine to people who need it, but it has never been necessary to cut plants to cook. They fall naturally from the weight of their own arms when a gust of wind comes in the evening, or when the cats use them as jungle-gyms.

Cultivating San Pedro is the single most important part of Josip's relationship with the plant. He explains:

> "When I harvest medicine, I can see the eyes of San Pedro. I can take his body in my two hands and ask him if he wants to be cooked to help somebody. Is there anybody in the world who can see the eyes of San Pedro and hold the body of San Pedro to

talk with him when he is already dry powder inside a plastic bag? There, the spirit of the plant dissolves like powder in water.

When we plant a cactus, we are growing medicine, a medicine of relationship and reciprocity. A medicine of freedom and love. Every San Pedro cactus is unique and has something to teach us.

When after years of care and trust a plant blooms flowers at last, the gifts we receive are pure medicine. We can witness how a thorn can become a flower, carrying a powerful message of transmutation. When a plant blooms, he can be ready to be cooked and become medicine himself.

After all this process of connection with the plant as it grows, we can be ready to serve medicine. We can understand at last the sacrifice the plant makes for us. We can take responsibility for harvesting and cooking a living being and keeping his spirit alive when we do it.

And this is why I say: grow medicine, serve medicine.

Grow medicine. And then. Serve medicine."

By 2020, the natural abundance of the cactus was overflowing the garden walls. The heads that naturally fell from the mature plants became gifts to friends, neighbors, and local archaeological sites. Josip's twenty-three years growing San Pedro had led us to the logical next step. It was time to plant on a larger scale.

In the midst of discussions about how to address the plant's sustainability crisis, we paid a visit to Josip's first San Pedro *maestro,* Felipe Pereda. Felipe is the Cultural Advisor and Wilka Umo Shaman of the Chimbote and Coishco Indigenous Community in North Peru. An activist for Indigenous rights and cultural preservation for over forty years, Felipe clarified and directed our initial ideas about gifting San Pedro and providing support for cultural heritage in Andean communities.

In 2021, Felipe, Josip, and I formalized our shared work to create a non-profit association in Peru. Huachuma Collective exists to empower Andean communities to plant San Pedro, and to support organizations, communities, and individuals who are protecting the wild plants.

Within 18 months, we had donated a thousand cacti from endangered populations to communities in North Peru. Josip took time in each habitat we visited to teach propagation and sustainable harvesting techniques. Felipe taught workshops on the traditional cultural uses of the plants. Community elders recalled stories about San Pedro from years past. Teenagers showed interest in the plants for their subversive potential. Just as Josip was inspired as a 15-year-old to become Felipe's apprentice because his San Pedro experiences led him to fascination with Peru's ancient cultures, young people today are similarly provoked by visions and intuitions received from San Pedro which connect them with their ancestors.

These early collaborations showed us how much the connection with living, growing Huachuma means to people in Andean communities. Cultivating the plant gives it value in the eyes of the people. The vast majority of people who grow San Pedro in Peru never drink it, but they recognize the value of its presence as a protective spirit which attracts good fortune. For them, the living plant has a value, an energy, even an aura which transcends mere beauty or utility. It was a sacred, protective plant of the ancestors, more auspicious when gifted than purchased.

San Pedro as a vehicle of connection to cultural heritage is not a new idea. Living cacti are often featured in archaeological sites and *pueblos* which make their living on cultural presence, such as Moche, Magdalena de Cão, and Huancabamba, where the plants are recognized as a living connection to the ancient world. In fact, San Pedro's role as a protector, guardian, and carrier of memory is so established in North Peru that it made us wonder about the wider implications of planting so many cacti, particularly in lands that ancient peoples held sacred. Could the very presence of San Pedro help to protect the memory of knowledge and cultural practices associated with it through the bottleneck of modernity and development? Could growing as many plants as possible in as many places as possible act as an almost mystically protective force to cultural heritage?

Planting, cultivating, harvesting, cooking, and drinking Huachuma takes on revolutionary dimensions when considered this way. The plants themselves become the vessels which protect and carry forward the memory of the past through difficult times. Most of what San Pedro once was to humanity is already gone, and what is left is held only in the living memory of the oldest plants and the wisest *maestros*. The tide of modernity drowns all but the sturdiest ships. These elders have made it through centuries of cultural and environmental loss, holding on as more and more was stripped away and forgotten, losing precious things that the world did not know how to value until they were gone.

Now, the future of wild San Pedro and its living cultures is in the hands of every single person who knows, loves, and listens to the plants. Advocating for the needs of the plants means preserving their cultural legacy in the Andes, and in turn, fortifying Andean culture means protecting the plants against extinction. As the masses froth for psychedelics, communities and individuals will rebuild reciprocal ways of relating to the plants and demonstrate them to the world. What has been lost cannot come back, but perhaps if we protect the roots and seeds that survive, they can regenerate and sprout once the danger has passed. San Pedro is nothing if not built for renewal.

In the days that followed the launch of Huachuma Collective, I fell into a fever. For three days in a mountainside motel in San Pedro habitat, I did not leave bed. Scenes from our travels flitted through my awareness. The plants visited in their creature forms: turquoise serpents, golden dragons, sharp-eyed pumas, bears that were also stars. I shivered and tossed, alternating between the sensation of floating high above the earth and of being sucked deep inside it, awake or asleep I did not know, in the present or the future I did not know. Behind closed eyes, my visions were flooded with colors.

A single San Pedro, purple-black and silent, stood at the head of the Valley of the Dragon. Its spines shone blood-red and translucent in the setting sun. The sky was shot with light, white and golden with pink at the edges, filling every crevice of the sleeping mountains. It was the only one. The only one left. I looked around in disbelief, deep grief filling my chest. The Last Guardian. The last.

Seven notes whistled, full and low. An ancient woman wrapped in woven cloth rocked by the fire, singing, remembering. Remembering. Bright jewels of songbirds and insects, long vanished, flitted around the edges of the firelight. The warm bulks of mammals that no longer walk the earth moved in the shadows. Extinct. Gone forever, except in San Pedro's memory. Except in San Pedro's song. The song came years ago, years before I knew what it meant.

Now, here on the mountainside with the last cactus, I knew. I could feel the vibration of it in my bones, bittersweet and unmistakable. A song of mourning. A song of honoring. A song of all that is long gone. Not a matter of bringing it back, but of remembering, so that something of its essence remains on earth, even to the end. All of the medicines together, singing their song at the end of the world.

Images from North Peru flashed before my eyes. Land mafias, gunning down Indigenous people for their properties. Tractors, flattening archaeological sites in the night so the corporations could keep growing tomatoes without interference from the Ministry of Culture. Uniformed children marching in lines while mining executives applauded. Money, so much money, passed under the table. Concrete and dust. Machetes and knives. The wisdom-keepers hiding. Fleeing. Silenced.

I staggered outside and vomited until there was nothing left.

The image of the Last Guardian stayed with me, a sentinel blinking a warning from the future. But in the days that followed, Josip and I made a discovery which forever changed how we understood the plants.

We were surveying a new habitat in a region where San Pedro is heavily affected by climate change. Most of the plants, even those that were very old and established, looked yellow-brown and desiccated, as though it had been years since they had received enough rain. Discouraged, we stopped at a makeshift market in the front room of a community member's home, hoping for a cold drink and conversation. Near the garden wall, encased on three sides by roughly poured concrete, was an ancient, spiny *E. peruviana.* We guessed it had been there before the house was built. By the account of the woman who sold us frigid Coca-Cola and crackers, the plant was at least a hundred years old. It was already a large adult in her earliest memories, and she was in her seventies now.

Today the plant was in full bloom, fifty flowers shining like bright-white egrets perched in a tree.

"May we take photos?"

Her eyes shone. "*Por supuesto que sí, adelante!*" Certainly, we could.

I stepped closer, touched the plant, introduced myself as I always did before raising my camera. Instead, I stayed frozen, hand pressed to the trunk, unable to believe what I was seeing.

Nestled like baby birds in the crevice between branching arms of the plant were thirteen tiny San Pedro seedlings, all less than a year old. A triad of thick branches formed a sort of platform where many husks of spent flowers and fruits had fallen and were now black and decaying. Long, woody spines crisscrossed over and around the platform of composting flowers, making it nearly impossible to see the delicate plants that were rooted there.

Silent tears flooded down my face, wetting my already sweat-soaked t-shirt. In all our surveys, we had previously found only two plants that were evidently seed-started. The poppy-seed-sized cactus seeds were so delicate and sensitive that we had believed their success rate in the wild to be one in a million, if that. I turned to Josip, unable to draw breath to speak.

He crossed the distance between us in two long strides. "Laurel, what is it? What's wrong?"

I pointed wordlessly.

"*Que- ahhhh. Ay, Dios mío. No puede ser.* It can't be."

"It is. *Amor.* Huachuma is a mother. She raises her own babies."

"I have never seen this before."

Two days later and a hundred miles north, we found another nest of San Pedro sprouts. And then another. Seedlings at every stage of development, hidden in the deepest recesses of the largest wild plants. I bloodied myself more than once, crawling inside sprawling San Pedro limbs like tree trunks to get a look at the little ones that grew there.

Perhaps it had been happening all along, all around us, this quiet raising of babies in the compost of flowers. But in those grace-soaked days, it felt as though Huachuma had decided at last to show her womb, her nursery, her secret rearing of life in the invisible places.

She had revealed herself as the Ark, quietly carrying the delicate sprouts of the next generation of plants in her protected center. She asked only that we care for her as she does what she has always done: buffer the extremes of change, and shield the most precious knowledge, memories, and visions of the future of life on Earth from those who would harm them.

BIBLIOGRAPHY

Cobo, Bernabé, and Francisco Mateos. 1956. "Obras del Padre Bernabe Cobo. ca. 1653." *Ed. Francisco Mateos 2.*

Davis, Wade. 1998. "Cactus of the Four Winds." *Shadows in the sun: Travels to landscapes of spirit and desire.* Island Press. 169-202.

Glass-Coffin, Bonnie. 2010. "Shamanism and San Pedro through time: some notes on the archaeology, history, and continued use of an entheogen in northern Peru." *Anthropology of Consciousness* 21, no. 1: 58-82.

Gorriti, Gustavo. 2000. *The Shining Path: A history of the millenarian war in Peru.* Univ of North Carolina Press.

Guerrero, Gomez. 2022. *RESOLUCION VICEMINESTERIAL N° 000252-2022-VMPCIC/MC.* Ministerio de Cultura de Perú. https://cdn.www.gob.pe/uploads/document/file/3845950/RVM%20252-2022-VMPCIC-MC.pdf.pdf?v=1668693714

Informe de la Autoridad Científica CITES Perú. 2013. "El San Pedro" o "Achuma": El género Echinopsis, Taxonomía, distribución y comercio." Ministero del Ambiente de Perú. https://www.minam.gob.pe/diversidadbiologica/wp-content/uploads/sites/21/2014/02/El-San-Pedro-o-Achuma-g%C3%A9nero-Echinopsis.-Taxonom%C3%ADa-disribuci%C3%B3n-y-Comercio.pdf.

Ostolaza, Carlos, Aldo Ceroni, Natalia Calderón, Esther Alvarez, Jonatan Zapata, Johanna Cortéz, and Lourdes Salinas. 2006. "Cacti of the Pativilca river basin, Lima, Peru." *Cactus World.* 117-128.

Ostolaza, Carlos, Aldo Ceroni, Jonatan Zapata, Johanna Cortéz, Lourdes Salinas, and Emilia García. 2007. "Cacti of the Cañete river basin, Lima, Peru: a research and conservation study." *Cactus World* 25, no. 4: 215-226.

Shakti, Yogini. December 2021. Post on the Facebook page "Spirit Events Sacred Valley."

Sharon, Douglas G., and Christopher B. Donnan. 1977. "The magic cactus: Ethnoarchaeological continuity in Peru." *Archaeology New York, NY* 30, no. 6: 374-381.

Sharon, Douglas. 2015. *Wizard of the four winds: A shaman's story, 2nd Ed.* The Free Press.

Vera Chilcon, Lenin Joel. 2016. "Estado de conservación de las poblaciones de trichocereus pachanoi, 'San Pedro,' en el refugio de vida silvestre Laquipampa, 2015." Universidad de Lambayeque.

The Harpy's Gift and the Jaguar's Curse: Mysteries from the Ethnobotany of Matsigenka Hunting Medicines in the Peruvian Amazon

Glenn H. Shepard Jr., PhD

Ethnobotanist | Medical anthropologist | Filmmaker | Museu Paraense Emilio Goeldi, Brazil

"I will discuss the case of Pascual, an old friend who described to me in horror how his use of Brunfelsia as a youth began turning him into a jaguar in his old age, and explore the concept of jaguar transformation more generally among the Matsigenka." —Glenn Shepard

In this essay Dr Glenn Shepard shares fascinating and intimate insights into the world of the Matsigenka people, illuminating many mysteries yet to be solved. This piece exemplifies the wonder, curiosity and awe that ethnobotany can hold as well as the abundance that we have to learn from different societies and people.

INTRODUCTION: A MYSTERY TALE

A 400 year-old English manor like St. Giles House is sure to inspire a sense of mystery, especially a murder mystery in the spirit of Agatha Christie: "Which ethnobotanist put foxglove from the garden into the Lion's Mane chai that killed the victim right after coffee break?..." Moreover, a sense of mystery is important to keep alive the curiosity that drives scientific inquiry. With such a distinguished group of presenters at ESPD55 like Dennis McKenna, Wade Davis, Mark Plotkin, Mark Merlin, Elaine Elisabetsky, Paul Stamets and others—formative figures in the disciplines of ethnopharmacology and ethnobotany—some younger people might feel a bit intimidated, as if all the most significant work has already been done, and there is nothing new left to discover. Therefore, in this paper I focus on a number of mysteries from my own research into the ethnobotany and ethnopharmacology of the Matsigenka people of the Peruvian Amazon, in the hopes of inspiring the next generation of ethnobotanists, ethnopharmacologists and anthropologists.

I have carried out fieldwork with the Matsigenka people of southern Peru for over 35 years. My initial research focused on ethnobotany, ethnoecology, shamanism, traditional medicine, grief and mourning and sensory anthropology (Shepard 1998a; Shepard 1999a, 1999b; Shepard et al. 2001; Shepard 2002a, 2002b; Shepard 2004). Later, I became involved in applied projects such as hunting management, resource sustainability and community-based ecotourism

(Ohl-Schacherer et al. 2007; Ohl-Schacherer et al. 2008; Shepard et al. 2010; Shepard et al. 2012). More recently, I have been involved in water, health and sanitation projects in several Matsigenka communities (Shepard 2018a). And yet as a result of a recent research breakthrough at the Field Museum of Natural History in Chicago (Thomas et al. 2021), I was drawn back into the mysteries of Matsigenka ethnobotany.

MYSTERY NO.1: THE MANU MYSTERY PLANT

The first mystery goes back many years. I spent January of 1997 identifying my plant collections from Peru at the Field Museum, and in the process nearly freezing to death in a winter blizzard.

"It was January in Chicago and I was spending the month at the Field Museum to identify a batch of plant specimens from the Peruvian Amazon. No tropical flower could have suffered as much from the contrast in climate as I did" (Shepard 2013).

There was one plant in particular that I was having trouble identifying. It is a very bitter plant highly valued by Matsigenka men as a purgative for improving hunting aim and skill. The plant is known in Matsigenka as *onya*, apparently a loan word from Spanish *uña* meaning "fingernail" due to the plant's long, conspicuous stipules. In addition to the distinctive stipules, the plant has an unusual orange-red "Japanese lantern" fruit capsule somewhat like *Physalis* (ground cherry). I had several complete, fertile collections but simply could not identify it, not even to the level of family. So, with tail between my legs, I went humbly to the world-renowned Field Museum botanist, Robin Foster, and said, "I know it's probably really obvious, but I just can't figure out what this is." But rather than laughing off my novice botanical skills, Robin got an awed look in his eye and said, "Aah! The mystery plant!. We have been collecting it for twenty years and haven't yet even identified it to family." With my faith in my botanical identification skills slightly bolstered, and my sense of mystery fully awakened (see Shepard 2013 for more on that story…) I put a question mark in my plant database where the botanical name should go and continued with my herbarium work.

Fast forward to October 2021, when after over fifty years of head-scratching, a team of tropical botanists lead by Robin Foster finally applied modern gene sequencing techniques and discovered that the "Manu mystery plant" in fact belonged to a previously unknown *genus* within the family of Picramniaceae (formally Simaroubaceae). The name of the new genus, *Aenigmanu*, means literally "Manu mystery," while the species name, *A. alvareziae* recognizes the Peruvian botanist who first collected it. In today's hyper-connected world, the discovery inevitably spawned dozens of sensational headlines on news sites throughout the world: "Solving decades-long mystery…", "Mystery plant finally declared a new species…" As I read through the reprint that Foster's team sent me, I found a short paragraph tucked away towards the end of the main text (Thomas et al. 2021, 1245):

"*Ethnobotany*—Reported to be used as an emetic hunting medicine by the Matsigenka (G. Shepard, pers. comm.). Common name (Matsigenka): 'Onya' (G. Shepard 1152)."

As is often the case, such "new discoveries" are not actually "new" so much as "new to science," preceded as they are by indigenous people's centuries-old knowledge and wisdom. It is also important to point out that *onya*, recently baptized as *Aenigmanu alvareziae*, is not technically a psychedelic plant, but rather an emetic, used by hunters to rid their bodies of impurities. Why, then, am I talking about an emetic plant in a conference dedicated to psychedelics? The fact is, the Matsigenka have no word that corresponds exactly to the Western concept of "psychedelic" or "psychoactive". The closest word in Matsigenka to this concept is *kepigari*, which is used to refer to all narcotic and psychoactive plants and substances. The word comes from the verbal root, *pega-* which in its most basic sense means to return, to turn around, or to spin on an axis: to go around and come back. By extension, and by adding different suffixes and prefixes, this root can be used refer to feelings of dizziness, nausea, intoxication and poison (Shepard 1998a, 2018b).

Thus, Matsigenka use the term *kepigari* to refer to shamanic hallucinogens and narcotics like ayahuasca, tobacco and *Brugmansia*, plants that literally make one dizzy, nauseous, and intoxicated. However, in the Matsigenka usage, the psychoactive effects of such substances are not separate from other forms of physiological toxicity such as purging, emetics and causticity. Thus *kepigari* can also be used to refer to emetic and purgative hunting medicines like *onya* as well as to deadly toxins like barbasco (*Lonchocarpus*) fish poison. In the West we use terms like hallucinogenic, psychedelic, psychoactive or entheogen which reinforce the mind-body duality which is foundational to the rationalistic, Cartesian scientific worldview. Psychonauts often want to control, minimize, or entirely eliminate "side effects" like physical nausea from the psychedelic experience. But for the Matsigenka, there is no such a thing as "side effects": the unpleasant effects of psychoactive plants like ayahuasca, tobacco and others are part and parcel of their intoxicating and curative power of *kepigari*: the poison and the medicine are one and the same.

In this sense, Matsigenka hunting medicines are the epitome of *kepigari*, since they include toxic, emetic, purgative and psychoactive plants that have the explicit purpose of cleaning out physical impurities from the hunter's body while putting the hunter into contact with the spiritual beings who control access to game animals. Typically, in the ethnobotanical literature such practices are referred to as "hunting charms" or "hunting magic." However, as Arthur Clarke once said, magic is just another word for technology. Matsigenka hunting plants are not magic or superstitious charms, but rather symbolically and pharmacologically charged medicines and biocultural technologies in the full sense of the word.

THE MATSIGENKA OF MANU BIOSPHERE RESERVE

The Matsigenka people speak a language belonging to the Arawakan family, the largest language family in South America. The extension of Arawakan languages in pre-colonial times reached from the Caribbean and possibly southern Florida all the way to southern Brazil. Indeed, the geographical range of the Arawakan language family is larger than the Inca empire (Aikhenvald 2012). The Matsigenka are the largest indigenous group of the Madre de Dios and Urubamba river region, a vast extent of nearly 10 million hectares of high-value tropical rainforest surrounding the core area of Manu Biosphere Reserve and National Park. Manu was Peru's first national park, established in 1973. Since then, the core area of Manu Park was integrated into a number of buffer zones into Manu Biosphere Reserve totaling about 1.8 million hectares, and recognized as a UNESCO world heritage site. Manu is a global biodiversity hotspot, famous for containing nearly 10% of Earth's total species diversity of birds (Terborgh et al. 1990; Beaudrot et al. 2016). Yet the Manu region is also a hotspot of linguistic and cultural diversity, including the Matsigenka, Yine, Nahua, Wachiperi, Amarakeri as well as isolated populations of Mashco-Piro and Nanti (Shepard et al. 2010).

Today, Manu is considered a global biodiversity refuge, sometimes referred to as a "Living Eden." However, in the past Manu was "ground zero" for one of the most notorious sites of rubber extraction in the Amazon, led by the infamous "King of Rubber" Carlos Fermin Fitzcarraldo. The isthmus of Fitzcarraldo, where he carried his legendary boat from one watershed into the other to open this inaccessible region to rubber extraction, is located at the headwaters of the Manu river. The original indigenous inhabitants of the Manu river were massacred, enslaved or died of diseases brought by the rubber tappers. The current Matsigenka population of Manu Biosphere Reserve are composed mostly of family groups that fled the violence of the Rubber Boom towards the Manu headwaters. These scattered groups were contacted by missionaries of the Summer Institute of Linguistics in the 1960s and settled in the village of Tayakome. With the establishment of Manu National Park in 1973, the missionaries were expelled from Tayakome, relocating their activities and about half of the population of Tayakome to the adjacent Camisea river outside of park boundaries (see Shepard et al. 2010 for a more detailed history).

Peruvian legislation permits the original indigenous habitants to continue residing in national parks, however they are subject to numerous restrictions. For example, the Matsigenka people residing in the two recognized native communities inside the restricted zone of Manu National Park are not allowed to cut lumber for sale or extract other resources commercially, and are prohibited from using firearms. For this reason, the Matsigenka still hunt mostly with bow and arrows through the present. This is one of the last regions in the Amazon where the indigenous population still hunts with traditional technology, besides isolated communities. For this reason, the Matsigenka maintain a wealth of traditional hunting practices and medicines (Shepard 2002b; Shepard et al. 2012).

MATSIGENKA HUNTING MEDICINES

Hunting plants are a significant aspect of the Matsigenka pharmacopoeia, constituting about 25% of the over 350 medicinal plant species I have collected in multiple communities (Shepard 1999a, 2002b). Collectively, these plants are known as *kovintsari inchashi*, "plants for good aim." Hunting is an exclusively male activity among the Matsigenka, and hunting medicines are considered a domain of male ethnobotanical knowledge. Hunting medicines were taught to Matsigenka shamans by the harpy eagle, providing them with good eyesight like eagles. Hunting medicines include emetic, purgative, narcotic and psychoactive plants that are used to improve men's ability to hunt game animals. Other plants in the category of "good aim medicine" are administered as eye drops, which cause a few minutes of intense stinging, like chili pepper or lemon juice squirted in the eye. After the stinging wears off, this treatment improves aim and visual acuity when hunting. The category of eyedrop plants is referred to as *kaokirontsi*, literally "bathing the liquid surface of the eye". The category includes several species of the genus *Psychotria* in the Rubiaceae family, related to *chacruna*, the DMT-containing plant that is mixed with ayahuasca vine to potentiate the psychoactive brew. The Rubiaceae is also the family of coffee and ipecac, and is generally known to be rich in alkaloids. Given the bioactive properties known from botanical groups like *Psychotria*, it seems likely that some of these plants may in fact increase visual acuity or manual dexterity (Shepard 1998b, 2011).

The category of Matsigenka hunting plants also includes emetic and purgative plants, like *onya* (*Aenigmanu*) as discussed above. (Note: although *Phyllomedusa* frogs occur in the region, the Matsigenka do not use their toxic secretions as a purgative/emetic stimulant for hunting, as found in nearby regions of the Peruvian and Brazilian Amazon; see Daly et al. 1992; Milton 1994). Emetic and purgative plants, typically described as "bitter" (*kepishiri*), "astringent" (*tineni*) or "pungent/painful" (*katsi*) help clean the body of impurities that interfere with the hunter's relationship with the spirit beings who control access to game animals. These spirit beings are known as the *Saankariite* (also written *Saangariite*), a word derived from the verbal root *saanka-* which refers to purity, cleansing, invisibility and erasure. *Saankariite* has been translated as "pure" or "invisible ones" (Rosengren 1998; Shepard 1999b, 2018b), or "invisible beings, good spirits, angels" (Snell et al. 2011). However, there are some additional nuances to the term that are discussed below.

The Saankariite raise the wild animals of the forest as pets, and release them for humans to hunt. For this reason, when a hunter wounds an animal with an arrow and the animal escapes and dies in the forest, the Saankariite smell the rotting carcass and get upset: "Who is wasting our bounty and letting it rot in the forest?". Also, if a hunter's wife is inattentive while cooking a pot of meat and lets the pot boil over, the foam that spills into the fire sends the odor of burnt meat wafting into the forest, which likewise angers the Saankariite. Menstrual blood has a smell described as being like rotten blood or carrion that is also offensive to the Saankariite. So, if a hunter is wasteful in his hunting practice, if his wife allows food to boil over or burn, or if the hunter has any contact with a menstruating woman, the smell of burnt or rotten meat or blood infuses the hunter's body. The Saankariite smell this odor from a distance and hide the game animals from him, so he won't even see any animals on the hunt. Thus, the question of "improving ones aim" goes beyond just good vision and manual dexterity, encompassing the spiritual dimension of human relationships with the natural and supernatural world.

A Matsigenka hunter "loses his aim" when his body becomes infused with the odor of carrion, burnt meat and rotten blood, a condition which leads him to become possessed with the "vulture spirit." Purgative and emetic plants serve to cleanse the body/soul of the carrion odor and vulture spirit that makes the Saankariite hide game animals from the hunter. Thus, hunting medicines like *onya* act to physically remove offensive odors, substances and spiritual effects from the body. Psychoactive plants are also important as hunting medicines among the Matsigenka, providing direct contact with the Saankariite in order to negotiate "deals" and exchanges for access to game animals and esoteric knowledge to improve hunting skills.

While 25% of Matsigenka medicinal plants consist of hunting medicines, another 25% are plants used by women to protect their children, especially newborn babies, from the vengeful attacks of game animals that have been killed by their husbands. Thus, the Matsigenka pharmacopoeia reflects a clear principle of gender balance and complementarity (Shepard 2002b). When a woman's husband kills an animal, that animal's spirit becomes angry and comes back to attack his child. The vengeful animal spirit manifests itself as a cloud of musky odor, like the gamey, garlicky odor of animal scent glands. This musky animal spirit frightens the baby, making it cry at night and become afflicted with vomiting, diarrhea or skin rashes. The Matsigenka word for this kind of affliction is *pugasetagantsi*, typically translated into local Spanish as *cutipa*, referring to revenge, returning an insult or "payback" for an act of aggression (Izquierdo et al. 2008).

To protect their children, Matsigenka women bathe newborn babies several times a day with a mixture of warm, fragrant herbs kept in a small clay pot, known as *ogaahare* ('her bathing pot'). The plants in this category are referred to generally as *okaatira ananeki* ('used by women to bathe babies'), and most are fragrant, including many species of the Myrtaceae, the family of guava and *Eucalyptus*, noted for their citrusy-fragrant leaves. The pleasant odor of these plants creates a fragrant force-field around the child that keeps the musky, pathogenic odor of game animal spirits at bay. Some of the plants included in this category have a sticky texture, which serves to adhere the fragrant herbal odor to the child's skin to ensure protection throughout the day and night.

The ethnobotany surrounding Matsigenka hunting practices thus incorporates the idea of gender complementarity in traditional knowledge while revealing an ecological feedback loop between humans, animals and spirit beings where the roles of predator and prey can sometimes become reversed. These complex interactions are expressed and transmitted through specific sensory experiences (taste, odor, texture, etc.), forming what I have described as a "sensory ecology" that integrates social, phytochemical and cosmological domains (Shepard 2004; Daly & Shepard 2019; Shepard & Daly 2022).

MYSTERY NO.2: 'TIS THE SEASON FOR AYAHUASCA

Ayahuasca, the psychoactive plant mixture used widely in Amazonian shamanism, is an especially important hunting medicine for the Matsigenka. The Peruvian word "ayahuasca" appears to be derived from Quechua language terms meaning "vine of the soul" or "vine of the spirits." The Matsigenka word is more to the point: *kamarampi* in Matsigenka means literally "vomiting medicine". The Matsigenka recognize at least eight wild and cultivated varieties of ayahuasca, most of which correspond to the botanical species *Banisteriopsis caapi*. They tend not to use the wild varieties in preparing the ayahuasca brew, preferring to use several cultivated varieties that are distinguished according to features such as vine and flower color, stem texture and variations in psychoactive and physiological effects. The Matsigenka prefer to harvest ayahuasca by breaking it by hand, and many of their cultivars are brittle and easy to harvest without using knives or machetes. In the past, it was considered an affront to the ayahuasca plant to cut it with a metal tool, though more recently, some have adopted this practice.

Although the Matsigenka value ayahuasca for its healing powers in shamanistic rituals, the main reason Matsigenka men in Manu drink ayahuasca is to improve their hunting abilities: "I take ayahuasca, the next day I go out and kill two monkeys". True to its Matsigenka name, "vomiting medicine," ayahuasca can sometimes cause violent physical purging (see Shepard 2015a). This aspect of the ayahuasca experience is valued within the broader realm of hunting medicines as a way of ridding the hunter's body of the "carrion odor" and associated "vulture spirit" that takes away his hunting ability. However, the ayahuasca experience also provides the Matsigenka with direct access to the Saankariite spirits.

The Saankariite are conceived of as numerous, joyous people, sometimes described as being small or "like children" who reside in an unimaginably distant realm, either "far off in the forest" or "up in the sky," living an immortal life of abundance and festivity (Shepard 2002a, 2018b). During the use of ayahuasca and other psychoactive plants, the Saankariite come "down from the sky" or from their distant realms to interact with shamans directly. Matsigenka shamans are said to cultivate a kind of twin "brother" (*ige*) among the Saankariite, such that during the ayahuasca ceremony, the two switch places: the spirit twin comes to the mundane world in the shaman's body while the shaman goes to the distant, invisible spirit world to gain power and esoteric knowledge (Shepard 1998a, 2010). Indeed, even as the Matsigenka shaman begins to boil ayahuasca in preparation for the ceremony, the spirit twin also begins to boil ayahuasca in the distant realm of the Saankariite.

The Matsigenka of Manu Park only take ayahuasca in the rainy season, from November through to June. This also corresponds with the main hunting season, when many forest fruits become ripe and animals fatten up. Matsigenka rarely if ever hunt large monkey species like the spider and woolly monkey during the dry season, because during those months the animals are "skinny" (*imatsatake*) and have little body fat, and hence less nutritional value (Shepard 2002b). Matsigenka hunters will sometime admit, "If it were up to me, I'd go ahead and kill a spider monkey in the dry season. But then my wife would get angry with me, 'Why did you kill this skinny monkey?!'" The practice of avoiding certain game animal species represents a kind of "saving," holding off on killing the animal to obtain more return on the effort. It also allows vulnerable game animal species a seasonal respite from hunting, especially during the dry season when they are more vulnerable due to nutritional stress. Such dietary avoidances are part of a suite of traditional concepts and practices that contribute to biodiversity conservation on indigenous lands (Estrada et al. 2022).

There is thus a clear association between ayahuasca use and hunting practices, both at the cosmological level and as a seasonal activity. However, there is a deeper reason why the Matsigenka use ayahuasca in the rainy season, but avoid it during the dry season. The small tree known as *puigoro* in Matsigenka (*Vernonia* sp.) is a member of the dandelion family that is related to the coyote bush. It is the most important seasonal indicator for the dry season in the Matsigenka ethnoecological calendar (Shepard and Chicchon 2001). Like the dandelion, the flowering of *puigoro* is soon followed by the formation of seeds borne on fluffy, feathery white pappi that float great distances in the air. The flowering and seed dispersal of *puigoro* peaks during the height of the dry season in July-August. The Matsigenka say that once *puigoro* flowers, the ayahuasca drinking season is over until the flowers have all fallen and the seeds all floated away, just as the *kanai* plant (*Triplaris americana*) begins to flower in October to indicate the beginning of the rainy season. The reason ayahuasca should not be consumed while *puigoro* is in bloom is that the dry season corresponds with the time when the Matsigenka set fire to their swidden gardens to achieve maximum burn. The Matsigenka say that the Saankariite, like the Matsigenka, also burn their gardens during the dry season. Thus, if one were to drink ayahuasca during the dry season while *puigoro* is in flower, the spirit world would be full of fires from the burning of the Saankariite swiddens. The wandering soul of the ayahuasca user could get caught in the flames and perish.

One might be tempted to associate the seasonal avoidance of ayahuasca with any number of social, dietary or symbolic factors. However, on one occasion when my hosts had prepared ayahuasca in late May just as the *puigoro* flowers were beginning to sprout their first buds, all of those at the session sensed a mysterious, hot breeze gusting from the horizon in all directions, a frightening experience as if we were surrounded by forest fires on all sides. When it was over, several of those present commented that ayahuasca drinking was definitely over for the season, since we all sensed the burning Saankariite gardens. Is it possible that the ayahuasca vine or the *Psychotria* admixtures in the brew undergo slight changes in chemical composition during the dry season, leading to different visionary experiences? Or had we just witnessed the burning of Saankariite gardens in the spirit world?

I will leave this question to the mystics and ethnopharmacologists as mystery number two.

MYSTERY NO.3: THE ANT, THE SHAMAN AND THE SCIENTIST

Although the Matsigenka consider the invisible Saankariite beings to live in an unimaginably distant place, far off in the forest or up in the sky, their existence is manifested in a local ecological habitat (Shepard et al. 2001). The shrub *Cordia nodosa*, a bristly tropical shrub related to borage (*Borago officinalis*), forms a mutualistic relationship with several species of ants. The *Cordia* plant offers the ants protective corridors of bristly hairs along its stems and swollen branch nodes, which the ants hollow out to make nests. In return, the ants protect the host plants from other insect predators and in some cases, clear out competing vegetation, creating notable clearings in the understory that the Matsigenka refer to as *okarapage*, "large forest edge". Local Quechua-speaking colonists refer to these clearings as "Devil's gardens" (*supay chacra*).

The Matsigenka recognize this mutualistic relationship between ants and the *Cordia* shrub: the Matsigenka word for the plant is *matyagiroki*, which means "arboreal ant shrub," where *matyaniro* refers generically to a number of ant species frequently encountered on plants and leaves, like *Allomerus*, *Azteca*, *Myrmelachista* and the miniature fire ant, *Wassmania*. Ants and other insects involved in such mutualistic relationships with plants are referred to generically as *iriite*, "its (i.e., the plant's) larvae," a term otherwise reserved for the larval stage of insects, and generally implying multiplicity, i.e., not a single larva but a large, almost uncountable number. Note, that, although the Matsigenka generally refer to plants using the inanimate noun form beginning in *o-* or *a-* (see Shepard 2018b), plants involved in mutualistic relationships with ants and other insects are referred to using the animate form beginning in *i-* or *ir-* (*iriite*). Thus, plant-insect mutualistic relationships for the Matsigenka are couched in ontogenic vocabulary, implying that the host plant is a kind of adult or "parent" to the fragile, multitudinous larval insect "children."

For the Matsigenka, the clearings found around *Cordia* plants are manifestations in the mundane world of the distant villages and gardens of the Saankariite. As noted above, the verb root, *saanka-* in Matsigenka refers to purity, cleanliness, transparency, invisibility and erasure, as in such words as *saankiari* "clean, transparent water" or *saankagantsi*, "to clean, fade, erase, disappear." However, the word Saankariite also incorporates the noun suffix *-iite* noted above, referring to insect larvae and mutualistic plant-insect relations. Thus, a more literal translation of Saankariite might be "invisible larvae," making a direct allusion to plant-insect mutualisms. A looser translation might be "invisible swarm" or "invisible multitude," in reference to the multitudinous, almost uncountable nature of larvae or insects involved in mutualisms such as the ants associated with *Cordia* (Shepard and Daly 2023).

The Matsigenka ethnoecological term *okarapage*, "understory opening, clearing" is often intoned in shamanic songs sung during ayahuasca sessions, known as *marintagantsi*, in contrast to the mundane *matikagantsi* tunes sung during manioc beer drinking fests. Matsigenka ayahuasca songs are chanted using a number of unique melodies and are only sung during ayahuasca intoxication (see Shepard 1998a; 2004; 2015a). *Marintaganst*i comprise a unique poetic genre that includes a suite of stock phrases as well as improvised lines that stimulate a call and response chorus between the lead singer and multiple other participants. The songs invoke the Saankariite and their distant realms, describe the giddy sensations of ecstasy, comment on the acquisition and transmission of ancient and esoteric knowledge, and depict the kaleidoscopic ayahuasca visions in poetic language as the blooming of colorful flowers. Matsigenka ayahuasca songs also include much archaic vocabulary, onomatopoeia, unique verb suffixes not used in other contexts and other non-ordinary language, making them difficult if not impossible to translate. Despite the presence of recognizable poetic language, much of the power of the Matsigenka ayahuasca songs is transmitted directly through their acoustic properties, rather than through normal linguistic signs (Shepard 2004). The Matsigenka say that ayahuasca songs come directly from the Saankariite, which is why they are difficult to remember in ordinary states of consciousness.

During the ayahuasca trance, Matsigenka shamans also use a musical bow known as *pegompi*, which resembles a one-string violin (Shepard 2015b). The word *pegompi* literally means "instrument of transformation," derived from the verbal root *pega-* which means to transform or to vanish. The Matsigenka say that the pegompi speaks the language of the Saankariite, a musical form of communication similar to bird songs that is harmonious and well-tuned (*poima*) with a "beautiful sound or odor" (*kametienka*). Like ayahuasca songs, the *pegompi* communicate with and call to the Saankariite by means of sounds that don't directly translate into language. By playing the pegompi and chanting ayahuasca songs, the Matsigenka call to the Saankariite in their distant realm and bring them close by, until the Saankariite themselves become part of the multivocal chorus of chanting.

Today, the Matsigenka mostly consume ayahuasca outdoors, far from any fires or artificial lights, or indoors in closed huts. However, in the past, Matsigenka shamans and their apprentices used to come to *Cordia* clearings to consume powerful psychoactive preparations such as tobacco paste, ayahuasca (*Banisteriopsis*), or the *Datura*-like toé (*Brugmansia*; Shepard 1998b, 2017). With the aid of such visionary plants, the shaman perceives the true nature of these mundane forest clearings: they are the villages and swidden gardens of the multitudinous, capricious, powerful but otherwise invisible Saankariite, who are unimaginably distant and inaccessible under ordinary states of consciousness. While in trance, the shaman enters the invisible village and develops an ongoing relationship with a spirit "brother" (*ige*) among the *Saankariite*, who can provide him or her with esoteric knowledge, news from distant places, healing power, artistic inspiration, auspicious hunting and even novel varieties of food crops or medicinal plants from their gardens (Shepard 1999b).

In 1996, Harvard PhD candidate Douglas Yu, then a student of the world-famous entomologist E.O. Wilson, visited me in the Matsigenka community of Yomibato to investigate the *Cordia*-ant colonies there as part of his doctoral thesis. Together with Matsigenka shaman Mariano Vicente, we went to a large *Cordia* clearing. Mariano explained his perspective on the ant-plant symbiosis and the shamanic significance of these clearings as reflections of Saankariite villages. As proof of this observation, Mariano pointed to raised scars around the trunk of a tree near the edge of the clearing and said, "See? These are the fire-marks from when the *Saankariite* burn their gardens. When the dry season comes, they burn their swidden gardens just like us."

Yu noticed that dozens of trees around this large stand of *Cordia* were pocked with similar scars. Intrigued, he cut into these formations with his pruning shears and found nests teeming with *Myrmelachista* worker ants that appeared to be galling the trunks to create additional housing, thus ensuring colony longevity. As detailed in *American Naturalist* (Edwards et al. 2009), this was the first recorded example of ants galling plants, thus resuscitating a pet theory of Richard Spruce's that Alfred Russel Wallace and later naturalists had rejected. This galling and colony-forming behavior, unique to *Myrmelachista*, was crucial in helping Yu fully characterize the ecological conditions shaping the mutualistic niche shared by three competing ant species. A long-standing ecological mystery, dating back to the early days of Amazonian botany and ecological science itself, was resolved thanks to the insights of a Matsigenka shaman.

In addition to this direct contribution to a scientific discovery, the striking synergies between scientific knowledge about the *Cordia* mutualism and Matsigenka concepts about an "invisible swarm" of multitudinous spirits living in vast villages suggests a fractal relationship between shamanic knowledge and observable ecological processes. Such shamanic observations are not merely abstract symbols or spiritual metaphors, but rather often relate to the living world as through a cosmological microscope, drawing non-arbitrary connections between microcosm and macrocosm, and relating ecological to cosmological processes. By holding the scientific perspective in one eye and the cosmological perspective in the other, we can imagine bringing both views into overlapping focus onto a novel, stereoscopic vista, and thus unveil a richer, more comprehensive and interesting landscape, somewhat analogous to what Ruth Ginsberg (1995) describes as the "parallax effect" in indigenous cinema (see Shepard & Daly 2023).

MYSTERY NO.4: CONFESSION OF A WERE-JAGUAR

Among the most important hunting medicines of the Matsigenka is a group of closely related species of *Brunfelsia*. Like *Datura*, *Brugmansia* and other "nightshades" (Shepard 2017), *Brunfelsia* belongs to the Solanaceae and is known to contain highly potent tropane alkaloids. It is known in Peruvian Spanish as *chirisanango*, based on a Quechua expression meaning "cold, chills." The name refers to the unusual perceptual effects caused by consuming the plant, resulting in a "pins and needles" tingling sensation in the extremities. At higher doses, the plant causes chills throughout the entire body and even convulsions. *Brunfelsia* is widely used in the Peruvian Amazon to treat arthritic and rheumatic pains. The Matsigenka say the plant was brought to them in ancient times by the harpy eagle as a powerful hunting medicine (Shepard 1998b, 2002b, 2011). Known for its anti-inflammatory properties, the plant also causes visions. To ensure their early development as hunters, young Matsigenka men often take a large dose of *Brunfelsia* and spend several days intoxicated and unable to walk due to the powerful tingling, shivering sensation. The Matsigenka say this tingling sensation in the fingers and feet, referred to with the onomatopoeic expression *tseki-tseki-tseki-tseki*, is an empirical expression of the harpy eagle's soul "infusing" or "contaminating" (*okitsirinkake*) the man's body.

Timothy Plowman's (1998) pioneering work on the taxonomy of the genus distinguished a number of species, and these seem to correspond in part with a number of distinctive folk species recognized by the Matsigenka including *sankenke*, *oshetopari* (literally "spider monkey root"), *pakitsapari* ("harpy eagle root"), *shimakoa* ("fish potion"), and *kaviniri*. I have collected several specimens of the first four folk species, however the final folk species *kaviniri* I have never collected, in part because the Matsigenka say it grows farther upriver in the highlands, and partly because they consider it to be an extremely dangerous plant, even to touch. Unlike the other folk species of *Brunfelsia*, which were brought to humanity by the harpy eagle, *kaviniri* belongs to the jaguar. Like the other species, *kaviniri* can turn a man into an excellent hunter, however he becomes such a good hunter that he also turns into a jaguar and begins killing and eating his fellow Matsigenka.

These observations about *kaviniri* are reinforced by the entry in Betty Snell's (Snell et al. 2011) Matsigenka dictionary:

> "Where the plant abounds, because it always grows in clusters, jaguars also abound... It is used to cure many illnesses, especially severe ones, but it must be used with great caution. In the visions it provokes, mostly jaguars are seen, and traditionally there were men who took it to turn themselves into jaguars. Many affirmed that when used frequently, the user's soul turns into a jaguar while asleep and goes out to attack people."

In 2013 I came face to face with a confessed were-jaguar. Pascual was a dear friend of mine from Tayakome who always brought me the most delicious pineapples. He was also a great storyteller and singer, with a gentle voice that was always on the verge of breaking into laughter. However, in his old age, he began turning into a jaguar. Around 2011, he began losing weight, suffered from disturbing dreams and, according to his wife, snored loudly in fits that sounded like a jaguar grunting. At the same time, a large jaguar began to appear on the path near his house, killing chickens and dogs.

Whenever a jaguar appears near a village, the Matsigenka always associate it with some old person who is turning into a jaguar (Shepard 2014). Normal jaguars live far away in the forest and hunt peccaries, but were-jaguars, humans who begin to "grow fur" (*maetagantsi*) and turn into jaguars, walk unafraid on paths near the village and kill dogs, chickens, and even children or adult people (Marris 2015). The verb *maetagantsi* means literally means "to grow fur," and is used to refer to people who are undergoing the process of jaguar transformation. The implication, well established in Amazonian conceptions about the body, is that the biological outer form of different beings can change and transform, while the underlying human essence remains the same (Viveiros de Castro 2004). Whereas jaguar transformation is considered by some indigenous societies to be a sign of great shamanic power, the Matsigenka consider it to be a curse, caused by excessive use of the *kaviniri* hunting medicine, among other factors (Shepard 2014).

Everyone in the village was talking about how Pascual was turning into a jaguar. I went to talk to him about it, and he admitted as much to me. He said:

"When I was young, they gave me *kaviniri* to drink. They said it would make me a great hunter. It did make me a great hunter. But no one warned me that in my old age, I would turn into a jaguar. Now I am an old man and have begun to grow fur. I am afraid to go to sleep at night, I have bad dreams. My wife is afraid to sleep next to me, she says I make jaguar noises. A jaguar has appeared in the village, and everyone knows it is me. I have already killed several chickens. I am afraid I'll kill my own grandchildren!"

In the neighboring village of Yomibato, a jaguar killed seven dogs, mauled two adults, and killed one child between 2014 and 2015. Everyone knew it was Pascual. He sought treatment from a local shaman during this time, who among other interventions had him eat honey. Since a jaguar's diet consists of raw flesh and blood, honey represents an entirely different kind of food, pushing Pascual towards more wholesome appetites. Pascual, who always loved to make wooden objects like oars, had carved dozens of small charms out of cedar wood known as *puirotyaki*, named after a kind of beetle (*puiro*) that is considered a good luck charm for children. Perhaps he thought the *puirotyaki* charms could help keep the jaguar transformation sickness at bay.

He achieved a temporary relief of his symptoms, but they came back after a time and he finally passed away in 2015. Like all people who die deaths considered uncanny, his family placed *taviri*, a tar-like resin made of stingless beeswax and sticky tree resin, into his nostrils before he was buried, in the hopes that the jaguar (which breathes through its nostrils) would smother when trying to come out of his dead body (Shepard 2002a). All of his possessions, including a huge collection of delicately carved *puirotyaki* charms, were buried with him, in the fear that any material possessions would attract the jaguar.

MYSTERY NO.5: CATTLE STAGGERS, ST. ANTHONY'S FIRE AND THE GINSENG OF THE AMAZON

Perhaps the most important category of hunting medicines, and indeed the most important medicinal plants in all the Matsigenka pharmacopeia, are the cultivated sedges (*Cyperus* spp.), known as *ivenkiki* in Matsigenka and *piri-piri* in Peruvian Spanish. Medicinal sedges used as hunting medicines include a large number of cultivated varieties that are difficult to tell apart from one another. Hunting sedge varieties are named after specific game animal species, as well as several fish species. When the man is in the forest about to shoot an arrow at the animal, he chews the dried sedge root (which has a bitter, aromatic flavor somewhat reminiscent of ginger and turmeric), then rubs the masticated root on his arms, hands, and on the bow and arrow. He will sometimes speak a quiet exhortation to the arrow to "Fly straight, straight into the monkey's heart!" (Shepard 1998b, 2011).

Again, reflecting the gender balance inherent in the Matsigenka pharmacopoeia, for nearly each named sedge variety used by men to improve their aim for specific game animal, there is also a named sedge variety used by women to protect their newborn children from the revenge inflicted by that animal's vengeful spirit. There are also dozens of other sedge varieties used for a wide range of medicinal and other cultural uses: to treat snakebites, to staunch arrow wounds, to treat headaches, to eliminate nightmares, to treat dizziness or insanity, to resolve conflicts between quarreling spouses, to improve a woman's ability to spin and weave cotton, to improve a person's singing abilities, and to calm down the behavior of a belligerent drunk. One dangerous variety is said to cause permanent madness. There is even the variety *sorarovenki* "solider sedge," that can be used to slip through military or police check points with being searched. Other varieties, cultivated exclusively by women, are involved in fertility, birthing and birth control: to ease a difficult childbirth, to avoid getting pregnant, to improve fertility, or to never get pregnant again (Shepard 1998b, 2011). *Tsoronivenki*, "rabbit sedge" is a wild variety related to the cultivated sedges that is said to cause a couple to have many babies with minimal time between pregnancies, like rabbits.

The sedges belong to the Cyperaceae, the same family as papyrus, used to make paper. The Cyperaceae is one of the botanical families with the lowest incidence of medicinal uses around the world, except in the Amazon, where cultivated sedges are widely used for any number of medicinal and cultural purposes (Tournon 1984; Milliken et al. 1999; Kujawska 2020; Kuijper 2021). How is it possible that a group of plants that mostly belong to the same botanical species is used to treat so many different illnesses and conditions? Their use as "charms" for hunting and other cultural uses typically makes ethnobotanists suspicious that such uses are merely symbolic or superstitious. However, research carried out by pioneering botanist Timothy Plowman and sedge expert Keith Clay revealed that cultivated sedges from the Amazon are in fact loaded with multiple ergot alkaloids, related to the fungus-derived toxins that first gave rise to LSD (Plowman et al. 1990). These sedges, like ergot-infested rye grains, are infected with a fungus belonging to the Claviceptaceae or "club-foot fungus" family. The fungus, known as *Balansia cyperii*, apparently confers protection against pathogens. As with ergot, *Balansia* infuses the infected plant tissues with toxic ergot-related chemicals, leading to the phenomenon known as "cattle staggers" in some ranching regions: cows eat infected sedge plants (or "nut grass") and become inebriated, sometimes falling and breaking a leg or drowning.

It appears that Indigenous Peoples across the Amazon have taken advantage of this naturally occurring fungal infection in sedges and used selective breeding to greatly increase the quantities of fungus and ergot alkaloids in the plants, to the point where the fungus destroys the flowers and fruit of the plant, making it entirely dependent on human cultivation. Indeed, the Matsigenka term for sedges, *ivenkiki*, is derived from the noun root *penki-* which refers to button-like sprouts. In place of a normal flower, fungus-infected sedges produce a greyish-white button (*openki*), rather like the texture and color of a small mushroom.

In light of this information, many Matsigenka medicinal uses of sedges are highly congruent with the physiological activity of ergot alkaloids, known to cause constriction of blood vessels (vasodilation), uterine contractions and psychoactive effects. Traditional uses for snakebite, arrow wounds and headaches are clearly related to the vasoconstrictive effects of ergot alkaloids. The vasoconstriction caused by consuming ergot-infected rye in the Middle Ages led to gangrene of the extremities, once referred to as "St. Anthony's fire." To this day, ergot is used in Western pharmaceutical medicine to treat migraines. Diverse Matsigenka uses associated with birthing and birth control also appear related to the effects of ergot on uterine contractions: since at least the 16th century, ergot has been used to facilitate childbirth or, in larger doses, to induce abortions (Hoffman 1978). Finally, diverse "magical" or "charm" uses, including hunting medicines as well as to help control emotions or improve other cultural abilities, might be related to the psychoactive and mood-altering effects of ergot alkaloids. These observations are not meant to "explain away" the complex understandings and practices around sedges found among the Matsigenka and numerous other Indigenous Peoples of the Amazon. However, these findings are certainly relevant in the "parallax" view suggested above for approaching the synergy between indigenous and scientific knowledge frames (Shepard & Daly 2023).

The widespread use of cultivated sedges by the Matsigenka and other Indigenous Peoples throughout the Amazon as a kind of panacea for multiple medicinal uses has led me to call it the "ginseng of the Amazon" (Shepard 2011). However, unlike ginseng, there is surprisingly little pharmacological or ethnobotanical research on sedges, although a number of recent anthropological studies have examined indigenous uses and understandings of these fascinating plants (Kujawska 2020; Kuijper 2021). I am extremely interested in pursuing additional research focusing on the multiple mysteries around the medicinal sedges of the Amazon, including domestication history, cultivation practices, the pharmacological properties of different cultivars and diverse indigenous conceptions about this extraordinary plant-fungus symbiosis.

THE NEXT MYSTERY: *VOYRIA*

Among the medicines used by Matsigenka hunters to improve their aim, I documented the tiny parasitic flower *Voyria*, which belongs to the African violet family. The delicate flowers, which litter the understory in golden-yellow clusters like fallen stars, have no leaves and produce no chlorophyll, but instead derive nutrients from neighboring plant roots. The Matsigenka gather a few *Voyria* flowers, which they call *turuivanto*, and crush them within a clean plant leaf and put a few drops in each eye. Like other Matsigenka eyedrop medicines (*kaokirontsi*), the treatment produces a few minutes of intense stinging in the eyes. Afterwards, the Matsigenka claim the benefit of increased visual acuity, better aim as well as the favor of the Saankariite in being able to see game animals hidden in the forest. There is a beautiful scene in the Discovery Channel documentary *The Spirit Hunters** showing Matsigenka shaman Mariano Vicente gathering and applying *Voyria* to the eyes of his grandson and to myself.

Though I was intrigued by the beautiful, delicate *Voyria* flowers, I never thought much again about this medicinal use until many years later, as I was reading Merlin Sheldrake's (2020) book *Entangled Life*. There, he discusses his research in Panama into the fungal endophytes involved in the nutrient exchange between *Voyria tenella*, a violet-flowered species that occurs in Central America, and adjacent plant roots. Might compounds produced through fungal endophytes also be involved in Matsigenka uses of *Voyria* flowers as hunting medicines,

---

* Discovery Channel documentary *The Spirit Hunters* (https://vimeo.com/11124916)

as appears to be the case for medicinal sedges? This is the next mystery I hope to explore, hopefully in collaboration with Merlin and so many other enthusiastic colleagues that I have met through the ESPD initiative.

Building on the contributions of pioneering ethnobotanists and ethnopharmacologists, many of whom were gathered at ESPD55, there is still so much work to be done! As I have shown with a few examples drawn from my research into Matsigenka hunting medicines, indigenous knowledge opens possibilities for multiple avenues of interdisciplinary and intercultural research that is relevant to contemporary issues in science and the humanities. As global political and economic forces increasingly disrupt ecosystems around the world, and as Indigenous Peoples suffer violence and dislocation at the hand of these same forces, it is urgent that scientists and Indigenous Peoples find mutually respectful ways to work together. There is no question that indigenous knowledge and practices contribute to biodiversity conservation around the world (Estrada et al. 2020). Thus, safeguarding indigenous territories, languages, practices, knowledge systems and beliefs is essential to global biodiversity conservation and climate stability. Indigenous knowledge systems reveal a more integrated worldview of relationship and reciprocal exchange between the cultural, natural and supernatural spheres. Indigenous and scientific knowledge frames and political and economic worldviews are clearly very distinctive, and in many ways appear entirely incommensurate. And yet as I have shown here, a "parallax view" allows us to hold both perspectives in focus to reveal new insights, as well as ever-deeper mysteries (Daly & Shepard 2019; Shepard & Daly in press).

ACKNOWLEDGEMENTS

In the first place, I thank the members of the Native Communities of Tayakome and Yomibato in Manu Biosphere for putting up with my incessant questions for so many years. In particular, I wanted to thank Mariano Vicente Kicha, Alejandra Cashiri, Cornelio Pascal Coshani, Ismael Vicente Shamoco, Merino Matsipango Shubirerini, Alejandra Araos, Mateo Italiano Toribio, and Cesar Avanti for their invaluable contributions to this work over the years. I acknowledge funding from the Wenner Gren Foundation, the National Science Foundation, the Leverulme Fund and the Brazilian National Research Council (CNPq) throughout various phases of research. I am especially thankful to Dennis McKenna for inviting me to ESPD, and to Annette Badenhorst for her tireless work organizing the seminars. I thank Nick and Dina Ashley-Cooper for opening their gorgeous estate at St. Giles House to all of us for ESPD55, to the staff for making us all feel at home, and to the generous donors who made the event possible. Finally, I thank Synergetic Press for publishing the complete ESPD series in such a handsome set of volumes.

BIBLIOGRAPHY

Aikhenvald, A.Y., 2012. *The Languages of the Amazon*. Oxford University Press, Oxford.

Beaudrot, L., Ahumada, J. A., O'Brien, T., Alvarez-Loayza, P., Boekee, K., Campos-Arceiz, A., Eichberg, D., Espinosa, S., Fegraus, E., Fletcher, C., Gajapersad, K., Hallam, C., Hurtado, J., Jansen, P. A., Kumar, A., Larney, E., Lima, M. G. M., Mahony, C., Martin, E. H., ... Andelman, S. J., 2016. Standardized assessment of biodiversity trends in tropical forest protected areas: The end is not in sight. *PLoS Biology*, *14*, e1002357–e1002357.

Daly, J.W., Caceres, J., Moni, R.W., Gusovsky, F., Moos, M., Seamon, K.B., Milton, K., Meyers, C.W., 1992. Frog secretions and hunting magic in the upper Amazon: Identification of a peptide that interacts with an adenose receptor. *Proc. Natl. Acad. Sci.* 89, 10960–10963.

Daly, L. and Shepard Jr., G.H. 2019. Magic darts and messenger molecules: Toward a phytoethnography of Indigenous Amazonia. *Anthropol. Today, 35*, 13–17.

Edwards, D.P., Frederickson, M.E., Shepard Jr., G.H. and Yu, D.W., 2009. A plant needs ants like a dog needs fleas: *Myrmelachista schumanni* ants gall many tree species to create housing. *American Naturalist, 174*, 734-740.

Estrada, A., Garber, P. A., Gouveia, S., Fernández-Llamazares, Á., Ascensão, F., Fuentes, A., Garnett, S. T., Shaffer, C., Bicca-Marques, J., Fa, J. E., Hockings, K., Shanee, S., Johnson, S., Shepard Jr., G. H., Shanee, N., Golden, C. D., Cárdenas-Navarrete, A., Levey, D. R., Boonratana, R., Volampeno, S., et al., 2022. Global importance of Indigenous Peoples, their lands, and knowledge systems for saving the world's primates from extinction. *Science Advances, 8*, eabn2927.

Ginsburg, F., 1995. The parallax effect: The impact of aboriginal media on ethnographic film. *Vis. Anthropol. Rev. 11*, 64–76.

Hofmann A. (1978). Historical view on ergot alkaloids. Pharmacology, 16 Suppl 1, 1–11.

Izquierdo, C., Johnson, A., and Shepard Jr., G.H., 2008. Revenge, envy and cultural change in an Amazonian society. In S. Beckerman & P. Valentine (Eds.), *Revenge in the Cultures of Lowland South America*, University of Florida Press, Gainesville, pp. 162–186.

Kuijper, I., 2021. The changing role of waste (*Cyperus* spp.) in Shipibo-Konibo culture. M.Sc. thesis in Ethnobotany, School of Anthropology and Conservation, University of Kent, UK.

Kujawska, M., Zamudio, F., Albán-Castillo, J., and Sosnowska, J., 2020. The relationship between a western Amazonian society and domesticated sedges (*Cyperus* spp.). *Econ. Bot., 74*, 292–318.

Marris, E., 2016. The anthropologist and his old friend, who became a jaguar. *National Geographic*, May 18, 2016. https://www.nationalgeographic.com/culture/article/160518-manu-park-peru-matsigenka-tribe-death-jaguar

Milliken, W., Albert, B., Goodwin Gomez, G., 1999. *Yanomami: A forest people*. Royal Botanic Gardens, London.

Milton, K., 1994. No pain, no game. *Natural History, 9*, 44–51.

Ohl-Schacherer, J., Shepard, G. H. J., Kaplan, H., Peres, C. A., Levi, T., & Yu, D. W., 2007. The sustainability of subsistence hunting by Matsigenka native communities in Manu National Park, Peru. *Conserv. Biol., 21*, 1174–1185.

Ohl-Schacherer, J., Mannigel, E., Kirkby, C., Shepard Jr., G. H., & Yu, D. W., 2008. Indigenous ecotourism in the Amazon: A case study of Casa Matsiguenka in Manu National Park, Peru. *Environmental Conservation, 35*, 14-25.

Plowman, T., 1998. A revision of the South American species of Brunfelsia. *Fieldiana Botany New Series, 39*, 1-135.

Plowman, T. C., Leuchtmann, A., Blaney, C., and Clay, K., 1990. Significance of the fungus *Balansia cyperi* infecting medicinal species of *Cyperus* (Cyperaceae) from Amazonia. *Econ. Bot., 44*, 452–462.

Rosengren, D., 1998. Matsigenka myth and morality: Notions of the social and the asocial. *Ethnos, 63*, 248–272.

Sheldrake, M., 2020. *Entangled Life: How Fungi Make Our Worlds, Change Our Minds and Shape Our Futures.* Random House, New York.

Shepard Jr., G.H., 1998a. Psychoactive Plants and ethnopsychiatric medicines of the Matsigenka. *J. of Psychoactive Drugs, 30*, 321–332.

Shepard Jr., G.H., 1998b. Gift of the harpy eagle: Hunting medicines of the Machiguenga. *The South American Explorer, 51*, 9–21.

Shepard Jr., G.H., 1999a. Pharmacognosy and the Senses in two Amazonian Societies. PhD thesis, Dept. Anthropology, University of California at Berkeley.

Shepard Jr., G.H., 1999b. Shamanism and diversity: A Matsigenka perspective, in: Posey, D.A. (Ed.), *Cultural and Spiritual Values of Biodiversity*. United Nations Environmental Programme and Intermediate Technology Publications, London, pp. 93–95.

Shepard Jr., G.H., 2002a. Three days for weeping: Dreams, emotions and death in the Peruvian Amazon. *Med. Anthropol. Q. 16*, 200–229.

Shepard Jr., G.H., 2002b. Primates in Matsigenka subsistence and worldview, in: Fuentes, A., Wolfe, L. (Eds.), *Primates Face to Face: The Conservation Implications of Human and Nonhuman Primate Interconnections*. Cambridge University Press, Cambridge, U.K., pp. 101–136.

Shepard Jr., G.H., 2004. A sensory ecology of medicinal plant therapy in two Amazonian societies. *Am. Anthropol, 106*, 252–266.

Shepard Jr., G.H., 2010. The secret shaman. In J. Eede (Ed.), *We are One: A Celebration of Tribal Peoples*. Quadrille/Survival International, London, pp. 130–131.

Shepard Jr., G.H., 2011. The hunter in the rye: Ergot, sedges and hunting magic in the Peruvian Amazon. *Notes from the Ethnoground*, Sept. 30, 2011. https://ethnoground.blogspot.com/2011/10/hunter-in-rye-ergot-and-hunting-magic.html

Shepard Jr., G.H., 2013. The sound of no Salinger. *Notes from the Ethnoground*, Jan. 27, 2013. https://ethnoground.blogspot.com/2013/01/the-sound-of-no-salinger.html

Shepard Jr., G.H., 2014. Old and in the way: Jaguar transformation in Matsigenka. Paper presented at the International Congress of Ethnobiology, Bhutan, June 2014. https://www.academia.edu/15538299/Old_and_in_the_way_Jaguar_transformation_in_Matsigenka

Shepard Jr., G.H., 2015a. Agony and ecstasy in the Amazon: Tobacco, pain and the hummingbird shamans of Peru. *Broad Street* 2, 5–20.

Shepard Jr., G.H., 2015b. Will the real shaman please stand up?: The recent adoption of ayahuasca among indigenous groups of the Peruvian Amazon, in: Labate B., Cavnar C. (Eds). *Ayahuasca Shamanism in the Amazon and Beyond*. Oxford University Press, New York, 16-39.

Shepard Jr., G.H., 2017. Toé (*Brugmansia suaveolens*): O caminho do dia e da noite, in: Labate, B.C., Goulart, S.L. (Eds.), *O Uso de Plantas Psicoativas Nas Américas*. Compania das Letras, São Paulo, 121-136.

Shepard Jr., G.H., 2018a. The awakening of the waters: Clean water, health and village sanitation in the Peruvian Amazon. *Notes from the Ethnoground*, Jan. 31, 2018. https://ethnoground.blogspot.com/2018/02/the-awakening-of-waters-clean-water.html

Shepard Jr., G.H., 2018b. Spirit bodies, plant teachers and messenger molecules in Amazonian shamanism. In D. McKenna, G.T. Prance, B. De Loenen, and W. Davis (eds.), *Ethnopharmacologic Search for Psychoactive Drugs II: 50 Years of Research (1967-2017)*. Santa Fe: Synergetic Press, pp. 70–81.

Shepard Jr., G. H., Chicchon, A., 2001. Resource use and ecology of the Matsigenka of the eastern slopes of the Cordillera Vilcabamba. In L. E. Alonso, A. Alonso, T. S. Schulenberg, & F. Dallmeier (Eds.), *Biological and Social Assessments of the Cordillera de Vilcabamba, Peru*. Conservation International, Washington D.C., pp. 164–174.

Shepard Jr., G.H. and Daly, L., 2022. Sensory ecologies, plant-persons, and multinatural
landscapes in Amazonia. *Botany, 100*, 83–96.

Shepard Jr., G.H. and Daly, L., 2023. Sensory ecology, bioeconomy and the age of COVID: A parallax view of Indigenous and scientific knowledge. *Top. Cogn.Sci.*, 15, 584-607.

Shepard Jr., G.H., Levi, T., Neves, E.G., Peres, C.A. and Yu, D.W., 2012. Hunting in ancient and modern Amazonia: Rethinking sustainability. *Am. Anthropol.*, *114*, 652–667.

Shepard Jr., G.H., Rummenhoeller, K., Ohl, J., Yu, D.W., 2010. Trouble in Paradise: Indigenous populations, anthropological policies, and biodiversity conservation in Manu National Park, Peru. *J. Sustain. For.* 29, 252–301.

Shepard, G.H. Jr., Yu, D.W., Lizarralde, M., Italiano. M. 2001. Rainforest habitat classification among the Matsigenka of the Peruvian Amazon. *Journal of Ethnobiology*, 21, 1–38.

Snell, B.A., Collants, A. Chavez P., I., Cruz K., V. Pereira C. J.E., 2011. *Diccionario Matsigenka-Castellano*. Serie Ling. Peruana No. 56, M.R. Wise (ed.). Lima: Instituto Linguistico de Verano.

Terborgh, J., Robinson, S., Parker, T. A. Munn III, C.A., and Pierpont, N. 1990. Structure and organization of an Amazonian forest bird community. *Ecol. Monogr.*, *60*(, 213–238.

Thomas, W. W., Hensold, N., Foster, R., Ree, R. H., and Soares Neto, R. L., 2021. *Aenigmanu*, a new genus of Picramniaceae from Western Amazonia. *TAXON*, *70*, 1239–1247.

Tournon, J., 1984. Investigaciones sobre las plantas medicinales de los Shipibo-Conibo del Ucayali. *Amazonia Peruana*, *5*, 91–118.

Viveiros de Castro, E.B., 2004. The Transformation of objects into subjects in Amerindian ontologies. *Common Knowledge*, *10*, 463–472.

From Huautla to Sibundoy: R.E. Schultes' Encounters with Psilocybin and Ayahuasca

Mark Plotkin, PhD, Brian Hettler, Pascual Gonzalez, and The Amazon Conservation Team

Ethnobotanist | Co-founder and President of the Amazon Conservation Team

Senior Manager of Mapping & Programs Support at the Colombia Office of The Amazon Conservation Team

Coordinator and Mapper for The Amazon Conservation Team |
*An organization that has partnered with more than 90 indigenous groups to map and improve management of almost 100 million acres of ancestral rainforest **

> *"Each time a medicine man dies, it is as if a library burned down."* —Mark Plotkin

Richard Evans Schultes was a pioneer in the field of ethnobotany, and was responsible for bringing awareness about different psychoactive plants from the Amazon to the West. This paper shares the fascinating history behind these adventures, and how they have sculpted the modern world of psychedelics today.

This paper is dedicated to the memories of three trailblazers of the Psychedelic Renaissance: Taita Salvador Chindoy, Maria Sabina Magdalena Garcia, and Dr. Valentina Wasson.

Richard Evans Schultes is widely considered the dominant figure in 20th-century ethnobotany. Applying what he learned from his indigenous teachers and guides, he helped bring awareness of peyote, psilocybin and ayahuasca to the outside world—before he turned 30 (!). And though Schultes is most widely known for his research on hallucinogens, he also carried out seminal investigations on coca, marijuana, hevea rubber and orchids.

Schultes' life and times have been chronicled by Davis (1993), Hettler (2022) and Plotkin (2017 et al; 2022). However, we now live in what has been termed the "Psychedelic Renaissance," in which every week seems to bring new articles, books, and research into the therapeutic poten-

* For more information see https://www.amazonteam.org/

tial of mind-altering substances that offer great promise in the treatment of such often intractable ailments as addiction, depression, and PTSD.

Given the ever-growing interest in entheogens—and the fact that Schultes was an organizer of the original 1967 ESPD Conference in San Francisco—we think it both timely and of benefit to the historical record to conduct a deeper dive into Schultes' original encounters with both psilocybin and ayahuasca.

MEXICO AND THE MAGIC MUSHROOMS

William Safford was an American ethnobotanist who published notable (and accurate) papers on two important hallucinogens: *Datura* and *Piptadenia*. However—in the course of his research—he made one major error: he claimed that the early Spanish chroniclers who reported the use of intoxicating mushrooms for divinatory purposes were incorrect (Safford, 1916; 1917). Safford believed that the Aztecs were simply misleading the members of the Catholic clergy so they could continue venerating and consuming their true sacrament, which was peyote.

While deeply researching peyote use for his undergraduate thesis at Harvard, Schultes had several compelling reasons to believe that Safford was mistaken. First, having studied peyote, he knew that it was a cactus with a distribution limited to a narrow range along the Texas—Mexico border. Second, he realized that even a layperson could easily distinguish between a dried mushroom and a dried cactus. Third, having immersed himself in the Spanish accounts of Aztec culture, he noted that several of these narratives were extremely accurate with respect to the knowledge of both the Aztecs and their conquerors. According to these chronicles, psychotropic mushrooms were served at the coronation banquets of Aztec emperors, where they were known as *teonanacatl*, the "flesh of the gods."

But the key to solving the mystery proved to be a serendipitous discovery that Schultes made while studying peyote specimens in the herbarium. He stumbled across a letter to Harvard Herbarium Director J.N. Rose from Blas Pablo Reko, an Austrian physician living in Guadalajara, Mexico, which stated:

> "...I see in your description of [peyote] that Dr. Safford believes this plant to be the "teo-nanacatl" of [Spanish chronicler] Sahagun, which is surely wrong. It is, actually, as Sahagun states, a fungus which grows on dung heaps, and which is still used under the same old name by the Indians of the Sierra Juarez in Oaxaca in their religious feasts..."

Schultes decided to study and document the economic botany of the Mazatec peoples of the region as his doctoral research, and headed south to Mexico in 1936. At the time, there were no reliable scientific accounts of any hallucinogenic mushrooms in the New World, much less documentation of mind-altering fungi being employed for healing and divination. Furthermore, the state of Oaxaca was relatively unknown and uncharted as well, with mountains that exceeded 12,000 feet that isolated at least some of the 16 indigenous groups from the outside world.

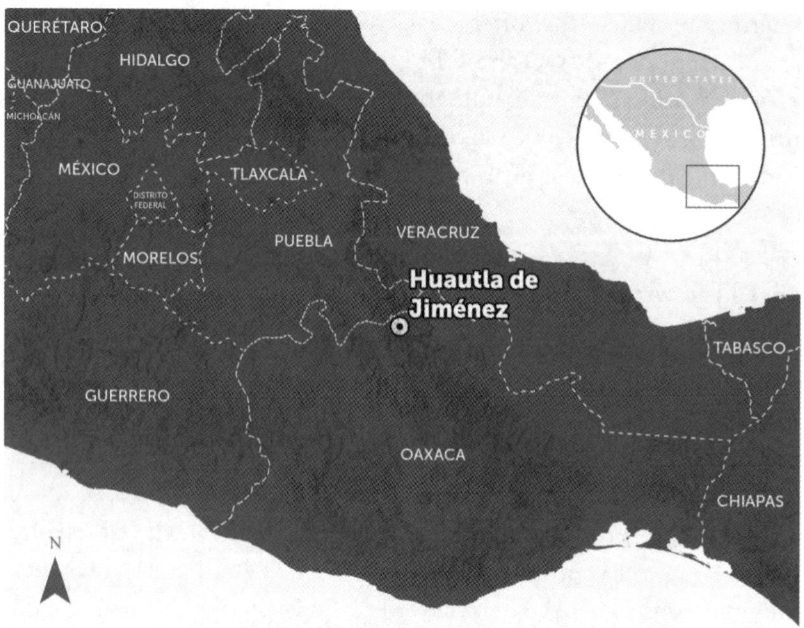

Fig. 1 Map of Huautla de Jimenez, the capital of the Mazatec peoples in the state of Oaxaca.

The Harvard grad student joined forces with Reko in Mexico City, and in July of 1938 the team traveled by train, mule and on foot to Huautla de Jimenez (Figure 1), the capital of the Mazatec peoples in the state of Oaxaca. There they were assisted in their quest by local shopkeeper José Dorantes. Local informants confirmed that these *Psilocybe* mushrooms—called *los niños santos* ("the little sacred ones") by the Mazatecs—were indeed considered objects of veneration and were a central pillar of both their religious and therapeutic practices. Schultes returned to Oaxaca the following year (1939) and confirmed that the mushrooms were employed for similar purposes by both the neighboring Chinantec and Zapotec peoples as well. The young scientist returned to Harvard to complete his dissertation and published two important papers on the magic mushrooms: one in the Harvard Botanical Museum Leaflets (1939) and the other in The American Anthropologist (1940). The groundbreaking importance of these papers would not be fully appreciated for decades to come.

Today, writers often attribute the western recognition of the magic mushrooms of Mexico to R. Gordon Wasson, an investment banker working for J. P. Morgan Jr.* who later became

* There is another little-known shamanic aspect to this history that involves the financier JP Morgan, Jr., the famous banker for whom Wasson was working in Manhattan when he first became intrigued by mushrooms. Morgan attended Harvard College where he prepared for a life in the business world, but he also studied mycology. Many years after he graduated, Harvard built the Farlow Herbarium to house their specimens of cryptogamic botany—that is, fungi and lichens. The university approached Morgan for financial support, and he made a substantial donation to the building that today still houses the magic mushrooms collected by both Schultes and Morgan's former employee Gordon Wasson (Pfister, 2018).

a Founding Father of the burgeoning field of ethnomycology. The notion that an investment banker in Manhattan decided to search hallucinogenic fungi in southern Mexico of his own volition is nonsensical and was never promulgated as such by Wasson. However, the means by which the mushrooms went from the Mazatecs to Schultes and Reko to Wasson and then to Albert Hofmann has seldom been recounted in detail prior to this paper.

An underappreciated but key figure in this story was Valentina Wasson, Gordon's wife. Tina, as she was more commonly known, was born and raised in Russia, and trained as a physician in London after her family fled the Russian Revolution in 1917. Ten years later, while hiking in the Catskills on their honeymoon, the couple encountered woodland mushrooms that Tina collected to cook and eat, while Gordon deemed them "poisonous toadstools" and refused to partake.

Witnessing how his wife not only survived but enjoyed her meal, Gordon's interest was piqued, and the couple embarked on a detailed study of how fungi had influenced the course of human history. This collaboration resulted in the classic text *Mushrooms, Russia, and History* (Wasson and Wasson, 1957). As part of their research, they contacted historians and anthropologists to gather information on the use of mushrooms in the past and during the present. One of the unsolved questions they hoped to answer was the role and identification of toxic mushrooms in the murder of the Roman Emperor Claudius in AD 54.

At the time that the Wassons were researching their book, the leading authority on the life of Claudius was Robert Graves, a poet and classics scholar who had written the brilliant fictional autobiographies *I, Claudius* (1934) and *Claudius the God* (1935). It was Tina who in 1949 had the idea to ask Graves if he could help them resolve the nearly 2,000-year-old cold case as to whether Claudius had been murdered with mushrooms, and if so, which species would have been employed.*†

Graves and the Wassons struck up a lively correspondence, and the most important exchange took place in 1952 when the Englishman sent the couple an article torn out of a pamphlet published by the pharmaceutical company CIBA, published in February of 1944. This short paper, penned by American anthropologist Robert Heizer, was titled "The Use of Narcotic Mushrooms by Primitive People," and focuses primarily on the use of *Amanita muscaria* in Siberia and *Psilocybe* in Mexico. Referenced as the two primary sources on the Mexico ethnomycology are Schultes' classic 1939 and 1940 papers on the subject. The actual copy of the pamphlet—now in the Harvard Herbarium Library archives—are annotated in Graves' handwriting: "My dear Gordon, perhaps too late for inclusion [in *Russia, Mushrooms and History*]; but useful? Most serendipitously, Robert."‡

---

* The results were published in the Harvard Botanical Museum Leaflets in 1972 by Gordon as "The Death of Claudius, or Mushrooms for Murderers".)

† Though Tina had passed away in 1958, in a letter dated 16 November 1968 to Gordon, Graves wrote: "How much we owe Tina; it was she who first wrote to me about mushrooms, remember?" (T. Riedlinger, pers. comm.).

‡ Prior to this exchange, few in the outside world knew or had any interest in magic mushrooms. And even today, most assume that there was some connection between Schultes and Wasson that brought psilocybin to the outside world. But here we can see that the "connective tissue" was Tina Wasson and Robert Graves, whose vital role in the story has been widely overlooked.

Thrilled and inspired by the evidence highlighted in the Heizer paper, the Wassons contacted Schultes for guidance and then set out for Huautla the following year (1953). On neither this visit nor on a second expedition the following year were the Wassons able to participate in a *velada*—a mushroom ceremony. In 1955, however, the now legendary Mazatec shaman Maria Sabina invited them to partake. Two years later (1957), Wasson penned an article detailing the experience that was published in the May 13, 1957 issue of *Life* magazine. The article, titled "Seeking the Magic Mushroom," proved to be an international sensation and led to an ever-increasing cavalcade of tourists to Huautla that continues to the present day.

Wasson began making annual expeditions to Oaxaca, often accompanied by the eminent French mycologist Roger Heim. Heim took some of the mushrooms back to France, where he was able to cultivate them. However, he was unable to isolate the active principal, and sent specimens to the renowned Swiss natural products chemist Albert Hofmann, now most widely known as the scientist who created LSD. In 1958, Hofmann was able to extract isolate and synthesize the active principle, which he named psilocybin.*

In an interview from Albert Hofmann by Stan Grof at Esalen in 1985 he said "And then, one day in the 1960s, I saw in the newspaper a notice that an American amateur mycologist and ethnologist, Gordon Wasson, and his wife had discovered mushrooms, which were used in a ritual way by the Indians. These mushrooms seemed to contain a hallucinogen that produced an LSD-like effect. Of course, I did not know who these ethnologists were, but I certainly would have been interested in investigating these mushrooms. Then, I got a letter from Professor [Roger] Heim, a French mycologist from the Sorbonne in Paris. Mr. Wasson and his wife, who had discovered this very old Mexican mushroom cult and had published information about the ritual use of these mushrooms, had sent him some botanical samples of the plant. They had asked him if he could examine the mushrooms and make precise botanical investigation. After Professor Heim completed the basic botanical work, he tried to isolate the active principle from the mushroom, but he did not succeed.... And so Professor Heim, who knew about the work we had done with LSD in Basel, asked me in a letter if I would be interested to take on this research.... Finally, we were able to isolate the active principles and it turned out to be two substances, which I named psilocybin and psilocin, because they had been isolated from *Psilocybe mexicana*... Gordon Wasson, who was a banker by profession and an amateur mycologist, was very impressed by the results. He did not know what active principles meant: for him it was the mushrooms that were the active agent. And he came to Basel to visit us and I showed him these active principles in a pure crystalline form.... Gordon was quite fascinated to see these crystals...." (*MAPS Fall Newsletter,* 2001).

---

* Schultes, Wasson and Hofmann have long been called the "founding fathers of ethnomycology." Most assume that Schultes and Hofmann knew each other before Wasson, a layman, came into the picture. Apparently, that was not the case, as Hofmann explained in one of the last detailed interviews he granted. That Wasson introduced Hofmann to Schultes—who then joined forces to coauthor *Plants of the Gods*, arguably the most important and influential book on hallucinogens ever written—represents a titanic contribution to the field of ethnobiology for which he must be credited. *Plants of the Gods* brought psycho-ethnopharmacology to the layman, but Schultes & Hofmann's monumental textbook *The Botany and Chemistry of Hallucinogens* was the first in depth scientific text of this topic.

Today, psilocybin is sweeping the world, offering so much therapeutic potential that mycologist Paul Stamets has deemed it the "Einstein Molecule". But there is one exceedingly important aspect to the magic mushroom story that is little known outside the mycological community. It is important to understand that all these psychoactive compounds are biodynamic—that they have an effect on the human body. For example, the burgeoning field of microdosing—in which amounts far too small to generate a psychedelic response are taken—purportedly offers curative effects for afflictions like depression, anxiety, and insomnia.

In one of his final and most important papers "Medicinal Chemistry's Debt to Ethnobotany" (1995), Albert Hofmann described how he and his colleagues employed the nucleus of the psilocybin molecule to develop an entirely new class of cardiac drugs, the first of which was known as Visken. This class of drugs—now known as beta blockers—have improved (and in fact saved) the lives of tens of millions. In Hofmann's words, "Without our investigations on the hallucinogenic Mexican mushrooms... Visken [and other beta blockers] would not have been developed."

AYAHUASCA AND THE NORTHWEST AMAZON

Today, ayahuasca is so ubiquitous that it can be purchased on the internet. This once obscure Amazonian liana—and the brew prepared from it and various admixtures—is celebrated and consumed from Israel to Indonesia to Istanbul, and every week seems to yield new reports of movie stars, famous athletes, and tech billionaires whose lives were changed by consuming this once sacrosanct and little-known brew.

The antiquity of ayahuasca use is impossible to determine with any certainty, but recent chemical analysis of Andean mummies proves that ayahuasca was being consumed at least a thousand years ago. And Schultes himself (1979) addressed this question:

> "There is a magic intoxicant in northwesternmost South America which the Indians believe can free the soul from corporeal confinement, allowing it to wander free and return to the body at will. The soul, untrammeled, liberates its owner from the everyday life and introduces him to wondrous realms of what he considers reality and permits him to communicate with his ancestors. The Kechua term for this inebriating drink—ayahuasca ("vine of the soul")—refers to this freeing of the spirit. The plants involved are truly plants of the gods, for their powers are laid to supernatural forces residing in their tissues, and they were the divine gifts to the earliest Indians on earth. *The drink employed for prophecy, divination, sorcery, and medical purposes, is so deeply rooted in native mythology and philosophy that there can be no doubt of its great age as part of aboriginal life* [italics by the author]."

Another question that remains unanswered is where both the ayahuasca vine and the ayahuasca ceremony originated. Constantino Torres, the leading authority on the early history of ayahuasca and hallucinogenic snuffs, unearthed vital clues that he presented in a paper at ESPD50 (2019). He found that one of the first detailed accounts was published in 1767 by the Jesuit missionary José Chantre y Herrera about ayahuasca use near the Marañón River in Amazonian Peru:

> "The [shaman] hangs his [hammock] in the middle or takes himself a bench or a small platform and next to it places a hellish brew called [ayahuasca], remarkably effective in depriving one of their senses. He makes a tea of the vine or bitter herbs, which after much boiling will become very thick. And it is so strong as to disrupt judgement in small quantities…"

In fact, all the early accounts of ayahuasca use come from the western Amazon: Maroni (1737) from the Rio Aguarico in Ecuador; Veigel (1755) from the Rio Napo, also in Ecuador; Wallace (1851) from the Rio Uaupés in Brazil, Spruce (1852) from the Rio Pastaza in Ecuador; Villavicencio (1858) also from the Rio Napo; Simson from the Putumayo of Colombia; Koch Grunberg (1904), also from the Uaupés; and MacCreagh (1926) from the Rio Tikie of Brazil*

Another significant person was Gordon MacCreagh, who was an extraordinary character: a soldier, writer, wild animal trader and seeker of the Lost Ark of the Covenant who travelled throughout tropical America, Africa, and Asia in the early 20th century. He was a member of the famous Mulford Expedition to the Amazon in 1921, which was led by botanist and pharmacist H.H. Rusby. MacCreagh published an extremely amusing account of the expedition in 1926, entitled White Waters and Black. Most important in the book, however, is a ten-page description of an ayahuasca ceremony which we believe is the most accurate and detailed account of what such a ritual may looked like in pre-Columbian times, and this report is widely overlooked in the ayahuasca literature.

Cumulatively, through location, these accounts appear to identify the center of origin as the northwest Amazon. However, recent investigations have shown that ayahuasca was also employed ceremonially in the Andean highlands in pre-Columbian times as well: analysis of mummy bundles by Miller et al (2019) revealed the presence of ayahuasca alkaloids in a grave of the Tiwanaku culture in Bolivia from 1000 AD and from an Inca grave in Peru by Socha et al (2022) from 1500 AD.

Despite the early and cursory accounts—mostly by missionaries and anthropologists—the detailed and scientific study of ayahuasca began with the arrival of Richard Schultes in the

---

* "Several writers—notably Spruce and the German anthropologist Koch-Grünberg—mention more than one 'kind' of caapi in the Vaupes basin. It was my good fortune in 1948 to be able to witness the preparation of, and to take a narcotic drink along an affluent of the Rio Tikie in north-westernmost Brazil. Specimens taken from a flowering vine, from the bark of which a cold-water infusion was made without the admixture of any other plants, were found to represent an undescribed species of a malpighiaceous genus closely allied to *Banisteriopsis—Tetrapteris methystica*. The beverage prepared from *Tetrapteris methystica* was a yellowish hue, quite unlike the coffee-brown colour characteristic of all preparations of *Banisteriopsis caapi* which I have seen. A small amount of stem material for chemical study that I gathered from the wild vine from which the type material came was lost in the overturning of my canoe. Consequently, nothing is known chemically of this kind of caapi. *That it is highly intoxicating, with effects very like those induced by Banisteriopsis, I can vouch from self-experimentation*" (italics by the author)."

Sibundoy Valley of Colombia in December of 1941. He had returned to Harvard after the Oaxaca expeditions, submitted his dissertation and received his PhD. Schultes then received a grant to study arrow poisons of Amazonia, since a compound from a South America curare formulation was becoming important in abdominal surgery. The young ethnobotanist would begin his Amazonian research in the Putumayo region, a territory in southern Colombia along the border with Ecuador and Peru exceptionally rich in both biological and cultural diversity*.

From the Colombian capital of Bogotá, Schultes headed south to the Andean city of Pasto. From there, he travelled by bus east along a road that followed what had been a pre-Columbian trail to reach the headwaters of the Putumayo River, the largest and most navigable river of the Colombian Amazon.

The headwaters of the Putumayo form in the remote Sibundoy Valley (Figure 2), a bowl-shaped depression on the eastern edge of the Colombian Andes. The valley is surrounded by four volcanoes, all of which reach over 12,000 feet. As such the valley is usually covered by clouds, receiving torrential rains that coalesce into the Putumayo as it runs east to join the main body of the Amazon River in Brazil. Because it sits near the narrowest stretch of the northern Andes and the lowest pass in the mountains, the Sibundoy has been a crossroads since the first humans arrived in the area. The Kamsa—the original inhabitants of Sibundoy—claim that they were the first people to enter Amazonia. And as they entered and began to explore Amazonia, they settled mainly in Sibundoy because it gave them ready access to the plants of both the Amazon and the Andes. The valley thus became a crossroads for trade as well as a sanctuary for healing plants: even in pre-Columbian times, itinerant healers would bring and trade medicinal species from other highland and Amazonian regions. So many of these healing plants were propagated there that Schultes concluded that Sibundoy harbored more hallucinogenic plants there than anywhere else in the world.

This original group—the Kamsá—speak a language unrelated to any other indigenous idioms, which tends to indicate a long period of isolation. The other indigenous group in Sibundoy is the Inga, who have a language related to Quechua, the language of the Incas. The two groups have very different origin stories but maintain similar modes of subsistence and healing methodologies. And their most essential plant for healing purposes is ayahuasca, whose central role in their culture is reflected in the Spanish term they use to describe it: "el remedio"—the medicine!

Schultes' mentor in Sibundoy was Salvador Chindoy, a renowned Kamsá medicine man (or *taita*, as the paramount shamans are called in this corner of Colombia) who was both well-known and well-regarded throughout the region. Like many an Amazonian shamans, Chindoy claimed that his knowledge was learned from the plants themselves, who spoke to him in dreams and visions. He told Schultes that ayahuasca was the ultimate medicine and the ultimate plant teacher. The only plant that featured nearly the same power, he said, was "borrachera," another

* In a highly unusual foreshadowing of future explorations, Schultes first heard of ayahuasca at the age of eight. Young Richard had contracted a severe stomach ailment and was bedridden for weeks. His father Otto—wishing to continue his son's education during his illness—went to the nearby East Boston Public Library and checked out Richard Spruce's classic 1908 account of his many years in South America, Notes of a Botanist on the Amazon and the Andes (1908) which he then read to the child. The book includes Spruce's short but memorable encounter with ayahuasca.

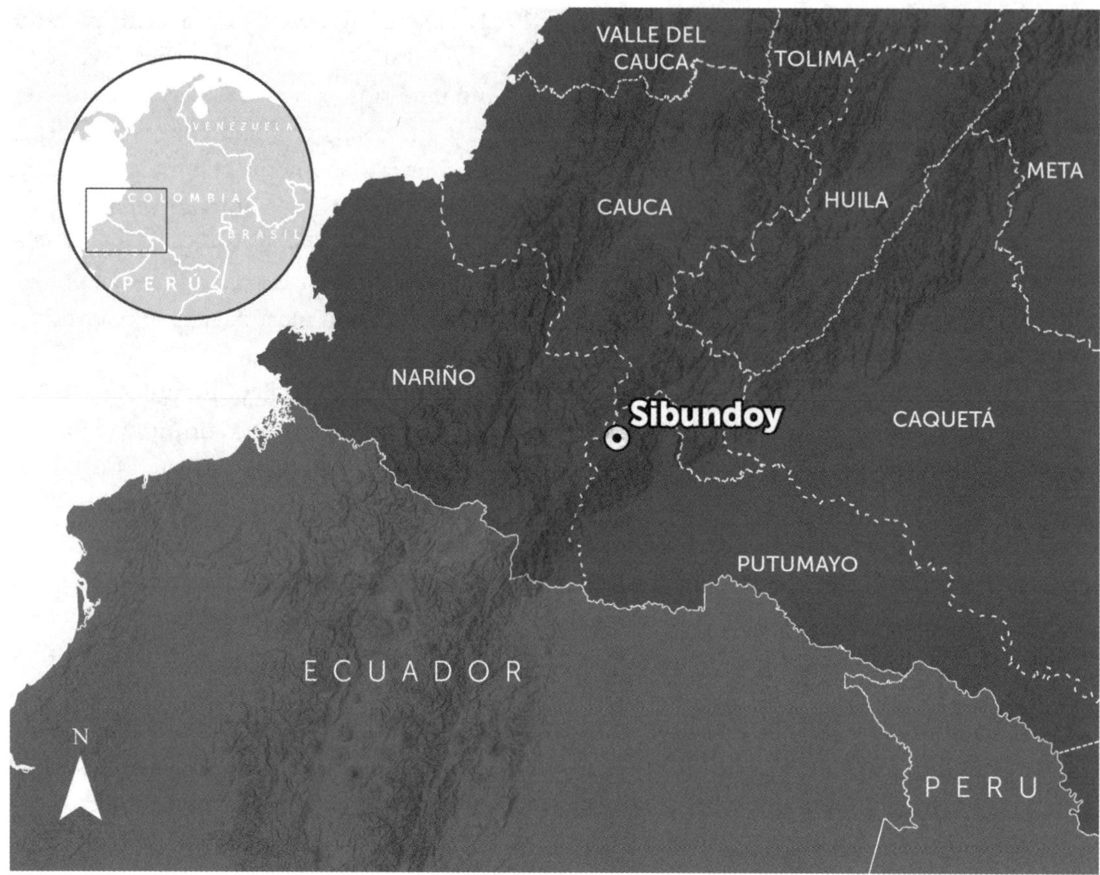

Fig. 2 Map of the Sibundoy Valley of Colombia.

powerful hallucinogen of the genus *Brugmansia* that is also widely propagated throughout the northern Andes as an ornamental as well. Such an important component of the Sibundoy pharmacopeia was this genus that Schultes counted 11 different varieties in use by the *taitas*.

Schultes' efficiency and effectiveness as an ethnobotanist in Sibundoy was turbocharged by his relationship with Pedro Juajibioy, Chindoy's nephew. Catholic missionaries had first arrived in the 1500s and they continued to yield strong influence centuries later. Juajibioy himself was a devout Catholic when he met Schultes, but the work and the ceremonies he undertook with both Chindoy and Schultes helped turn him into both a skilled botanist and a revered healer as he accepted and embraced traditional knowledge and methodologies. And he became a much sought-after guide and teacher for many ethnobotanists like Wade Davis, Luis Eduardo Luna and Timothy Plowman who followed in Schultes footsteps and worked, collected, and studied in the Sibundoy.

From Sibundoy, Schultes headed east in early 1942 to the territory of the Kofán peoples where he could initiate his studies of arrow poisons and continue his study of ayahuasca.* In an echo of the delayed reaction to his research into the magic mushrooms of Mexico, Schultes published the initial results of his ayahuasca studies in the Harvard Botanical Museum Leaflets, and the world ignored his findings for decades. However, after time these same findings reverberated across the globe.

To his last days, Schultes predicted that other mind-altering substances awaited discovery by the scientific world, but the race was on to protect these species and the indigenous cultures who could best teach us how to employ them. He was one of the organizers of the original ESPD Symposium in 1967, and since then not only have powerful new (to science) therapeutic compounds (like iboga and kratom) come to light, but we also now know that understudied creatures (like frogs) and ecosystems (like coral reefs) can also yield novel compounds. At the same time, we are witnessing new applications for some of the substances that Schultes helped bring forward, such as treatment for PTSD and asthma, uses not known to Schultes' indigenous teachers and guides.

The lessons and legacy of Richard Evans Schultes remain valid: that Mother Nature is an almost inexhaustible source of therapeutic compounds; that Indigenous Peoples are both the best teachers about and best stewards of these ecosystems; and that protecting this biocultural legacy is in everyone's self-interest.

Since the two previous ESPD conferences, the world has awakened a bit more to these lessons, especially with respect to entheogenic substances like ayahuasca and magic mushrooms.

Nonetheless, the destruction of primary forests and indigenous cultures proceeds at a rapid pace as well. The challenge of protecting this biocultural legacy remains.†

ACKNOWLEDGEMENTS

The authors would like to express their appreciation to Denise Castronovo of the Harvard Herbarium and Tom Riedlinger for their research assistance.

BIBLIOGRAPHY

Burroughs, William S. 1963. *The Yagé Letters*. City Lights Books.
Davis, Wade. 1996. *One River*. Simon and Schuster.
Graves, Robert. 1935. *Claudius the God*. The Albatross.
Graves, Robert. 1934. *I, Claudius*. Vintage Books.

---

* To learn more about the Kofán people and ayahuasca read our paper "Intellectual propery rights issues in community-based participatory research: The case of the Sucumbíos Kofán Yajé (Ayahuasca)" by David F. Rodríguez-Mora, MS.

* A Schultes conundrum- he often told colleagues and journalists that he never "got off" on ayahuasca, memorialized in a comment to William Burrough's in his book, The Yage Letters (1963): "That's funny, Bill—all I saw was a few colors!" This avowal is demonstrably untrue: in an earlier paper, I quoted Pedro Juajibioy describing the first time Schultes took ayahuasca, which was in Sibundoy with Pedro's uncle Salvador Chindoy (Plotkin et al., 2017). Following is another account, based on Schultes' experience with the Bara Maku people in Brazil (Schultes, 1957).

Heizer, R. 1944. "The Use of Narcotic Mushrooms by Primitive Peoples." CIBA Bulletin, (Vol. 5): pp. 1713-1716

Hofmann, Albert. 1955. "Medicinal Chemistry's Debt to Ethnobotany." In *Ethnobotany: Evolution of a Discipline*, (editors: R.E. Schultes and S. von Reis), Timber Press, pp. 311–319.

MacCreagh, Gordon. 2001. *White Waters and Black*. University of Chicago Press.

Miller, Melanie J., et al. 2019. "Chemical Evidence for the Use of Multiple Psychotropic Plants in a 1,000-Year-Old Ritual Bundle from South America." *Proceedings of the National Academy of Sciences*, vol. 116, no. 23, pp. 11207–11212., https://doi.org/10.1073/pnas.1902174116.

Pfister, D. R. 2018. "Gordon Wasson—1898–1986" *Mycologia*, (80)1, pp 11–13., https://www.tandfonline.com/doi/pdf/10.1080/00275514.1988.12025491

Plotkin, M. 2022. "Richard Evans Schultes." *Harvard Magazine*. 2022, pp. 40-41.

Plotkin, M., B. Hettler and W. Davis. 2018. "Viva Schultes!: A Retrospective" In *The Ethnopharmacologic Search for Psychoactive Drugs*, (editors: G.T. Prance and D. McKenna) Synergetic Press, pp. 95–120

Riedlinger, Thomas J. 1990. *The Sacred Mushroom Seeker*. Dioscorides Press.

Safford, W. 1915. "Identification of Teonanacatl of the Aztecs." Address to the Botanical Society of Washington DC.

Safford, W. 1916. "Identity of cohoba." *Journal of the Washington Academy of Sciences*. 1916 (6): pp. 547-562.

Schultes, Richard Evans. 1937. "Peyote and Plants Used in the Peyote Ceremony." *Botanical Museum Leaflets, Harvard University*, vol. 4, no. 8, 1937, pp. 129–152., https://doi.org/10.5962/p.236321.

Schultes, Richard Evans. 1939. "Plantae Mexicanae II: The Identification of Teonanacatl, a Narcotic Basidiomycete of the Aztecs." *Botanical Museum Leaflets, Harvard University*, vol. 7, no. 3, pp. 37–56., https://doi.org/10.5962/p.295127.

Schultes, Richard Evans. 1940. "Teonanacatl: The Narcotic Mushroom of the Aztecs." *American Anthropologist*, vol. 42, no. 3, pp. 429–443., https://doi.org/10.1525/aa.1940.42.3.02a00040.

Schultes, Richard Evans. 1938. "The Appeal of Peyote (*Lophophora williamsii*) as a Medicine." *American Anthropologist*, vol. 40, no. 4, pp. 698–715., https://doi.org/10.1525/aa.1938.40.4.02a00100.

Schultes, Richard Evans. 1957. "The Identity of the Malpighiaceous Narcotics of South America." *Botanical Museum Leaflets, Harvard University*, vol. 18, no. 1, pp. 1–56., https://doi.org/10.5962/p.168508.

Schultes, Richard Evans, and Albert Hofmann. 1987. *Plants of the Gods: Origins of Hallucinogenic Use*. A. Van Der Marck Editions.

Socha, Dagmara M., et al. 2022. "Ritual Drug Use during Inca Human Sacrifices on Ampato Mountain (Peru): Results of a Toxicological Analysis." *Journal of Archaeological Science: Reports*, vol. 43, 2022, p. 103415., https://doi.org/10.1016/j.jasrep.2022.103415.

Spruce, Richard. 1908. *Notes of a Botanist on the Amazon and the Andes*. Macmillan.

Torres, Constantino. 2018. "From Beer to Tobacco: A Probable History of Tobacco and Yagé." In *The Ethnopharmacologic Search for Psychoactive Drugs*, (editors: G.T. Prance and D. McKenna) Synergetic Press, pp. 36–54.

Wasson, R. Gordon. 1955. "Seeking the Magic Mushroom." *Life* magazine, pp. 100-102, 109-113.

Wasson, R. Gordon. 1972. "The Death of Claudius or Mushrooms for Murderers." *Botanical Museum Leaflets, Harvard University*, vol. 23, no. 3, pp. 101–128., https://doi.org/10.5962/p.168556.

Wasson, Valentina and R. Gordon Wasson. 1957. *Mushrooms, Russia, and History*. Pantheon.

Wasiwaska Research Center—An Ethnopharmacological Plant Repository in Southern Brazil

Luis Eduardo Luna, PhD, and Dale Millard

Director of Wasiwaska | Anthropologist | Author

Naturalist | Ethnobotanist

"We will present an overview of the institution and the creation of the ethnobotanical garden, the history, ethnography, botany, pharmacology and cultivation of some important species, as well as some of our observations with regard to apparent symbiotic relationships amongst certain of the plants and animals in the garden."

—Dale Millard and Luis Eduardo Luna

This paper shares the creation of an Ethnopharmacological Plant Repository in Southern Brazil. It is a presentation of a collaborative project to establish a collection of sacred and medicinal plants at Wasiwaska Research Center in Florianópolis, Brazil.

ABSTRACT

The Wasiwaska Ethnobotanical Garden, located in Florianópolis on the island of Santa Catarina, in southern Brazil, is part of the Wasiwaska Research Center for the Study of Psychointegrator Plants, Visionary Art and Consciousness, created in 2001 by Colombian/Finnish anthropologist Luis Eduardo Luna and Brazilian cultural manager Adriana Rosa. The garden, to a great extent is the result of the advice and collaboration of South African naturalist Dale Millard, who during his visits to the institution, helped design and develop the space largely around agroforestry principles. Land use incorporates three main activities, botanical collection and preservation, agroforestry and food production, and reforestation. A private botanical garden comprises around four hundred species that surround the house and adjacent buildings. These species represent a unique collection of many rare and poorly known fruit trees as well as sacred and medicinal plants. The botanical garden gradually extends towards an independent project, which aims to reforest a patch of former Coastal Atlantic Forest (Mata Atlántica). This place lost its primary vegetation due to several hundred years of occupation by colonists originally from the Azores islands who cultivated manioc, sugar cane and coffee. We will present an overview of the institution and the creation of the ethnobotanical garden, as well as some of our observations regarding apparent symbiotic relationships amongst certain of the plants and animals in the garden.

INTRODUCTION BY LUIS EDUARDO LUNA

The creation of an ethnobotanical garden was an idea Terence McKenna and I shared when back in 1971 we spent two months together at Villa Gloria, a humble wooden house my parents had 14 kilometers from Florencia, in the Colombian Amazon. He was traveling with his then partner Erica Niesfeld, while I was having holidays in my native town after seven years of absence spent in Spain. Terence was then writing *The Invisible Landscape*, which he co-authored with his younger brother Dennis. He was under the spell of their extraordinary adventure at La Chorrera, some months earlier, and I was an avid listener. In Villa Gloria we had our very first *yajé* experience. Kalmán, a Hungarian friend who lived in Florencia, had acquired some *yajé* (*Banisteriopsis caapi* + *Diplopterys cabrerana*) he had got from Don Apolinar Jacanamijoy, an Ingano *taita** who had moved with his family from the Mocoa area. The four of us drank the *yajé*, an experience that came to define the path I followed later in life. It triggered in me a great curiosity to know about the use of sacred plants by some of my ancestors. I am a mestizo, and so partially an *indio*. With the years I came to the realization that it is impossible to understand Amerindian cultures without reference to the importance they give to plants capable of notable body-mind modifications.

Terence and Erica bought a small plot near Villa Gloria with the idea of creating a plant repository. Unfortunately, soon after this, the area of the Department of Caquetá, of which Florencia is the capital, came under the crossfire between the army, *guerrilleros*, and cocaine traffickers, not at all a safe spot for *gringos*. The project was therefore abandoned.

I spent the summer of 1973 with Terence (and Erica) in Berkeley and maintained copious correspondence with him for many years. In 1979 I went back to Florencia to see my parents, and had my second *yajé* experience, this time under the guidance of Don Apolinar himself. I was discovering Amerindian epistemology, a way of knowing that recognizes mind in nature, the world being conceived as populated by non-human animal, fungal and plant persons. I decided to make a film about Don Apolinar, but he died before I was able to arrive there with the equipment. I went to visit Terence in his home in the Bay Area, who told me he had heard about an ayahuasca (*Banisteriopsis caapi* + *Psychotria viridis*) tradition around Iquitos, in the Peruvian Amazon. He had been given three names, one of them Don Emilio Andrade Gómez, of whom I made the film *Don Emilio and His Little Doctors* (1981), and who became my friend and teacher. He was the first person who mentioned to me the concept of plant teachers: tobacco, ayahuasca, *toé* (*Brugmansia* sp.), and other plants, if taken under appropriate conditions of special diet and isolation, may teach about this and other worlds. In 1986 I found a similar idea in the Sibundoy Valley of the Colombian Putumayo, where the garden of medicinal and sacred plants around the houses of the *taitas* is considered *el jardín de la ciencia* (the garden of science).

In 1983 I went to see Dennis, Terence's brother, who was finishing his doctoral dissertation at the Department of Botany of Vancouver University. We became close friends, collaborating through the years in various projects, one of them the collection of plants from the Peruvian Amazon for *Botanical Dimensions*, the institution Terence and his then wife Kat Harrison, had created in 1985 on the Big Island of Hawaii. I personally delivered a basket of several species,

* *Taita* is a local name for indigenous traditional healers

among them a large package of seeds and several dozens of specimens of *Psychotria viridis*, which later proliferated on the property. Dennis was the person who introduced me to Pablo Amaringo (1943-2009), a Peruvian painter and former *vegetalista* who was living in Pucallpa, the second city of importance of the Peruvian Amazon. Our collaboration resulted in the book *Ayahuasca Visions: The Religious Iconography of a Peruvian Shaman*, and the creation in 1988 of the Usko-Ayar Amazonian School of Painting, which had as its main goal the artistic documentation of the flora and fauna of the Amazon region. The school created its own ethnobotanical garden, but it had to be abandoned when we were threatened by members of *Senderoso Luminoso* (the *Shining Path*), an armed communist guerrilla organization. With funds provided originally by the school and by *Seeds of Change*, an organic food and seed company created by Gabriel Howearth and Danny Ausubel, the *Sachamama Ethnobotanical Garden* was created near Iquitos, originally with the collaboration of fourteen students from the Usko-Ayar school, who opened trails for a month, each student with the task of producing a portrait of one of the plants in the garden. It was a magnificent collection exhibited in 1994 at the Capital Children Museum, later renamed The National Children Museum, in Washington DC.

In 1992 I got a two-year position as a visiting professor at the Department of Anthropology at the Federal University of Santa Catarina, in Florianópolis, on the island of Santa Catarina. Since 1979 I was a senior lecturer of the Department of Modern Languages at the Swedish School of Economics in Helsinki (now The Hanken School of Economics). Before that I had spent seven years in Norway, where I taught Spanish and Latin American literature at Oslo University. My first degree was from Universidad Complutense de Madrid. I arrived in Florianópolis with my Finnish partner and our two boys, ages two and four. Our third child, a baby girl, was borne in Brazil, which meant that as a father of a Brazilian citizen, I could apply for a permanent position at the Department of Anthropology, which I got. After a divorce I had to choose between staying alone in Brazil to pursue an academic career, or returning to Finland to my old position, and being close to my children. I went back to Helsinki, but I had already purchased a piece of land where I had planned to create a little institution where I could invite people in my field of research and develop the old dream of an ethnobotanical garden. I traveled back and forth between Helsinki and Florianópolis, until my retirement from the Hanken School of Economics in 2012. With the invaluable contribution of my Brazilian wife Adriana Rosa, we built the house and the garden, creating what became Wasiwaska, Research Center for the Study of Psychointegrator Plants, Visionary Art, and Consciousness, where we organize 2-3 interdisciplinary seminars every year (www.wasiwaska.org). The ethnobotanical garden and our adjacent reforestation project are now our focus of attention.

INTRODUCTION BY DALE MILLARD

I have always been interested in nature and growing plants as far back as I can remember. I had a growing cacti and succulent collection by age 7. I was forever getting into trouble with my parents for going missing or not coming home. I was usually searching for succulents such as stapeliads, scorpions, frogs, and snakes in the blocks of wilderness, interspersed between suburbs of Johannesburg in South Africa. Later, in my teens, during the weekends, I would ride my bicycle as far as I could, often up to 100 kilometers, to get into undisturbed wilderness. To my parents' dismay, I would often return with my collections, many of which were highly venomous. We are thankfully all still here!

After school I went on to work in nature reserves adjoining the Kruger National Park, though at that time many private reserves had already dropped their fences, unifying the reserves under much broader conservation programs. I then went on to become curator of herpetology at the Swadini Reptile Research Center. During this time, I made friends who allowed me access to the private reserves and the giant Kruger National Park. I lived alone in an old farmhouse, on the banks of the Blyde River near the town of Hoedspruit. The house, organized through my employers, was surrounded by a high voltage electric fence to keep the animals out of the garden. That fence was a curse for me, especially as the three access gates were locked with old padlocks and chains. Returning from work in the evening on my motorbike, especially in the rain, when trying to get a key into the locks, nearly always resulted in my being shocked. I soon planned where I could get over the fence on foot by placing step ladders against the fence, insulated by an old rubber conveyor belt. It was my highway into nature, with all the animals, and from here I would often walk a short two kilometers to work, and back. I really cherished having, what seemed as the whole of wildest Africa in my backyard. By this time, I had already discovered psychedelics, mostly LSD, MDMA, mushrooms, marijuana, and brief experimentation with ketamine as I had it available in my fridge at work to anesthetize animals. After my work with reptiles, I went on to do community work in the villages, surrounding Manyeleti Game Reserve. Manyeleti means "the place of the stars" in the local Xitsonga language. During the apartheid years, this formed part of the old homeland of Gazankulu, inhabited mostly by Tsonga people. The area was still under the tribal authority of the Mnisi and Mathebula family. The Tsonga are people very close to nature, with their surnames and clan names all referring to animals. The chief's wife, Lina Mnisi, took a special interest in my work, and although totally unnecessary I was ascribed two old men as my security guards who stayed on the same property, Lot Mathebula and Edward Nkabinde. Both were former poachers, and through accompanying them through the bush, I soon discovered they were master trackers. I realized they had a way of reading the landscape and extracting information that was totally invisible to most people. Their ability to follow animal tracks and the detailed information accessed seemed to be almost "Supernatural". They could tell which species, the direction it went, the time of day, its sex, age, speed, and behavior, all from studying the ground, and they could even do this when all traces had seemingly vanished. I tried to learn as much as I could from these friends and refine what I was able to see. This time spent was very formative for me in that it totally changed the way I observe and interpret nature. I had become immersed in a world that was far more about pattern recognition than rational language, as is indeed the way of most animistic societies.

From there, I went to live in the foothills of the Maluti mountains, on a beautiful farm called Rustlers Valley. It was here that I originally came to meet Luis Eduardo Luna through a rather peculiar array of coincidences that happened in South Africa well over 20 years ago, when I had followed a girlfriend of mine at the time to Rustlers Valley. I did not know that I would end up becoming a shareholder spending many precious years living in that valley. There was this guy, whom I had not heard of, Terence Mckenna, who had been giving talks downstairs from where I was staying. The talks were on plants, already a passion of mine, though these were described to me as magical plants which intrigued me. I had never been exposed to whole communities of folk who were into this! Some weeks later I remember walking into the restaurant and meeting both Bill Mollison the permaculturist, and Luis Eduardo Luna. Terence had told Luis Eduardo about this place Rustlers Valley and recommended he visit! And little did I know at that time that I would go on to pursue a lifelong interest in psychoactive plants, permaculture, and agroforestry.

Rustlers Valley is adjacent to Mautse Ancestral Valley, an ancient valley that can no longer be used as a sacred site and home of *sangoma* healers and their ancestral spirits. In a tragic story, the healers who lived in caves were all evicted, and the land sold.. Mautse was a place for pilgrims, healers, and their patients to be in close contact with their ancestral spirits, so they may receive direction and be healed. The *Sangomas* of Mautse were from many different tribes making it an absolute goldmine of ethnographic knowledge and a place for me to learn about medicinal plants and the cultures who use them. An exceptional woman named Nontobeko Magenganene or Monica in English, offered to share her knowledge! Monica was a Zulu Mndau prophet, meaning her ancestors lived in water. Accessing them often involved entering strong trance states and being submerged to experience this utopian otherworldly dimension. I was fortunate to be able to introduce Luis Eduardo Luna and his wife, Adriana Rosa to Monica and her world. Monica was totally instrumental in inspiring my passion and work with medicinal plants. Monica was absolutely a very wise soul and extremely generous teacher. We remained close years until she left this plane to become an ancestor herself.

My curiosity and passion for nature, medicinal plants and traditional cultures intensified when I started traveling and living in different parts of the world, namely Africa, Southeast Asia, and Brazil. My experiences with sacred plants and mushrooms taken in environments such as forests and game reserves among the animals greatly deepened both my appreciation and understanding of the natural world.

In a roundabout way, I owe it to Terence that I got to meet Luis Eduardo Luna and came to be involved with the ethnobotanical garden at Wasiwaska. Luis had told me of his project in Florianópolis, Brazil and together with the help of his wife Adriana Rosa and her late father Geraldo we began collecting, germinating, and planting species.

DESIGN, INSPIRATION AND LAND USE

The project has developed organically over the years and is forever growing and evolving. The main intentions, guiding the design and planning, are to provide an aesthetically beautiful and species rich garden that is productive in organic food and medicine, which we and our staff consume. We also swap the produce with friends or donate our excess. Accessibility to high quality agrochemical free food and availability to healthcare is becoming not only fashionable but necessary, as the world is increasingly dependent on chemically fertilized and nutritionally poorer plant species.

The areas of main production are situated in a satellite pattern with interconnecting paths leading through the native forest. We try to disturb the native vegetation as little as possible. Our satellite gardens are achieved largely through clearing of alien pines *Pinus elliottii*, and when large trees get taken down by winds. We plant these areas with native forest and fruit species. We aim to maintain a living gene bank, a growing collection of interesting, rare fruits, medicinal and sacred plants.

The garden is meant to inspire and educate visitors into the marvels of medicinal plants and poorly known fruits. The plants are labeled, though this job is never complete, down to family and species level. There are many paths that one can explore, and this provides us with good daily exercise. The garden is vitally important in our own understanding, learning and experimentation with plants. It allows us to observe most of the plants through their entire life cycles from germinating seeds, till they bare their own seeds.

The garden exists on old manioc and coffee grounds. The soil is not very rich in nitrogen and is mostly deep red poorly drained clays throughout the property. Rain falls both in summer and winter, and both extremes of long dry and long wet periods are experienced on the island. It has been a challenge to grow such a diverse collection of plants from different habitats and places, though it has been a unique learning opportunity and a true pleasure to see a forest garden maturing to production that was mostly planted from seed.

Many challenges were experienced along the way including tornados, and the remarkably intelligent native leaf cutter ants, *Acromyrmex* sp. that surely know when new species are being planted in their territories. Often one arrives in the morning to find a treasured species totally bare and leafless. As they are a native species and we are outnumbered, we have learnt that one will never win the battle against them, our solution has been, *keep planting more*!

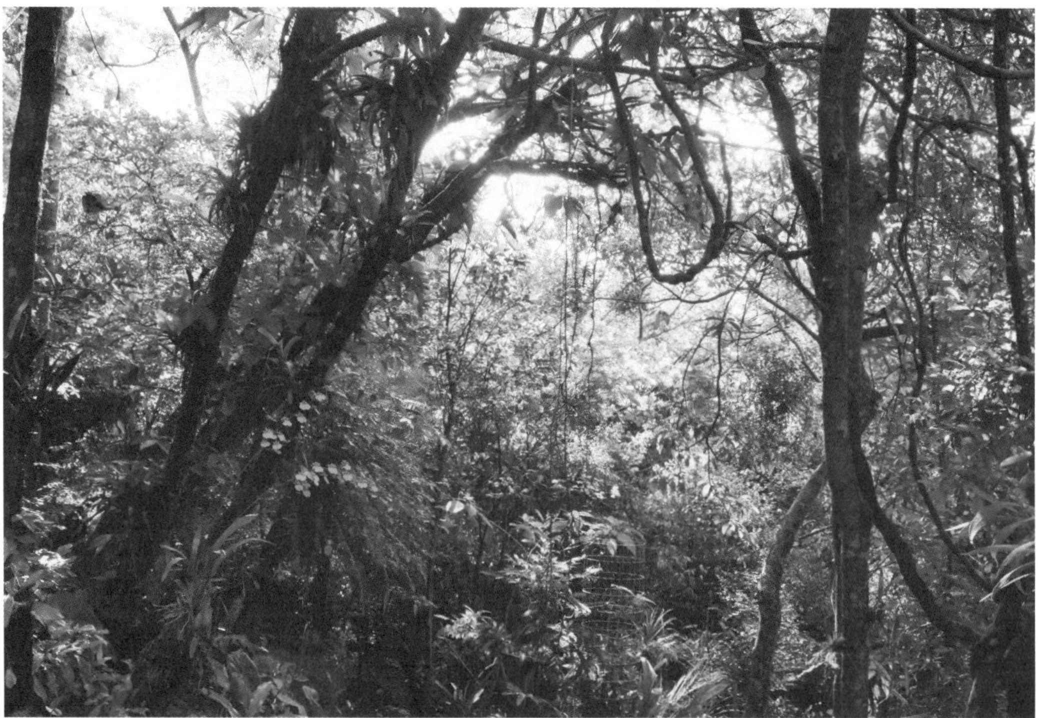

Fig.1 The Wasiwaska Ethnobotanical Garden. Partial view. *Photo Mauricio Tolosa*

THE PLANTS

It is beyond the scope of this article to catalog the entirety of the collection or to present comprehensive details regarding plant species, which may be accessed elsewhere through existing literature publications, or online resources. Rather we are attempting to share some of our own experiences and observations not mentioned in the literature, many of which came to our attention through entering relationships by cultivating these amazing plant beings.

MEDICINAL GARDEN

A large percentage of the collection consists of medicinal and ethnobotanically interesting plant species from many of the main medical systems throughout the world. There are too many to mention here, though medicines we use from the garden regularly for personal well-being included:

Tumeric (*Cucurma longa*)—We grow several medicinal gingers of the Zingiberaceae family, rich in antioxidants, anti-inflammatory compounds, and to support liver function.

Ashwagandha (*Withania somnifera*)—The famous Ayurvedic herb which has adaptogenic, anti-inflammatory, and neuroprotective properties.

Petiveria alliacea known in Brazil as *guinea*, and *mucura* or *anamú* in the Peruvian Amazon, is a very useful antibiotic, anti-inflammatory and anti-cancer medicine. Its seeds are easily dispersed and attached to passing-by human and non-human animals.

Guaco (*Mikania glomerata*) leaves make a great tea for colds and flu. It is a strong bronchodilator with anti-inflammatory, antimicrobial and anti-anxiety properties.

Andrographis paniculata. Due to the spread of the SARS CoV-2 virus, we decided to grow this extremely valuable antiviral medicine from Southeast Asia. Andrographis has several published studies showing multiple mechanisms blocking viral entry and replication of SARS CoV-2. We use it for infections instead of antibiotics. It is one of the most bitter of all plants, so we do not add it to the morning smoothie!

Medicines such as *chanca Piedra*, *Phyllanthus niruri* and the toothache plant *Spilanthes acmella* are locally very abundant so there is no need to grow them.

The medicinal garden is used to educate visitors and friends and provide the ingredients for the decoctions and tinctures we take as our medicine.

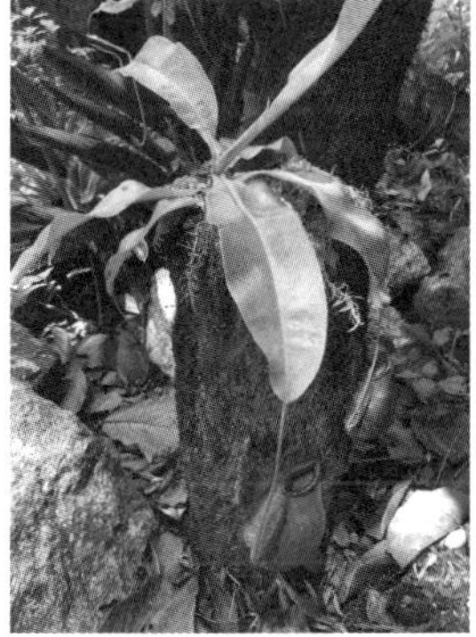

Fig.2 Nepenthes ampullaria (hybrid). *Photo L.E.Luna*

NEPENTHES COLLECTION

We have started a small collection of S E Asian Pitcher plants or *Nepenthes* species, which we grow close to the main house so we can observe them, while they feed on insects that might otherwise feed on us! *Nepenthes* are fascinating and remarkable for their evolutionary adaptations. Most species are adapted to attracting and feeding off insects, such as *Nepenthes rafflesiana*, which we have recently acquired. A very similar species through divergent evolution, now recently classified as *Nepenthes hemsleyana* (previously *Nepenthes rafflesiana truncata*), has in certain populations in Borneo, evolved its pitcher structure to become the home of a small species of woolly bat, which uses the modified pitcher lid as an antennae structure unable to echolocate and find its way home through the forest. The plant benefits through nutrients from the bat's droppings. Other species such as *Nepenthes iowii*, also from Borneo have evolved their pitcher structures to become a toilet for tree shrews and birds that come to feed from its nectarines, which are specialized structures that produce a sugary substance under the lid. One can only wonder, how and in what time frame the evolutionary changes and dietary preferences take place? Others, like *Nepenthes ampullaria* which we are also growing, are adapted for growing at the base of other plants and survive mostly through feeding on fallen leaf matter. We hope we can grow more species from this wonderful genus in the future.

ORCHID COLLECTION

Brazil and the mid-Atlantic Forest is home to an impressive array of beautiful orchid species. We grow many species such as the native *Cattleya.* We have also *Bifrenaria, Epidendrum* and *Vanilla* as epiphytes on trees and rockery around property. Their beautiful floral displays add greatly to the aesthetics of the garden. Once established on the trees, they require little maintenance and provide long lasting colourful flowers.

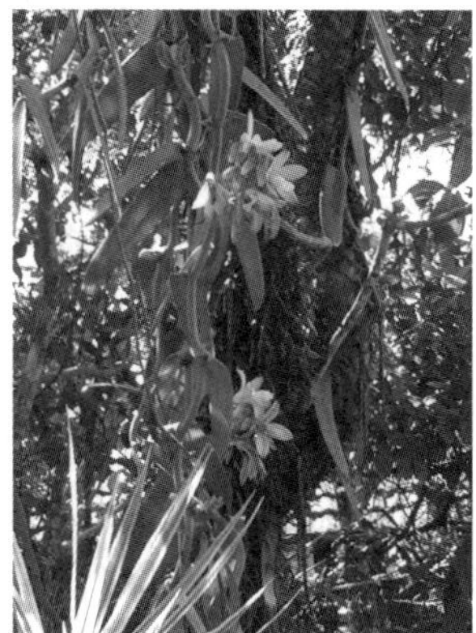

Fig.3 Vanilla chamisonnis. *Photo L.E.Luna*

SACRED PLANT COLLECTION

Banisteriopsis caapi

The collection in the Wasiwaska Ethnobotanical Garden started with a handful of seeds of *Banisteriopsis caapi* sent to us from a friend living in Acre, in the Brazilian Amazon. We expected to receive some cuttings for vegetative reproduction, but a phone call clarified that we should grow Banisteriopsis from seed if we are to get strong healthy plants, with more expansive root systems. Once germinated, the small plants were placed randomly in the garden, but later we had to move some of the plants to other areas, as *Banisteriopsis* easily overwhelms other plant species nearby. We currently grow two varieties of *Banisteriopsis caapi*, called *tucunacá* and *caupurí* according to the taxonomy developed by the UDV (*União do Vegetal*), one of the religious Brazilian organizations that use ayahuasca as a sacrament. *Tucunacá* has smooth stems, while *Caupurí* presents internodes along the stem. This was the variety first described by Richard Spruce in 1852. We also have a third variety which is a hybrid between the two. It is hoped with time we can collect more *Banisteriopsis* species and varieties of medicinal importance.

One of the main limitations working with heavy clay soils is sourcing enough organic matter for compost and mulching. Much of the organic matter for our garden is the exceptional biomass from the fallen leaves of our old *Banisteriopsis caapi* vines. It is often said this plant prefers well drained soils though with time we have observed that this species also grows very well on clay soils. The finely netting root system is fantastic as a soil stabilizer preventing erosion.

As *Banisteriopsis* is a high value medicine and wild populations are threatened due to the ever-increasing demand, due to the widespread use of ayahuasca as a medicine throughout the world, it is important both for the conservation of the species and for the wellbeing of humanity that sustainable agricultural production models are achieved in the near future. We have experimented with growing this species alongside suitable host tree species. The choice of host tree species must take into account several criteria. The tree when mature must be able to provide the support for one of the largest of lianas. It should be fast growing, to keep ahead of the fast-growing vines. They should be tall to make good use of vertical space for photosynthesis. They should be strong and flexible enough to withstand the drag of strong winds.

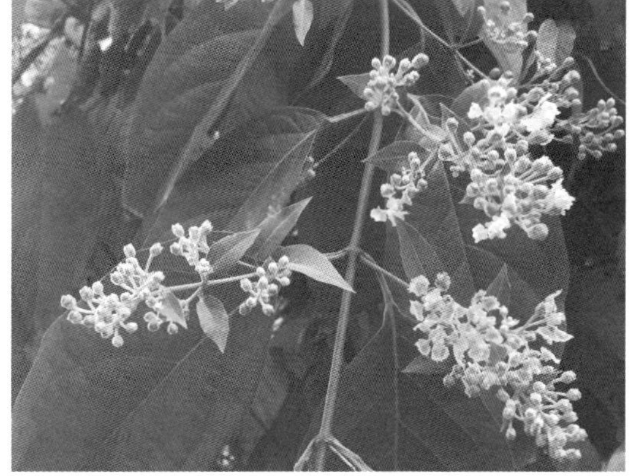

Fig.4 *Banisteriopsis caapi* flowers.
Photo L.E.Luna

We have discovered two ideal Fabaceous deciduous species to host our *caapi* vines, and both are Brazilian species. One is the gigantic *garapuvú* (*Schizolobium parahyba*), a very fast-growing pioneering species from the surrounding Mid Atlantic forest. The second species is *Enterolobium contortisiliquum* or *pacara* earpod tree from eastern Brazil and throughout much of South America. The latter species has a symbiotic relationship with certain soil bacteria that form nodules on the roots and fix atmospheric nitrogen. Some of this nitrogen is utilized by the tree, though some can also be used by other plants growing nearby.

Planted in this way, they make ideal companion guilds in an agroforestry system, and provide ideal vertical production of vine stem and biomass from leaves. It has been most interesting to observe the relationships that develop between caapi and its host tree, as one realizes that the vine could very easily smother the top of the tree with its own leaves, placing the tree in the dark and thus photosynthesis would not be possible. Yet they appear to grow harmoniously with extreme respect to each other's spatial use of light and the distribution of weight support is complementary to maintain balance.

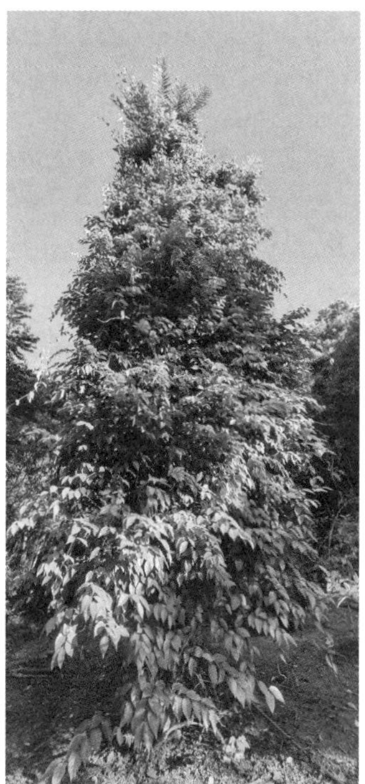

Fig.5 *Banisteriopsis caapi* growing on a garapuvú (Schizolobium parahyba) tree.
Photo L.E.Luna

With time these tree and vine combinations often merge, with the base of the vine absorbed into the lower trunk of the tree, protruding from the tree like an umbilical cord. They become vertical biodiversity ecosystems and we have observed insects and birds making use of these. Many species of the spectacular butterflies on the island use these structures in the garden for basking to warm their bodies in the morning before flying. Further research should be undertaken to establish which other tree species make good candidates for this purpose. On the island, the vines flower within two weeks of the first onset of cold weather,

weather that does not occur in *caapi*'s native Amazonia. Vines harvested at this time, when boiled and reduced, produce an intensely sweet syrup tasting of honey and chocolate.

PSYCHOTRIA GARDENS

Psychotria viridis is the main species used in the preparation of the sacred medicinal beverage, ayahuasca. Three areas are designated for growing *Psychotria viridis*. The original garden near the main house was grown from plants sent to us from the same friend who sent us the *Banisteriopsis* seeds. Two varieties were sent which we cloned through leaf and stem cuttings and were regarded as being potent in alkaloids relative to the number of foveolae, also called domatia, appearing on the underside of the leaves. This is association between the psychoactive potency of the plant and the number of those structures is apparently made by practitioners in the Amazon. Though still not confirmed analytically, it is well known that much variation in dimethyltryptamine (DMT) occurs amongst genetic varieties and species. Personal observations with growing this species over time reveal that higher levels of DMT are reached in the summer months, and much like its relative coffee, if nurtured when young with plenty of nitrogen rich compost and water, it can be grown in full sun, positively affecting tryptamine levels in the leaves.

There are many species of *Psychotria* in the surrounding forest, such as *Psychotria pernitida*, with delicate waxy, tubular flowers that attract several species of hummingbirds. Some years ago, we found a specimen of *Psychotria carthaginensis* growing on the eastern part of the island, a species also important in the preparation of ayahuasca. A cutting from that collection has now matured and has flowered in the garden allowing for positive identification.

Ololiuqui (*Rivea corymbosa*), *Argyrea Nervosa* and *Ipomoea violacea*

Rivea corymbosa has a long history of use as a sacrament amongst the Aztecs in pre-Hispanic times. It is a large woody vine of the Convolvulaceae with spectacular bursts of white flowers

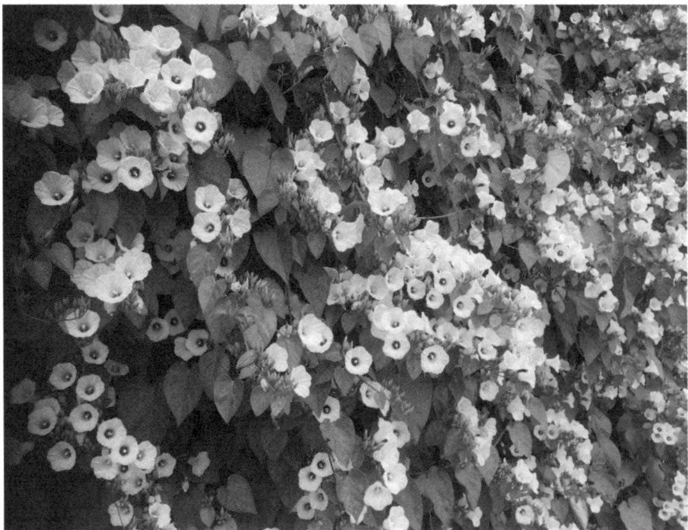

Fig.6 Flowers of ololiqui (Turbina corymbosa). *Photo L.E. Luna*

which attract large numbers of bees to their nectar. Like other Convolvulaceae, it expands rapidly and needs to be held in check. We planted it along a stone wall, and now it covers the wall completely. We have also planted *Argyreia nervosa*, a very large perennial vine, along the fence. These vines upon maturity produce breathtaking displays of dark pink flowers. We also grow morning glories (*Ipomoea violaceae)*, adding bright blues to the garden in summer.

Diplopterys cabrerana

Diplopterys cabrerana, known in Colombia as *chagropanga* or *chiliponga* is a Malpighian vine with high levels of tryptamines in its leaves. The combination of *Banisteriopsis caapi* and the leaves of *D. cabrerana*, either brewed or as a cold infusion, is known under the name *yagé* by several indigenous communities of the Colombian and Ecuadorian Amazon.

We have several *Diplopterys* vines growing throughout the property. Once established they produce a lot more foliage for medicine than *Psychotria viridis*. It almost seems as if the plant enjoys being harvested. We have been experimenting with this plant over the last five years with hope that we can come up with qualitative phenomenological analysis showing differences of experience between the more commonly consumed ayahuasca (*Banisteriopsis caapi* + *Psychotria viridis*) and *yagé* (*Banisteriopsis caapi* + *Diploptery cabrerana*). We are still awaiting flowering and seeds from our vines. The surrounding forest and indeed much of Brazil has a plethora of Malpighian species, practically all of which remain unstudied regarding their chemistry and potential medicinal use.

Brugmansia aurea

One of the truly magnificent plants in the garden is *met-kwai borrachero*, the jaguar's intoxicant, in the terminology of the Kamsá of the Sibundoy Valley in the Colombian Putumayo. In Spanish it is known as *culebra borrachero*. Richard Evans Schultes named it *Methysticodendron amesianum*,

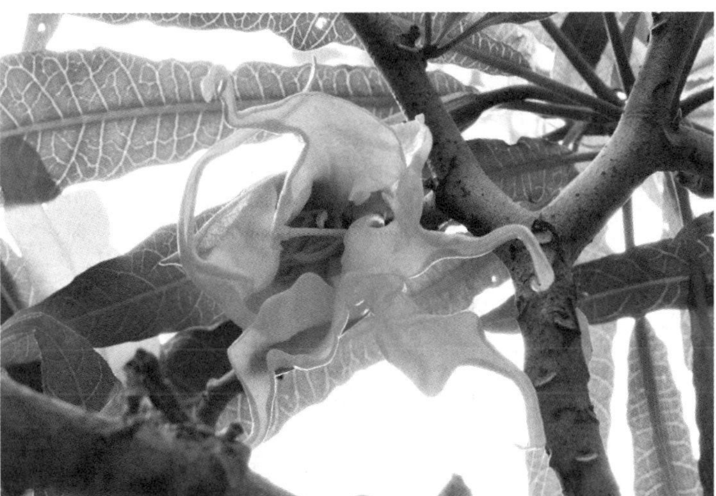

Fig.7 Flower of Brugmansia aurea. *Photo Mauricio Tolosa*

placing it in its own genus, because of its morphology. Not only its flowers but also its leaves are very different from the other species of this genus: they are long (sometimes exceeding 50 cm), thin, asymmetrical, and slightly curved, the edges always with varied undulations, like those of a key. Some contort strangely and turn their backs towards the sky. The *culebras* in our garden are all cloned from the same plant. When given ample feeding and water, they seem to flower continuously, six or seven times per year. The *culebra* twisted white flowers exhale a deep and haunting fragrance. Some of its petals seem to take a ballet step; others are confused in the interlacing of stamens. In addition to providing us with beauty, our *culebra* alerts us when the garden lacks water, because then its branches faint from fatigue. Schultes's name for this plant remained for many years until it was accepted as a genetic mutation of *Brugmansia aurea*, a specific and powerful chemotype with a higher concentration of tropane alkaloids than the other *Brugmansia*, jealousy preserved over generations. According to Schultes, the *taitas* of the Kamsá and Inganos of the Sibundoy use it in important cases of divination, prophecy or therapy, its effects lasting up to four days, including periods of total unconsciousness.

Anadenanthera colubrina and *A. peregrina*.

Anadenanthera is a genus of the family Fabaceae, with a wide distribution on the South American continent and in the Greater Antilles. We have in our garden beautiful specimens of *Anadenanthera colubrina* var. *cebil*, and *Anadenanthera peregrina*, var. *peregrina*. The very first book written in the Americas in a European language was by the friar Ramón Pané, who under the orders of Christopher Columbus on his second voyage (1494) made a careful description of the use of *cohoba* (*A. peregrina*) among the Taino of the island of Hispaniola (now Santo Domingo/

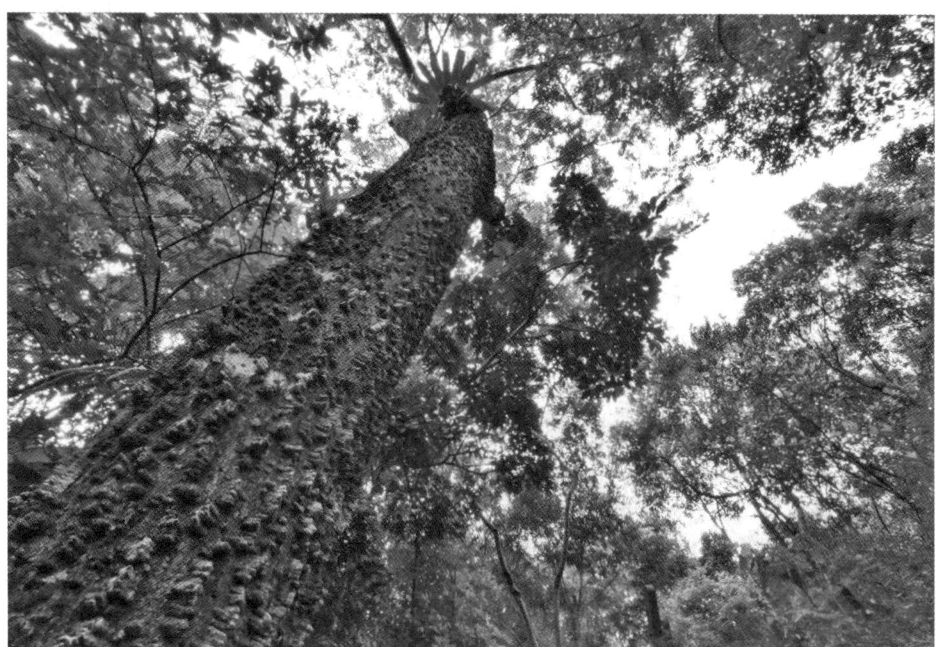

Fig.8 *Anadenanthera colubrina. Photo Mauricio Tolosa*

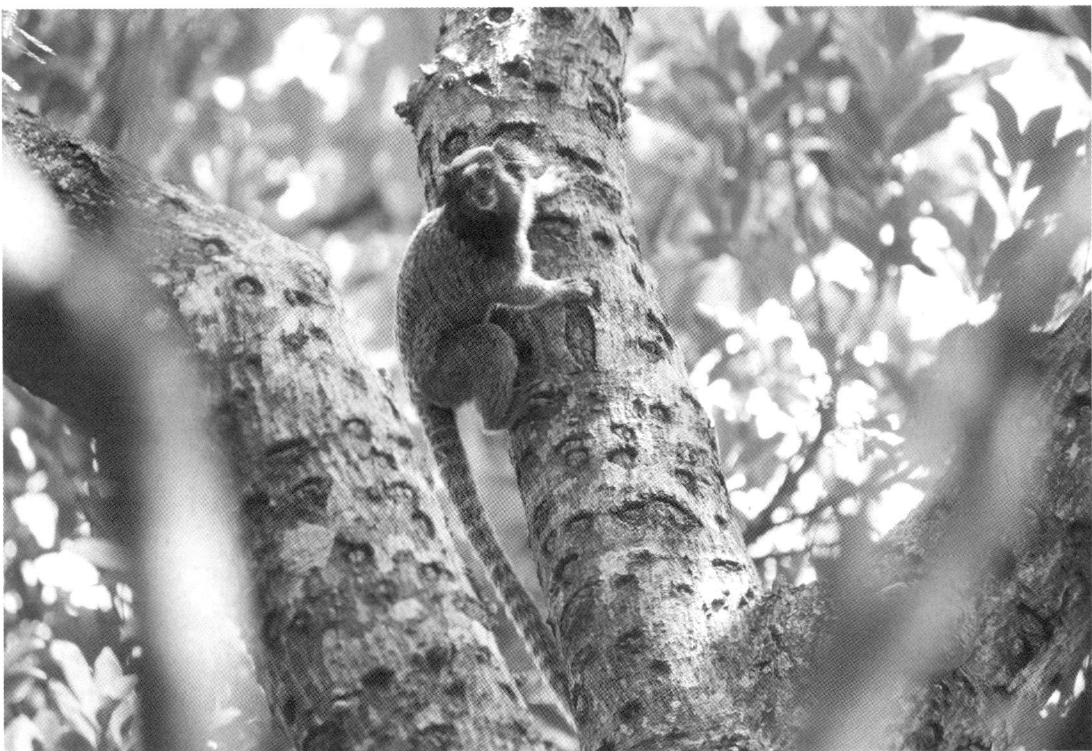

Fig.9 Marmoset monkey Callithrix jacchus, on an *Anadenanthera colubrina* tree. *Photo Dale Millard*

Haiti), who either snuffed or smoked its powdered seeds. They contain bufotenine and dimethyltryptamine (among other chemical compounds), both of which are powerful psychedelic alkaloids. The use of *Anadenanthera* snuffs has been widespread among indigenous cultures of South America and the Greater Antilles for thousands of years. Today its use is still common among many indigenous cultures, including, but not limited to the Guahibo, the Piaroa, and the Wichí. Carbon dating of archaeological evidence in the form of snuffing tubes, smoking pipes, and artistic representations of *Anadenanthera* use in Latin America and the Greater Antilles date back to more than 4000 years ago. *A. colubrina* was one of the sacred plants of Tiwanaku, one of the most important pre-Inca South American cultures (see Torres & Rebke 1996).

Our main specimens of *A. colubrina* were planted around sixteen years ago. The largest one is now about ten meters high. It possesses a rugged imposing trunk at times populated by small bromelias. *Anadenanthera* are well suited agroforestry species. They are fast growing, nitrogen fixing and are deciduous, meaning they are bare in winter, allowing light penetration for other species.

A very curious and ongoing observation concerns a small species of marmoset monkey *Callithrix jacchus*, known locally in the Guarani language as *Sagüi*. The *Sagüi* are not originally native to Florianópolis, and were introduced in the past through the pet trade. Although they are considered an invasive species by the conservation authorities, as they compete with native species and are avid nest robbers of bird eggs, they are largely left alone by humans to carry on with their monkey business on the island. They live in small families averaging nine to twelve members in the surrounding forests and suburban gardens. *Sagüi* are tolerated by most island inhabitants, likely due to their apparent perceived "cuteness"! This species displays very complex social, breeding, and feeding behaviors. Communication is achieved through various staring gazes, facial expressions, whistles, calls and scent marking. It is truly a wonder of nature that such a small animal species with a brain the size of a walnut demonstrates such a degree of complex behaviors and even a wide spectrum of emotions.

Much of their original habitat, the Cerrado of Northeastern Brazil has been developed by humans, largely around agricultural use. The Cerrado is still the second largest vegetation type in Brazil next to the Amazon, with a mere 21 percent of its original vegetation intact. These monkeys have now adapted and mastered a different, and wetter type of forest. The Sagüi, like most marmoset monkeys are considered to be "gummivores" (Power, 2009), which means that a large percentage of their diet, between twenty to seventy percent, depending on the season, consists of tree gums or exudates, for which they have complex gut flora for digestion. They also feed on fruits, making them both a frugivore and gummivore species. They have specialized sharp incisors for biting holes through the bark of trees to get at this latex.

These monkeys have always been regular visitors to the garden. One afternoon approximately 4 years ago, we noticed a family biting holes in the large *Anadenanthera colubrina* var. *cebil*, a native of the Cerrado. We soon realized that they would visit this tree every morning and every evening with great enthusiasm to get this treat. As this species is a well-known ancient psychoactive species rich in tryptamines, for which its seeds are used in snuffs, we were wondering if the monkeys received any benefits other than dietary from this practice. This genus is known to be rich in tryptamines and limited analyses have also detected several beta carbolines in this genus (Torres and Repke, 1996). Whilst we were pondering this idea of whether or not the monkeys could be getting stoned, they systematically began targeting other high tryptamine species. Next was *Mimosa tenuiflora* and then the *Acacias*. The resulting bite marks on the tree originally seemed highly destructive to the trees, and driven to save our specimens, we engaged in a kind of psychological warfare with the *Sagüi*, placing mirrors and balloons, using aposematic colours found in nature, black, white, and red, that were painted with threatening eyes and expressions. It worked!—for about a month, and then we realized that the monkeys do not seem to harm the trees excessively, perhaps even pruning the branches, to allow light for other plants. We may never know what the monkeys in our garden are up to in targeting these tryptamine rich species, though it is peculiar that the only other species where we have observed this behavior is in *Porcelia macrocarpa*, Annonaceae, commonly known as the Monkey's banana as they also feed off its fruit. Although this species is not known to contain tryptamines of interest to date, it would be an interesting species for analysis with this regard as other Annanoaceous species have been found to contain interesting new tryptamine amides (Yang-Chang Wu et al,2005)

JUREMA (*MIMOSA TENUIFLORA*)

Forgotten in a drawer for several years, we found two seeds of *Mimosa tenuiflora*, a small tree from the Brazilian Northeast. One of the seeds germinated, so we were able to see its progress, its leaves closing at night as if sleeping. Our *jurema* is now a mature five-meter-high tree that has gone through quite an ordeal. We discovered one afternoon to our great disappointment, that a bark beetle (*Curculionidae sp.*) had totally ring-barked our only specimen. We were able to save the *Jurema* by reconnecting the cambium layers through a technique known as bridge grafting. The insect came back and made yet another ring. Armed with a torch, Dale caught the perpetrator at night. The tree is not at its best in this climate, as it prefers drier ecosystems.

The bark of *Mimosa tenuiflora* as well as *Mimosa ophtalmocentra*, not yet in our garden, contains high concentration of DMT (N-N-dimethyltryptamine). A drink called *jurema* has been used by at least twenty ethnic groups. Its oldest reference is from an 18th century inquisitorial document: as other sacred indigenous medicines, it was considered an instrument to communicate with the devil. *Jurema* is often associated with the concept of *ciencia do índio* (Indian science), referring to the sacred and secret knowledge of some ethnic groups. *Jurema* was later adopted in *candomblé*, and other Afro-Brazilian religious cults. For a monograph on this plant see Samorini, 2016.

KAVA KAVA (*PIPER METHYSTICUM*)

Kava kava is an ancient cultigen originating in the South Pacific Islands, The roots are widely chewed as a euphoriant and used in ceremonies throughout Polynesia. There are potentially hundreds of Kava cultivars today. As Kava does not form seeds, and is grown from vegetative cuttings, these different cultivars and chemotypes have largely developed regionally over time from selections and not through breeding. The different varieties can contain vastly different profiles of the active kavalactones, with some being intoxicating and sedating, whilst others more uplifting and euphoric. Other cultivars, such as those from Vanuatu being especially potent and useful as analgesics for pain. In the forest around us is another Piperaceae species *Piper mikanianum*, whose roots are rich in asarone and which is morphologically almost identical to *kava-kava*.

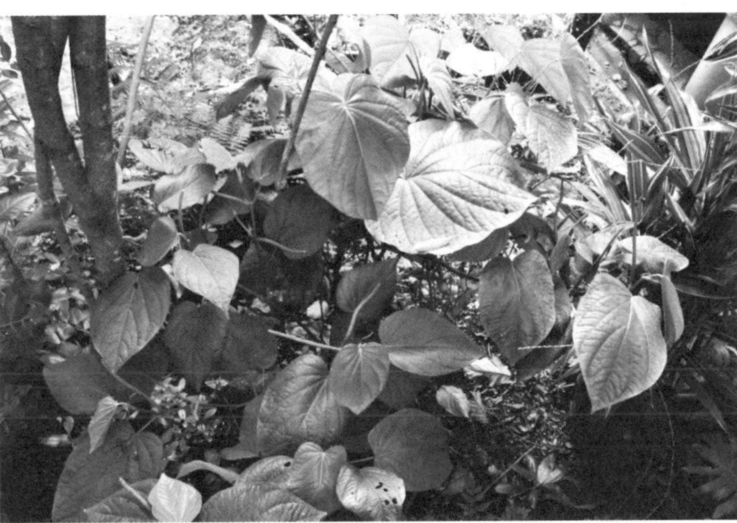

Fig.10 Kava kava (*Piper methysticum*). *Photo L.E. Luna*

CACTI AND SUCCULENTS

We maintain a small collection of cacti and succulents. Our region is not suited to many cacti species which typically prefer dry conditions. We experience some problems in winter, with the combination of cold and wet conditions causing some of our cacti to rot. Due to this many of our cacti are in pots that can be moved, and we are currently in the process of building a small cacti conservatory greenhouse dedicated to these plants. We grow peyote (*Lophophora williamsii*) and several *Echinopsis* species such as San Pedro cactus *Echinopsis pachanoi* and *Echinopsis werdermannianus*, which is a large columnar cactus from Bolivia very closely related to *E. terscheckii* though it may be synonymous with *Echinopsis taquimbalensis var. wilkeae* according to the expert Keeper Trout. The *Lophophora* collection began from just two plants that were grafted onto *Echinopsis* and *Pereskia. Lophophora* are slow growing and may take as long as 15 years in the wild to reach sexual maturity. With this grafting process, we can produce plants that flower and produce seed in under five months. Peyote plants and even seeds have become prohibitively expensive. This was a successful way to produce seed in a short space of time so that we may grow more of these plants.

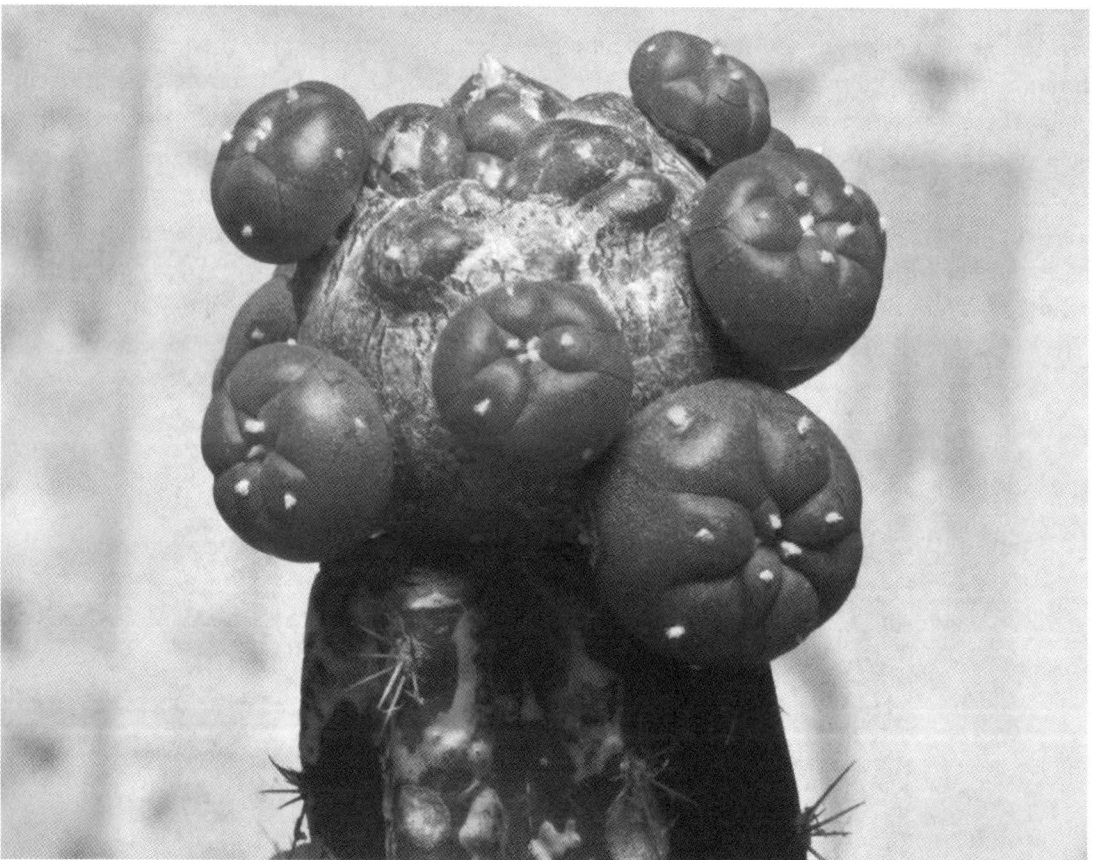

Fig.11 Peyote (Lophophora willamsii) growing on San Pedro cactus (Equinopsis pachanoi).
Photo Dale Millard

STIMULANTS

Stimulants have been used by humans for millennia, to increase mental acuity, physical endurance and for pleasure. We have some of the important ancient stimulants growing in the garden. Mate (*Ilex paraguariensis*), coffee (*Coffea arabica*), khat (*Catha edulis*), and cacao (*Theobroma cacao*). Previous attempts to grow tea (*Camellia sinensis*) and *guaraná* (*Paullinia cupana*) were unsuccessful. We hope in the future we could replace these species and expand our collection of these plant allies.

FRUITS

The agroforestry section harbors most of our fruit species. Apart from the well-known fruits such as bananas, mangoes, cashews, litchi, guavas, citrus, and avocados we aim to collect and grow more of the lesser known or rare fruit species, the collection is forever expanding in this regard with delicious flavours not available in the shops.

The native Atlantic Coastal Forest has a large diversity of poorly known and delicious fruits mostly from the Myrtaceae or Guava family. We make a special effort to grow and collect these native species which we then use in reforestation. Some of the more unique and interesting fruits grown are *jabuticaba* (*Plinia cauliflora*) also known as the Brazilian grape tree. These trees produce an abundance of black shiny round fruits directly from the trunk and branches. The flesh of the fruit is held under pressure by the skin, so that they literally burst with flavour upon eating. *Grumixama* or Brazilian cherry (*Eugenia brasilensis*) is practically extinct in the wild, as its former range is in the district of São Paulo. *Cambucá* (*Plinia edulis*) is another rare Myrtaceous fruit. We have a large, beautiful specimen planted about eighteen years ago, which gave its first fruits only six years ago.

We like to collect the Clusiaceae for their exotic delicious fruits. We have mangosteen (*Garcinia mangostana*) from Indonesia, *bacuparí* (*Garcinia brasiliensis*) from the local forest and *Mammea americana* from the Antilles, all in this family. We experiment continuously with what we are able to grow at our latitude. We have planted two *Theobroma* tropical species from the Amazon, and although we may be too far south to grow these species, our trees are healthy and we are hopeful that upon maturity, they will set fruit. One is the chocolate or cacao (*Theobroma cacao*), the other *cupuaçú*, a highly perfumed fruit with a creamy pulp that is almost addictive. It also produces a very high-quality chocolate.

We also collect Annonaceous fruits such as *atemoya*, a delicious hybrid between *Annona cherimola* and *Annona squamosa* with few seeds, as well as *graviola* (*Annona muricata)* and *Annona montana*. As cross pollination is possible between certain species in this family. It is hoped that soon we will be able to produce our own unique fruits through hybridization.

WILDLIFE

Apart from the monkeys, we receive regular visitors in the form of animals and birds to the garden. We are ideally situated for this as we are very close to the ocean, with its marine species and birds. We overlook the mouth of the Ratones river, running through a vast mangrove wetland,

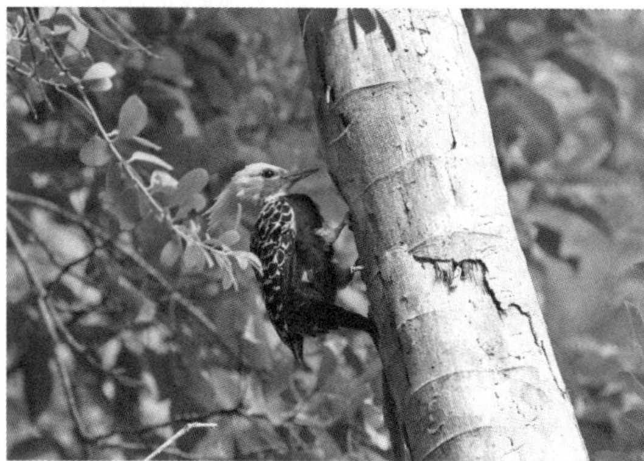

Fig.12 Blonde crested woodpecker (Celeus flavescens). *Photo Mauricio Tolosa*

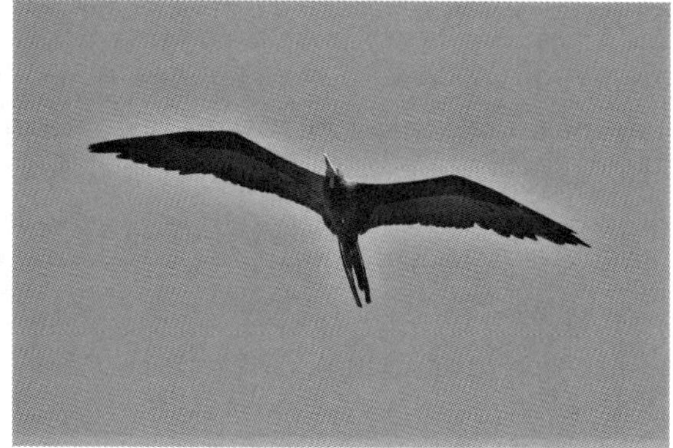

Fig.13 Frigatebird (Fregata magnificens). *Photo Mauricio Tolosa*

encompassing several different ecotones. The island has an impressive 530 recorded bird species making it a birding paradise. Populations and sightings of many species have clearly increased as the garden and agroforestry project has matured. We see far more birds, especially as we now have large trees such as the guarapuvú, close to the main house, which act as a kind of airport for birds such as channel-billed toucan (*Ramphastos vitellinus*) searching for the fruit of some our palm trees, with their disproportionately heavy beaks that send them swooping down upon take off, before they gain any altitude. These trees are also daily roosts for the *urubú* or black vultures (*Coragyps atratus*) and Brazilian turkey vultures (*Cathartes aura ruficollis*), with bright red heads. These birds have exceptional smell and if one is close enough or can zoom in on their heads, it is possible to see a clear window running directly through their nostrils. The common *potoo* (*Nyctibius griseus*) can be heard at dusk with a very distinct call that drops in crescendo. Finding them in the day is a lot trickier as diurnal hours are spent totally motionless pretending to be a branch. Mornings and evenings we hear the loud calls of long-tailed *chalalacas* (*Ortalis vetula*) that spend part of their time feeding on the fruits of our treetops. Fast running *saracuras do mato* (*Aramides saracura*), of astonishing and varied songs, come to feed with our chickens. Sometimes hundreds of magnificent frigatebirds (*Fregata magnificens*) can be seen hovering in the overhead skies. Burrowing owls (*Athene cunicularia*) are a common species living in small families in holes in the ground. Amethyst woodstar (*Calliphlox amethystina*), violet capped woodnymph (*Thalurania glaucopis*), Blonde crested woodpeckers (*Celeus flavescens*), blue fronted parrots (*Amazona Aestiva*) are all frequently encountered in the garden.

Crab eating foxes (*Cerdocyon thous*) are regular visitors from the adjacent mangroves. They are not closely related to regular fox species and are peculiar in that they show little fear of humans. Rather they are curious. We have experienced them coming within a meter of us, and they often follow us at a little distance when we are walking in the forest. We have two small rivers flowing through the property. These are homes to Brazilian snake necked turtles (*Hydromedusa maximiliani*) and the waters are teaming with *pitu* or bristled river shrimp (*Macrobrachium olfersii*).

Living within this Coastal Atlantic Forest comes with occasional surprises. We are forever finding *gambás*, white eared possums (*Didelphis aurita)* and the much smaller species called *kweka* or Brazilian gracile possums (*Gracilianus microtarsus*) in our houses. These we carefully remove and return to the forest. We also have lots of Argentine black and white *tegu* (*Tupinambis merianae*) which are the largest lizards in the Americas and several species of snakes, of which only two species on the island are venomous, most being totally harmless. We have also encountered several of the magnificent *serpente tigre* also called *caninana* (*Spilotes pullatus*) is a large nonvenomous snake, growing over two and a half meters, with bright yellow and black markings. It has excellent eyesight, is mostly arboreal and actively forages during the day for birds and small mammals. We occasionally find painted coral snakes (*Micrurus corallinus*) which are both the most beautifully marked and most venomous of all coral snakes, having both a presynaptic and postsynaptic neurotoxic venom. The other venomous species occurring on the island is the legendary *jararaca* (*Bothrops jararaca*) new world lancehead viper whose venom was the original source of the class of blood pressure drugs known as angiotensin converting enzyme (ACE) inhibitors (Mladic et al. 2017) taken by over thirteen million people worldwide. The first drug of this type was released under the brand name Captopril. Two other venomous species to keep an eye out for when working in the garden are the Brazilian wandering spider (*Phoneutria nigriventer*) which likely possesses the most studied venom of all spiders, a very complex mix of peptides. A rather bizarre side effect of this venom is priapism in human males, sparking great interest in the development of erectile dysfunction drugs (Peigneur, et al. 2018). The other venomous species to watch out for is a caterpillar *Lonomia obliqua,* the larvae of a *Saturniid* moth that has escaped out of the Amazon with the lumber industry. It has a potent venom causing both coagulation and bleeding problems. Although antivenom is produced by the Butantan Institute in São Paulo for all these species, accidents are extremely rare and fatalities even less so. One should always take precautions! Left alone they are generally not a problem for humans, and most incidents are in dogs that chase after the snakes.

CONCLUSION

It is very difficult to estimate the true value of gardens such as this. With growing geopolitical instability and climate change access to good quality organic food and medicine is far from guaranteed. These gardens are a legacy for the future and only become more productive with time, but provide educational and inspirational value too. The garden also contributes to horticultural research through the pioneering propagation and production of species. This includes two tree species for the successful propagation of *B. caapi*, the grafting of peyote, as well as the identification of new varieties and possibly species through close observation.

Thanks to generous donations we were able to build a stone path that snakes through the garden and forest, giving access to areas which were previously almost totally out of reach. We also acquired four beehives of local of mandaçaia stingless bees (*Melipona quadrifasciata quadrifasciata*) to contribute to the pollination of our plants. We have already seen the difference, as the number of flowers of several of the species in the garden has increased. We are planning to have many more beehives, perhaps up to twenty of various species, to place along the stone path. We also would like to add railings along the path to facilitate access for people with walking difficulties, children and elders. We would like to finish the cacti and succulent house, for which we have already built the basic structure, but funds are needed to add a lasting transparent roof, glass walls, and solar panel. One more wish is to have proper metal plates with the identification of around 400 species in our ethnobotanical garden. Our ambition is to create a magnificent center of tropical and subtropical species for preservation, research, and sharing to other similar centers.

The pandemic forced us to stay in one place, giving us the opportunity to experience two full non-interrupted cycles. The time of the *pitangas*, the time of the guavas, the time of the avocados, the time of the citrus, the time when the vanilla and other orchids are blooming, and the deep perfumed of our *Calliandras* and our *dama da noite* (lady of the night, *Cestrum nocturnum*) permeates the garden. As the fruits come, so do the birds, the monkeys, the bats, the lizards, the bees, and the butterflies. A garden is always a place of sudden encounters and surprises. The plants manifest themselves in various ways along the seasons, sensitive to draughts and rainy periods, appearing and disappearing, growing fruits, and flowers, climbing, making alliances with insects or other plants, at times competing straightforwardly in the search for light. Our garden is an endless source of knowledge and joy, best approached when the chatter of words is dimmed and we are open to pure perception, when we become like plants and enter their time in silence.

BIBLIOGRAPHY

Mladic M, de Wall T, Burgraff L, Slagboom J, Somsen G, Niessen W, Manjunatha, Kool J. 2017. Rapid screening and identification of snake venoms using at-line nanofractionation LC-MS. *Analytical and Bioanalytical Chemistry.* 409(25): 5987–5997

Peigneur S, De Lima M, Tytgat G. 2018. *Phoneutria nigriventer* venom: a pharmacological treasure. *Toxicon* 151: 96-110.

Power M, 2009. *American Journal of Primatology* 71: 957-963

Samorini G. 2016. Jurema. La pianta della visione. Dai culti del Brasile alla psiconautica di frontera. Shake Edizioni, Milano. ISBN 9788897109433.

Torres C.M. and Repke, D. 1996. Anadenanthera. Visionary Plant of Ancient South America. The Haworth Herbal Press, New York, London.

Wu, YC, Chang, FR and Chen, CY. 2005. Tryptamine-derived amides and alkaloids from the seeds of *Annona atemoya*. *Journal of natural products* 68(3: 406-408.

Hydrosphere

Psychoactive Allies of the Waters

Farming Marine Sponges for Psychoactive Compounds

Zak Kulberg

Marine scientist | Marine bioprospector

"Marine sponges are known to produce a variety of compounds with activity on the serotonin receptors 5-HT$_{2A}$ and 5-HT$_{2C}$, similar to other psychedelics. Many of the compounds from the sea with this activity are tryptamines, like those from psychedelic plants and fungi, with a tendency to possess the element bromine."- ZAK KULBERG

The ocean holds vast potential for medicines and psychoactive compounds. This paper explores the possibilities of marine sponges as a source of such molecules, and processes which can potentially yield them.

ABSTRACT

Compounds with aromatic amine cores, such as tryptamine and phenethylamine alkaloids are often responsible for the neuroactivities of marine sponge extracts in bioassays for drug discovery. Neuromodulating tryptamine (and phenethylamine) derivatives in marine sponges can be applied to develop new psychoactive substances, for the treatment of mental health conditions such as anxiety and depression. Metabolism in the sessile pre-nervous system of marine sponges, with their diverse array of chemical defenses (some of which are psychoactive), provides clues into the ecological production of powerful bioactive compounds. Do these psychoactive substances from the sea give us the opportunity to participate in an ecological phenomenon that has guided the evolution of neurochemical consciousness? Or do sponges simply protect themselves with these compounds to prevent the glue of other organisms from sticking to their surface? In this work, directed biotransformation was explored to theoretically increase the production of brominated tryptamine derivatives and other alkaloids in farmed marine sponges. This research was conducted to trigger the production of known and unknown psychoactive substances and uncover the molecular biology of their biosynthetic pathways. Theoretically, a psychoactive tryptamine or phenethylamine derivative may increase in concentration in a marine sponge after incubation in an appropriate precursor (ie. tryptamine, tryptophan, phenethylamine, phenylalanine, bromide salts). This paper considers the application of biotransformation and modern analytical approaches to psychoactive bioprospecting strategies.

INTRODUCTION

For over a millennium, beginning in the 6th century, soporific sponges were used to apply surgical anesthesia by inhalation or absorption through the nasal membrane. These were sea sponges impregnated with psychoactive plant concoctions varying from opium to hashish, hemlock, and henbane. Anesthesia from soporific sponges was eventually replaced by nitrous oxide, ether and chloroform (Juvin and Desmonts, 2000). By the mid-1800's, sponges wet with ether in glass inhalers were used for similar purposes (Haridas and Bause, 2013).

There is no clear historical use of sponges for their alkaloids to get "high," although 5-bromo-N,N-dimethyltryptamine (6) which is found in multiple sea sponges, is discussed as a theoretical psychedelic by Alexander Shulgin in *TiHKAL* (1997) and reviewed by Hamilton Morris in his *VICE Magazine* article Sea DMT (Morris and Wallach, 2013).Various YouTube creators and trip reports share experiences consuming this compound, however this is not the only tryptamine from marine sponges with indications of psychoactivity.

In the 1980s, research by Jochen Gartz (Gartz, 1989a, 1989b) used directed biotransformation* to demonstrate that the yield of tryptamine psychedelic psilocin from fruiting mycelia of *Psilocybe cubensis* increased hundreds of times (from 0.01-0.15 % weight to up to 3.3% weight) by exposing the mycelia to high concentrations (25 mM) of tryptamine HCl (Table 1). A reduction in the amount of psilocybin was explained as potentially due to lower amounts of phosphate in the growth media. Additional data also showed that the mycelia converted the substrate N,N-diethyl-tryptamine into the corresponding 4-hydroxy derivative (Gartz, 1989b). One biotransformation step appears to be N-methylation, while another is hydroxylation of the 4 position on the tryptamine indole system.

Flush #	% Psilocin dry weight	% Psilocin dry weight	% Psilocybin dry weight	% Psilocybin dry weight
	Treated with Tryptamine [25 mM]	No tryptamine added	Treated with Tryptamine [25 mM]	No tryptamine added
1	2.1	-	0.01	0.55
2	3.3	0.01	0.02	0.48
3	2.8	0.02	0.2	0.51
4	3.1	0.09	0.07	0.46
5	2.9	0.15	0.13	0.61

Table 1: Percentage of psilocin or psilocybin in fruiting mycelia of *Psilocybe cubensis* with or without exposure to tryptamine, modified from Gartz (1989a).

Briefly, biotransformation seeks to supply the building blocks for biosynthetic reactions. The amino acids tryptophan and phenylalanine/tyrosine are starting points in humans for the biosynthesis of neurotransmitters serotonin and dopamine/noradrenaline, respectively. The receptors (GPCR's) of these endogenous compounds play major roles in the processes of psychoactive

* Biotransformation is the alteration of a drug or compound.

drugs. These neurotransmitters are synthesized through multiple steps including a common decarboxylation by the enzyme L-aromatic amino acid decarboxylase (AAAD) (Christenson et al., 1972). Relatives of this enzyme may also play a role in the biosynthesis of psychoactive alkaloids as part of biosynthetic gene clusters. There may be a variety of tryptophan decarboxylating enzymes in microbes or sponges responsible for part of the biotransformation of tryptophan derivatives, like the non-canonical aromatic amino acid decarboxylase (PcncAAAD) found in *Psilocybe cubensis* (Torrens-Spensce et al., 2018). However, so far, metagenomic data analysis from 5 of the sponges the author cultured in Okinawa, Japan indicates an absence of annotated aromatic amino acid decarboxylase sequences. Evolutionarily, serotonin production may have negatively impacted the survival of sessile sponges by triggering settlement of fouling organisms. Halogenase enzymes are responsible for the bromination* of many biologically actie alkaloids (Agarwal et al., 2017), and are detected in many sponge associated microbes (Bayer et al., 2013). Indeed, tryptophan halogenases have been studied for their contribution to brominated tryptamine derivatives (Gutleben et al., 2019). Brominated dopamine derivatives in marine organisms likely play a role in the inhibition of tyrosine hydroxylation pathways during the formation of glues from fouling organisms, and do not necessarily play roles in neurotransmission.

Serotonergic drugs tend to be composed of tryptamine derivatives. This chapter will briefly detail some of the known serotonergic compounds found in extracts of marine sponges. This includes brominated tryptamine derivatives with psychoactivity indicated by affinities for serotonin receptors, particularly (but not exclusively) 5-HT_{2A} and 5-HT_{2C}, such as bromo-aplysinopsin derivatives 6-bromoaplysinopsin (9) and 6-bromo-2'-de-N-methylaplysinopsin (10), and the brominated compounds, barettin (33) and 8,9-dihydrobarettin (34). A more encompassing technical review on the pharmacology of psychoactive marine natural products from sponges mentioned above was co-authored by Mark Hamann (Kochanowska-Karamyan and Hamann, 2010), who previously headed the USDA natural product repository and has collaborated with the National Institute of Mental Health's Psychoactive Drug Screening Program to bioassay 5-bromo-N,N-dimethyltryptamine (6) and other halogenated DMT derivatives (5, 7) (Ibrahim et al., 2017).

BROMINATED TRYPTAMINES

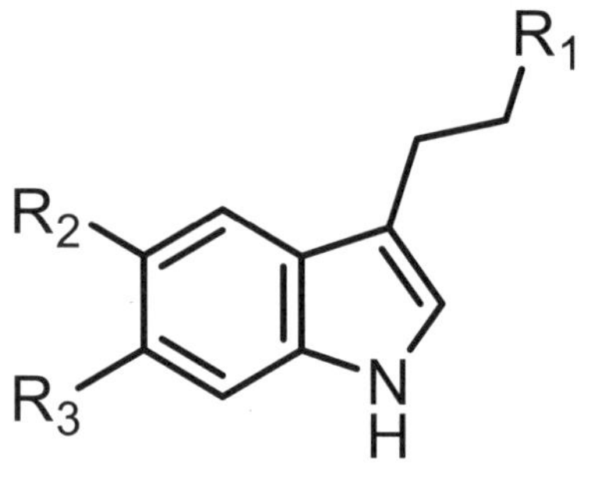

Alexander (Sasha) and Ann Shulgin showcased psychoactive tryptamine and phenethylamine derivatives in their books *TiHKAL* (1997) and *PiHKAL* (1991), respectively. *TiHKAL* described a variety of tryptamine derivatives containing the element bromine [5,6-dibromo-N,N-dimethyltryptamine (1) , 5,6-dibromo-tryptamine (2), 5,6-dibromo-N-methyl-tryptamine (3), 5-bromo- N,N-dimethyltryptamine (6)] known to be produced by marine sponges (*Smenospongia auria, Smenospongia echin, Polyfibrospongia maynardii*).

R_1 R_2 R_3 N H

* When something is "brominated" it is treated with bromine. One or more bromine atoms are introduced, typically in place of a hydrogen atom.

Sasha went on to write "I had the fantasy of trying to scotch the rumor I'm about to start, that all the hippies of the San Francisco Bay Area were heading to the Caribbean with packets of Zig-Zag papers, to hit the sponge trade with a psychedelic fervor."

	Compound	R_1	R_2	R_3
1	5,6-Dibromo-N,N-dimethyltryptamine	$N(CH_3)_2$	Br	Br
2	5,6-Dibromotryptamine	NH_2	Br	Br
3	5,6-Dibromo-N-methyltryptamine	$NH(CH_3)$	Br	Br
4	N,N-Dimethyltryptamine	$N(CH_3)_2$	H	H
5	5-Chloro-N,N-dimethyltryptamine	$N(CH_3)_2$	Cl	H
6	5-Bromo-N,N-dimethyltryptamine	$N(CH_3)_2$	Br	H
7	5-Iodo-N,N-dimethyltryptamine	$N(CH_3)_2$	I	H

Table 2 Structures 1-7: Tryptamine derivatives. Structures 1-3 and 6 are brominated tryptamines present in sponges.

Hamann et al. authored US patent 8,268,856, "Method to use compositions having antidepressant anxiolytic and other neurological activity and compositions of matter". They reference their work on the 5-bromo-N,N-dimethyltryptamine (6) and 5,6-dibromo-N,N-dimethyltryptamine (1) composition of three sponges: *Verongula rigida*, *Smenospongia aurea*, and *Smenospongia cerebriformis* (Kochanowska et al., 2008). Their later collaboration (data shown in Table 2), tested 5-bromo-N,N-dimethyltryptamine (6) and various halogenated DMT derivatives (5,7) binding affinities to serotonin receptors with NIMH PDSP (Ibrahim et al., 2017).

Receptor	Compound 4 Ki (nM)	Compound 5 Ki (nM)	Compound 6 C Ki (nM)	Compound 7 D Ki (nM)	Controls	
					Ergotamine Ki (nM)	Methysergide Ki (nM)
5-HT_{1A}	110.0 ± 17.0	5.5 ± 0.4	9.6 ± 1.1	130.0 ± 16.0	0.17	14
5-HT_{1B}	66.0 ± 9.0	66.0 ± 5.0	19.0 ± 2.0	43.0 ± 5.0	0.3	2.5
5-HT_{1D}	29.3 ± 3.7	14.0 ± 1.0	2.6 ± 0.32	8.5 ± 1.38	0.3	69
5-HT_{1E}	>10,000	356.0 ± 34.0	398.0 ± 30.0	310.0 ± 33.0	19	237
5-HT_{2B}	145.0 ± 13.0	7.8 ± 0.7	27.0 ± 1.0	98.0 ± 4.0	1.9	0.1
5-HT_{3}	5,187 ± 883	1,325 ± 125	1,374 ± 212	4,486 ± 804	>10,000	>10,000
5-HT_{5A}	>10,000	408.0 ± 54.0	1,038 ± 110	1,254 ± 197	-	>10,000
5-HT_{6}	189.5 ± 32.5	30.0 ± 2.0.0	22.0 ± 2.0	198.0 ± 20.0	12	52
5-HT_{7}	77.0 ± 16.0	7.2 ± 0.6	8.3 ± 0.9	116.0 ± 13.0	1,291	30

Table 3 Halogen derivative binding affinities to serotonin receptors with NIMH PDSP, modified from Ibrahim et al. (2017).

BROMINATED APLYSINOPSINS

A variety of compounds called aplysinopsins, named after the sponge *Thorecta aplysinopsis* (Kazlauskas et al., 1977), show various affinities for the serotonin receptors 5-HT$_{2A}$ and 5-HT$_{2C}$, reflecting probable psychoactivity. Some of these compounds are brominated. Table 5, modified from Bialonska and Zjawiony (2009), shows structures, source sponges, and psychoactive targets of aplysinopsins, or in several cases, compounds found to affect the symbiosis between a sea anemone and clown fish (Murata at al., 1986). The modified table does not include sources of aplysinopsins aside from sponges, such as *Tubastraea* corals and the anemone *Radianthus kuekenthali*. Aplysinopsin derivatives were assessed for structure activity relationships by Cummings et al. (2010).

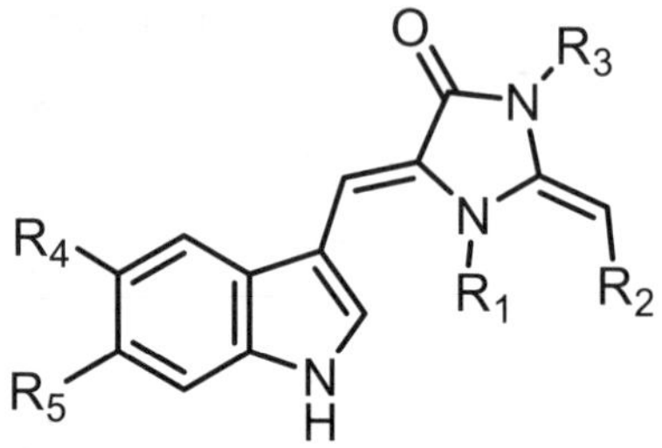

Aplysinopsin Numbering System (E form dominant in nature)						
	Compound	**R_1**	**R_2**	**R_3**	**R_4**	**R_5**
8	Aplysinopsin	CH_3	H	CH_3	H	H
9	6-Bromoaplysinopsin	CH_3	H	CH_3	H	Br
10	6-Bromo-2'-de-N-methylaplysinopsin	H	CH_3	CH_3	H	H
11	Methylaplysinopsin	CH_3	CH_3	CH_3	H	H
12	5,6-dibromo-2'-demethylaplysinopsin	H	H	CH_3	Br	Br
13	N-3'-Ethylaplysinopsin	CH_3	CH_2CH_3	CH_3	H	H
14	5-Bromo-4'-demethylaplysinopsin	CH_3	H	H	Br	H
15	5-Fluoroaplysinopsin	CH_3	H	CH_3	F	H
16	5-Chloro-4'-demethylaplysinopsin	CH_3	H	H	Cl	H
17	5,6-Dichloro-4'-demethylaplysinopsin	CH_3	H	H	Cl	Cl
18	5-Fluoro-4'-demethylaplysinopsin	CH_3	H	H	F	H
19	6-Fluoro-4'-demethylaplysinopsin	CH_3	H	H	H	F
20	6-Chloro-4'-demethylaplysinopsin	CH_3	H	H	H	Cl
21	4'-demethylaplysinopsin	CH_3	H	H	H	H
22	5-Bromo-4'-ethylaplysinopsin	CH_3	H	CH_2CH_3	Br	H
23	5-Chloroaplysinopsin	CH_3	H	CH_3	Cl	H
24	5-Bromoaplysinopsin	CH_3	H	CH_3	Br	H
25	5-Iodo-4'-ethylaplysinopsin	CH_3	H	CH_2CH_3	I	H
26	6-Fluoroaplysinopsin	CH_3	H	CH_3	H	F
27	6-Chloroaplysinopsin	CH_3	H	CH_3	H	Cl
28	5,6-Dichloroaplysinopsin	CH_3	H	CH_3	Cl	Cl
29	4'-Ethylaplysinopsin	CH_3	H	CH_2CH_3	H	H
30	6-Fluoro-4'-ethylaplysinopsin	CH_3	H	CH_2CH_3	H	F
31	6-Bromo-4'-ethylaplysinopsin	CH_3	H	CH_2CH_3	H	Br

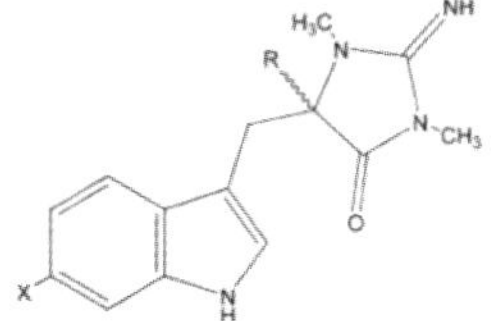

Structure of Aplysinopsin 32			
	Compound	X	R
32	1',8-dihydroaplysinopsin	H	H

Table 4 Structures 8-32. Aplysinopsins.

Compound	Source	Receptor activity and behavior
(8) Aplysinopsin	Thorecta sp. sponge Great Barrier Reef Australia [1] *Verongia spengelli* sponge—Florida Keys (Hollenbeak and Schmitz, 1977) *Dercitus sp.* sponge—Caribbean (Djura and Faulkner, 1980) *Smenospongia aurea* sponge—Caribbean (Tymiak and Rinehart, 1980) *Dictyoceratida* sponges (Bergquist and Wells, 1983)	Induces symbiosis between sea anemone and anemone fish [20] Induces symbiosis between sea anemone and anemone fish (Murata at al., 1986).
(9) 6-Bromoaplysinopsin	Tubastrea coccinea coral Hawaii [15] *Smenospongia aurea* sponge—Caribbean (Tymiak and Rinehart, 1980) [18] *Smenospongia aurea* sponge—Jamaica (Hu et al., 2002) *Smenospongia aurea* sponge—Florida Keys (Kochanowska et al., 2008)	Serotonin receptors modulator [6] Antiplasmodial [6] Induces symbiosis between sea anemone and anemone fish [20] Induces symbiosis between sea anemone and anemone fish (Murata at al., 1986) 5-HT_{2A}, (Ki μM): 2.0; 5-HT_{2C}, (Ki μM): 0.33; 5-HT_{2C} Selectivity: 6 (Hu et al., 2002)
(10) 6-Bromo-2'-de-N-methylaplysinopsin	*Smenospongia aurea* sponge—Jamaica (Hu et al., 2002) *Hyrtios erecta* sponge—Japan (Aoki et al., 2001)	Inhibitor of nitric oxide synthase (Aoki et al., 2001) 5-HT_{2A}, (Ki μM): >100; 5-HT_{2C}, (Ki μM): 2.3; 5-HT_{2C} Selectivity: >43 (Hu et al., 2002)
(11) Methylaplysinopsin	Aplysinopsis reticulata sponge - Australia [9] *Smenospongia aurea* sponge—Jamaica (Hu et al., 2002)	Inhibits monoamine oxidase (MAO) and displaces serotonin from receptors (Baird-Lambert et al, 1982).
(12) 5,6-dibromo-2'-demethylaplysinopsin 5,6-dibromo-2'-demethylaplysinopsin	*Hyrtios erecta* sponge—Japan (Aoki et al., 2001)	Inhibitor of nitric oxide synthase (Aoki et al., 2001)
(13) N-3'-Ethylaplysinopsin	*Smenospongia aurea* sponge—Jamaica (Hu et al., 2002)	5-HT_{2A}, (Ki μM): 1.7; 5-HT_{2C}, (Ki μM): 3.5; 5-HT_{2C} Selectivity: 0.5 (Hu et al., 2002)
(32) 1',8-Dihydroaplysinopsin	*Thorectandra sp.* Sponge - Indo-Pacific reefs (Segraves and Crews, 2005)	Induces symbiosis between sea anemone and anemone fish (Murata at al., 1986).

Table 5 Source sponges and psychoactive targets of aplysinopsins8-13, and 32.

Table modified from Bialonska and Zjawiony (2009)

Cummings et al. (2010) created a clear structure activity relationship (SAR) for aplysinopsins (8,9 and 14-31) and their activities on 5-HT1A, 5-HT_{2A}, and 5-HT_{2C} serotonin receptors (Table 5). The SAR's show an increased specificity for the 5-HT_{2C} receptor for non-fluorine halogenation substitutions at the 6 carbon (Table 6). The double bond from the 8 to 2', just like in barettin (33), also seems to connotate 5-HT_{2C} receptor preference. All compounds were screened at 3 μM except 6-Bromoaplysinopsin, which, due to poor solubility, had to be screened at 1 μM.

Compound	% Displacement		
	5-HT_{1A}	5-HT_{2A}	5-HT_{2C}
(8) Aplysinopsin	0 +/- 1	47 +/- 3	0 +/- 7
(9) 6-Bromoaplysinopsin	1 +/- 3	8 +/- 1	46 +/- 8
(14) 5-Bromo-4'-demethylaplysinopsin	6 +/- 2	0 +/- 5	0 +/- 5
(15) 5-Fluoroaplysinopsin	4 +/- 3	10 +/- 1	0 +/- 6
(16) 5-Chloro-4'-demethylaplysinopsin	9 +/- 3	9 +/- 1	0 +/- 6
(17) 5,6-Dichloro-4'-demethylaplysinopsin	4 +/- 2	0 +/- 4	10 +/- 5
(18) 5-Fluoro-4'-demethylaplysinopsin	0 +/- 3	0 +/- 1	19 +/- 6
(19) 6-Fluoro-4'-demethylaplysinopsin	0 +/- 4	6 +/- 4	1 +/- 8
(20) 6-Chloro-4'-demethylaplysinopsin	1 +/- 2	0 +/- 3	0 +/- 6
(21) 4'-demethylaplysinopsin	0 +/- 6	0 +/- 2	6 +/- 10
(22) 5-Bromo-4'-ethylaplysinopsin	0 +/- 0	9 +/- 3	18 +/- 10
(23) 5-Chloroaplysinopsin	9 +/- 2	22 +/- 4	43 +/- 11
(24) 5-Bromoaplysinopsin	18 +/- 2	37 +/- 1	64 +/-5
(25) 5-Iodo-4'-ethylaplysinopsin	15 +/- 1	35 +/- 2	46 +/- 6
(26) 6-Fluoroaplysinopsin	2 +/- 3	79 +/- 3	0 +/- 5
(27) 6-Chloroaplysinopsin	3 +/- 3	0 +/- 5	49 +/- 5
(28) 5,6-Dichloroaplysinopsin	0 +/- 4	12 +/- 2	79 +/- 4
(29) 4'-Ethylaplysinopsin	0 +/- 3	50 +/- 2	0 +/- 5
(30) 6-Fluoro-4'-ethylaplysinopsin	0 +/- 1	86 +/- 1	0 +/- 5
(31) 6-Bromo-4'-ethylaplysinopsin	0 +/- 1	0 +/- 8	49 +/- 10

Table 6 Displacement activity of aplysinopsins on 5-HT_{1A}, 5-HT_{2A} and 5-HT_{2C} serotonin receptors. *Table modified from Cummings et al. (2010)*

Compound	Binding affinity (K_i nM)		K_i selectivity ratio 5-HT_{2A}/ 5-HT_{2C}
	5-HT_{2A}+/- SEM	5-HT_{2C}+/- SEM	
(8) Aplysinopsin	598 +/- 53	14,451 +/- 5893	0.041
(9) 6-Bromoaplysinopsin	ND	2202 +/- 674	>45
(26) 6-Fluoroaplysinopsin	235 +/- 42	2114 +/- 203	0.11
(27) 6-Chloroaplysinopsin	ND	166 +/- 55	>602
(28) 5,6-Dichloroaplysinopsin	ND	46 +/ 8.6	>2170
(29) 4'-Ethylaplysinopsin	655 +/- 94	8323 +/- 2911	0.079
(30) 6-Fluoro-4'-ethylaplysinopsin	173 +/- 42	5230 +/- 858	0.033

Table 7 This table shows "Binding affinity and selectivity ratio for aplysinopsins 8,9 and 26-30. Compound affinities for cloned human serotonin 5-HT_{2A} and 5-HT_{2C} receptor subtypes (n=3). ND = not detected at highest concentration tested. For those affinity values that could not be determined at the highest concentration tested, an affinity of >100,000 nM is assumed for the purpose of the selectivity calculations." *The table is modified from Cummings et al. (2010)*

BROMINATED BARETTINS

The marine sponge *Geodia barretti* produces the brominated tryptamines barettin (33) and 8,9-dihydrobarettin (34), which showed greater activity on the serotonin receptor 5-HT2C over 5-HT_{2A}, and activity only on the 5-HT_{2C} receptor, respectively (Table 7) (Hedner et al., 2006).

33	Barettin	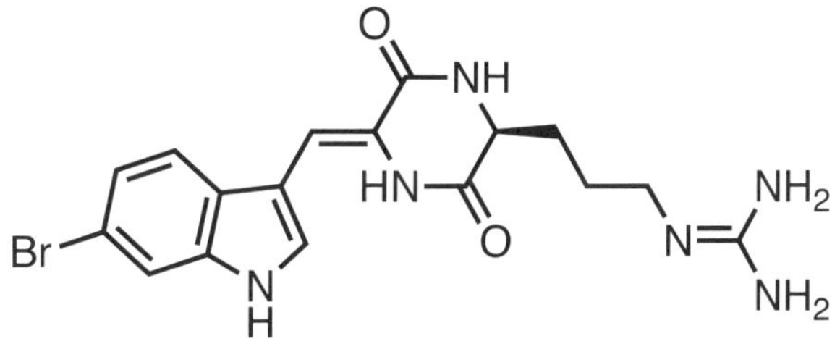
34	8,9-Dihydrobarettin	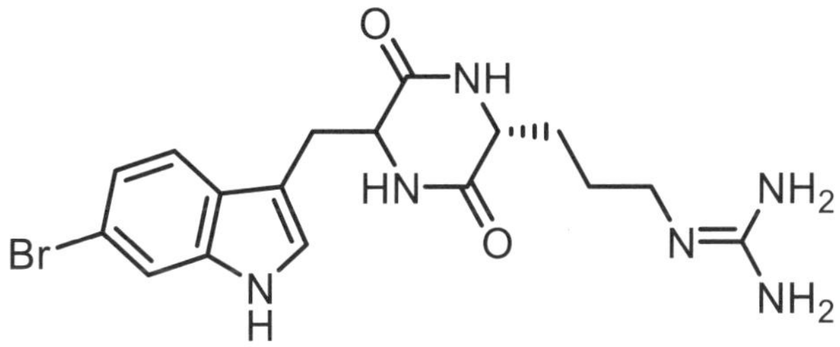

Table 8 Structures 33-34. Barettin and 8,9-Dihydrobarettin. *Hedner et al., 2006*

Receptor	K_i[µM]			
	(33) Barettin	(34) 8,9-Dihydro barettin	5-Hydroxytryptamine	Methysergide-Selective ligand[b]
5-HT_{1A}	>10	>10		
5-HT_{1D}	>10	>10		
5-HT_{2A}	1.93 +/- 0.59	>10	0.69 +/- 0.1	0.01 +/- 0.003
5-HT_{2C}	0.34 +/- 0.14	4.63 +/- 0.13	0.020 +/- 0.004	0.0025 +/- 0.001
5-HT_{3A}	>10	>10		
5-HT_4	1.91 +/- 0.12	>10	0.50 +/- 0.07	0.031 +/- 0.01
5-HT_{5A}	>10	>10		
5-HT_6	>10	>10		
5-HT_{7A}	>10	>10		

Table 9 This table shows "Binding activity of barettin, 8,9-dihydrobarettin, 5-HTP, and methysergide on different serotonin receptors. Affinities of Barettin (33), 8,9-Dihydrobarettin (34) , 5-Hydroxytryptamine, Methysergide (5-$HT_{2A, 2C}$) to the 5-HT_{2A}, 5-HT_{2C}, and 5-HT_4 Receptors Expressed in HEK-293 Cell Membranes (data presented as a mean +/- SEM with three independent experiments performed in triplicate). *[1,2-^{3}H]5-Carboxamidotryptamine used for 5-$HT_{1A,1D,5A,7A}$:[*N*-methyl-^{3}H]LSD used for 5-$HT_{2A,2C,6}$:[9-methyl-^{3}H]BRL-43694 used for 5-HT_{3A}: [*N*-methyl-^{3}H]GR11308 used for 5-HT_4. [b] Methysergide (5-$HT_{2A,2C}$): tegaserod (5-HT_4)." *This table is from Hedner et al., (2006)*

GELLIUSINE A

A final example of serotonergic brominated tryptamine derivatives from marine sponges is (+/-) gelliusine A (35), found in the New Caledonian sponge, *Orin spp.*.

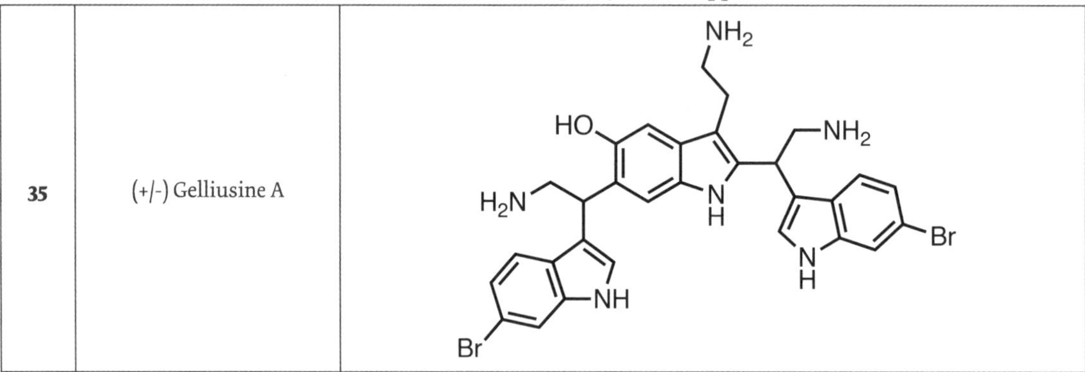

Table 10 Structure 35: (+/-) Gelliusine A.

UNKNOWN PSYCHOACTIVITY AND MARINE NATURAL PRODUCT STRUCTURE BASED INSPIRATION

The brominated tryptamine compounds (1-3) from sponges listed by Alexander Shulgin in *TiHKAL* (1997) also have other anticancer, antibiotic, and anti-inflammatory activities (Mollica et al., 2012). Beyond serotonergic activity, many brominated and non-brominated tryptamine alkaloids from sponges show anticancer and antiviral activity, clearly indicating the importance of the marine environment for inspiring new medicine (Dembitsky, 2002; France et al., 2014; Pauletti et al., 2010; Thomas et al., 2010; Sagar et al., 2010). Though many compounds have been discovered through antibacterial, antifungal, anticancer, and antiviral bioactivity guided assays, seldom are the compounds tested for psychoactivity. Moreover, discovery of a compound based on other bioactivities does not exclude that a compound possesses psychoactive properties.

An annual review on marine natural product chemicals is published in the journal *Natural Product Review*, which reviews all new marine natural product compounds published in the past year. For example, Figure 1 shows that 247 of the 677 compounds referenced for the 2003 review (Blunt et al., 2003) were from sponges. The diversity of marine natural product compounds in these reviews spans the space of potentially psychologically active alkaloids with brominated tryptamine, beta-carboline, phenethylamine, and pyrrole cores, as well as structures for other unique and diverse alkaloids (Blunt et al., 2005). The author was particularly inspired by such structures in the 2003-2005 reviews while surveying coral reef in Samoa, Tokelau, Kiribati, Tuvalu, and Fiji aboard the RV Heraclitus, and thereafter visiting editors of the reviews in New Zealand.

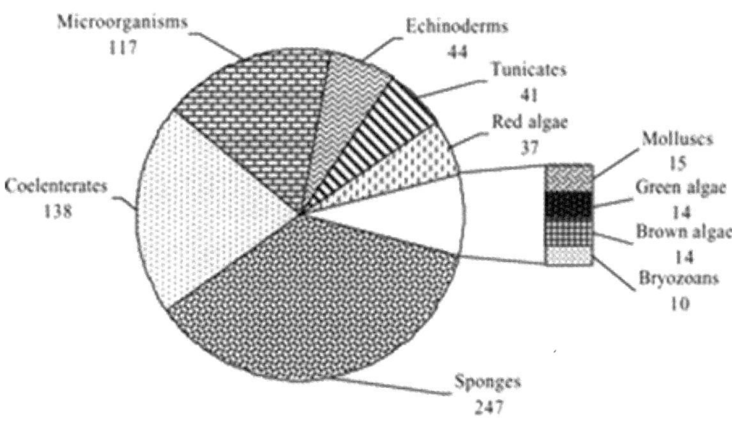

Fig. 1 Taxonomic breakdown of compounds referenced in the 2003 Marine Natural Products review. *Blunt et al. 2003*

MATERIALS AND METHODS

Biotransformation and the Support of Universities and Pearl Farms

Marine sponges were collected and cultured in collaboration with pearl farming companies Atlas Pearl in Raja Ampat, Indonesia (2010-2011) and Ryukyu Shinju in Ishigaki and Iriomote, Okinawa, Japan (2012, 2014-2016). While working at the Atlas Pearl oyster farm in Raja Ampat, Indonesia, an area in the epicenter of the Coral Triangle's marine biodiversity, 81 sponge samples were collected and some were cultivated. The samples from Atlas Pearl were extracted at Udayana University in Bali and tested by 3 Master's students to observe the inhibition of hatching brine shrimp eggs. Though no psychoactivity bioassay was available, this paved the way to work with additional pearl farms and universities for future research.

Biotransformation experiments were conducted in Okinawa, Japan at the Okinawa Institute of Science and Technology (OIST; 2012-2014) and at the University of the Ryukyus (2014-2016) using marine sponges sampled from the Ryukyu Shinju pearl farm pearling longline in Ishigaki Island.

The research served to develop a methodology using a single sponge from Ryukyu Shinju pearl farm in Ishigaki Island, which at that time was unidentified (later 28s DNA sequencing matched this sponge to the genus *Mycale* using BLAST). Sponges from the Ryukyu Shinju pearl farm site in Funauki Bay were collected, and hundreds of sponge cuttings were grown from dozens of broodstock. Part of the research focused on finding possible sponges for mariculture production of extractable compounds with market values. There are market values for both bath sponges and compounds known to be produced based on the taxonomic identification of the sponges farmed, such as manzamine A, aeroplysinin-1, manoalide, aaptamine, and swinholide A.

Farming sponges for psychoactive substances may be more practical through mixed mariculture. Aside from pearl farms, the author has collected and grown sponges with a coral restoration project, the electrical Biorock® (Pemuteran, Bali, and Gili Trawangan, Lombok, Indonesia), and PT Karamba fish farm near Komodo Island, Indonesia.

The sponge farming trial at Ryukyu Shinju in Iriomote tested various substrates such as nets, cages, and threaded lines, as well as depths. Sponges were hung from the pearling longlines and suspended on nets from the seafloor with empty water bottles as floats. The farmed sponges provided data on growth and survival, as well as serving as replicate samples for biotransformations and their molecular biology. A major factor in sponge survival was minimal tissue damage and sufficiently large cutting size. Sponge survival and growth varied between sponge types. Tissue regeneration and rounding was observed from cuttings. Ideally, for biotransformation experiments a sponge cutting can be placed in a small container with the precursor compounds of interest without damaging additional tissue, and replicate cuttings from the same individual can be used for multiple substrates.

The author is currently (2022-2023) employed by Nusantara Pearl Group in Morotai and Tual, Indonesia, developing a corporate social responsibility program for culturing coral and sponges. It is foreseeable to test serotonergic compounds from sponges as inducers of spawning in hatchery reared experiments.

RESULTS & DISCUSSION

Biotransformation and Substrates

Beyond the sole use of tryptamine, its metabolic precursor L-tryptophan was compared to enzymatically inactive D-tryptophan. Sodium bromide salt was also used in the incubation/biotransformation experiments with and without tryptophan and phenylalanine in the hope of upregulating production of brominated alkaloids. A number of other metabolic building blocks, such as dopamine, indole and indoleacetic acid, were also used in an attempt to trigger the production of possibly psychoactive phenethylamines and indole derivatives. The list of biotransformation substrates included the neurotransmitters GABA and glutamate, and the polyketide synthase substrate malonic acid. Glucose was systematically added in an attempt to supply additional energy for the reactions. In addition to biotransformation, it was hoped that supplying sponges with the neurotransmitters GABA, glutamate, and dopamine, and the neurotransmitter precursors phenylalanine and tryptophan, that mRNA sequencing would uncover primitive neurotransmission-like processes. However, mRNA quality was insufficient for sequencing except for indoleacetic acid, sodium bromide, and the control. The compounds tested with LC-MS for biotransformation in sponge tissues were indole, indoleacetic acid, sodium bromide, dopamine, glutamic acid, GABA, malonic acid, and glucose.

The solubility of each compound and pH (indoleacetic acid and indole) had to be taken into account when designing the molar concentration of the incubation treatment, as well as the effect on solubility of the filtered and sterilized seawater. Biotransformation's were conducted on freshly cut sponge tissue in 50 mL falcon tubes for between 0-5 hours, and either frozen immediately on liquid nitrogen (for co-extraction of mRNA) or dry ice.

Sponge Identification and Sponge Microbial Symbiont Metagenomes

Conversely from chemo-typing, sponge taxonomic identification allows some background research on known compounds already detected in various sponges. The presence of some compounds may be inconsistent, and this is thought to be in part due to production by microbial symbionts in the sponge tissue rather than the sponge itself. Identifying sponges can be tricky. Methods of identification often include DNA barcoding and taxonomy based on spicules, which are skeletal components formed out of calcium carbonate or silica. Sponges from Indonesia and Okinawa were sent as taxonomic voucher specimen with photos and diving GPS coordinates to sponge taxonomist Dr. Nicole de Voogd at Naturalis Natural History Museum in Leiden and University of Amsterdam. Okinawan sponges were identified in part with the local expertise of the author's host, marine natural product chemist Dr. Junichi Tanaka at University of the Ryukyus. *Hyrtios erecta* was identified, collected, grown, and extracted in both Indonesia and Japan ("Sponge B"). This sponge is known to produce the serotonergic brominated aplysinopsin 6-bromo-2'-de-N-methylaplysinopsin (10), nitric oxide synthase inhibitor 5,6-dibromo-2'-demethylaplysinopsin (12) (shown in Table 5), as well as additional brominated tryptamines and brominated quinolones (Aoki et al., 2001).

Biotransformation and LC-MS detection

Biotransformation versus control crude extracts were monitored at OIST using LC-MS, comparing absence versus presence of metabolic products and relative M/Z peaks intensity of metabolites detected in controls. Ideally, stable isotope labeled tryptamine and L-tryptophan could be used to confirm incorporation into transformed compounds, by detecting M/Z peaks, indicating the difference in isotope weights; unfortunately, this was beyond budget. Liquid chromatography mass spectrometry (LC-MS) for "Sponge E" provided proof of concept that biotransformation's, or at least detectable changes in metabolite production, were taking place. However, it should be noted, for reasons that lay with the institution and outside the power of the author, M/Z values were cut off below 300, severely limiting the detection of many compounds of interest. LC-MS M/Z peaks were used to search corresponding known marine natural product compounds from the databases MarinLit and AntiMarin. These databases pair mass spectrometry and NMR data with compounds from the sea, allowing for a general search of matching values of known compounds from LC-MS data of crude sponge extracts. John Blunt and Murray Munro of Canterbury University in New Zealand, previous lead editors of the annual review on *Marine Natural Products*, developed MarinLit as a database of marine natural products, making it convenient to search known compounds by taxonomy, taxonomy by known compounds, NMR peaks by known compound, known compounds by M/Z values, and all related publications. Very few M/Z values matched in the MarinLit and AntiMarin databases, the most notable match being tryptophan diketopiperazine. The directed biotransformation with marine sponges did produce increased diversified metabolites and M/Z values of increased intensities, indicating increased concentrations.

Since many psychoactive compounds from the sea are brominated (Dembitsky, 2002; Pauletti et al., 2010), the raw data was searched for the characteristic double isotope peak M/Z patterns of brominated compounds with isotope peaks of bromine, which provided many candidates.

Biotransformation and TLC/pTLC

At the University of the Ryukyus (2014-2016) farmed sponges Sponges A-D from Ryukyu Shinju pearl farm in Funauki Bay, Iriomote and Sponge E from the Ishigaki farm, provided proof of concept that biotransformation reactions were occurring. They visualized using thin layer chromatography (TLC) with ultraviolet light to detect the absence versus presence of metabolic products, and the relative intensity of fluorescence of metabolites present in both the control samples and directed biotransformation experiments. Preparatory TLC (pTLC), was also practiced to prepare small quantities of compounds detected with fluorescence. This provided further proof of detectable changes in metabolite production, serving as a means to isolate compounds for high resolution mass spectrometry without the use of liquid chromatography. However, the intensity of the fluorescence can be deceiving in terms of the actual quantity of compound present for detection by other means.

As a sidenote, indoles and tryptamines, which are aromatic compounds, tend to be fluorescent under UV, and additional double bonds tend to increase light interactions. The neurotransmitters serotonin, dopamine, noradrenaline, and adrenaline, all aromatic amines, fluoresce under UV light when condensed with formaldehyde, which in fact was an early advent in imaging neurons in formaldehyde treated brain tissue (Falck et al., 1982; Corrodi and Jonsson, 1967; Falk, 1962). Formaldehyde and other aldehydes can condense with tryptamines into beta-carbolines and with phenethylamines into isoquinolines, which may be easier to visualize than the initial compounds.

Biotransformation and mRNA and DNA Sequencing of Sponges

Perhaps, by feeding an organism the appropriate precursor for biotransformation it can also detectably upregulate biosynthetic genes and trigger gene cluster expression. Additional mRNA and DNA sequencing provided metatranscriptomic (Sponge E) and metagenomic data (Sponges A-E) for annotated and unannotated sequences. This can potentially uncover metabolic pathways of interest in the host organism and its symbiotic microbes.

Biotransformation may serve as a means to mine the biosynthetic transcriptome of sponges and other organisms of interest. After mRNA was extracted, the transcripts were sequenced with Illumina sequencing from 3 samples of a large sprawling sponge, "Sponge E", found on the Ryukyu Shinju Ishigaki pearl farm, of the probable genus *Mycale.* Due to mRNA extract quality, only the control, sodium bromide, and indoleacetic acid treatments were sequenced. Unique mRNA transcripts and robust changes in the expression levels of the 3 conditions were compared and annotated with BLAST and KEGG attempting to uncover enzymatic biosynthesis pathways.

Had other treatment types given higher quality mRNA, this process may have helped elucidate processes related to neurotransmitter metabolism in the pre-nervous system and alternative metabolic pathways producing secondary metabolite alkaloids. However, this would only work for poly-A tailed eukaryotic mRNA and not mRNA of bacterial origin. To my knowledge *Mycale* type sponges do not produce tryptamine or phenethylamine alkaloids, although LC-MS data did indicate diversified metabolic products when fed the biotransformation precursors. Possible metabolic engineering using mRNA transcripts for compounds which have high value to humanity but are difficult to synthesize, may be considered for as a long-term goal of sustainable production as an alternative to wild collection, farming methods, and synthetic organic chemistry.

Sponges A-E were exposed to biotransformation experiments in 2014-2015 were preserved in alcohol and eventually, in 2022, full metagenomic DNA, 28s ribosomal DNA (for sponge), and 16s ribosomal DNA (for microbial taxonomic identification) was sequenced using Illumina at the University of California, San Francisco (UCSF). The 28s DNA sequences were compared to known sequences of sponge DNA in the Basic Local Alignment Search Tool (BLAST) database from the National Center for Biotechnology Information (NCBI), revealing the closest relatives of the 5 sponges, the taxonomy of which was used to search additional background information on possibly related natural product chemistry.

Three out of the five sponges with sequenced 28s DNA revealed best matches to other sponges known to produce varieties of tryptamine and/or phenethylamine derivatives. "Sponge B," identified before sequencing as *Hyrtios erecta*, was related to *Thorectandra excavates*, and more distant sponges of the *Thorectandra* genus known to possess a 6-bromo-aplysinopsin derivative (Khushi at al., 2021), as well as *Fascaplysinopsis reticulata*, known to possess a non-brominated aplysinopsin (50) and other aromatic indole alkaloids shown in Table 11 (Wang et al., 2019). "Sponge C" 28s DNA closely matched with *Aaptos aaptos*, which produces the tricyclic phenethylamine/isoquilonine derivatives called aaptamines (51-53), Table 12, known for various receptor activities (Table 8), such as delta and mu opioid receptor agonism (Johnson et al., 2017), dopamine receptor antagonism (Luyao et al., 2021), anticancer (Dyshlovoy et al., 2014), antifungal, and antiviral activities (Yu et al., 2014). "Sponge D" was closely related to two sponges known to produce aromatic alkaloids, *Verongula rigida* (Table 14), and *Pseudoceratina arabica* (Table 15). *Verongula rigida*, as discussed in Table 14 and referred to in US patent 8,268,856, is known to possess 5,6-dibromo-N,N-dimethyltryptamine (1/54), 5-bromo- N,N-dimethyltryptamine (6/55), 6-bromoaplysinopsin (9/57), and various indole derivatives, such as the brominated tryptamine derivative makaluvamine O (60), the brominated beta-carboline derivative arborescidine C (58), and 5,6-dibromoabridine (59) (Kochanowska et al., 2008). The brominated alkaloid veranamine (61), also from from *Verongula rigida*, has in-vivo antidepressant activity and selectivity for the 5-HT2B serotonin receptor (Kochanowska-Karamyan et al., 2020). *Pseudoceratina arabica* is known to possess various brominated phenethylamine derivatives (62-65) such as moloka'iamine (63), noted to have some parasympathetic activity (Luparello et al., 2020; Badr et al., 2008).

Additionally, 28s DNA sequencing data indicated several eukaryotic symbionts such as dinoflagellates, which may be responsible for some secondary metabolites in sponges. The probable producers of many secondary metabolites found in sponges are microbial. The metagenomic data is still under analysis.

47	Homofascaplysin B	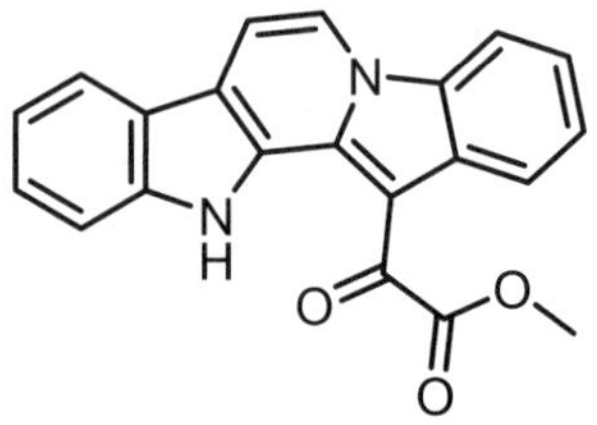 N H O O O
48	Secofascaplysin	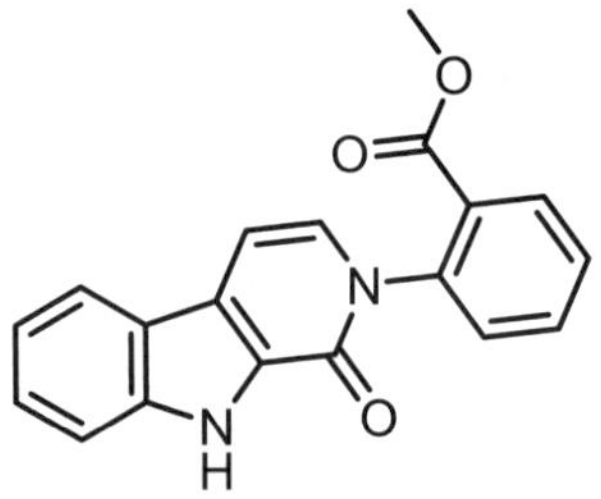 O O N N H O
49	4-Bromo-2-pyrido[3,4-b]-2-ylbenzoic acid	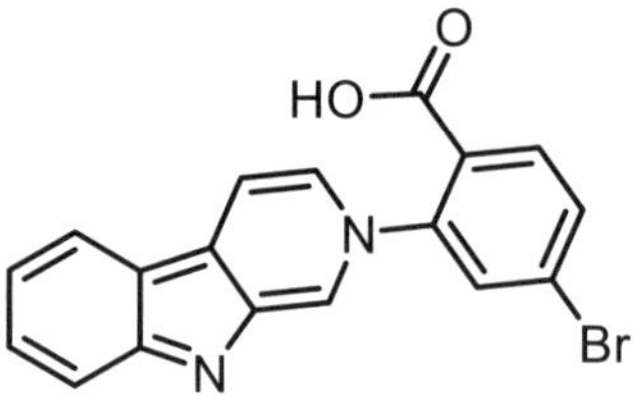 O HO N N Br
50	Oxoaplysinopsin	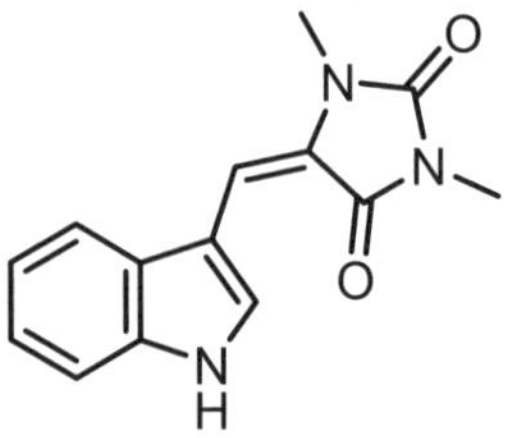 O N N O N H

Table 11 Structures 47-50. Alkaloids from *Fascaplysinopsis reticulata*, Closely Related to Sponge B.

51	Aaptamine	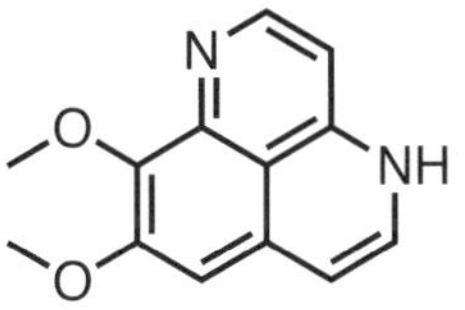
52	9-Demethyl aaptamine	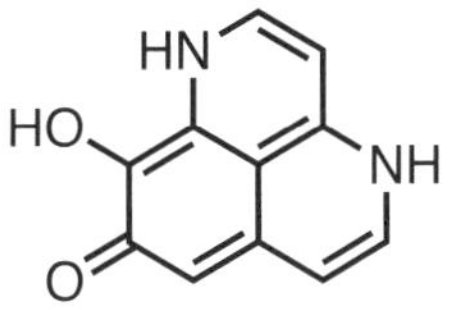
53	Demethyl(oxy)-aaptamine	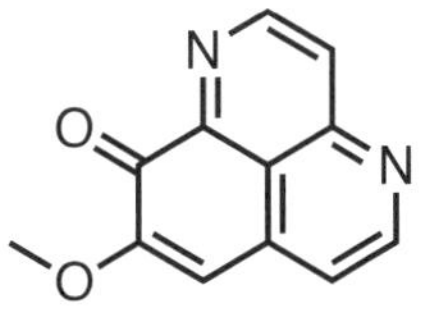

Table 12 Structures 51-53. Alkaloids from *Aaptos aaptos*, Closely Related to Sponge C.

Compound	(Johnson et al., 2017)	(Luyao et al., 2021)
(51) Aaptamine	Delta Opioid Receptor Agonist (OR, EC50 5.1 μM) Mu Opioid Receptor Agonist (μ-OR, EC50 10.1 μM)	α-Adrenoreceptor Antagonism (ADRA2C, IC_{50} 11.9 μM) β-Adrenoreceptor Antagonism (ADRB2, IC_{50} 0.20 μM) Dopamine Receptor D4 Antagonism (DRD4, IC_{50} 6.9 μM).
(52) 9-Demethyl aaptamine	Delta Opioid Receptor Agonist (OR, EC50 4.1 μM)	
(53) Demethyl(oxy)-aaptamine	Delta Opioid Receptor Agonist (OR, EC50 2.3 μM)	

Table 13 Opioid, Dopamine, and Adrenoreceptor Activities of Aaptamines 51-53.

54	5,6-Dibromo-N,N-dimethyltryptamine	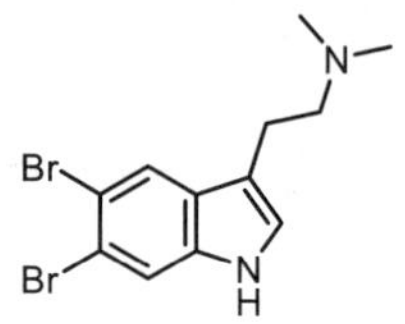
55	5-Bromo-N,N-dimethyltryptamine	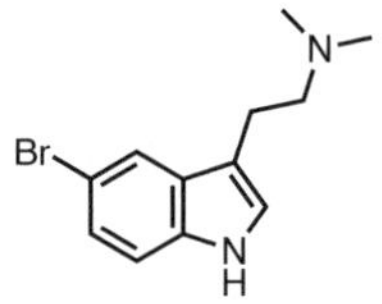
56	Aplysinopsin	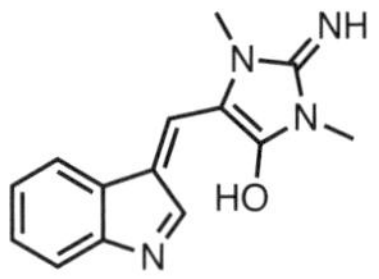
57	6-Bromoaplysinopsin	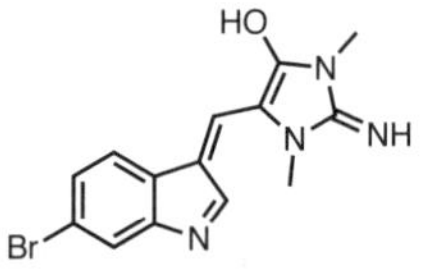
58	Arborescidine C	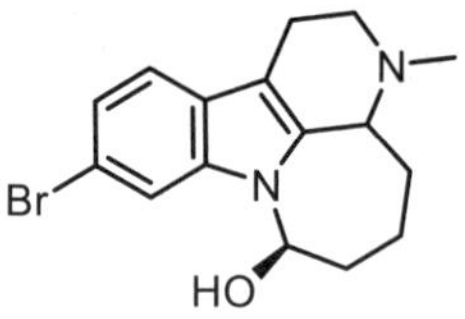
59	5,6-dibromoabrine	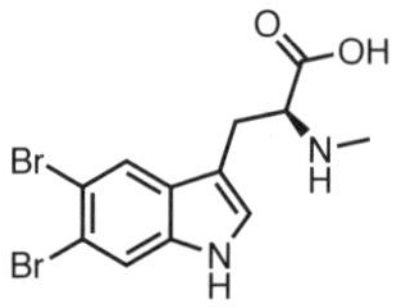
60	Makaluvamine O	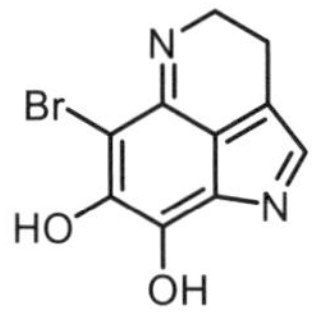
61	Veranamine	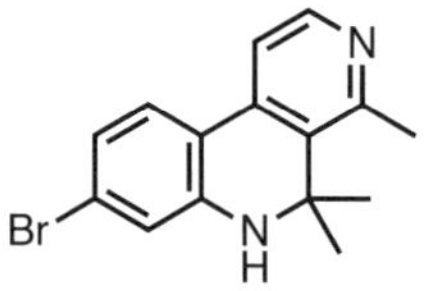

Table 14 Structures 54-61. Alkaloids from *Verongula rigida*, Closely Related to Sponge D.

62	Hydroxymoloka'iamine	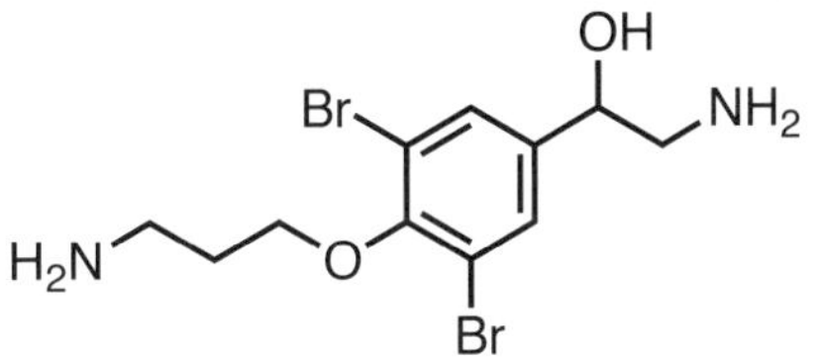
63	Moloka'iamine	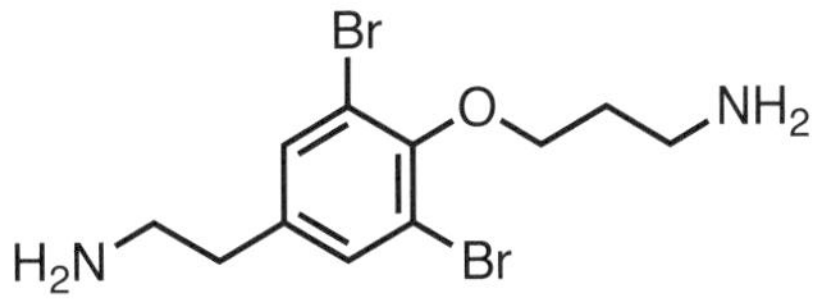
64	Ceratinamine	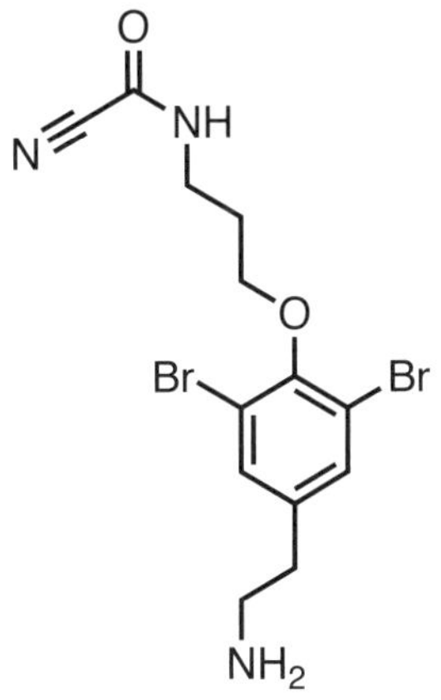
65	Psammaplysin-A	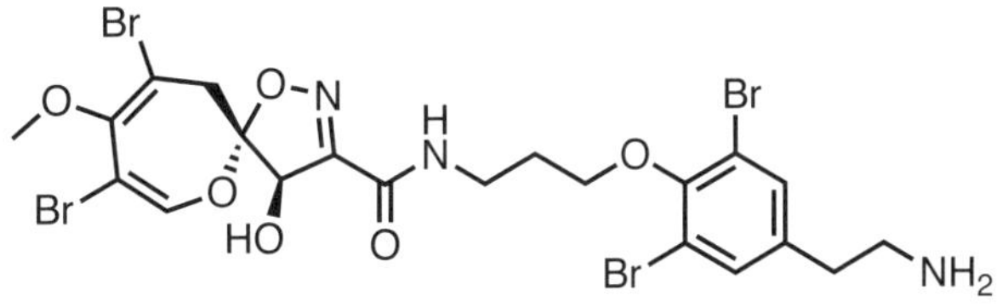

Table 15 Structures 62-65. Alkaloids from Pseudoceratina arabica, Closely Related to Sponge D.

CONCLUSION

The findings of this work show that biotransformation with tryptamines and other biosynthetic precursors can diversify and amplify mass spectrometry detection of small molecules from sponges, and that the resources for drug discovery from marine sponges have not been exhausted. Farming marine sponges for psychoactive drug discovery experiments may provide new drug leads for treating mental health conditions like depression and anxiety. The National Institute of Health's Psychoactive Drug Screening Program tests a wide variety of *in vitro* serotonin and catecholamine GPCR targets for bioassays associated with mental health conditions. This would be the ideal collaboration to explore the psychoactivity of crude extracts, pTLC band extracts, and HPLC fractions of control versus biotransformation experiments with sponges and other marine drug producing organisms. After drug discovery, sustainable supply becomes an issue for offering the active pharmaceutical ingredient of interest, and when this may not be easily synthesizable, other methods of production such as farming, microbial culture, and genetic engineering of biosynthetic pathways may rely on the techniques explored in this paper. The author is developing a CSR program with Indonesian communities and a pearl farm chain to grow sponges for chemical extracts, culture algae to test for the production of beta-carbolines from *Acanthostrongylophoa ingens* and aaptamine from an *Aaptos* sponge, and preparing *Hyrtios erecta* and *Aaptos aaptos* sponges for biotransfomation experiments with tryptamine and phenethylamine.

ACKNOWLEDGEMENTS

The author would like to thank the organizations Atlas Pearl, Ryukyu Shinju, Udayana University, Okinawa Institute of Science and Technology (OIST), University of the Ryukyus, City College of San Francisco, and Dr. Xiangpeng Li in the lab of Dr. Adam Abate at University of California, San Francisco. Many professors, technicians, and bioinformaticians at OIST made data acquisition possible. Dr. Nicole de Voogd was available for consultation in some capacity at each step of the way without an authored publication. Dr. Mark Hamann is appreciated for his feedback on the paper. The author thanks Gabrielle Bangay for redrawing chemical structures to be in consistent format.

BIBLIOGRAPHY

Agarwal, V., Miles, Z.D., Winter, J.M., Eustáquio, A.S.., El Gamal, A.A., Moore, B.S., 2017. Enzymatic Halogenation and Dehalogenation Reactions: Pervasive and Mechanistically Diverse. *Chem Rev., 117*(8):5619-5674.

Aoki, S., Ye, Y., Higuchi, K., Takashima, A., Tanaka, Y., Kitagawa, I., Kobayashi, M., 2001. Novel neuronal nitric oxide synthase (nNOS) selective inhibitor, aplysinopsin-type indole alkaloid, from marine sponge Hyrtios erecta. *Chem Pharm Bull* (Tokyo), *49*(10),1372-4.

Badr, J.M., Shaala, L.A., Abou-Shoer, M.I., Tawfik, M.K., Habib, A.A., 2008. Bioactive brominated metabolites from the red sea sponge *Pseudoceratina arabica. J. Nat. Prod. 78*(8), 1472-1474

Baird-Lambert, J., Davis, P.A., Taylor, K.M.,1982. Methylaplysinopsin: a natural product of marine origin with effects on serotonergic neurotransmission. *Clinical and experimental pharmacology & physiology, 9*(2), 203–212.

Bayer, K., Scheuermayer, M., Fieseler, L., Hentschel, U., 2013. Genomic mining for novel $FADH_2$-dependent halogenases in marine sponge-associated microbial consortia. *Mar Biotechnol (NY)., 15*(1):63-72.

Bergquest, P.R., Wells, R.J., 1983. Marine natural products: chemical and biological perspectives. Shauer, P.J., Ed., Academic Press: New York (1983). Vol. V. p 1.

Bialonska, D., Zjawiony, J.K., 2009. Aplysinopsins—Marine indole alkaloids: chemistry, bioactivity and ecological significance. *Mar. Drugs, 7*, 166-183.

Bifulco, G., Bruno, I., Minale, L., Riccio, R., Calignano, A., Debitus, C., 1994. (+/-)-Gelliusines A and B, two diastereomeric brominated tris-indole alkaloids from a deep water new caledonian marine sponge (*Gellius* or *Orina* sp.). *Journal of natural products, 57*(9), 1294–1299.

Blunt, J.W., Copp, B.R., Munro, M.H., Northcote, P.T., Prinsep, M.R., 2003. Marine natural products. *Natural product reports, 20*(1), 1–48.

Blunt, J.W., Copp, B.R., Munro, M.H., Northcote, P.T., Prinsep, M.R., 2005. Marine natural products. *Natural product reports, 22*(1), 15–61.

Christenson, J.G., Dairman, W., Udenfriend, S. 1972. On the identity of DOPA decarboxylase and 5-hydroxytryptophan decarboxylase (immunological titration-aromatic L-amino acid decarboxylase-serotonin-dopamine-norepinephrine). *Proc. Natl. Acad. Sci. USA. 69*(2), 343-7.

Djura, P., Stierle, D.B., Sullivan, B., Faulkner, J., Arnold, E.V., Clardy, J., 1980. Some metabolites of the marine sponges *Smenospongia aurea* and *Smenospongia* (.ident.*Polyfibrospongia*) *echina. The Journal of Organic Chemistry. 45*(8), 1435-1441.

Corrodi, H., Jonsson, G. 1967. The formaldehyde fluorescence method for the histochemical demonstration of biogenic monoamines a review on the methodology. *Journal of Histochemistry & Cytochemistry, 15*(2), 65-78.

Cummings, D.F., Canseco, D.C., Sheth, P., Johnson, J.E., Schetz, J.A., 2010. Synthesis and structure-affinity relationships of novel small molecule natural product derivatives capable of discriminating between serotonin 5-HT1A, 5-HT2A, 5-HT2C receptor subtypes. *Bioorg Med Chem.18*(13), 4783-92.

Dembitsky, V.M., Brom- i ĭodsoderzhashchie alkaloidy morskikh mikroorganizmov i gubok [Bromo- and iodo-containing alkaloids from marine microorganisms and sponges]., 2002. *Bioorg Khim. 28*(3), 196-208. Russian.

Djura, P., Faulkner, D.J., 1980. Metabolites of the marine sponge *Derictus sp. J. Org. Chem. 45*, 737-738.

Dyshlovoy, S.A,, Fedorov, S.N., Shubina, L.K., Kuzmich, A.S., Bokemeyer, C., Keller-von Amsberg, G., Honecker, F., 2014. Aaptamines from the marine sponge Aaptos sp. display anticancer activities in human cancer cell lines and modulate AP-1-, NF-κB-, and p53-dependent transcriptional activity in mouse JB6 Cl41 cells. *Biomed Res Int.* 2014, 469309.

Falck, B., 1962. Observations on the Possibilities of the Cellular Localization of Monoamines by a Fluorescence Method. *Acta Physiologica Scandinavica. Suppl.* 197, 1-25.

Falck, B., Hillarp, N.A., Thieme, G., Torp, A., 1982. Fluorescence of catechol amines and related compounds condensed with formaldehyde. *Brain Res Bull. 9*(1-6), xi-xv.

França, P.H., Barbosa, D.P., da Silva, D.L., Ribeiro, Ê.A., Santana, A.E., Santos, B.V., Barbosa-Filho, J.M., Quintans, J.S., Barreto, R.S., Quintans-Júnior, L.J., de Araújo-Júnior, J.X., 2014. Indole alkaloids from marine sources as potential leads against infectious diseases. *Biomed Res Int.* 2014, 375423.

Gartz J., 1989. Biotransformation of Tryptamine in Fruiting Mycelia of *Psilocybe cubensis. Planta Med. 55*(3), 249-50.

Gartz J., 1988. Biotransformation of Tryptamine Derivatives in Mycelial Cultures of *Psilocybe.(2nd International Symposium on "New Bioactive Metabolites from Microorganisms", Gera (GDR). 1988*, May 2-7.

Gutleben, J., Koehorst, J.J., McPherson, K., Pomponi, S., Wijffels, R.H., Smidt, H., Sipkema, D., 2019. Diversity of tryptophan halogenases in sponges of the genus Aplysina. *FEMS Microbiol Ecol. 95*(8):fiz108.

Hamann, M.T., Kochanowska, A.J., El-Alfy, A., Matsumoto, R.R., Boujos, A., 2012. Method to use compositions having antidepressant anxiolytic and other neurological activity and compositions of matter. US patent number 8,268,856.

Haridas, R.P., Bause, G.S., 2013. Correspondence by Charles T. Jackson containing the earliest known illustrations of a Morton ether inhaler. *Anesth Analg.* 117:1236–40

Hedner, E., Sjögren, M., Frändberg, P.A., Johansson, T., Göransson, U., Dahlström, M., Jonsson, P., Nyberg, F., Bohlin, L., 2006. Brominated cyclodipeptides from the marine sponge *Geodia barretti* as selective 5-HT ligands. *J Nat Prod. 69*(10):1421-4.

Hollenbeak, K.H., Schmitz, F.J., 1977. Aplysinopsin: Antineoplastic tryptophan derivative from marine sponge *Verongia spengelii. Lloydia. 40*, 479-481.

Hu, J.F., Schetz, J.A., Kelly, M., Peng, J.N., Ang, K.K., Flotow, H., Leong, C.Y., Ng, S.B., Buss, A.D., Wilkins, S.P., Hamann, M.T., 2002. New antiinfective and human 5-HT$_2$ receptor binding natural and semisynthetic compounds from the Jamaican sponge *Smenospongia aurea. J. Nat. Prod. 65*, 476-480.

Ibrahim, M. A., El-Alfy, A.T., Ezel, K., Radwan, M.O., Shilabin, A.G., Kochanowska-Karamyan, A.J., Abd-Alla, H.I., Otsuka, M., Hamann, M.T., 2017. Marine Inspired 2-(5-Halo-1H-indol-3-yl)-N,N-dimethylethanamines as Modulators of Serotonin Receptors: An Example Illustrating the Power of Bromine as Part of the Uniquely Marine Chemical Space. *Marine drugs, 15*(8), 248.

Juvin, P., Desmonts, J.M., 2000. The ancestors of inhalational anesthesia: the Soporific Sponges (XIth-XVIIth centuries): how a universally recommended medical technique was abruptly discarded. Anesthesiology., 93(1), 265-9.

Jimenez, C., Quinoa, E., Adamczeski, M. Hunter, L.M., Crews, P., 1991. Novel sponge-derived amino acids. 12. Tryptophan-derived pigments and accompanying sesterpenes from *Fascaplysinopsis reticulata. The Journal of Organic Chemistry. 56*(10), 3403-3410.

Johnson, T.A., Milan-Lobo, L., Che, T., Ferwerda, M., Lambu, E., McIntosh, N.L., Whistler, J.L., 2017. Identification of the first marine-derived opioid receptor "Balanced" agonist with a signaling profile that resembles the endorphins. *ACS Chem. Neurosci. 8*:473–485.

Kazlauskas, R., Murphy, P.T., Quinn, R.J., Wells, R.J., 1977. Aplysinopsin, a new tryptophan derivative from a sponge. *Tetrahedron Lett.*1, 61-64.

Khushi, S., Salim, A.A., Elbanna, A.H., Nahar, L., Capon, R.J., 2021. New from Old: Thorectandrin Alkaloids in a Southern Australian Marine Sponge, *Thorectandra choanoides*. *Mar Drugs. 19*(2), 97.

Kobayashi, J., Ishibashi, M., Nagai, U., Ohizumi, Y., 1989. 9-Methyl-7-bromoeudistomin D, a potent inducer of calcium release from sarcoplasmic reticulum of skeletal muscle. *Experientia. 45*(8), 782-3.

Kochanowska, A.J., Rao, K.V., Childress, S., El-Alfy, A., Matsumoto, R.R., Kelly, M., Stewart, G.S., Sufka, K.J., Hamann, M.T., 2008. Secondary metabolites from three Florida sponges with antidepressant activity. *J Nat Prod. 71*(2), 186-9.

Kochanowska-Karamyan, A.J., Araujo, H.C., Zhang, X., El-Alfy, A., Carvalho, P., Avery, M.A., Holmbo, S.D., Magolan, J., Hamann, M.T., 2020. Isolation and Synthesis of Veranamine, an Antidepressant Lead from the Marine Sponge *Verongula rigida*. *J Nat Prod. 83*(4),1092-1098.

Kochanowska-Karamyan, A.J., Hamann, M.T., 2010. Marine indole alkaloids: potential new drug leads for the control of depression and anxiety. *Chem Rev. 110*(8), 4489-97.

Luparello, C., Mauro, M., Lazzara, V., Vazzana, M., 2020. Collective Locomotion of Human Cells, Wound Healing and Their Control by Extracts and Isolated Compounds from Marine Invertebrates. *Molecules. 25*(11), 2471.

Luyao, H., Luesch, H., Uy, M., 2021. GPCR Pharmacological Profiling of Aaptamine from the Philippine Sponge *Stylissa* sp. Extends Its Therapeutic Potential for Noncommunicable Diseases. *Molecules (Basel, Switzerland), 26*(18), 5618.

Morris, H., Wallach, J., 2013. Sea DMT. *Vice Magazine*, March 26, 2013. https://www.vice.com/en/article/znqdve/sea-dmt-000481-v20n3

Mollica, A., Locatelli, M., Stefanucci, A., Pinnen, F., 2012. Synthesis and bioactivity of secondary metabolites from marine sponges containing dibrominated indolic systems. *Molecules. 17*(5), 6083-99.

Murata, M., Miyagawa-Kohshima, K., Nakanishi, K. Naya, Y., 1986. Characterization of compounds that induce symbiosis between sea anemone and anemone fish. *Science, 234*, 585-587.

Nakamura, H., Kobayashi, J., Ohizumi, Y., Hirata, Y., 1982. Isolation and structure of aaptamine a novel heteroaromatic substance possessing α-blocking activity from the sea sponge *Aaptos aaptos*. *Tetrahedron Lett. 23*, 5555–5558.

Nakamura, Y., Kobayashi, J., Gilmore, J., Mascal, M., Rinehart, K.L., Jr., Nakamura, H., Ohizumi, Y., 1986. Bromoeudistomin D, a novel inducer of calcium release from fragmented sarcoplasmic reticulum that causes contractions of skinned muscle fibers. *J Biol Chem. 261*(9):4139-42.

Ohizumi, Y., Kajiwara, A., Nakamura, H., Kobayashi, J., 1984. Alpha-adrenoceptor blocking action of aaptamine, a novel marine natural product, in vascular smooth muscle. *J Pharm Pharmacol. 36*(11), 785-6.

Pauletti, P.M., Cintra, L.S., Braguine, C.G., da Silva Filho, A.A., Silva, M.L., Cunha, W.R., Januário, A.H., 2010. Halogenated indole alkaloids from marine invertebrates. *Mar Drugs. 8*(5), 1526-49.

Sagar, S., Kaur, M., Minneman, K.P., 2010. Antiviral lead compounds from marine sponges. *Mar Drugs. 8*(10), 2619-38.

Segraves, N.L., Crews, P.J., 2005. Investigation of brominated tryptophan alkaloids from two Thorectidae sponges: *Thorectandra* and *Smenospongia*. *Nat. Prod. 68*, 1484-1488.

Segraves, N.L., Lopez, S., Johnson, T.A., Said, S.A., Fu, X., Schmitz, F.J., Pietraszkiewicz, H., Valeriote, F.A., Crews, P., 2003. Structures and cytotoxicities of fascaplysin and related alkaloids from two marine phyla—Fascaplysinopsis sponges and Didemnum tunicates,

Tetrahedron Letters, 44(17), 3471-3475.

Shulgin, A.T., Shulgin, A., 1997. *TIHKAL: The continuation*. Transform Press, Berkeley, CA.

Shulgin, A., Shulgin, A., 1991. *PIHKAL: A chemical love story*. Transform Press, Berkeley, CA.

Thomas, T.R., Kavlekar, D.P., LokaBharathi, P.A., 2010. Marine drugs from sponge-microbe association--a review. *Mar Drugs. 8*(4), 1417-68.

Torrens-Spence, M.P., Liu, C.T., Pluskal, T., Chung, Y.K., Weng, J.K., 2018. Monoamine Biosynthesis via a Noncanonical Calcium-Activatable Aromatic Amino Acid Decarboxylase in Psilocybin Mushroom. *ACS Chem Biol., 13*(12):3343-3353.

Tymiak, A.A., Rinehart, K.L, Jr., 1980. Constituents of morphologically similar sponges. *Tetrahedron. 41*, 1039-1047.

Van Lear, G.E., Morton, G.O., Fulmor, W., 1973. New antibacterial bromoindole metabolites from the marine sponge *Polyfibrospongia Maynardii*. *Tetrahedron Letters, 14*(4), 299-300.

Van Maarseveen, J.H., Scheeren, H.W., De Clercq, E., Balzarini, J., Kruse, C.G., 1997. Antiviral and tumor cell antiproliferative SAR studies on tetracyclic eudistomins. II. *Bioorg Med Chem. 5*(5), 955-70.

Wang, Q., Tang, X.L., Luo, X.C., de Voogd, N.J., Li, P.L., Li, G.Q., 2019. Aplysinopsin-type and

Bromotyrosine-derived Alkaloids from the South China Sea Sponge *Fascaplysinopsis reticulata*. *Sci Rep. 9*(1), 2248

Yu, H.B., Yang, F., Sun, F., Li, J., Jiao, W.H., Gan, J.H., Hu, W.Z., Lin, H.W., 2014. Aaptamine Derivatives with Antifungal and Anti-HIV-1 Activities from the South China Sea Sponge *Aaptos aaptos*. *Marine Drugs. 12*(12), 6003-6013.

Mycosphere

Mycelial Universe of Psychoactive Fungi

Revisiting the Mckenna Stoned Ape "Theory" and the Ever-Evolving Case of Its Plausibility for Stimulating Neurogeneration

Paul Stamets

Mycologist | Author and Speaker | Medical researcher

> *"We need to have a paradigm shift in our consciousness. If we don't get our act together, and come in commonality and understanding with the organisms that sustain us today, not only will we destroy those organisms, but we will destroy ourselves."*—PAUL STAMETS

A transcribed speech edited by Paul Stamets on the history and potential of psychedelic fungi.

I'm humbled to be around so many kindred spirits and great minds. Thank you deeply Dennis and the McKenna Academy and to all of you. I am going to take you through a short history of psilocybin use and emerge into what I think are new horizons of extraordinarily exciting research. This is my journey with psilocybin, but I'm only one knowledge keeper in a continuum of knowledge keepers. This is not one individual story, this is the story of all of us as a community.

There are archaeological suggestions of the use of psychoactive mushrooms: for example the Mesoamerican Mayan mushroom stones; the Aztec culture was well documented using psilocybin mushrooms, and cave paintings from northern Algeria 7000 years ago which depict mushrooms and bees. As many of you know, psilocybin mushrooms were preserved in honey, an ancient tradition that even persists today and in Central America and Mexico. In Greek mythology in 400 BCE, this stone relief features Demeter giving Persephone a mushroom before she enters into the autumnal underworld, for her to reemerge in the spring. We only know of the history of psilocybin mushrooms in Paleolithic times or in ancient times, through the artists who rendered these works. Artists play an important role in preserving the knowledge of the past, in many cases before written language. These are archaeological echoes of what may well have been representations of psychoactive mushroom use. Today, it is so important to give tribute to Indigenous Peoples, especially to Maria Sabina, who in 1955 opened up her doors for Gordon and Valentina Wasson. This historic encounter sparked a new awareness, scientifically and culturally in psilocybin mushrooms.

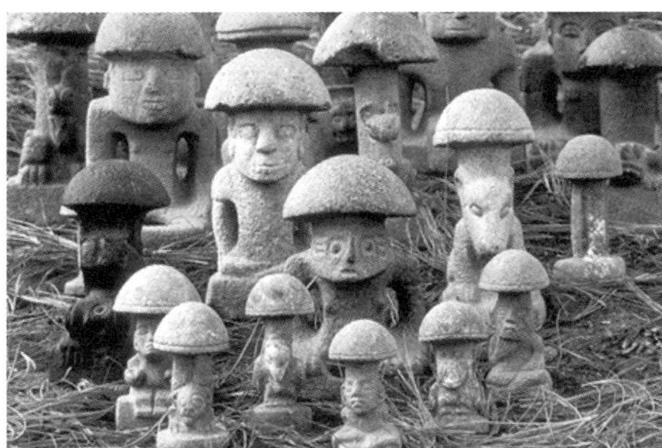

Fig. 1 Mayan mushroom stones. Photograph by Grant Kalivoda.

Valentina Wasson was not only a physician but a mycologist. When Valentina and Gordon were on a honeymoon in the Adirondacks in upstate New York, as they walked down a trail, they encountered a beautiful fruiting of mushrooms. Tina was so excited she ran to the mushrooms with glee and excitement, whereas Gordon was horrified. They had just married, and it is from that dialectic and their lifelong ethnomycological study began. They coined the terms "mycophobia" and "mycophilia". Unfortunately, Valentina Wasson died in 1958. She was of Russian heritage and grew up in a culture that was extremely mycophilic, whereas Gordon (who was of English heritage) grew up in a largely mycophobic society. In that region of Oaxaca where Maria Sabina practiced, they were using three primary species: *Psilocybe caerulescens, Psilocybe mexicana* and *Psilocybe zapotecorum*. The Wassons worked with the French mycologist Roger Heim, and their collaboration led to the co-publication of a monograph called *Les Champignons Hallucinogene du Mexique,* in which was described many species new to science, but not new to the indigenous people. A pivotal moment in the re-emergence of knowledge was when, in 1957, copies of Life Magazine arrived in the mailboxes of millions of Americans with a complete color field guide to many psilocybin mushrooms and the wondrous descriptions of Gordon Watson's experience with curandera Maria Sabina. This was sadly to the detriment of Maria Sabina and her village, as an influx of tourists began to arrive. These rituals had been kept hidden for centuries, as they were brutally persecuted during the Spanish conquest. However, Wasson revealed these secrets to the world and Oaxaca has not been the same since (Gerber et al., 2021).

MY CHILDHOOD MEMORIES: HOW I BECAME A MYCOLOGIST AND A PSYCHONAUT

I want to give tribute to my father and my mother, and my brother John. These individuals have been hugely influential in my life. I grew up in a in a large house, in a scientific family. We had a complete laboratory in the basement. This laboratory was a reasonable size and had three or four rows of shelves full of chemicals, glassware, scales and microscopes. My brother John was 5-6 years older than me. He was a serious scientist, a chemist. I was the youngest one in my family. I adored my own oldest brother and I wanted to hang with him all the time, but I think he felt I was a nuisance in the laboratory, distracting him from his serious work.

Since my father served on the aircraft carrier the Intrepid during World War II, he got the aircraft carrier radio, the main radio from that ship. We had it in our basement. My brother John would allow me to sit and explore coded messages originating from spies behind the Iron Curtain. I strung about a 200-foot-long copper wire with glass insulators to be able to get long wave radio signals from afar. I would listen to coded messages for hours. Just being in the presence of my brother meant a lot to me.

My brother John went to Yale to pursue chemistry. My older brother Bill went to Cornell. My twin brother and I were left unsupervised with John's laboratory in the basement. I remember eagerly looking up experiments that said "Danger do not bring near a flame". One time, we had a massive explosion in the laboratory and my mother came run running down to check on me. Fortunately, the blast force was directed away from me. After that I developed a new found respect for the chemicals John amassed.

John eventually became my tripping buddy. We journeyed together a lot. Previously I had become so excited about the work that he was doing at Yale on neurophysiology. He had come back from Mexico and Colombia with these incredible stories of tripping on psilocybin mushrooms. At one course at Yale, his textbook was *Altered State of Consciousness* edited by Charles Tart, University of California, Davis. I asked for it and he lent me this book while on spring break. I immersed myself into this treatise. My best friend, Ryan, who I was hanging with all the time, saw my interest in this book and asked if he can borrow it. I consented provided he gave it back in about a week as my brother was going back to the university. A week passed and soon my brother was returning, so I kept on bugging Ryan to please give me back my brother John's book. John was asking me for it, and pressuring me. Finally, I just got really upset "Ryan, I need the book back now. He's leaving." I said Ryan replied, "I can't give it back to you. My father found it and burned it." I could not believe Ryan's father burned my brother's book. I am ashamed to tell my brother what had happened. He was very disappointed. Thereupon I realized, wow, if this resulted in Ryan's father, an authoritarian figure, reacting in such a way, then I definitely wanted to focus on this subject.

I went on to immerse myself in the field of mycology. I spent an enormous amount of time in the University of Washington Science Library in the basement where most of the journals that had pages on Psilocybe mushrooms ripped out. I eventually was invited into Dr. Daniel Stuntz's lab at the UW who had an intact collection of journals. I had entered Evergreen State College working under the guidance of Dr. Michael Beug. Together, we received legal Drug Enforcement Administration (DEA)coverage for doing psilocybin mushroom research with another student, Jeremy Bigwood. I focused on taxonomy, cultivation and microscopy. My work led to the publication my first book in 1978, *Psilocybe Mushrooms & Their Allies* at the age of 23. That's almost 45 years ago. The image in Figure 2 is when I presented my book to my mother, who graciously loved me dearly but nervously accepted my peculiar interest in this subject. My brother John, of course, expressed a mixture of pride and amusement that his younger brother came out with a book and psilocybin mushrooms, a subject he kindled in his little brother.

Another book that greatly influenced me was *The Crack In The Cosmic Egg* by Joseph Chilton Pearce. The focus of the book was when you immerse yourself into a subject deeply for years, revelations come to you almost intuitively, escaping the gravity of cognitive reductionist thinking.

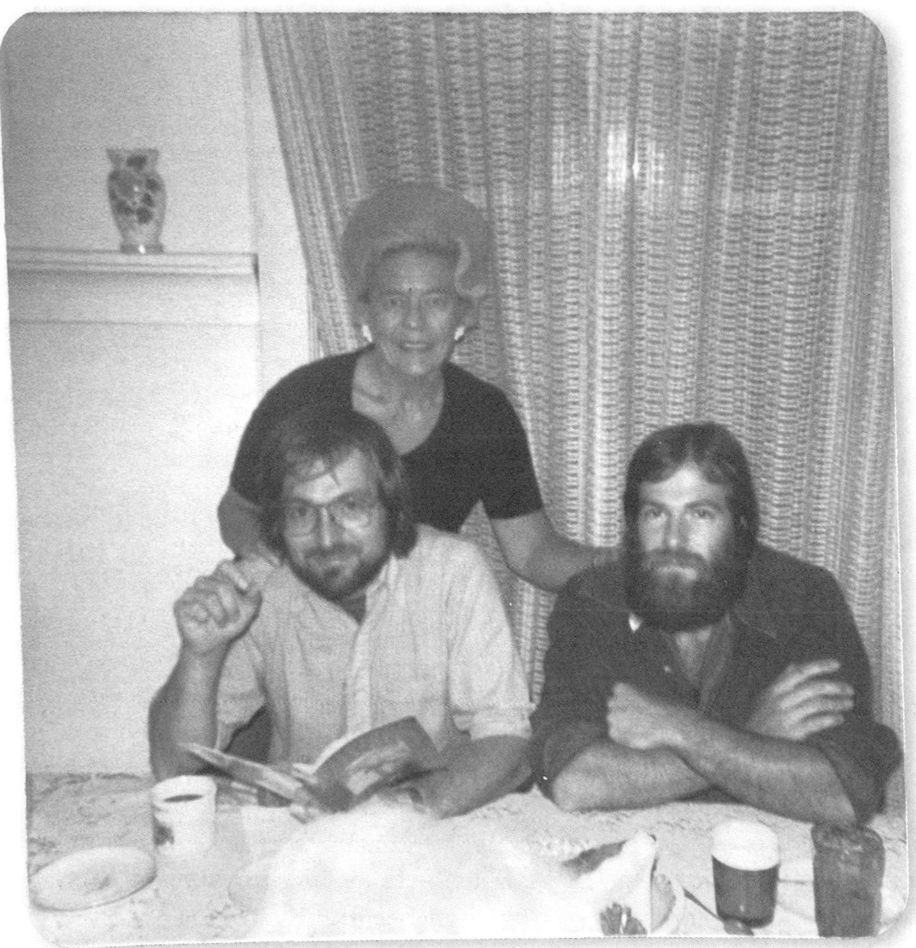

Fig. 2 In 1978, I presented to my mother and brother John my just published book on psilocybin mushrooms—*Psilocybe Mushrooms & Their Allies.*

It's a sudden eureka moment of just intuitive realization. These are not the origins of your own thinking. These are the origins of the milieu in which you've immersed your focus, and it's like nature is channeling you this wisdom. I feel this is how my life has been propelled.

Dr. Alexander Smith was a mycologist and one of my mentors. Like my father, he also asked me for psilocybin mushrooms late in life. I turned them both down, and I denied their requests even though they were hugely important male mentors in my life. Alexander Smith published many new to science psilocybin mushrooms. When I asked them: "If I said yes and consumed psilocybin mushrooms with you, would your wives agree to do them with us?" They both said, no, absolutely not. I replied that I don't want to be responsible for you having a life changing decision near to the end of your life. This experience will be be very difficult for you to explain to your partners. It could shake the very foundations of your religious beliefs. It could change your whole view of reality. I don't want that responsibility of creating a divide in your relationship. So I said, if your wives would take the mushrooms with me together, then I will do it. Since they both declined, I declined. Moreover, I would leave on my travels directly thereafter. I felt a responsibility to help them process the experience for days afterward. Since I wouldn't be there for them, I realized this was not the right set and setting.

These two experiences helped me focused on my life's philosophy and the fact that I have an important responsibility. Thereupon, I came up with the phrase "Nature provides, I don't". When you give psilocybin, or sacrament, or a psychotropic to somebody else, you own part of that experience. You have a responsibility for the therapy. I believe you incur a responsibility to be a good therapist, psychologist or psychiatrist to help people assimilate and process this extraordinary experience. Giving someone such a powerful substance and then to walk away from it, I think, is irresponsible.

There are four mycologists who have been most influential in my career. Dr. Alexander Smith from the University of Michigan, who some consider to be the father of American mycology, and who published widely on new species of Psilocybe. Dr. Daniel Stuntz from the University of Washington had a species named after him: *Psilocybe stuntzii*. Catherine Scates, a self-taught mycologist, had a huge influence. And most importantly, Dr. Michael Beug from the Evergreen State College. Michael received a Drug Enforcement Administration license which covered my and Jeremy Bidgood's work on psilocybin mushrooms in 1977 and years thereafter. I could legally collect and cultivate psilocybin mushrooms. About every third person that came up to me I suspected was an undercover DEA agent, so I guarded my privilege of possessing psilocybin very carefully. We now live in a liberal state of acceptance of psychedelics right now, and especially mushrooms. It has become the zeitgeist of our times. But back then, we lived in a high state of paranoia. It was a time of anti-war protests, the time subsequent to Nixon weaponizing the drugs and creating the war on drugs, which was a politically and racist motivated strategy. They are able put in the same bucket African-Americans, environmentalists, anti-war protesters and the LGBQT communities, and the feminist movements. Nixon and his cronies realized the so-called 'war on drugs' was a very convenient excuse to suppress the majority of their more liberal political opponents.

I went on to publish four species of Psilocybe mushrooms. One was *Psilocybe azurescens*, one of the most potent species in the world with more 2-3% psilocybin. Another is *Psilocybe liniformans* var. *americana*, an extremely rare species, *and Psilocybe cyanofibrillosa*. In 1977, we initiated a series of annual psilocybin mushroom conferences. In 1979, we co-organized a the first MycoMedia mushroom conference on the coast of Oregon and invited Stephen Pollock, MD, Dale Leslie, Jeremy Bigwood, Jonathan Ott, and the Mexican mycologist Dr. Gaston Guzman —who subsequently completed a monograph on the genus Psilocybe.

Thereupon, we sponsored psilocybin centered mushroom conferences over 20 years. In 1998 there was a renowned conference in Amsterdam. Albert Hofmann, Sasha & Ann Shulgin, myself and many other experts. Later, when I realized that because I'm a Deadhead and knew Ken Kesey, the Merry Pranksters, but I also knew Sasha Shulgin and Andy Weil and many other psychedelic scientists and medical doctors, that I was uniquely at an intersection of these two camps. So, I decided to do The Millennium Mushroom Conference in 1999, bringing together Ken Kesey, The Merry Pranksters and the bus with the psychedelic scientists at Breitenbush

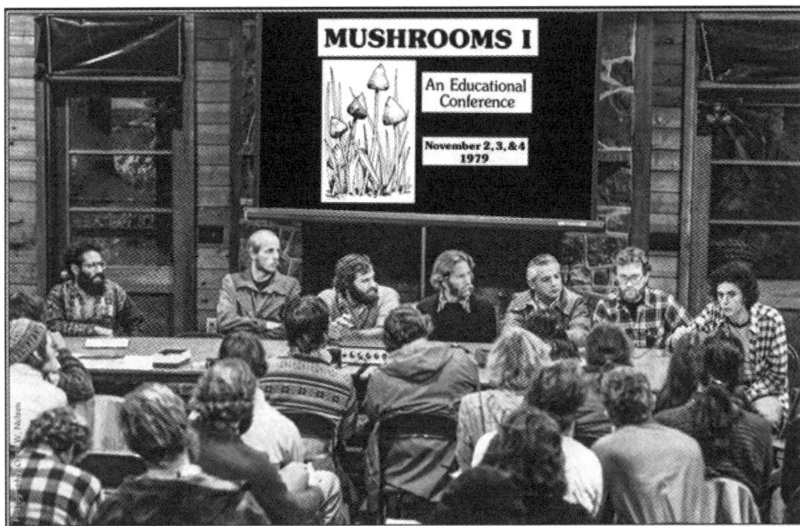

Fig.3 Mushrooms I panel in Florence, Oregon, 4th November 1979. In the image is Steve Pollock, M.D, James Q. Jacobs, Paul E. Stamets, Dale T. Leslie, Gaston Guzman, PhD, Jeremy Bigwood and Jonathan Ott. *Photograph by Chris W. Nelson*

Hot Springs in Oregon. We had nearly 30 speakers and about 120 people. Financially it was a disaster: I lost about $50,000. However, in retrospect, it was the most wonderful investment I've ever made. On Halloween night we had a pageantry of psychonauts dressed up as animals, fairies and wizards. I lost control of the conference. A cauldron containing a half dozen species of psilocybin mushroom became "witches brew" from which most attendees drank from. So many attendees brought in wild collected Psilocybes which were carefully identified before being added to a massive vessel of tea. The magic potion tea was enriched with *Psilocybe semilanceata, P. cyanescens, P. baeocystis, P. callosa, P. cyanofibrillosa, P. pelliculosa* and the yet-to-be-named *Psilocybe azurescens.* Psilocybin inspired our collective artistic creativity. This event will go down in history as one of the greatest epic gatherings of psychonaut's. This ESPD55 conference is a continuum of these gatherings where knowledge keepers are coming to pass on our experiences to the next generation. Coincidentally, with all of these conferences psychedelic art is featured and continues to be so to this day.

I went on to publish seven books and am now working on a new one. However, Terence & Dennis Mckenna, along with Kat Harrison and Jeremy Bigwood published *Psilocybin Magic Mushroom Grower's Guide* under the pseudonyms "Oss & Oeric". This was the book that had the greatest influence in showing people how to grow psilocybin mushrooms on a small scale. Psilocybin mushrooms created a novel source of scholarship funds, where people in colleges throughout the United States and Europe grew small amounts of psilocybin mushrooms in their closets and their dormitory rooms to help support their academic endeavors.

Terence and Dennis, prior to this time, about a decade before their cultivation book, proposed The Stoned Ape Theory, undoubtedly stimulated by the writings of Richard Evans

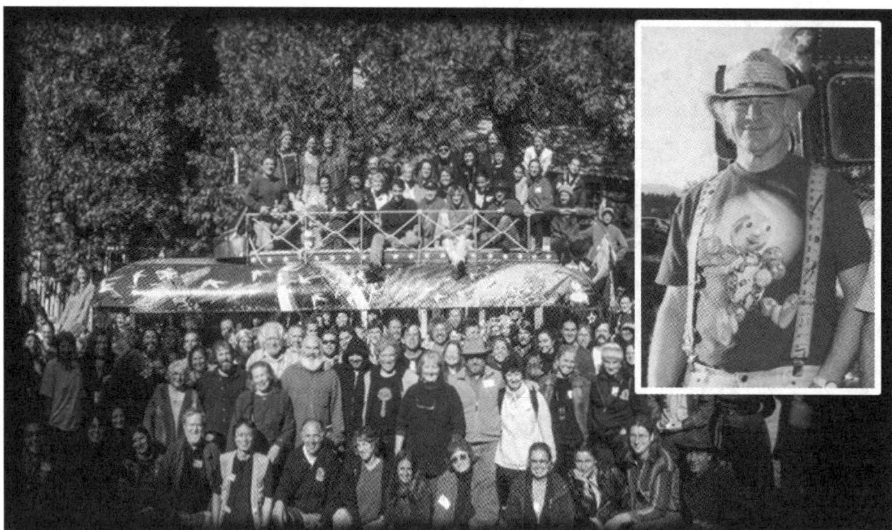

Fig. 4 The 1999 Millenium Mushroom Conference. The man in the image on the right is Ken Kesey. *Photograph by William Stamets*

Schultes, R. Gordon Wasson, Weston La Barre and Mircea Eliade, many of whom experienced psilocybin mushrooms inducing profound altered states of consciousness. I suggest to you that the Stoned Ape Theory was then a hypothesis*. A hypothesis is the idea that is not currently substantiated by fact but by conjecture. A theory is when a hypothesis evolves into an idea substantiated by fact, but also not necessarily proven. These books, along with Andrew Weil's *The Natural Mind*, Ken Kesey's *One Flew Over the Cuckoo's Nest*, Gary Menser/s *Hallucinogenic and Poisonous Mushrooms Field Guide*, Sasha and Ann Shulgin's *Tikhal* and *Pikhal* fueled the interest of psychonauts worldwide. Ken Kesey and I became friends. When we first met, Ken told me "Paul, I don't know shit about mushrooms. People bring them to me all the time, expecting me to be a mushroom expert. The one species I do know well is Liberty caps." So, Ken Kesey relied upon me for species identification and we developed a nice bond. Moreover, I was brought into the Kesey's immediate and extended family whose mantra was built upon love, art, play, tolerance, and respect. And they were friends of the Grateful Dead, whose music accompanied me on many of my explorations.

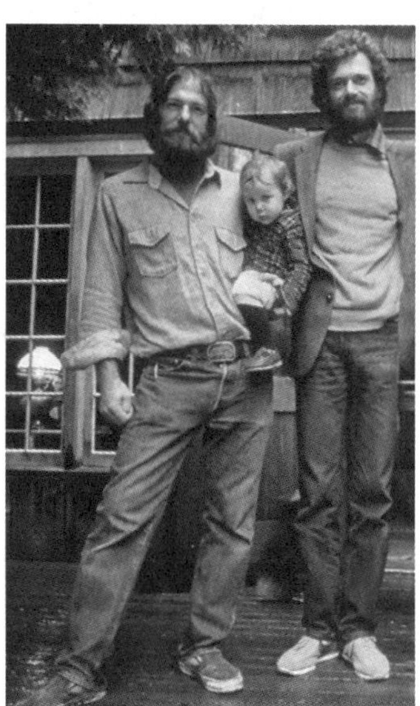

Fig.5 Paul Stamets, LaDena Stamets, Terence McKenna at the Breitenbush Hot Springs, Oregon 27th of October 1983. *Photograph by Chris W. Nelson*

* A hypothesis is "a proposition or proposed explanation made on the basis of limited evidence as a starting point for further investigation." (Future Learn 2022).

"THE STONED APE HYPOTHESIS"

Let's look at the Stoned Ape Hypothesis. There was a sudden enlargement of the human of the hominid brain about 2 million years ago that expanded substantially 2 to 3 times from that of our predecessor species. *Homo sapiens* (us) are a recent evolutionary species. We're only about 200,000 years old which is quite remarkable as our ancestors' brain underwent this rapid increase in cranial capacity during a time of dramatic climate change. Climate change forced our species to adapt and create new skill sets absolutely necessary for survival. What else sparked the sudden expansion of the hominid brain? Terence and Dennis hypothesized that our ape-like ancestors' repeatedly ingesting psilocybin mushrooms stimulated new neurons to form, enlarging our brain's capacity and skillsets for survival.

As our hominid ancestors descended from the trees, they followed and hunted ungulates and other animals. If you are tracking animals, you're looking for footprints and dung. They would encounter mushrooms in the dung. *Psilocybe cubensis* grows in the dung of cows, zebras, elephants and numerous other species in Africa. These golden mushrooms can be quite large and seen from afar. Most primates are grub eaters, eating larvae as a protein source. Aging *P. cubensis* is often thriving with larvae, and most primates eat maggots. In fact there are 22 primates, 23, when you count humans, that consume mushrooms for food. With so many primates who are documented using mushrooms and larvae for food, it speaks to a deep historical foundation of the intersection of primates and mushrooms. They saw them as essential foodstuffs. The Goldi monkey in Bolivia, for example, in the Amazon eats ~12 times his body weight per year. So, this is just not an incidental interaction with fungi- fungi are a mainstay of the foodstuffs of many primates.

Logically our hungry hunter-gathering ancestors would seek dung dwelling mushrooms out as a food source—but the psilocybin species imparted a dramatically powerful secondary effect, stimulating the brain with visions. These visions would be shared with those you consumed the mushrooms with. Brain neurons would be stimulated to grow. At the time and to this day, Mckennas' hypothesis was roundly dispelled by scientific critics as being ridiculous—a stoners dream, roundly disregarded by "serious scientists". Of course, stoners celebrated this concept and thought, "Yes, but of course!". Psilocybin myconauts know from their experiences with psilocybin mushrooms that they expand consciousness. Most psychedelically naïve critics still to this day have no clue.

Is this idea indeed so preposterous? Let's consider this in a broad view. For millions of years, our ancestors would be, in the forest. Tracking animals by scouting for dung, *Psilocybe cubensis* would be an obvious potential source of nutrition. Consuming this mushroom would not happen once or twice, but millions upon millions of times over millions of years. Epigenetics describes the influence of external influences on the genomics of an organism with genes coding responses from repeated stimuli to ensure better survival. Psilocybin meets this criterion as an epigenetic stimulant.

Those who have collected *Psilocybe cubensis*, aka golden tops, can see these from hundreds of feet away, they are so obvious. While tracking animals, our hominid ancestors would inevitably and frequently encounter *Psilocybe cubensis*. These foragers would likely share this newfound soft food with family members who are also hungry. We may never know. However, the hypothesis that psilocybin stimulates neurogeneration using today's modern analytical methods is now testable. I think we can preliminarily prove it and increasingly so in the future. *Psilocybe cubensis*, to this day, remains the most consumed psilocybin mushroom in the world. With such widespread use, the data sets are becoming more robust than ever before. This species is easily grown in manure-based substrates and is especially easy to grow on sterilized grains.

I want to address the importance of the morphology with psilocybin mushrooms. They are ideally harvested when they are young: when the spore generating gills are immature. At this stage, the cap flesh is very thick. But what happens in a matter of a few hours is the caps expand and the cap flesh thins, transforming by extending the gill surfaces upon which increasing spore production ensues. Spores contain no psilocybin and there is a bio-transformation of these substantial amounts of the psilocybin rich flesh into psilocybin-less spores. All of this happens in a matter of a few hours. Many people are allergic to mushroom spores, and they can exacerbate problems with asthma. Since adverse reactions are critically important in terms of public safety, mushrooms should be harvested at an adolescent stage when the partial veils are intact. Fruitbodies with closed veils can fully expand to flattened caps in a matter of a few hours. The veils fall to become a membranous annulus—a ring around the stem. Out of caution, *Psilocybe cubensis* is best harvested and consumed when the veils are closed, and the gills are still covered. Some amateurs think the bigger the mushroom is, the better- this is not true. There's a reapportionment of the flesh going into thinner, less dense gill tissue. Even though the mushrooms appear larger, the density decreases and so despite morphologically appearing bigger the masses remain the same or even less with maturity due to the prolific exodus of spore mass.

Let's look at some of the data that's been published recently in the past ten years. Here's a survey of prisoners, inmates, approximately 480,000 people surveyed. When they did this, they completed a survey and a questionnaire where they asked about their use of drugs. Very interestingly, psilocybin use was associated with a 27% decrease of larceny, 22% decrease odds of property crime had an 18% decrease in violent crime* (Jones et al., 2022). Critics could say association is not necessarily causation, but it can be. Psilocybin use showed a reduction of intimate partner to partner violence—if one of the partners had a past history with psilocybin. Overall, these meta studies show that psilocybin use is associated with the reduction again of violence, criminal and anti-social behavior. I speculate that if there was a dating app and you're looking at your romantic prospects, a really important question is "have you tripped on psilocybin before?". If yes, you advance.

There are 120 clinical studies registered at www.clinicaltrials.gov ongoing right now and only one or two are using mushrooms. The overwhelming focus is psilocybin, the molecule. There's a massive disconnect between real world use and clinical studies. I think it's no exaggeration to say the following: More than 99% of the use of psilocybin is in the form of psilocybin mushrooms and a tiny percentage is using the pure molecule. The vast disparity of real-world use versus the reductionist thinking of using just the molecule is biased in order to get FDA approval. This is a glaring disparity we see currently in psilocybin clinical science: the dialectic of the natural product world view versus the single molecule point of view.

On April 7th, 2023, a meta observation study showed that psilocybin was the only psychedelic associated with lower odds of opioid use disorder. Opioid use disorder (OUD) is a huge

---

* To learn more about this topic see "Psychedelics and the Prevention of Interpersonal Violence: The Role of Emotion Regulation" by Michelle St. Pierre, MA, PhD and Zach Walsh, PhD.

problem across the world. OUD has affected my family. To overcome shame, to overcome guilt, pain, PTSD, emotional trauma, tragedy, users find solace using opioids. Opioid users are vilified by society, further shaming them and reducing their self-image. So, what do they do? They use more opioids. When you have a family member addicted to opioids, it affects not just the user, it affects the family, your friends, your neighbors, your village, your city, your state, your province, your country, the world. The expense to society is tremendous to us all, overwhelming the court systems, law enforcement and health providers.

Psilocybin is different. The evidence strongly suggests that psilocybin reduces crime. Psilocybin reduces violence. Psilocybin makes nicer people. Like another pebble in the pond, but this pond is one of positivity. When you resolve the trauma and you kick opioids, and become a nicer person, a better partner, you are more empathetic, you transform into a force of good trying to downregulate anger of other people. You try to reach out a hand of friendship and understanding. With this pebble in the pond, there's emanations of goodness from you to your family, to your neighbors, to your village, to your city, your province, to your state, your country, and to the world. The difference between the negative and the positive is extraordinary. The number of resources that can be saved, reducing stress on our governments and expenses to society are difficult to overstate. Think of it: psilocybin mushrooms are in our heritage today at a time critical that they can have an enormous impact, helping us resolve many of the critical issues that we face. Today we have converging tragedies of the Commons. Psilocybin is uniquely positioned to reconcile many of these negative forces.

OUR RESEARCH

I want to delve into some of the research we've been doing. I came up with a combination of admixtures known as "The Stamets Stack". I stack it with niacin because niacin is a vasodilator and psilocybin is a vasoconstrictor. I thought, that with greater dilation, more psilocybin could be delivered via the blood vessels. Niacin also excites the nerve endings. Those of you who've taken high doses of niacin feel it in about 15 minutes, you start flushing red, your skin itches, your clothes feel abrasive. Since neuropathies oftentimes present themselves as the deadening of the toes and the fingertips from vasoconstriction and the consequential dieback of nerves, I thought that with vasodilation and excitation of the nerve endings, niacin could help deliver the psilocybin's neurogenic benefits. By adding lion's mane mushrooms (*Hericium erinaceus*), one of the best studied medicinal mushrooms in the world, the erinacine rich mycelium of this species could augment regeneration myelin on the axons of the nerves and stimulate production of nerve growth factors (NGF). There are at least four clinical studies published on Lion's Mane.* I hypothesized stacking these three together would have many synergistic advantages. Moreover, high doses of niacin could act as a deterrent like Antabuse is to alcoholics should there be legal constraints on microdosing for over the counter products provided to consumers.

When microdosing with psilocybin mushrooms, the addition of 25 to 50 milligrams of niacin is just at the sub-flushing range for most people. If you have ten times that much niacin,

* See www.mushroomreferences.com for scientific research on various mushrooms.

the adverse reaction from flushing becomes very uncomfortable. So, the idea was how can we convince the FDA to allow access for microdosing for the masses? I think that's adding niacin as an adversant is one additional advantage. You could also use low doses of ipecac, capsaicin , etc. but niacin uniquely provides a multiplicity of benefits. This stack could enhance macrodosing *and* microdosing with psilocybin. I know personally from experience that niacin enhances the psilocybin experience.

There are two common protocols for microdosing. One is the Jim Fadiman's protocol, and the one protocol that I came up with which is 4-5 days on and then 2 to 3 days off. Jim Fadiman's protocol is dose on one day, then followed by 2 days of no dosing. I asked, Jim, how do you come with your protocol? He said "I just made it up." I said, "Yeah, I just made mine up too." We both share that there needs to be a break so your receptors can reset, become re-sensitisized, so when they are again washed with psilocybin and psilocybin analogs, they can be re-stimulated for neurogeneration.

I do a lot of *in vitro* tissue culture in the lab, running many cell lines (strains or verities, aka phenotypes). We have over 700 fungal strains in our culture library. We are growing mycelium en masse constantly, with tens of thousands of kilograms grown per month. We intimately understand senescence—the loss of a strain's viability—and the importance of keeping cell lines young. We are keenly focused on the pace of cell divisions and how to accelerate mycelium in its production of downstream daughter cells.

Many of you may not know if you over culture mycelium, it senesces, losing networking and new tip forming abilities. The analogy I can make is that when the mycelium is young, it's like the netting of a nylon sock but if you over propagate it, it becomes like that of a tennis net. The mycelial fabric loses its interconnections and the density of forking and networking cells. If you titrate 25 milligrams for 30 days at one milligram per day for 25 of those 30 days, you're giving those cells that are dividing a constant, albeit low level exposure to a neurogenic agent as opposed to dosing all at once, in one session, at 30 mg. The half-life of psilocin is 1.8 hours. In one day, there is about 1/10,000th of psilocin in your serum and receptor occupancy is vastly reduced. I thought, titrating psilocybin over time so new regenerating neurons, like the growth of mycelium, could enhance in its longer-term cell growth. This allows for better neurogeneration, hypothetically, than one super strong dose. I think the analogy of growing mycelium and neurons has merit.

Dr. Pamela Kryskow, Eesmyal Santos-Brault, Kaitlin Harvey (the two founders of Quantified Citizen) and myself came together with others, co-designing an app which you can download now*. The app was designed to study microdosing behavior and is fully vetted and approved by Canadian medical ethic experts. All data is anonymized, so you own your personal data. We wanted to see what the characteristics were of the users that were engaged, by asking people to go to the app, and log microdosing habits for that day. This can include details such as what you are taking (mushrooms, LSD, DMT), the amount you consumed, and the characteristics of the formula that you were taking. Then there's challenge tests, cognitive tests, memory tests, hearing tests, visual acuity tests, etc… and then you record your progress (or non-progress) over time. We announced this when I was on the Joe Rogan podcast and that got a lot of people involved. We ended up having

* You can download this app Android and iOS Apple devices via www.microdose.me

more than 8000 people participate for our first analyzed data set. Now we have more than 24,000 subscribers, and literally millions of data points. Much of this data has yet to be analyzed.

An extraordinary metric in our first study group is that we had more non-micro doses (n = 4653) than micro doses (n = 4050), a relatively even-weighted population. This also impressed the peer reviewers at Nature, the publishers of *Scientific Reports.* We published our meta observational survey on November 18th, 2021, and it was the third most downloaded article in *Nature Scientific Reports* that year (Rootman et al., 2021). This is a comprehensive data set which has undergone revisions to become even more robust today. It compares sex, sexual preferences, income, ethnicities, mental health status and motivations for microdosing.

In the Quantified Citizen microdose app, there are basically three different metrics of dosage ranges of psilocybin mushrooms that are grouped as follows:

Low Dose	<.10 grams	16% of respondents
Med Dose	.10–.30 grams	72% of respondents
High Dose	>.30 grams	12% of respondents

88% of users consumed 10-30 grams of *Psilocybe cubensis*, the species used approximately 90% of the time. Many ongoing clinical studies that are investigating psilocybin are using the equivalent of about three grams of *Psilocybe cubensis*, equal to 30 milligrams at 1% concentration of psilocybin in this species. The "Hero's Journey" is generally considered to be approximately 5 grams of mushrooms or 50 mg of pure psilocybin.

Psilocybin content can substantially differ due to the species, maturity of fruitbodies, substrate, length of storage and other conditions. In total 78% of the respondents were using 1/10th to 1/3rd of a dried psilocybin mushrooms, 39% of the people who were stacking were using the Stamets Stack, 5%, for instance, were using chocolate and 90% were using *Psilocybe cubensis.*

What follows is some of the preliminary data for more than 8000 participants. With the stack in terms of mood and mental health, there was a substantial reduction in depression, which was highly significant in terms of improving mood on the PANAS scale (Positive and Negative Affect Scale). The P value* of significance for PANAS was extraordinarily low: p= <.00001 and alleviating depression in the DASS21 scale (Depression and Anxiety Stress Scale) a more modest, yet significant P=< 0.05. This data was very positive, showing that microdosing with the stack helped alleviate these two mood disorders compared to non-microdosers. Microdosers with psilocybin in any form also showed significant benefits.

When we published our first paper on microdosing, the critics came out of the woodwork:

* "The P value is defined as the probability under the assumption of no effect or no difference (null hypothesis), of obtaining a result equal to or more extreme than what was actually observed. The P stands for probability and measures how likely it is that any observed difference between groups is due to chance. Being a probability, P can take any value between 0 and 1. Values close to 0 indicate that the observed difference is unlikely to be due to chance, whereas a P value close to 1 suggests no difference between the groups other than due to chance. Thus, it is common in medical journals to see adjectives such as "highly significant" or "very significant" after quoting the P value depending on how close to zero the value is." (Dahiru et al., 2011)

"What about expectancy and the placebo effect?". The weirdest criticism is one about this was not a placebo-controlled study. This is an observational study and of course not blinded. People know what they're doing. People *expected* that this will help them resolve depression, they heard about it, read about its positive outcomes, so expectancy is valid factor that could skew the results. Dr. Pamela Kryskow and I have had discussions about this. She's a medical doctor and the head of the Psychedelic Association of Canada. We went back and forth about these criticisms. I asked "don't we have a test that's beyond subjectivity?" and she replied "Yes, we have a motor skill test: the "tap test". When we tasked our statisticians to examine the scores of participants reporting on this psychomotor test, we found a signal that was remarkable.

The finger tapping test registers how often you can tap two alternating forefingers fingers on a surface in 10 seconds. Tapping ability typically decreases with age, during midlife. This test is used specifically for measuring Parkinson's, Alzheimer's, dementia, and traumatic brain injury. There's a steady decline in tapping frequency with Alzheimer's, dementia and Parkinson's patients as they lose the ability of coordination from progressive neurodegeneration.

To test motor skills, we selected people aged 55 years and older. In doing this we saw a signal, a signal was so strong that the statisticians who are coauthors stated "We found something, but we have a hard time believing the data". So, they re-analyzed this data using three statistical analytical techniques. The results survived re-analysis. The data here shown here that in 30 days of individuals using the Stamets Stack, the performance of the finger test went from 48 to 68 taps in 10 seconds with a very substantial p value significance, p=0.04. This means there is one chance in 250 that the signal is random. The non stackers were non-significant in their tapping ability as well as the people who were doing psilocybin in any other form or combination. It's just the people who are combining psilocybin mushrooms, lion's mane and niacin. This result shows a substantial increase in psychomotor performance. We published these results in a second paper, also in Nature: Scientific Reports (Rootman et al., 2022a, Rootman et al., 2022b).

Our discussions naturally gravitated to discussions as the possible modes of action to explain the significant increase in finger tapping agility. I'm not a neurologist, but I again went down the wormhole of neurology and neurodegeneration. We found there's very good *in-vitro* tests for identifying new drugs for neurogeneration. I have personally spent more than $1 million on the data that you're about to see. This has been a concerted effort with seven of my scientists and a great team of people at Fungi Perfecti, LLC* under my leadership.

We focused on MAPk (Mitogen Activated Protein kinases). These are actually proteins that bind with receptors on the nerves. They are stimulated by NGF (nerve growth factors) and BDNF (brain derived neurotropic factors). NGF's stimulate neurogeneration and differentiation. BDNF stimulates neurogenesis, newborn nerve cells. Compounds that bind with JAK1 receptors are neuro anti-inflammatories, like interleukin-10 (IL-10). Cell growth can be associated with inflammation so to have this added effect is important. The four terms of art here are neurogenesis (newborn nerve cells), neurogeneration (nerves growing), neuroregeneration (nerves may begin to atrophy and then commence regrowth) and then neuroplasticity, which leads to synaptogenesis with more nodes of crossing between neural networks.

---

* Visit www.fungi.com for more information on Fungi Perfecti LLC

At clinicaltrials.gov, a site where all clinical trials must be registered for any new drug or therapy to be eventually considered by the FDA, there are 125 clinical trials using psilocybin and 12 of these use niacin as their positive, placebo control. Why? The clinicians chose niacin because in about 15 minutes the patients will feel something, at about the same time the onset of symptoms are felt with psilocybin. With niacin, people soon become hot, red and itchy. These studies purportedly are abiding the to "gold standard" of the double blind, placebo-controlled study framework. But, in fact, the study becomes unblinded in 15 minutes when the niacin group soon realizes that they got the niacin placebo. A principal investigator in one of these studies confessed to me it is ridiculous that they used niacin as an opposite reaction to psilocybin as all the patients could determine that they received the niacin placebo or the active drug.

What I am suggesting is to use niacin *with* psilocybin. Some of our synergy data shows that with the stack with niacin, there is a five time increase in the expression of nerve growth factors binding to these proteins that lead to neuronal generation. At the equivalent of 3 milligrams of psilocybin, we have synergy of psilocybin and niacin far more than their cumulative, additive effects. At the equivalent of 10 milligrams of psilocybin and niacin, the synergy coefficient is 6.4. Synergism is a form of the entourage effect. When looking at the addition of an extract from lion's mane mycelium, containing erinacines, the active neurostimulating constituent, we find augmented synergy. Each of these components, at high dilution, show no activity in stimulating these receptors. But, when these three elements are combined, they show synergistic stimulation. When the components have no effect individually, but when combined, they do, this is termed Maximum Calculable Value (MCV). Notably, this is ~1/1000 of a standardized therapeutic dose. We can show activity stimulating these receptors across a wide spectrum of concentrations across numerous neuroreceptors, of not only psilocybin but many of the psilocybin tryptamines, including baeocystin, nor baeocystin, and nor psilocin. These inter-related tryptamines individually and in combinations stimulate fields of receptors coding for neurogeneration.

The stack has the added advantage of enhancing the entourage effects. The most exciting receptor protein by far is TrkB. TrkB is stimulated by BDNF which cause stem cells to differentiate into newborn neurons in the hippocampus. Moreover, several recent articles in neuroscience underscore that BDNF is important also treating depression by enhancing neuroplasticity.

Often times breakthroughs in science come from people thinking outside of their box of expertise. I think I have found something that is paradigm shifting. Not only that the combination of these tryptamine analogs stimulate nerve growth factors, but the admixtures of niacin and lion's mane mycelium further potentiate neurological benefits above baselines.

All of this needs to be validated with controlled clinical studies. But we have evidence empirically from the tap test, and from the in vitro data that you've seen. Moreover, we have recent data with nerve cells growing *in vitro* showing neurite outgrowth from the Stamets stack. These three silos of evidence justify the clinical trials that my team is about to embark upon.

I want to propose to you that we are no longer the *Homo sapiens* or the past 200,000 years. Terence and Dennis McKenna's Stoned Ape Hypothesis is now truly elevated to a testable theory. It is time for us to evolve into a new species. I'm proposing that this new Latin binomial be *Homo ascendis*. We are at a crossroads in our evolution. We are in the most dire of times. A majority of the species in the fossil record are species that have become extinct. Extinction is a natural course of evolution, and we are now facing, I believe, an extinction level event. We have uncontrolled climate change –climate chaos. We have zoonotic disease vectors: bird flu, COVID, monkeypox and new emergent pathogens threatening humanity. We have viral storms now common coming at us from multiple angles as we lose biodiversity, as we increasingly pollute the environment, as we lose food, biosecurity as diseases spread, as wars proliferate. We are a time we need to reinvent the human species.

I think psilocybin makes nicer people.

Psilocybin reduces violence. Psilocybin can help us overcome addiction. Psilocybin can make us more peaceful and harmonious citizens, not from a threatening totalitarian overlord, but from within. Psilocybin can help us respect and honor biodiversity, Indigenous wisdom, science, and spiritual freedom. We are at a most critical time. I think the psilocybin will increase our collective cultural and innate intelligence, so we can create the inventions that are so needed for us to survive and to thrive. We need to invent new solutions that can help us overcome the impending calamities of our own making. The bases are loaded, folks, and nature bats last. This is our moment in history to make a course change. All of you can help champion our evolution into the next level of human. It is up to us to do this, and we *can* do this. I think psilocybin is one way for that success.

Thank you very much.

BIBLIOGRAPHY

Dahiru, Tukur.2011. "P-Value, a True Test of Statistical Significance? A Cautionary Note." Annals of Ibadan Postgraduate Medicine, March 3, 2011. https://www.ajol.info/index.php/aipm/article/download/64038/51838.

Future Learn. 2022. "Updates, Insights, and News from FutureLearn | Online Learning for You." FutureLearn. October 25, 2022. https://www.futurelearn.com/info/courses/academic-research-methodology/0/steps/190710#:~:text=A%20more%20modern%20definition%20of,starting%20point%20for%20further%20investigation.

Gerber, Konstantin, Inti García Flores, Angela Christina Ruiz, Ismail Ali, Natalie Lyla Ginsberg, and Eduardo Ekman Schenberg.2021. "Ethical Concerns about Psilocybin Intellectual Property." *ACS Pharmacology & Translational Science* 4, no. 2 (January 1, 2021): 573–77. https://doi.org/10.1021/acsptsci.0c00171.

Jones, Grant M, and Matthew K. Nock. 2022. "Psilocybin Use Is Associated with Lowered Odds of Crime Arrests in US Adults: A Replication and Extension." *Journal of Psychopharmacology* 36, no. 1 (January 1, 2022): 66–73. https://doi.org/10.1177/02698811211058933.

Mushroomreferences.com—a Curated List of References Relevant to Physicians,

Scientists and the Intellectually Curious." n.d. Mushroomreferences.com. https://mushroomreferences.com/.

Rootman, Joseph, Pamela Kryskow, Kalin Harvey, Paul E. Stamets, Eesmyal Santos-Brault, Kim P. C. Kuypers, Vince Polito, Francoise Bourzat, and Zach Walsh. 2021. "Adults Who Microdose Psychedelics Report Health Related Motivations and Lower Levels of Anxiety and Depression Compared to Non-Microdosers." *Scientific Reports* 11, no. 1 (November 18, 2021). https://doi.org/10.1038/s41598-021-01811-4.

Rootman, Joseph, Maggie Kiraga, Pamela Kryskow, Kalin Harvey, Paul E. Stamets, Eesmyal Santos-Brault, Kim P. C. Kuypers, and Zach Walsh. 2022a. "Psilocybin Microdosers Demonstrate Greater Observed Improvements in Mood and Mental Health at One Month Relative to Non-Microdosing Controls." *Scientific Reports* 12, no. 1 (June 30, 2022a). https://doi.org/10.1038/s41598-022-14512-3.

Rootman, Joseph, Maggie Kiraga, Pamela Kryskow, Kalin Harvey, Paul E. Stamets, Eesmyal Santos-Brault, Kim P. C. Kuypers, and Zach Walsh. 2022b ."Author Correction: Psilocybin Microdosers Demonstrate Greater Observed Improvements in Mood and Mental Health at One Month Relative to Non-Microdosing Controls." *Scientific Reports* 12, no. 1 (July 28, 2022b). https://doi.org/10.1038/s41598-022-17428-0.

Reports of Psychoactive Boletes

Colin Domnauer, Doctoral Candidate, and Bryn Dentinger, PhD

Curator of Mycology at the Natural History Museum of Utah and an Associate Professor in the School of Biological Sciences at the University of Utah

Ethnobiologist Mycologist | University of Utah

> *"Despite the numerous and suggestive reports, the identity of psychoactive boletes remains a mycological mystery. In this presentation, the history of psychoactive bolete reports is compiled together, our scant sum of knowledge on the topic is summarized, and future directions for research are suggested."* —COLIN DOMNAUER

INTRODUCTION

For more than half a century, the existence of certain species of mushrooms in the family Boletaceae* possessing psychoactive properties has been rumored, with independent ethnographic reports emerging from Papua New Guinea and China. In both cases, local inhabitants describe consuming a type of bolete mushroom, followed by the occurrence of various hallucinations, generally characterized by a perception of being surrounded by an abundance of colorful, diminutive creatures—clinically referred to as "lilliputian hallucinations". Despite numerous and suggestive reports, the identity of psychoactive boletes remains a mycological mystery. To this date, no rigorous scientific studies have been performed that conclusively reveal the taxonomic identity or active chemical constituents of this unstudied group of psychoactive mushrooms. Here, the history of psychoactive bolete reports is compiled together, our scant sum of knowledge on the topic is summarized, and future directions for research are suggested.

MUSHROOM MADNESS IN PAPUA NEW GUINEA

Less than a decade after introducing the western world to the existence of "magic mushrooms" through his groundbreaking article in *Life* magazine in 1957, ethnomycologist R. Gordon Wasson, accompanied by mycologist Roger Heim and anthropologist Marie Reay, embarked on a similar journey to Papua New Guinea (PNG), although the magic mushroom he was seeking in this case was never ultimately determined. The expedition was spurred by the emergence of various ethnographic reports which had made the intriguing claim that, upon consuming a certain type of mushroom, the native inhabitants of the Wahgi Valley, PNG would occasionally

* Also known as "Boletes"; mushrooms with caps, stalks, and a sponge-like layer under the cap.

develop "mushroom madness", an apparent psychotropic intoxication characterized by wild, abnormal behavior.

The earliest known written reference to mushroom madness in PNG comes from no less than the first outsider to live amongst the native inhabitants of the Wahgi Valley, a missionary, Father William Ross, who in 1934 writes: "The wild mushroom called nonda makes the user temporarily insane. He flies into a fit of frenzy." (Ross, 1934, 351). Although admittedly vague, it is interesting how this claim of a psychoactive mushroom in PNG was made 5 years prior to Richard Evans Schultes' publication describing a "narcotic" mushroom in Mexico (Schultes, 1939) yet attracted much less attention. A much more substantial documentation of this phenomenon was provided by anthropologist Marie Reay, who after spending 15 months living amongst the Kuma people in the mid-1950s would produce the most detailed descriptions of the "mushroom madness" we have today (Reay, 1960; 1977). She first observed this strange phenomenon herself in 1954, when the natives suddenly began to exhibit a variety of abnormal behaviors including dancing, running amuck, rapid alterations in mood, and an overall stark change in demeanor which they attributed to their consumption of certain mushrooms called nonda (Reay, 1959, 188; Reay, 1977, 58).

In the native Kuma language, the phrase to describe one under the influence of the nonda mushrooms is "komugl tai". "Komugl" refers to the ear, likely signifying deafness, or the inability to comprehend, while "tai" is the name for the bird of paradise. In this context, "tai" would be specifying the shivering dance the bird of paradise performs as its colorful plumage is unveiled. Thus, Reay explains the translated meaning as "shivering madness", and she comments on the metaphorical significance: "In birds and in humans, shivering signaled a transformation from ordinary, everyday behavior to special, out-of-the ordinary behavior that was nevertheless expected and appropriate in context. Both men and women underwent fits of shivering when they were about to exhibit the outlandish behavior of Komugl Tai." (Reay, 1977, 56).

Reay would continue to recount additional details from her experiences witnessing the mushroom madness over a series of articles, offering a more thorough illustration of the apparent subjective effects encountered by those under the mushroom's influence: "[He] began to experience lilliputian hallucinations, seeing bush demons flying about his head. The demons were allegedly buzzing about his head when he heard a strange and terrible noise inside his ears... he was rapidly losing all power to focus his vision. Some reported having double vision, and in any case, it was easy for him to lose his way.... The disturbance of hearing and eyesight was frightening and confusing" (Reay, 1977, 55). Other psychological effects included rapid alterations in mood with greater emotional expression. Reay also noted the manifestation of several physical conditions such as difficultly with muscle coordination, "alternating sensations of extreme heat and cold", "double vision, exaggerated shivering, and intermittent aphasia" (Reay, 1960, 137; Reay, 1977, 58). The general attitude of onlookers was one of wariness when the madness was in its most intense phase, and a teasing playfulness when the severity of symptoms was less intense (Reay, 1977, 58). Interestingly, she notes how mushroom madness was never intentionally pursued, was neither envied nor ashamed, but rather was simply regarded as an accidental affliction (Reay, 1977, 63).

With their interest piqued at the possibility of describing yet another psychoactive mushroom new to science just five years after the isolation of psilocybin, Wasson and Heim spent nearly a month in PNG in late 1963, with Wasson conducting ethnographic interviews of local populations while Heim made mycological collections in the surrounding forest. By the end of their time, they had aggregated approximately 400 different species of local mushrooms. From this sum, Wasson and Heim then compiled a catalog of seven candidate species that the Kuma had indicated were responsible for inducing the "mushroom madness", six of which belonged to the family Boletaceae.

Following the expedition, one of these species, *Boletus manicus*, was sent to the laboratory of Swiss chemist Albert Hofmann for chemical analysis. Hofmann was of course a world-expert in this matter, famous for his invention of LSD and discovery of psilocybin from the Mazatecan mushrooms; if anyone could decipher the chemical underpinnings of "mushroom madness", it was Hofmann. Indeed, only a few years had passed since 1958 when Roger Heim supplied Hofmann with specimens *Psilocybe mexicana* which led to the isolation of psilocybin. And thus, in 1963, they were hoping to achieve similar results, only this time with a completely different purportedly psychoactive mushroom- *Boletus manicus.* However, in this instance, the results of his chemical investigations were not as fruitful, as he was unable to isolate any active principles. While Hofmann was able to detect the presence of three unidentified indole substances, they were in trace quantities "too low to allow structural studies" (Thomas 2003, 393). In fact, given such a low concentration, if any of these unidentified indolic substances in *B. manicus* are indeed responsible for the psychoactive effects, they would have to be at least as potent as LSD (Thomas, 2003, 394). Of course, the active substance could just as likely be some other chemical class.

However, Heim and Wasson noted the dubious nature of this list of potential psychoactive species, as various Kuma informants provided discordant information as to which species were responsible, with one man even claiming that every mushroom could cause madness (Heim and Wasson, 1965, 26). To add to the confusion, the Kuma also stated that only some individuals would be affected, and only during certain times of the year. Moreover, it was reported by Reay that the effects of mushroom madness were markedly different between men and women. In an earlier account, she notes "The men seem to go berserk...the women feel like dancing" (Reay, 1960, 139). Furthermore, men would only be affected for a few hours, while the effects for women could last multiple days (Reay, 1977). Thus, there are many facets of the mushroom madness that seem to defy solely pharmacological explanation.

Given these perplexing accounts, coupled with a lack of definitive chemical evidence, Reay, Wasson, and Heim concluded that the "mushroom madness" phenomenon in PNG was in fact nothing more than a culturally institutionalized drama, a sanctioned act allowing for the display of normally culturally restrained behavior, while "the mushrooms—or at least most of them—do not seem to cause physiological effects leading to madness" (Heim and Wasson, 1965, 30; Reay, 1960, 139).

Nonetheless, Reay later hypothesized that this may not have necessarily always been the whole truth, suggesting perhaps at one time there was once a pharmacological agent in use, but over time "genuine outbreaks of mushroom madness later became culturally institutionalized acts (in which the mushrooms were no longer necessary) ... 'The most stereotyped psychotic syndromes may in the natural course of events alter symptomologically along with changes in society, its mores, and the Zeitgeist.'" (Reay, 1977, 74; Yap, 1974 as cited in Reay, 1977). She further supports this reasoning by noting how "during every manifestation of Komugl Tai, bystanders would discuss whether one or two men were genuinely komugl [poisoned] or simply 'pretending'" (Reay, 1977, 74). Indeed, Reay mentions that individuals were not held responsible for their actions when under the influence of the mushroom madness. (Reay, 1960, 138). It therefore stands to reason that perhaps this once genuine phenomenon could have, at least in part, been co-opted and imitated by individuals seeking an excuse to perform culturally impermissible activities, offering "an unparalleled opportunity for social catharsis" as Reay (1960, 139) writes.

That being said, it seems inadequate to regard all aspects of the mushroom madness as a cultural construction or a mere figment of imagination. As is the case when attempting to decipher the details of any ethnopharmacological mystery, the observations are best explained when we consider the intersection of pharmacologically active substances within a given cultural context of beliefs and practices. It is naïve to attempt to ascribe the behavior following the consumption of a psychoactive substance as originating solely from either the chemistry of the natural product itself on the one hand, or from cultural imagination on the other; the resultant experience is of course influenced by both pharmacological factors as well as cultural predispositions, often categorized as the set, setting, and dosage (Alpert et al, 1964). Relations to and perceptions of natural phenomena are extremely fluid and culturally dependent, specific to a given language and worldview which function as a unique filter through which meaningless sensation is translated into meaningful sense. Put more simply, "In traditional cultures, set is shaped primarily by the worldview that all individuals share... The contents of the visions, in other words, are shaped by culture" (Rätsch, 2005, 22). Weil and Rosen (1983, 25) also write of this inseparable intertwinement between the subjective and objective aspects which shape drug experiences: "Set and setting together can modify pharmacology drastically. Therefore, talking about the effects of drugs in the real world is not so simple. Effects of drugs are relative to particular people, places, and times." And lastly, in her memoir reflecting on 45 years of researching the cross-cultural uses of hallucinogens, anthropologist Marlene Dobkin de Rios states her similar conviction that "culture determines the stereotyping of hallucinatory visions" (Dobkin de Rios, 2009, 63). Therefore, as in the case of the mushroom madness of PNG, the visible expressions of a cultural phenomenon purported to involve a psychoactive substance are unlikely to be entirely accurate indications of purely pharmacological activity, but they are also unlikely to be entirely attributable to cultural fabrication.

In 2003, roughly 40 years after the expedition of Wasson, Heim, and Reay, a team of researchers conducted follow up interviews with the same local populations in PNG. They noted how most knowledge of the subject has unfortunately been lost, with the last known incidence of "mushroom madness" occurring in the 1980s, and only the elders capable of recalling the phenomenon: "An old man, probably in his nineties, reported his experience under the influence of the mushrooms: He saw tiny people with mushrooms around their faces. They were teasing him and he was trying to chase them away." (Treu & Adamson, 2006, 7). Interestingly, the specific details of this man's subjective experience closely resemble Reay's initial explanation of the effects, both referencing the manifestation of lilliputian hallucinations.

To this day, the identity of the supposed psychoactive boletes in PNG remains elusive. Indeed, to Reay, Heim, Wasson, and Hofmann, the very existence of psychoactive boletes became doubtful. Since that time, no mycological research has been conducted on the topic. However, more recently, the plausibility of these earlier claims has been reinvigorated by an accumulating body of new evidence for psychoactive boletes, emerging not from PNG, but now 5000km away in Yunnan, China.

HISTORY OF PSYCHOACTIVE BOLETE REPORTS IN YUNNAN

It was half a century after Hofmann had failed to find any substance from *Boletus manicus* when published reports began to surface from Yunnan that certain frequently encountered blue-staining bolete mushrooms were known to produce hallucinations if undercooked. Remarkably, the qualitative effects recounted by those poisoned by the psychoactive boletes in Yunnan closely matched the details of the symptoms reported to result from the nonda bolete mushrooms of Papua New Guinea. In both cases, the experience was engendered by an undercooked blue-staining bolete and was said to be characterized by inducing "lilliputian hallucinations", a perception of numerous diminutive figures appearing in one's surrounding environment.

In 1991, a team of Chinese psychologists published an analysis of 300 cases of "*Boletus speciosus*" (a North American species that is unlikely to occur in China) poisoning gathered from the records of Yunnan Province mental hospital. Here again, a regular subjective experiential theme was noted amongst those poisoned by the boletes: "all the poisoned patients complained of lilliputian hallucinations and claimed that they saw little people and animals moving about everywhere: they saw them on their clothes when they were dressing and saw them on their dishes when eating; the hallucinations were even more vivid when their eyes were closed" (Linchu and Kuang, 1991, 6).

Linchu and Kuang (1991) provide a suite of clinical information which may aid speculation as to the pharmacologic nature of the active substance(s) in the boletes, although the veracity of these claims cannot be confirmed. These details include onset time ("6-24 hours after ingestion"), duration ("lasting days to weeks"), physiological symptoms ("constipation, urinary retention, loss of appetite"), and psychological symptoms (hallucinations, stupor, "difficult to distinguish from schizophrenia", "able to more or less give expression to feelings, especially inner emotions, that they would not ordinarily display") (Linchu and Kuang, 1991). Despite these apparently severe conditions, none of the 300 cases were reported to result in death. Interestingly, the researchers also noted that the patients' EEGs were "similar to those under the influence of LSD", which subsequently returned to a normal baseline following the remission of their symptoms (Linchu and Kuang, 1991, 7). Lastly, the antipsychotic Thorazine® (chlorpromazine) was given to patients suffering most severely and did in fact control their symptoms. Based on all these observations, they conclude by labelling the active chemical in the bolete as a "psychotomimetic", with no further explanation.

The researchers also conducted questionable experiments administering "liquid extracts" (solvent unspecified) of the mushroom to a monkey and dog; the observed effects in the animals included "abnormal behavior", a blank stare "of inquiry and fright", "gazing fixedly and angrily", and the inability to fall asleep (Linchu and Kuang, 1991, 7). At first glance, this change in demeanor appears to support the presence of some bioactive substances in the boletes. However, an equally plausible explanation for these effects could be made without any reference to mushrooms, as similar outcomes would likely have resulted in the absence of active chemicals given the fact that the extract was administered as an enema.

The next major publication to reference the psychoactive boletes of Yunnan was written in 2008 by mycologist David Arora. Based off his time travelling in Yunnan, he shares his encounters with the blue-staining boletes known locally as "xiao ren ren" (小人人), or "jian shou qing" (见手青), which translate as "little people" and "see hand blue", a reference to their hallucinogenic capabilities and blue bruising, respectively. The hallucinogenic capabilities are well-known within the mycophilic communities of Yunnan who hold these mushrooms in high esteem, though not for the psychoactivity per se. In fact, Arora notes, the psychoactive effects are not something most people in Yunnan ever intentionally pursue but are rather an accidental consequence of improper cooking (Arora, 2008). Curiously, this was precisely the same case with the boletes from PNG: "It was stressed by our sources that the mushrooms were never sought in order to experience mind-altering effects. In fact, mushrooms were collected for their value as a food source, and side effects occurred as a coincidence if certain species were part of the meal" (Treu & Adamson, 2006, 7). Similarly, these blue-staining boletes in Yunnan are prized for being a delectable edible and are commonly sold throughout wild mushroom markets in Yunnan. With a savory onion odor, meaty texture, and rich umami flavor, they are frequently utilized in restaurant dishes and rural household dinners, alike*. In fact, jian shou qing boletes are even more popular than the well-known choice edible porcini mushrooms (*Boletus meiweinuiganjun*, *B. bainugan*, *B. shiyong*) (Pérez-Moreno et al., 2020, 51; Dentinger & Suz 2014).

Arora (2008, 152) provides an illustrative account of a professor from Yunnan retelling his experience of seeing the little people one night after dinner:

"It was in a restaurant. I asked for stir-fried mushrooms and just as I was getting ready to leave, after eating them, I noticed moving colors and shapes. I wasn't worried. My first thought was, 'Oh, they must not have cooked the mushrooms enough—I'll be able to see the xiao ren ren! But it was disappointing—there were no xiao ren ren to be seen. I looked everywhere—at the walls, the tables, the floor, outside. But then, I don't know why, I lifted the tablecloth just a little and peeked under—ohhhh—a lot! Hundreds of xiao ren ren, marching like soldiers. And even more curious, when I lifted the tablecloth higher the heads came off and stuck to the bottom of the cloth and the bodies kept marching in place [on the surface of the table]. I put down the tablecloth and looked at my watch. Then I looked under the tablecloth again. I did this many times, at two-minute intervals and each time they were there, marching and grinning". "I measured them, too," the professor added. "They were 2 cm high." (Arora, 2008, 542).

There are many striking parallels to be drawn between the purported psychoactive boletes in Papua New Guinea and Yunnan. In both independent cases continents apart, local people enjoy consuming a blue-staining bolete mushroom as a food source. Occasionally, due to unintentional undercooking, a suite of psychophysiological symptoms may develop, most notably that of lilli-

* For more information on this see our paper "Ethnopharmacology of Psychoactive Substances in Chinese Culture" by Jonathan Lu.

putian hallucinations, visions of tiny creatures which have been characterized as "bush demons" in PNG or "xiao ren ren" in Yunnan (Reay, 1977, 59; Arora, 2008, 541).

WHAT ARE LILLIPUTIAN HALLUCINATIONS?

Lilliputian hallucinations are a clinically defined type of visual syndrome characterized by the perception of numerous diminutive human, animal, or fantasy figures inhabiting one's ordinary surroundings. The term, coined in 1909 by French psychiatrist Raoul Leroy, originates from Jonathan Swift's novel *Gulliver's Travels*, specifically referencing the land of Lilliput, a fictional island populated by tiny humans less than 15cm tall.

Lilliputian hallucinations are distinguished from more well-known forms of perceptual distortion such as micropsia or "Alice in Wonderland" syndrome, whereby normal everyday objects appear to be distorted in size. Lilliputian hallucinations, on the other hand, involve the appearance of hallucinated figures within an otherwise unchanged perceptual environment. While the ordinary objects composing one's surroundings are left unaltered, there is now the notable novelty of an abundance of fantastical diminutive figures inhabiting one's field of perception. Curiously, such lilliputian hallucinations have been noted to possess some general characteristic features which apparently manifest to different patients with amazing consistency. These typical attributes have been classified into general qualitative categories such as abounding in numerosity (often hundreds or thousands in number), being highly mobile (often jumping, dancing, or marching), colorful, "rendered in exquisite detail", and of course, being of diminutive stature, on average measuring 10-30cm tall (Blom, 2021). Moreover, they are virtually always (97% of the time) described as being three-dimensional and life-like, a "reality-grounded projective hallucination" realistically inhabiting the physical world for example by "marching under real doors, and climbing on real chairs and tables, while generally respecting the laws of gravity and three-dimensional space." (Blom, 2021, 627). Aggregated reports have demonstrated these diminutive creatures may appear in the form of "tiny men, women, children, gnomes, imps, or dwarfs, often strikingly dressed as harlequins, clowns, dancers, soldiers, peasants, 'mandarins', 'caftan wearers', and so on." (Blom, 2021, 629). Nonetheless, despite the fact that the subjective experience of lilliputian hallucinations has been described in exquisite detail and with extraordinary consistency across a range of demographics and conditions, the mental processes underlying this peculiar phenomenon remain poorly understood.

Since its initial description in the early 20th century, lilliputian hallucinations have been recorded to arise from an extremely diverse set of medical conditions. Reviewing this century of clinical data in the published psychiatric literature, Blom (2021) aggregates 226 case studies of lilliputian hallucinations, providing the most comprehensive and quantitative analysis of the phenomenon to date. Compiling all the various conditions historically referenced to induce lilliputian hallucinations, it was found that the most frequently ascribed causes were alcohol withdrawal, macular degeneration, psychotic disorders, CNS lesions, and psychoactive drugs (Blom, 2021, 630). However, there are currently no known conditions that, in and of themselves, invariably and reliably elicit lilliputian hallucinations; rather, lilliputian hallucinations are clinically regarded as an unpredictable, occasional byproduct that may emerge within a diverse set of central nervous system afflictions. Expectedly, the current lack of any known causal agent capable of consistently generating lilliputian hallucinations is a major reason why the precise mechanisms behind this phenomenon remain largely indecipherable. Perhaps these supposed psychoactive boletes which appear to generate lilliputian hallucinations with remarkable regularity may yield valuable insight into the inner workings of a mysterious aspect of the human mind.

DIFFICULTY PINPOINTING ACTIVE SPECIES

In addition to the abundance of anecdotal evidence, there is an equal abundance of perplexing points which makes pinpointing the mysterious bolete difficult. For one, the name "jian shou qing" appears to be applied to all blue-staining boletes in general, rather than to a specific species. Arora estimates there are nearly 20 species of blue-staining boletes being sold in the markets, yet "...people tend to assign the xiao ren ren quality to many or all blue-staining boletes." (Arora, 2008, 540). This linguistic imprecision obviously creates ample room for taxonomic misidentification. The high number and speciose nature of boletes in Yunnan also makes difficult any attempt to establish any clear links between species names and properties; morphological similarities often cause different species to be mistakenly conflated together. For example, a recent DNA analysis of mushrooms being sold across markets in Yunnan was able to identify 158 distinct species, while local vendors had identified and labelled only 41 different species names (Zhang et al., 2021). Clearly, different mushrooms are being referred to under a single name. Further amplifying this effect is the fact that multiple species are often mixed together in a single meal, such that any attempt to retroactively identify the exact species responsible for poisonings is often muddled.

Another reason for the confusion is because there are several Boletaceae species that may produce diverse poisoning symptoms ranging from gastrointestinal upset to hallucination. However, these are often all indiscriminately bundled together under the single blanket term of "poisonous boletes". In other words, drastically different symptoms as well as entirely different species may be regularly conflated. These linguistic ambiguities coupled with the high Boletaceae species diversity in Yunnan makes accurately discerning the identity of the supposed psychoactive species an extremely arduous task. Given the inconsistencies of the current reportage, we should not expect to obtain a reliable source of information on this topic until more systematic research is conducted.

This confusing situation is clearly illustrated by the dissimilitude amongst recent written references to Yunnan's psychoactive boletes. For example, an article reviewing a decade of mushroom poisonings in Hong Kong reported a case of hallucinations induced by a bolete mushroom in the genus *Tylopilus*. Specifically, in reviewing 13 cases of bolete poisoning, 11 had manifested as solely gastrointestinal symptoms, while the other two cases had hallucinogenic symptoms without any reported gastrointestinal upset. Notably, in both these two psychoactive cases, the boletes had been purchased from Yunnan. The symptoms in these two psychoactive bolete cases were summarized as follows: "The first patient presented with numbness and weakness in all four limbs, dizziness, and malaise after mushroom consumption. The time of symptom onset was not documented, and symptoms resolved on the same day as mushroom consumption. No mushroom sample was obtained for identification. The second patient developed dizziness, malaise, and visual hallucination 10 hours after mushroom consumption. Her symptoms resolved 48 hours post-ingestion. The causative mushroom was identified as *T. nigerrimus*,* an inedible bolete." (Chan et al, 2016).

Next, in 2021, as part of their annual appraisal of recorded mushroom poisonings, the China CDC provided a species list of boletes involved in poisoning incidents, only one of which was noted for its psychotropic effect: "Nine boletes (*Baorangia major*, *B. pseudocalopus*, *Boletellus indistinctus*, *Heimioporus gaojiaocong*, *H. japonicus*, *Neoboletus venenatus*,† *Rubroboletus sinicus*, *Suillus pinetorum*, and *Tylopilus neofelleus*) causing gastroenteritis and one (*Lanmaoa asiatica*) causing psycho-neurological disorder were identified from poisoning incidents" (H. Li et al 2021). Another recent publication has suggested that the hallucinogenic jian shou qing boletes include "*Butyriboletus roseoflavus*, *Lanmaoa asiatica*, and *Sutorius magnificus*", and that these may also cause gastrointestinal upset (Pérez-Moreno et. al, 2020). There are also discussions of Yunnan's psychoactive boletes that have surfaced via the hundreds of Chinese news articles written over the past decade, virtually all of which make drastically different statements, despite being presented as scientific fact, regarding the taxonomic identity, psychophysiological properties, and active chemical constituents of Yunnan's hallucinogenic boletes. With claimed culprits spanning half a dozen genera, inconsistencies in the supposed symptoms, and a bewildering variety of speculated bioactive molecules, clearly more research is needed.

WHAT IS *LANMAOA*?

Within the amalgamation of references to hallucinogenic boletes, the most commonly mentioned species name is *Lanmaoa asiatica*. *Lanmaoa* is a recently segregated genus of mushrooms in the Boletaceae family defined by a thin hymenophore (spore-bearing layer of tightly arranged vertical "tubes" on the underside of the cap), light yellow flesh that slowly stains pale blue when damaged, and the microanatomy of the cap surface. Many species have a distinct savory odor described as being similar to bouillon or onion. In Yunnan where it is regularly consumed, *L. asiatica* is heralded as one of the most delectable edible mushrooms. In fact, interestingly, the holotype collection‡ of *L. asiatica* was acquired from a street market in Yunnan. *L. asiatica* is the type species of the genus *Lanmaoa* and is known from montane pine forests exclusively in Yunnan. While the currently constructed phylogeny of the *Lanmaoa* genus indicates closely related species of *L. asiatica* also exist in North America (Figure 1), there has been no claims that any of these close relatives are psychoactive. Before any such questions regarding the identity or properties of psychoactive species can evaluated, the first necessary step where research must focus is to expand the current phylogeny of *Lanmaoa* by constructing a robust taxonomic foundation upon which future collected specimens can be confidently placed and identified. This task is rendered difficult by the immense diversity of Chinese boletes and current paucity of available genetic sequences.

---

* Current name is *Retiboletus nigerrimus*

† Current name is *Sutorius venanatus*

‡ A holotype is the original voucher specimen designated when a species is first described.

In their 2021 report, the Chinese CDC commented on this knowledge gap, specifically referring to the unexamined psychoactive properties of *Lanmaoa asiatica*, stating "When causing poisoning, this species could cause hallucinations. It is different from species containing psilocybin, its toxicity is still unclear and needs further studies." (H. Li et al. 2021). In 2022, *L. asiatica* was included in the list of Yunnan's poisonous mushrooms making their collection, sale, and consumption supposedly prohibited. Nevertheless, they continue to be sold and eaten; numerous news articles appear every week during the mushroom season in Yunnan discussing someone's hallucinatory experience after eating jian shou qing boletes. Moreover, this mushroom has a long and supposedly safe history of being consumed by local people for decades, if not centuries. The current contradictions thus raised by placing this commonly consumed mushroom in the same category alongside verifiably deadly toxic mushrooms is simply an indication of the need for more scientific research on this topic.

The precise identity of *Lanmaoa asiatica* remains somewhat ambiguous. Morphological identification is often inadequate due to insufficiently distinct features that allow it to be reliably

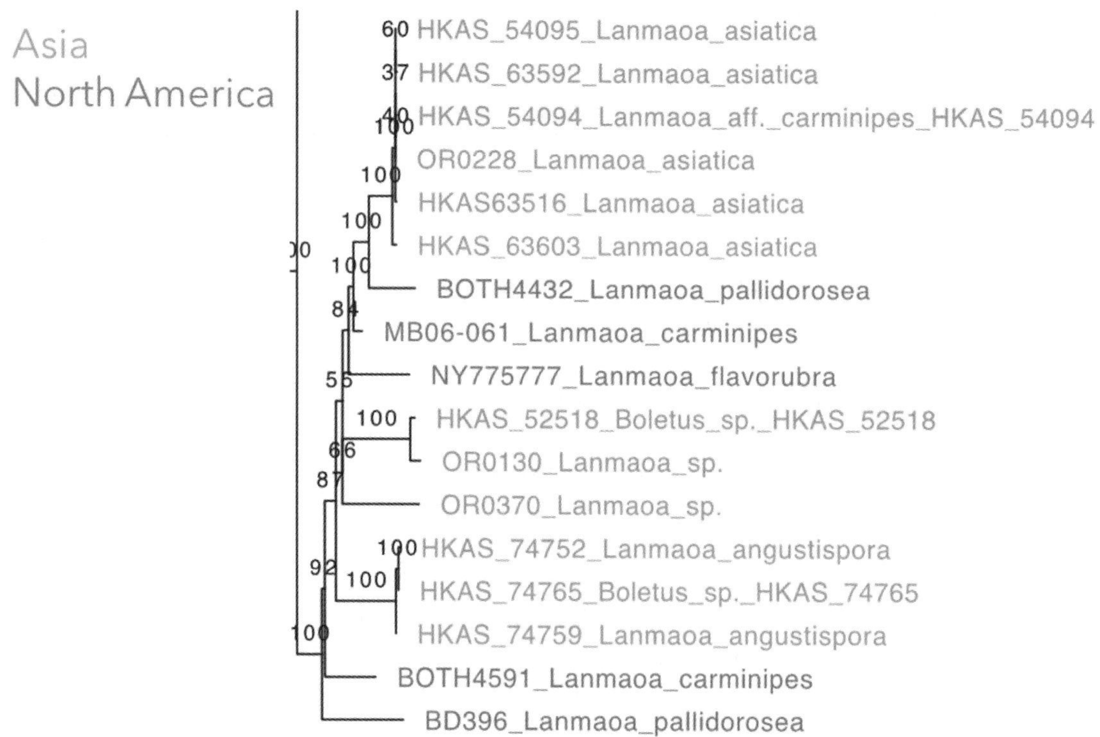

Fig.1 Maximum likelihood phylogeny of *Lanmaoa* spp. inferred using DNA sequences of the large subunit ribosomal RNA gene (28S) indicates closely related species of *L. asiatica* present in North America. The sequence labeled HKAS_54094 is from the holotype of *L. asiatica*.

distinguished from closely related species. Unfortunately, a DNA barcode sequence* from the type collection is not available to authenticate newly collected material. Moreover, cryptic species are commonplace in fungi, which may further obfuscate the true identity of the causal agent of the psychoactive intoxications. Illustrating this point, only a single ITS barcode sequence labeled as *Lanmaoa asiatica* is available in public DNA sequence databases, which is not derived from authenticated material (i.e. a type or specimen determined by the species' author). Similarly, a whole genome labeled as *L. asiatica* is also available, derived from a different specimen (also not authenticated) than the DNA barcode was generated from. Upon extracting the DNA barcode from the genome and comparing it to the existing DNA barcode, the sequences are only 97% similar. This level of similarity is often used as a proxy for different species (Nilsson et al. 2008), suggesting the samples used for the DNA sequences are from two taxa. Which one is correct: the one represented by the single DNA barcode, the one represented by the genome, both, or neither?

GENOMIC INSIGHTS?

The search for novel natural products has evolved as new genomic technologies have made it possible to sequence entire genomes at a relatively low cost. Searching for novel biosynthetic genes that generate natural products ("genome mining") is now common practice in natural product discovery (Nett 2014). In *Fungi*, natural product biosynthetic genes tend to be physically clustered in the genome (Keller 2019), making their identification more apparent. Using the fungal version of the popular biosynthetic gene cluster (BGC) mining software antiSMASH (Blin et al. 2021), we searched the putative *L. asiatica* genome for BGCs. Fifteen BGCs were detected, including six predicted to produce terpenes, seven predicted to produce nonribosomal peptides, and one each predicted to produce either a nonribosomal peptide or terpene, and a polyketide. There were little to no similarities to known BGCs and most of the predicted biosynthetic genes are uncharacterized (annotated as "hypothetical protein"). Notably, no indole-producing BGCs were predicted, inconsistent with the potential of tryptamine alkaloids such as psilocybin as a potential causal agent of psychoactivity. In fact, using reciprocal best hits (RBH; Tatusov et al. 1997) with BLAST (Altschul et al. 1997), the closest homologs in the putative *L. asiatica* genome of the decarboxylase gene from the psilocybin biosynthetic pathway (PsiD; Fricke et al. 2017), were highly divergent (data not shown). Similarly, using RBH, the closest homologs in the putative *L. asiatica* genome to the glutamate hydroxylase gene (IboH) and the cytochrome P450 gene (IboC) representing the first and last enzymatic steps in the biosynthesis of ibotenic acid (the psychoactive agent in *Amanita muscaria* and related mushrooms; Obermaier & Müller 2020) were also highly divergent. If this genome is, in fact, derived from the mushroom that causes the reported psychoactive effects in Yunnan, then it appears unlikely that the pharmacological activity can be attributed to the only known psychoactive compounds from mushrooms, the prodrugs psilocybin and ibotenic acid. However, it must be stressed that the identity of the

* A DNA barcode is a sequence from part of the genome that enables species identification. For Fungi, this is the ribosomal internal transcribed spacers (ITS) (Schoch et al. 2012).

organism from which the genome is derived, as well as that of the true source of psychoactivity, remains frustratingly and confusingly obscure.

THE NEED FOR MORE RESEARCH IN YUNNAN

The importance of resolving these taxonomic uncertainties is most clearly demonstrated by the extreme prevalence of their unfortunate consequences: unintentional mushroom poisoning. From 2010 to 2020, mushrooms were the leading cause of foodborne illness and death in China with over 10,000 poisoning incidents resulting in 788 deaths (W. Li et al., 2021). As shown in Figure 2, these concerns were most highly concentrated in Yunnan province, with the most outbreaks, illnesses, and deaths in all of China, at 40.0%, 43.6%, and 41.0%, respectively (W. Li et al., 2021).

Mushroom poisoning is becoming an increasingly frequent occurrence each year. The year 2020 alone saw twice as many mushroom poisoning events in China as 2019; 102 different species were involved in these poisoning incidents, 24 of which were species completely new to science (H. Li et al., 2021). The discovery of new species of mushrooms in Yunnan is rapidly on the rise, specifically in the family Boletaceae (Figure 3). In the past decade (2010-2019), 429 new to science species of large fungi (mushrooms + lichens) were discovered in Yunnan Province (Zhang et al., 2021, 2). In 2022, the China CDC commented on this growing, intertwined problem by declaring that "more taxonomic work is needed, and more new species will be hopefully discovered. The low level of awareness of mushroom poisoning, in contrast to the high species diversity in China is a huge challenge for mushroom poisoning control and prevention." (H. Li et al., 2022). These escalating trends provide a clear rationale for, and demonstrate the urgency and importance of, conducting mycological research focused on studying potentially toxic species of bolete mushrooms.

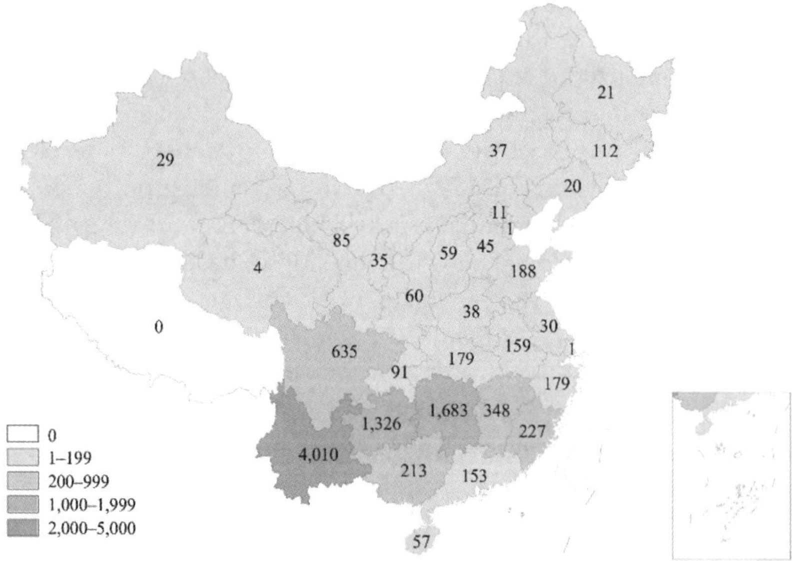

Fig.2 Number of recorded mushroom poisoning cases in China by province, from 2010-2020. Yunnan has the highest frequency of any province, responsible for nearly half of the entire country's poisoning events. *From Figure 2 in W. Li et al., 2021*

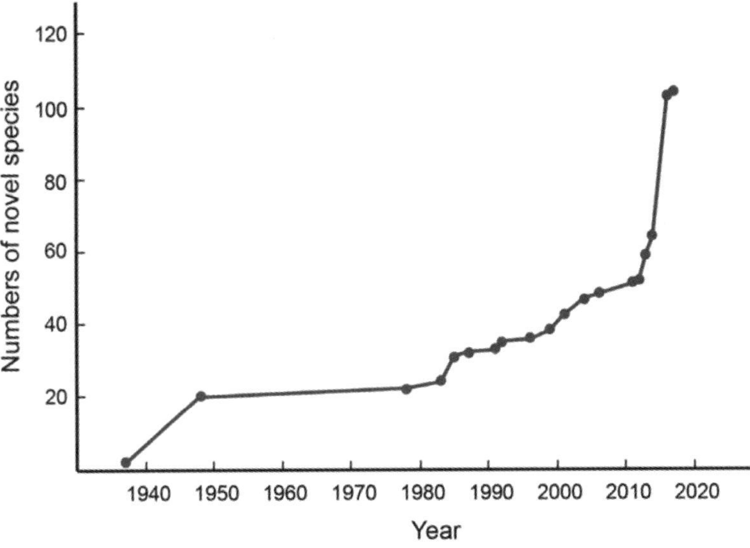

Fig.3 Number of novel Boletaceae species discovered each year in Yunnan in rapidly increasing in recent years. *Taken from Figure 1 from Feng and Zhuliang (2018)*

These issues are especially concentrated in Yunnan. Sometimes referred to as the "Kingdom of Wild Fungi", Yunnan is one of Earth's 34 biodiversity hotspots, a unique natural environment home to an estimated 40% of the world's edible mushrooms (approximately 900 species) as well as a rich culture of prolific mushroom use (Zhuliang, 2002; Feng and Zhuliang, 2018). Despite the hundreds of species of wild edible fungi found and sold in Yunnan, the region remains vastly understudied mycologically, as "little is known about the geographic structuring, cryptic speciation, and even the number of species of mushrooms that are frequently consumed by the local people" (Zhang et al., 2021). For example, one recent study collected 3585 specimens of mushrooms sold in markets across Yunnan province; based on their experience, local sellers were able to identify 41 different species within this sample set; however, molecular data (ITS sequences) revealed four times as much diversity to be present (158 distinct species) (Zhang et al., 2021). Moreover, of these species being openly sold in street markets, half (51%) were unassignable to currently described species, one-third had no known edibility data, a handful were in fact known to be poisonous, and others still were red listed as endangered species (Zhang et al., 2021). These findings clearly demonstrate the need for a more refined understanding and documentation of mushroom species diversity in Yunnan. The current absence of any standards for the selling of wild mushrooms in these markets, coupled with the poorly understood species diversity, creates the current dangerous situation of unregulated collection, sale, and consumption of potentially poisonous or endangered species. Perhaps expectedly, these facts occurring within an active culture and economy surrounding wild edible mushrooms synergize together to result in an abnormally large number of mushroom poisoning occurrences.

Moreover, this is not only affecting local populations in Yunnan, but consumers around the globe. As recent research has demonstrated, the unfortunate result of improper taxonomic delineation and identification is that poisonous species of mushrooms are found mixed in commercially sold packages, despite being labelled and marketed as "edible porcini", for example (Dentinger & Suz, 2014; Cutler II et al., 2021). This poses an obvious hazard for global food safety and regulation. In fact, analysis of one package revealed half a dozen different species to be contained, some previously undescribed to science, most with unknown edibility data, and none of which corresponded to the content claims of the seller. Customer testimonials of these tainted products include concerning statements such as "I was poisoned by these. Never been so sick in my life" and "Avoid these, you are gambling with your life..." (Cutler II et al., 2021). Despite notifying the merchant of these findings, these items remain for sale.

Unlike with cultivated edible mushrooms grown on a controlled farm, edible mushrooms such as the boletes are exclusively collected in the wild and are thus more susceptible to being mistakenly mixed with similar species before being sold to unsuspecting consumers. The importance of this issue is evidenced by the magnitude of China's global trade of wild edible fungi as roughly 50,000-80,000 tons surpassing over $100 million USD are exported each year (Pérez-Moreno et al, 2020, 21; Wang et al., 2022). Notably, mushrooms in the family Boletaceae account for roughly 20% of this annual revenue, the vast majority of which come from Yunnan (Wu and Lu, 2006).

For all these reasons, resolving the taxonomic uncertainties and toxicological profiles of commonly sold blue-staining boletes in Yunnan is a task of utmost importance. Underlying all these range of issues is an insufficiency of basic mycological research being conducted, which is an essential requirement in a region with such a high diversity, consumption, and exportation of wild edible fungi as Yunnan.

CONCLUSION

The current evidence for the existence of psychoactive boletes is anecdotally abundant yet scientifically insubstantial, leaving much left to be known. Independent reports of strikingly close qualitative resemblance have emerged from Papua New Guinea and Yunnan, China over the past century. In both cases, continents apart, local people have reported that following the consumption of an undercooked blue-staining bolete mushroom, hallucinogenic effects particularly distinguished by the perception of lilliputian hallucinations are known to result. However, to date, there have been no scientific studies to conclusively determine the taxonomic identity of the mushroom(s) involved or their active chemical constituents. While local people in Yunnan continue to frequently consume this bolete, it has simultaneously become listed by local authorities as a prohibited toxic species to be avoided. Such contradictions and lack of consensus surrounding the basic facts of the matter indicate the current insufficient level of available knowledge regarding the toxicity of this mushroom. It is a concern of not only local and global food safety, but of basic mycological research with potentially valuable applications in other fields. While much remains shrouded in mystery, one thing is certain: there is an urgent, growing demand for reliable scientific information on this topic, a statement echoed by the Chinese CDC in 2022, and which our future research will seek to provide.

BIBLIOGRAPHY

Alpert, Richard, Timothy Leary, and Ralph Metzner. 1964. *The Psychedelic Experience: A Manual Based on the Tibetan Book of the Dead*. Vol. 1. https://doi.org/10.5694/j.1326-5377.1965.tb71965.x.

Altschul, Stephen F., Thomas L. Madden, Alejandro A. Schäffer, Jinghui Zhang, Zheng Zhang, Webb Miller, and David J. Lipman. 1997. "Gapped BLAST and PSI-BLAST: a new generation of protein database search programs." *Nucleic acids research* 25, no. 17: 3389-3402.

Arora, David. 2008."Xiao ren ren: the "little people" of Yunnan." *Economic botany* 62, no. 3: 540-544.

Blin, Kai, Simon Shaw, Alexander M. Kloosterman, Zach Charlop-Powers, Gilles P. Van Wezel, Marnix H.

Blin, Kai, Simon Shaw, Alexander M. Kloosterman, Zach Charlop-Powers, Gilles P. Van Wezel, Marnix H.

Medema, and Tilmann Weber.2021. "antiSMASH 6.0: improving cluster detection and comparison capabilities." *Nucleic Acids Research* 49, no. W1: W29-W35.

Blom, Jan Dirk. 2021. "Leroy's elusive little people: A systematic review on lilliputian hallucinations." Neuroscience & Biobehavioral Reviews 125: 627-636.

Chan, C. K., H. C. Lam, S. W. Chiu, M. L. Tse, and F. L. Lau. 2016. "Mushroom poisoning in Hong Kong: a ten-year." *Hong Kong Med J* 22, no. 2: 124-30.

Cutler II, W. Dalley, Alexander J. Bradshaw, and Bryn TM Dentinger.2021. "What's for dinner this time?: DNA authentication of "wild mushrooms" in food products sold in the USA." *PeerJ* 9: e11747.

Dentinger, Bryn TM, and Laura M. Suz.2014. "What's for dinner? Undescribed species of porcini in a commercial packet." *PeerJ* 2: e570.

De Rios, Marlene Dobkin. 2009. *The psychedelic journey of Marlene Dobkin de Rios: 45 years with shamans, ayahuasqueros, and ethnobotanists*. Simon and Schuster.

Feng, Bang, and Zhuliang Yang.2018. "Studies on diversity of higher fungi in Yunnan, southwestern China: A review." *Plant diversity* 40, no. 4: 165-171.

Fricke, Janis, Felix Blei, and Dirk Hoffmeister.2017. "Enzymatic synthesis of psilocybin." *Angewandte Chemie International Edition* 56, no. 40: 12352-12355.

Heim, Roger, and R. Gordon Wasson.1965. "THE'MUSHROOM MADNESS'OF THE KUMA." *Botanical Museum Leaflets, Harvard University* 21, no. 1: 1-xx.

Li, Haijiao, Hongshun Zhang, Yizhe Zhang, Jing Zhou, Yu Yin, Qian He, Shaofeng Jiang et al. 2021. "Mushroom poisoning outbreaks—China, 2020." *China CDC weekly* 3, no. 3: 41.

Li, Haijiao, Hongshun Zhang, Yizhe Zhang, Jing Zhou, Yu Yin, Qian He, Shaofeng Jiang et al. 2022. "Mushroom Poisoning Outbreaks—China, 2021." *China CDC weekly* 4, no. 3: 35-40.

Li, Weiwei, Sara M. Pires, Zhitao Liu, Jinjun Liang, Yafang Wang, Wen Chen, Chengwei Liu et al.2021. "Mushroom poisoning outbreaks—China, 2010–2020." *China CDC weekly* 3, no. 24: 518.

Keller, Nancy P. 2019. "Fungal secondary metabolism: regulation, function and drug discovery." *Nature Reviews Microbiology* 17, no. 3: 167-180.

Nilsson, R. Henrik, Erik Kristiansson, Martin Ryberg, Nils Hallenberg, and Karl-Henrik Larsson. 2008. "Intraspecific ITS variability in the kingdom Fungi as expressed in the international sequence databases and its implications for molecular species identification." *Evolutionary bioinformatics* 4: EBO-S653.

Nett, Markus.2014. "Genome mining: concept and strategies for natural product discovery." *Progress in the Chemistry of Organic Natural Products 99*: 199-245.

Obermaier, Sebastian, and Michael Müller. 2020."Ibotenic acid biosynthesis in the fly agaric is initiated by glutamate hydroxylation." *Angewandte Chemie* 132, no. 30: 12532-12535.

Pérez-Moreno, Jesús, Alexis Guerin-Laguette, Roberto Flores Arzú, and Fu-Qiang Yu. 2020. *Mushrooms, Humans and Nature in a Changing World: Perspectives from Ecological, Agricultural and Social Sciences*. Springer Nature.

Rätsch, Christian. 2005. *The Encyclopedia of Psychoactive Plants: Ethnopharmacology and Its Applications*. Park Street Press.

Reay, Marie. 1959. *The Kuma: freedom and conformity in the New Guinea Highlands*. Carlton, Melbourne UP.

Reay, Marie. 1960. ""Mushroom Madness" in the New Guinea Highlands." *Oceania* 31, no. 2: 137-139.

Reay, Marie.1977. "Ritual madness observed: a discarded pattern of fate in Papua New Guinea." *The Journal of Pacific History* 12, no. 1: 55-79.

Ross, William.1936. "Ethnological notes on Mt. Hagen tribes (mandated territory of New Guinea). With special reference to the tribe called Mogei." *Anthropos* H. 3./4: 341-363.

Schoch, Conrad L., Keith A. Seifert, Sabine Huhndorf, Vincent Robert, John L. Spouge, C. André Levesque, Wen Chen et al. 2012. "Nuclear ribosomal internal transcribed spacer (ITS) region as a universal DNA barcode marker for Fungi." *Proceedings of the National Academy of Sciences* 109, no. 16 : 6241-6246.

Schultes, Richard E. 1939. "The identifications of teonanácatl, a narcotic basidiomycete of the Aztecs." *Botanical Museum Leaflets, Harvard University* 7: 37-55.

Tatusov, Roman L., Eugene V. Koonin, and David J. Lipman.1997. "A genomic perspective on protein families." *Science* 278, no. 5338 (1997): 631-637.

Thomas, Benjamin.2003. "Boletus manicus heim." *Journal of psychoactive drugs* 35, no. 3: 393-394.

Treu, Roland. 2006. "Ethnomycological Notes from Papua New Guinea." 2006. https://auspace.athabascau.ca/handle/2149/1669.

Yap, Pow-meng.1974. *Comparative psychiatry: A theoretical framework.* Vol. 3. published for the Clarke Institute of Psychiatry by University of Toronto Press.

Wang, Ran, Mariana Herrera, Wenjun Xu, Peng Zhang, Jesús Pérez Moreno, Carlos Colinas, and Fuqiang Yu.2022. "Ethnomycological study on wild mushrooms in Pu'er Prefecture, Southwest Yunnan, China." *Journal of Ethnobiology and Ethnomedicine* 18, no. 1: 1-24.

Weil, Andrew, and Winifred Rosen. 1983. *From chocolate to morphine.* New York: Houghton Mifflin Company.

Wu, J. C., and H. Lu. 2006. "Prospect of wild edible mushrooms industry and suggestions for industry development in Yunnan." *J West China Fore Sci* 35, no. 2: 154-8.

Zhuliang, Yang.2002. "On wild mushroom resources and their utilization in Yunnan Province, Southwest China." *Journal of Natural Resources* 17, no. 4: 463-469.

NEUROSPHERE

Psychoactive substances at the brain/mind interface

It's High Time for Science

Bruce Damer, PhD

Astrobiologist | Institute Director and Chief Scientist at BIOTA

> *"Long a tool for artists and musicians, could psychedelics refined with endogenous practices yield a high-octane fuel to advance science and engineering? If so, this capability will come just in time to tackle the hard problems of human and planetary survival."*
>
> —BRUCE DAMER

Speculations on the foundations, research, and practices of psychedelics as catalysts of creative problem solving in science, engineering, and leadership

ABSTRACT

A few months after the criminalization of LSD in California in May 1966, a groundbreaking pilot study carried out by Willis Harman and colleagues was published. Harman and his team had administered doses of LSD and mescaline to a group of 23 professionals including engineers, a mathematician, and an architect. Participants then worked on their chosen problems, with useful and in some cases highly innovative solutions reported by over half of the study group. Extraordinary states of consciousness have generated inventions and fueled scientific discovery from far back into our ancestry on the plains of Africa. The ingestion of psychoactive substances to produce visionary insights is commonplace throughout our history but their study as tools for problem solving in technical fields is emerging from a nearly six-decade hiatus. This essay reviews the 20th Century history of psychedelics as "mind manifesting" tools for creativity, and speculates on the connection between extraordinary or 'genius' levels of creativity and neurological states induced using psychedelics. Exemplars of such creative capacities are given and some new terms introduced. The author concludes by describing in depth his own creative experience working on a solution to a key problem in science: how did life begin on the Earth, four billion years ago? Some questions and proposals surrounding the return to the clinical study and work practice of psychedelics in technical fields are offered and the case for this new direction is made in our time of increasingly complex global challenges.

PERSONAL PREAMBLE

I took the opportunity during my talk at the ESPD55 meeting to fully and publicly *step out of the psychedelic closet* reporting my own use of psychoactive compounds both for my own healing but also as tools for my profession. I was not without feelings of trepidation as there is a taboo for 'drug use' in many professional fields, including the "hard" sciences. Indeed, many organizations carry out screening for drug use or will not employ those who admit use of psychedelics, still a criminal offense in much of the world. At the age of 60 with much of my original contributions to science, computing, and the space exploration field already under my belt, I chose to *come out* and become an advocate. Despite the reputational risk entailed, I still hope to be able to continue to work with colleagues and institutions.

I believe that any price I am obligated to pay will be outweighed by the potential benefits to society, and that I can serve as an example for young people entering problem-solving careers. Perhaps some of them will experiment as I have done and find more effective routes to their own 'way to genius.' I am a passionate believer in this doorway to the elevated intellect and believe it will be essential for us to pass through the challenging keyhole soon to be presented by a planetary ecosystem convulsing from the effects of human activity. Should we not investigate any tools or practices which can help us meet such a daunting challenge?

The legalization and normalization of the use of psychedelics within the medical establishment is imminent thanks to efforts of organizations like MAPS and Heffter Research Institute. As MAPS founder Rick Doblin often reminds us, the reason this is now happening is that *people stood up to be counted.* Cultural mainstreaming of psychedelics is also well underway. Thought leaders such as Michael Pollan (2018) described "how to change your mind" through psychedelics and covered the Harman study in his recent TV series of the same name. It may therefore be the right time to invite the underreported and underground users of psychedelics in science, engineering and leadership to step forward, share their story, and build a platform to evaluate and develop a "fourth path" of psychedelic research and practice.

INTRODUCTION

> *gen·ius*
> */ˈjēnyəs/*
>
> *From Latin, 'attendant spirit present from one's birth, innate ability or inclination', from the root of gignere 'beget'.*

Perhaps more than any other thing that we humans do, it is moments of creative genius that have laid down the stepping stones to the remarkable and functional complexity of our civilization. Genius is perhaps the most potent change agent for our future as well. Its mysterious action will likely determine if we survive and thrive or, frankly, go extinct. When did the first stroke of genius occur? Genius probably emerged as a capacity baked into our *Homo* ancestors. Sometime around a million years ago one of us struck a hard rock against a chunk of glassy flint to make a cutting tool and was impressed by the expected spray of sparks. In a flash of original insight, that ancestor understood that these sparks were like tiny fires. Testing this insight, they struck the flint again over a clutch of dried grass and smoke appeared, and then flames. Shared and packaged, like magic, fire then became on-demand and portable. With flint in hand, a cooked food diet grew our bodies and brains and we spread out to successfully settle much of the Earth.

The hypothesized discoverer of fire exhibited all the traits of genius at work: coming in with a level of experience and an innate curiosity; open to questioning a common phenomenon; engaging in a rapid association of disparate things including rock, sparks, grass and flame; being able to receive a novel insight; formulating and carrying out an experiment to test that insight; and finally, to *'beget'* the invention by transforming it into a routine practice for others. Countless scientists, engineers and leaders throughout history have experienced their own flashes of insight that have been called genius, once they have been landed into practical solutions which alter many aspects of our lives. We are awestruck by the generative power of genius, and have come to count on its appearance, yet it is still largely a mystery how and from whence it comes. Science has only recently begun tackling the question of how similarly elevated states of mind are made manifest. The investigation of the supercharged mind is moving into hyperdrive with the development of powerful new tools. One of these is whole-brain real-time imaging, and another, the well-prepared use of psychedelic substances. If we can crack the code of the catalysts of high creativity, we will increase our capacity to deal with challenges of climate change and the vicissitudes of the human psyche. Indeed, investing seriously in such a technology may spark a *Century of Genius*.

A growing literature from scholars studying the lives and character of history's geniuses has dispelled old myths and produced new frameworks around the phenomenon. Imaging of the brains of highly creative people in one early test group, authors from the Iowa Writers' Workshop, gave us a hint of which brain regions may be involved during flashes of insight (Andreasen, 2005). Studies of family background and environmental influences as well as genetic disposition have also given us a broad brush on who might have an innate capacity for genius (Simonton, 2004). Lastly, the tools and knowledge afforded to billions of us through the Internet offer the chance for unleashing genius in greatly increased ways. Our collective genius may therefore be poised for a leap in expression, especially if we provide it some nudges along the way. A quick Internet search finds only sparse reporting of major scientific, technical and leadership breakthroughs aided by the use of strongly psychoactive compounds. Perhaps psychedelics might have not actually played much of a role, if as suggested from the above definition, genius arises through an '*attendant spirit present from one's birth, innate ability or inclination*'.

There may be, however, a vast pool of unreported use of these compounds to unlock extraordinary creative states, all cloaked under the veil of academic reputational risk and company drug testing. Under the radar, tens of thousands (or more) of professionals have been using these psychoactive compounds purportedly to boost their workplace problem solving ability. Employees at leading tech companies, biomedical entrepreneurs, and crypto-financiers covertly share notes about their macro and micro-dosing regimens. Company retreats immerse C-level leadership in plant medicine ceremonies to derive innovative new business strategies. If this pool of use can be sampled and the data compiled, scientific and clinical studies completed, and best practices defined, the use of psychedelics may be validated and enter a normalized, legal and well-supported use in society. If this happens, we may obtain a vital new tool for our future and, as the Beatles song suggested, our collective prospects could be lifted with *a little help from our friends*.

At the May 2022 ESPD55 meeting to which this volume is dedicated, I called for both the *validation* and *valorization* of the use of psychedelics in the fostering of genius. In other words, it may well be *high time* to start the scientific study of these compounds and other practices in problem solving.

I believe we now stand on the brink of what could be called a *fourth path* of psychedelic science and practice which just might become the most impactful on our collective future. The *first path* of the use of psychoactive compounds comes from the dawn of human history, with their ceremonial use in family, tribe, village and as a core sacramental technology behind the rise of cities and civilizations. The *second path* began in the 19th Century and blossomed in the mid-20th as a doorway to individual exploration and growth with major impacts on the arts, philosophy and spirituality. A *third path* has emerged both within the indigenous homelands and western clinical settings employing these powerful compounds as therapeutics in the realm of healing and human psychology.

THE MIND MANIFESTING POWER OF PSYCHEDELICS

Surprisingly, this proposed *fourth path* is not new, it traces its roots back seventy years to the very dawn of psychedelic culture in the mid-20th Century. Many of the first experiencers of mescalin, LSD and psilocybin immediately noticed a profound enhancement of perceptual and mental acuity. Instinctively, they felt that such states could portend a great future as a tool for the scientific and technical arts. In fact, the very term "psychedelic" was coined by Humphrey Osmond in 1957 derived from the Greek words ψυχή psychḗ 'soul, mind' and δηλείν dēleín 'to manifest', for "mind manifesting," implying that psychedelics might enable hitherto underutilized potentials of the human mind (Weil and Rosen, 1993).

One newspaper article published just after John F. Kennedy's 1963 announcement that America would place a man on the moon reported: *NASA to use LSD to Train Lunar Astronauts* (Damer, 2011). In his seminal yet largely forgotten article published as the opening salvo in the first issue of the first academic journal dedicated to psychedelics, Harvard's *Psychedelic Review* (1963), philosopher Gerald Heard asked "Can this Drug Enlarge Man's Mind?" Heard opens with:

> *"Narcotics numb it [the mind]. Alcohol unsettles it. Now a new chemical called LSD has emerged with phenomenal powers of intensifying and changing it — whether for good or ill is a subject of hot debate."*

It is worth digging into a bit more of Heard's intuitive sense of LSD's value to society (with my **emphasis**):

> *"Can LSD provide any **assistance to the creative process**? Even when given under the best of conditions, it may do no more than "give an experience." Thereafter the subject must himself work with this **enlarged frame of reference**, this **creative schema**. If he will not, the experience remains a beautiful anomaly, a gradually fading wonder...*
>
> *What, then, should be done about it?*

> *It is the unique* ***quality of attention which LSD can bestow*** *that will or will not be of benefit. Intensity of attention is what all* ***talented people must obtain or command if they are to exercise their talent. Absolute attention*** *— as we know from, for example, Isaac Newton's and Johann Sebastian Bach's descriptions of the* ***state of mind in which they worked****—is the* ***most evident mark of genius functioning****."*

Psychiatrist Frank Barron (1962, 1965) took Heard's beautifully rendered intuition and called for testing such creative applications. , To rise to Barron's challenge, engineer Willis Harman engaged in trials with LSD with professionals including engineers, physicists, mathematicians, an architect, a furniture designer, and a commercial artist. In the landmark paper "Psychedelic agents in creative problem-solving: a pilot study" (Harman et al., 1966) the authors summarized their results:

> *"Based on the frequently reported* ***similarities between creative and psychedelic (drug-induced, consciousness-expansion) experiences****, a preliminary study was conducted to explore the effects of psychedelic agents (LSD-25, mescaline) on* ***creative problem-solving ability****. Twenty-seven professionally employed males were given a single psychedelic experience in 1 of 7 small groups (ns = 3 or 4) following extensive selection and preparatory procedures. This drug-induced problem-solving session was* ***carefully structured*** *with particular focus on establishing Ss' expectancies and a* ***psychosocial milieu conducive to creative activity****. Tentative findings based on tests of creativity, on subjective reports and self-ratings, and on the utility of problem solutions suggested that, if given according to this* ***carefully structured regimen, psychedelic agents seem to facilitate creative problem-solving, particularly in the "illumination phase."*** *The results also suggest that various degrees of increased creative ability* ***may continue for at least some weeks*** *subsequent to a psychedelic problem-solving session."*

That same year of 1966, both California and Nevada governors outlawed the manufacture, sale, and possession of the LSD effectively shutting down Harman's program, his psychedelic research center at San Francisco State College and enforcing a nearly fifty-year hiatus in this compelling direction in the use of psychedelics. One of the authors of the Harman study, a young Jim Fadiman, went on to start the microdosing movement in the 2000s (Fadiman and Korb, 2019).

It seems to me that it is indeed high time for the scientific, business and practitioner communities to take up where Harman and colleagues left off and restart this promising path of the use of psychedelics for the Human future. Others including Sessa (2008) and Baggott (2015) have made a similar call. As of this writing I am happy to report that the return to clinical study of the creative problem-solving potential of psychedelics has resumed, with an exacting and much larger scale pilot study carried out in the Netherlands (Mason et al. 2021) which I will return to later.

SETUP

A new field of inquiry often requires new terminology and a refiguring of older definitions, so I would like to propose the following language.

Endo and Exo

"Endo" is a shorthand term I have come to employ, signifying "from within" or endogenous, paired with the term and "exo" or "entering in from outside", or exogenous. Visionary states which manifest as trip-like "takeovers" or "downloads" in awake states but without the ingestion of substances could be termed "endo-trips." Exo-trips would be those which are catalyzed by a drug, or also by a brain-changing practice such as breathwork. As I will report later, in my case I found a way to employ an artful combination of endo and exo practices to good effect. Problem solvers and others with strong innate imaginations probably already possess strong capacities for visualization so they can build and inhabit many "endo castles in the sky." The reports of Harman's subject group suggest that those already trained in endo-tripping were greatly aided by the addition of an exo-element.

Micro and Macro

Bournemann (2020) provides an exhaustive review of the literature surrounding the burgeoning practice of "microdosing" popularized by 1966 Harman study co-author James Fadiman (Fadiman, 2019). Microdosing is described by scientists as 'sub-perceptual doses of a psychedelic, usually defined as between one tenth and one twentieth of a normal dose (Fadiman and Korb 2019). In addition, these authors offered a web site and survey in which hundreds of participants sent in narrative reports in which approximately 80% of accounts were positive or neutral in content, while other qualitative studies summarized by Bournemann charted negative effects and others attested to an improvement of creativity. Quantitative and interview studies were carried out using surveys with parameters such as focus and productivity, to investigate many anecdotal claims made as the microdosing movement got its start in Silicon Valley companies. Macrodosing studies in a clinical setting have only recently started up after the long hiatus since Harman's work and will be covered below.

Set → Setting → Setup

The memorable terms "set and setting" were developed by early psychedelic pioneers such as Al Hubbard and popularized by Timothy Leary. In preparing for a psychedelic session, it was proposed that the experiencer ought to have two aspects in hand: "set" (i.e., mindset comprised of thoughts, expectations, and mood) and "setting" (the environmental and social environment). As Harman's pilot study suggests in their "carefully structured regimen" and as treated later in this essay, it might be warranted to add a third term to this equation: "setup." Setup would encompass the preparation of minds with a problem or design to be considered, methodologies to engage in the creative work while under the influence of a psychedelic, and tools and practices to land workable solutions later. Setup is related to and could also incorporate Betty Eisner's concept of "matrix" which she describes as: "consideration of the environment from which an individual originally comes, in which the individual currently lives during the time of the sessions, and, if changed, to which the individual returns after successful therapy--the everyday living space" (Eisner, 1997).

Decrypting the Genius OS

It is valuable to take a trip into neurological pin-ball to track where creative thoughts might originate, bounce around, reflect off other thoughts and end up depositing their balls of novel insight. Putting aside proposals that consciousness might dwell outside of the brain and body or is plugged into a greater "conscious field" or as Aldous Huxley mused in The Doors of Perception, a "mind at large" (1954) lets visit the neuroscientific endeavor to map the creative process within our skulls. Modern efforts to read the boot code of the creative operating system began with the work of Nancy Andreasen et al. (2005) who suggested that there were distinct regions of the brain which became more active and interconnected when members of the renowned Iowa Writer's Workshop where given word association tests in a brain scanner.

Girn et al. (2020) add the psychedelic spin to this emerging creativity inquiry in their recent extensive review "Updating the dynamic framework of thought: Creativity and psychedelics." One key point they bring up is that in some cases, the "subjective sense of creativity enhancement does not match the actual 'quality' of insights or realisations under the drug—as judged by others." This 'epistemic innocence' of the psychedelic experience (Letheby, 2016) leads some to attribute more novelty and importance to an insight gleaned on a psychedelic exo-trip. This can also happen on an endo-trip without the sense of expansion brough on by drugs, suggesting that the practitioner must be capable of being their own critic, observing any and all "downloads" with more than one grain of salt. In technical fields, the skeptical requirement is baked-in to the dictum to test, repeat, and test again (and preferably with independent verification). Therefore, the genius OS best come equipped with its own built-in debugger!

As for the operation of the OS itself, glimmers of the operating modules and algorithms are beginning to surface in brain-imaging studies, some carried out with the use of psychedelics. Carhart-Harris and Friston (2010) proposed that "the action of psychedelics on primary process thinking and its hypothesized relationship to changes in brain function, [operates] particularly in relation to the default-mode network" (or DMN). A recently proposed model called the "dynamic framework of thought" by Christoff et al. (2016) "focuses on the competing forces of constraint and variability on thought [viewing] creative generation as a relatively unconstrained mode of thought that is similar, in that sense, to dreaming." Theoretical support enters at this point to propose an ambitious mechanistic model for drug action on creative ideation by Carhart-Harris and Friston (2019) excerpted from Girn et al.:

> *"This model, couched in terms of hierarchical predictive coding and the Free Energy Principle (Friston, 2010), proposes that psychedelics elicit their characteristic effects by decreasing the precision-weighting of high-level priors (e.g., beliefs or assumptions) which are encoded by high-level aspects of brain function, such as by the default network and other regions of association cortex… Thus, as a result of a decrease in the weighting of these high-level priors during the psychedelic experience, low-level inputs are liberated from top-down constraints and are more available to conscious awareness. In effect, this is viewed to broaden the volume and breadth of available sensory and mnemonic content and increases the potential for 'out of the box' ideas, novel insights, and new perspectives."*

As is apparent, decoding the OS of creative processes, let alone the specific server calls of genius, is an endeavor in a nascent state with decades of work ahead.

GENIUS IN THE SCANNER

Perhaps most compelling and largest recent human subject trial seeking causal pathways between psychedelics and creativity is a groundbreaking study completed by Mason et al. (2021). This work represents the resumption of the work begun in a preliminary way by Willis Harman and coworkers (1966, 1970). This new generation of investigators used a 21st Century framework surrounding the question of how the creative process works. The authors comment that "Over the years, a number of anecdotal reports have accumulated suggesting that the consumption of serotonin agonist (5-HT-2A receptor) psychedelic drugs (Nichols, 2016), like lysergic acid diethylamide (LSD), psilocybin, and mescaline, can enhance creativity (Baggot, 2015; Sessa, 2008).". However, they add that "although there has been much historical interest in the ability of psychedelics to enhance creative capacity, the scientific literature is largely lacking.". With new receptors in hand and with real-time brain imaging data from 60 individuals, the authors proceeded to quantify these anecdotal reports employing emerging models of creative thought processes:

> *"Although arguably difficult to define, the creative process has been viewed as a dynamic process (Manesh et al. 2020; Runco 2019), requiring shifting between different modes of thought in order to reach an end result (Guilford 1967). These modes include divergent thinking (DT), which consists of generating novel and original ideas, and convergent thinking (CT), the subsequent evaluation of generated ideas in regards to their usefulness and effectiveness."*

The study was carried out at the University of Maastricht in the Netherlands to test the hypothesis of Kuypers (2018) who predicted that given previous studies which demonstrated "a decrement in the functional connectivity in parts of the DMN… after administration of psychedelics (Carhart-Harris et al. 2012; Palhano-Fontes et al. 2015)… a consequence of this effect being enhanced cognitive flexibility and creative thinking (Carhart-Harris et al. 2014)."

The authors' conclusion forms a wonderful and compelling link from the anecdotal reports and early studies to 21st Century, experimental neuroscience. Briefly, they found:

> *"…that psilocybin induces time- and construct-related differentiation of effects on creative thinking, suggesting that psychedelics could be a novel tool to investigate underlying neural mechanisms of the creative process (Girn et al. 2020; Kuypers 2018). In addition, these findings add some support to the historical claims that psychedelics can influence aspects of the creative process, reducing conventional, logical thinking, and giving rise to novel thoughts, but emphasizes the distinction between spontaneous and deliberate creative cognition, as well as acute and persisting effects of the drug."*

At the time of the writing of this chapter a clinical trial of LSD and creative thinking carried out at the University of Campinas in Brazil was published (Wießner et al. 2022) suggesting that the return of the study of psychedelically enhanced higher creative states is well underway.

WALKING IN THE FOOTSTEPS OF GENIUS

In his book *Origins of Genius* (1999), Dean Simonton summarizes the characteristics of typical creative geniuses from the accumulated literature as people who "[are] open to diverse experiences, display exceptional tolerance of ambiguity, seek out complexity and novelty, and can engage in defocused attention" (p. 87). Simonton goes on to state that such "creators" also tend to be more introverted than extroverted, and can appear remote, withdrawn or perhaps anti-social, while oftentimes exhibiting a rebellious, nonconventional independence. To make their breakthroughs and land them into products in the world, creative geniuses are persistent in overcoming obstacles and setbacks and flexible in altering their strategies, applying a great deal of concentrated hard work to problems. Of course, we might also ask: what *kind of creative intelligence* are we considering here? Howard Gardner famously diverged from the field of intelligence studies' singular focus on cognitive abilities (problem solving) to propose a Theory of Multiple Intelligences (Gardner, 2011). Gardner and Hatch (1989) argued that "while problem solving is recognized as a crucial component, the ability to fashion a product, to write a symphony, execute a painting, stage a play, build up and manage an organization, carry out an experiment is not included, presumably because the afore-mentioned capacities cannot be probed adequately in short-answer tests.". To broaden the definition Gardner introduced eight different types of intelligences consisting of: Linguistic, Logical/Mathematical, Spatial, Bodily-Kinesthetic, Musical, Interpersonal, Intrapersonal, and Naturalist. The details of each of these special capacities of gifted people will not be taken up here, but should be considered as we seek genius beyond the furled brow of the mythical lone thinker scribbling on their blackboard.

Charles Darwin, the instigator of my field of the origin of life as well as evolutionary biology itself, is perhaps one of the greatest of scientific geniuses. Albert Einstein, Marie Curie, Francis Crick, and many others fit the bill for genius based upon the impacts they have had on their scientific fields, and on the entire human enterprise. Technical geniuses who were well known for their flashes of insight leading to world-changing innovations included Nikola Tesla, Thomas Edison, and more recently for the sheer volume of transformative products, the design partnership of Steve Jobs and Jony Ive at Apple.

Mathematician Ralph Abraham, a longtime colleague and neighbor of mine is an exemplar of the transformative power of psychedelics to redirect an intellectual career (and also a way of life). In an article entitled Mathematics and the Psychedelic Revolution (Abraham, 2008) he describes his visionary downloads enabled in part with high doses of LSD which launched a new branch of mathematics. He also argues that psychedelics also influenced Silicon Valley's technology innovators and their products of which we would all agree are modern time's epitome of sparks of genius which have lit up the world:

> *"There is no doubt that the psychedelic evolution in the 1960s had a profound effect on the history of computers and computer graphics, and of mathematics, especially the birth of postmodern maths such as chaos theory and fractal geometry. This I witnessed personally. The effect on my own history, viewed now in four decades of retrospect, was a catastrophic shift from abstract pure math to a more experimental and applied study of vibrations and forms, which continues to this day."*

Technology journalist John Markoff covered this history in a wonderfully researched and widely read book *What the Dormouse Said: How the Sixties Counterculture Shaped the Personal Computer Industry* (Markoff, 2005). Starting in the vacuum tube and transistor era of the 1950s and '60s, he chronicles the engineers and business leaders who were heavily influenced by what I would like to suggest in this context we might call 'elixirs of constructive vision.' I personally explored this connection having amassed one of the largest private collections of vintage computer hardware and documents in my DigiBarn Computer Museum (Damer, 2011). In an adjacent room in my barn sits Timothy Leary's extant library, news archive, record collection and personal effects. I was deeded these materials in 2011 by Denis Berry, co-trustee of Leary's Futique Trust for my support in helping find a home for his core archives at the New York Public Library. Hodges (2019) chronicled Leary's foray into software including his Mind Mirror series which I have in my collection alongside computers like those that Leary would have used. In many ways, the tonnage of these archives speaks to the creative power of the combination of silicon with the 'dirty pictures,' chemist Alexander "Sasha" Shulgin's name for scribbled diagrams of potent psychoactive compounds. Sasha, also based in the Bay Area of Northern California, was in a way the digital age's *alchemist*, synthesizing and testing compounds such as MDMA, 2CB and hundreds more (Shulgin et al. 2011). Not surprisingly he recorded his work on early personal computers, the first of which he donated to the DigiBarn.

Steve Jobs and Francis Crick along with Nobelist Cary Mullis (Mullis, 2000; Markoff, 2005; Fadiman, 2011) used LSD as a mind opening experience which forever changed their creative processes. Jobs reported in (Isaacson, 2009) that LSD "reinforced my sense of what was important—creating great things instead of making money, putting things back into the stream of history and of human consciousness as much as I could."

TWO SCIENTISTS, TWO TALES OF FLASHES OF INSIGHT

Dean Simonton (2004) proposes a framework for genius which engages discovery within the zeitgeist of the times when ideas are ripe to appear. He covers efforts to map variations of genius as analytical or intuitive and the many theories of the cognitive action, including free and flat associative hierarchies which characterize highly creative people. These individuals can move from convergent (focused mind) thinking to divergent (mind wandering) approaches in which many associative variations can be tried, increasing the odds of finding that one rare unique connection.

One such example of a novel innovation arising from remote associations of rather different things occurred to my colleague David Deamer one day in 1989. For months Dave had been playing with four themes in his head: planar membranes (his specialty), ion channels across them, DNA and RNA nucleic acid molecules, and the "Coulter" cell counter. He had set himself the task of figuring out how to get DNA and RNA to pass through a membrane. While driving in Oregon these disparate things assembled in a flash into a functioning molecular machine. Dave pulled over to the side of the road and sketched out a specially shaped pore which forms a tunnel in the membrane through which a strand of nucleic acid is being pulled, each base making up the strand pausing, and then moving on (Fig. 1, left). An electric current across the mem-

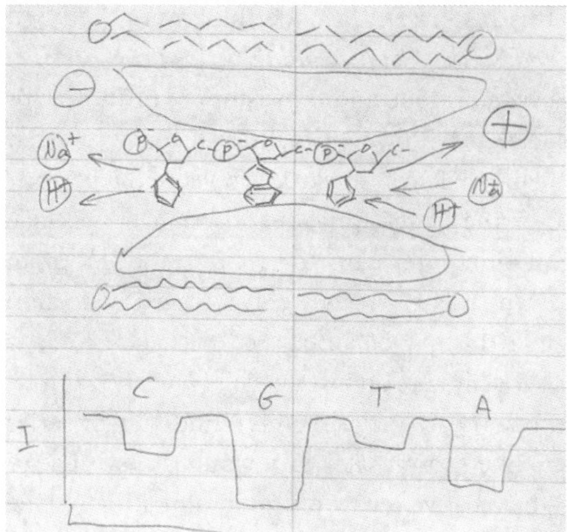

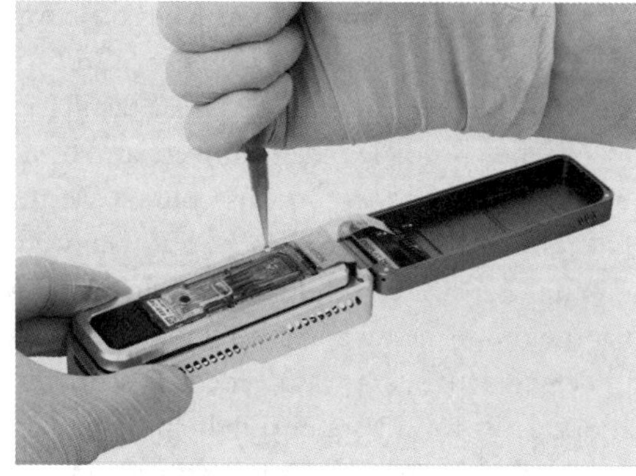

Fig. 1 David Deamer's 1989 sketch of his flash of insight (left) which led to the invention of nanopore sequencing (above), an important new medical technology. *Images courtesy David Deamer and Oxford Nanopore*

brane could record which base was transiently blocking the pore, yielding a voltage interruption carrying the unique signature of which base it was. Dave knew it was truly something novel, and sensed it was a viable design that would work well in practice. Like Einstein's famous utterance surrounding his vision of a man falling from a rooftop (Einstein, 1920) that led to General Relativity, this was one of the "happiest thoughts" of Dave's life. Fifteen years later the founders of a company in Oxford, UK read his article on the idea and approached him to develop it into a new medical technology, the nanopore sequencer. Today Dave's flash of insight is embodied in a thousand-dollar gene sequencing device you can hold in your hand, replacing a half million-dollar refrigerator sized cabinet (Fig. 1, right).

It should be noted that Dave's experience occurred without the ingestion of any substances at all, and spontaneously arose while in the setting of a mundane private activity: driving through the countryside. In his case, decades of previous training and laboratory experience created the *setup* for this beautiful, and workable solution to appear seemingly out of the ether (Damer 2019).

As we continue this exploration of a few examples of states of high creativity in science and technology, we can probably now offer a tentative reply to the question "what is the genie called genius?" Perhaps it is a rare entity comprised of an admixture of innate ability, intelligence, and persistence, with extant environmental conditions and some dumb luck thrown in. Hardly absent from this formulation is the requirement that genius comes to "the prepared mind" (suggested in a personal conversation with the author by neuropsychopharmacologist David Nutt at ESPD55). Therefore, the arising of these extraordinary outputs from the human intellect requires a substantial input from the societal surrounds and personal preparation, the setup. Dave and I share the capacity for mind to generate spontaneous flashes of insight and I will next detail my own experience which generated a possible scenario (and testable hypothesis) for a big question in science—the origin of life.

HIGH TIME FOR A SCIENTIST

Around the age of thirteen I watched a TV biography of Albert Einstein and was fascinated by his ability to mentally enter into an inner world of physics, experiencing highly visual journeys which led to his proposals for the theory of relativity. He called these *Gedankenexperimente* (thought experiments) and perhaps the most famous is Einstein's description of "chasing a beam of light" at the age of sixteen (Norton, 2013). In the early spring of 1976 while walking in the sagebrush-dotted hills near my family home in Kamloops, British Columbia, Canada I experienced what I interpreted to be my first scientific thought experiment, and this was to guide me the rest of my life. Bending down to study a mariposa lily emerging from the just-thawed ground, I was suddenly awestruck by the beauty of its trillium shape and asked the question: how can such a complex thing emerge from a much simpler thing, a bulb in the soil beneath? Standing up I looked out upon the sweeping river system that meets in our town, with all the plants and trees extending from the pocket desert to the beginning of the northern boreal forest in the distance. My mind tried to count up all of these emerging life forms and posed another question: where did all of this come from, was there a common bulb, or seed somewhere deep in the past from which they all sprouted? I probed back through time trying to travel to that origin point, smiled and felt excited that I had found the question that really fascinated me: how did life itself begin?

I felt a deep sense of happiness descend upon me as I committed to work on this problem, sensing that it might take a long time, perhaps as much as ninety years. Being then fourteen, I thought that could mean that I might be over a hundred years old before a convincing solution emerged, but this was plausibly within the realm of my lifetime. When I began to walk back toward my parents' home I was suddenly confronted by a vision, not from my imagination but arriving from somewhere else. A geometric apparition was seemingly hanging in front of my eyes but yet clearly still operating from within my head. It was a moving bundle of balls, connected by sticks, somewhat like the Tinker Toy sets I played with as a younger kid. It was my first thought experiment, or "download", just in time to guide my newly minted life's mission. I was a bit taken aback by its proximity and vividness but chose to just give it my full attention. I first studied its movement, trying to "get inside it" and deduce what orderly process, such as a gear box, might be driving its motion. My inquiry into its inner workings woke up the bundle and prompted it to direct the following mental missive to me: "figure out how I made a copy of myself!". Taking this in, my mind went to the scene of an automobile factory, with cars moving along an assembly line. I turned my attention back to the apparition with a bit of skepticism around its statement, offering: "it seems to me that for copies of a machine to be made, you need a much bigger machine like a factory to make them, and I don't see a bigger machine anywhere, it's just you floating there!". I walked over to a cliff and gazed out over into a deep creek-cut canyon. The bundle reappeared and gave me one more nudge, offering a response to my challenge: "It's a good point, but not the right answer, so work on it!" . The apparition then winked out. I was grateful for its brief appearance and guidance and I looked forward, feeling very contented to engage in the years and decades of inquiry that now lay ahead. Of course, as a teenager I had no model for what has just happened, and no reason to be skeptical. I was open to the possibility that such things could happen (and still am). Perhaps wisely, I did not share this experience with anyone realizing that someday, after a long journey of inquiry, and with some solid results in hand, that it might be time to share what had happened with the seeming entity with which I conversed that day. Perhaps a new question we might all now want to ask of such apparitions is: "*so, exactly where do you come from?*"

Setting Up

Decades later, after earning degrees in computer science, a first job coding an entire graphical user interface, writing "artificial life" programs, hosting conferences on early life on Earth, helping organize and innovate the first avatar-inhabited virtual worlds, and a decade of simulation and design projects for NASA, I had worked on so many surrounding aspects of the origin of life question that I felt ready to tackle it head-on. In 2008 I began work on a PhD, building and running an environment called the Evolution Grid (or EvoGrid) to simulate complex interactions within diffuse atomistic soups. Searching for ways to speed up bond formation, the EvoGrid was an attempt to computationally characterize how things got complex in the universe. What our team concluded was that all of cosmic evolution (stars to elements to planets, and then to life itself) might follow a mathematical formulation called stochastic hill climbing in which objects become co-joined on one step and stay together long enough to reach higher ones (Damer, 2011; Damer et al. 2012). I playfully refer to this as the "cosmic wiggle" harkening back to Terence McKenna's "cosmic giggle" which I personally heard him enunciate, setting the stage for our creative investigations (described later in this chapter):

> *"To contact the cosmic giggle, to have the flow of kazooistry begin to give off synchronistic ripples, whitecaps in the billows of the coincidental ether, if you will. To achieve that, a precondition is a kind of unconsciousness, a kind of drifting, a certain taking-your-eye-off-the-ball, a certain assumption that things are simpler than they are, almost always precedes what Mircea Eliade called 'the rupture of plane' that indicates that there is an archetypal world, an archetypal power behind profane appearances."* (McKenna 1998)

All this preparatory work became much more grounded when in 2009 I met David Deamer, who became my mentor and colleague and invited me to join his department at UC Santa Cruz. Dave has decades of experience in a field called *membrane biophysics* and made some key discoveries including the previously described nanopore sequencing, and another that membranes, the boundary structures of cells, form from materials present in ancient meteorites which would have been delivered to the Earth four billion years ago (Deamer, 1985). Dave and I began regular meetings for tea and discussions of origin of life science in which he trained me and introduced the issues and personalities of this central field of Astrobiology, and brought me into scientific meetings and organizations. Without his mentorship and kind critiques of my "big picture" ideations, there would have been no path to transmute any of my visionary downloads into plausible scientific scenarios with testable predictions. This is a clue to how we can land the products of creative bursts in the real world, or whether they are destined for the dustbin (see Genius Lost later in this essay). These years of tea times, reading hundreds of journal articles, struggling with new terminology and methodology in a dozen fields, and a clear commitment constituted the "setup" step for me which was a fecund feedstock for my next flash of insight.

The question of life's origins has a 150-year scientific history, beginning with a sentence in a letter from Charles Darwin to his friend J.D. Hooker (1871):

> *"But if (& oh what a big if) we could conceive in some warm little pond with all sorts of ammonia & phosphoric salts,—light, heat, electricity & etc. present, that a protein compound was chemically formed, ready to undergo still more complex changes [..]"*

This Darwinian scribble is the source of the catchy phrase "warm little pond" which has entered into public consciousness. It is the great scientist's only known writing about the question of the origin of life. Less well known is the second part of his sentence that a "protein compound" must form, "ready to undergo still more complex changes.". Proteins are one of the building blocks of life, composed of linear chains of linked amino acids. Darwin intuitively understood that they were important, and that for life to first begin, they must somehow be synthesized and then be able to undergo evolutionary cycles generating longer, more complex proteins. In the 21st Century we describe this process as an away-from-equilibrium chemical system. Darwin's guess has until recently been largely overlooked in our field. It turns out to have been extremely prescient and has guided the scenario we have developed working with colleagues around the world. We situated a key stage in *abiogenesis* (another term for the origin of life) in an updated version of the warm little pond: a little hot spring pool subject to cycles of filling, drying and refilling. A few years before we met, Dave and his graduate students had discovered that if they dried down mixtures of the building blocks of another key polymer of life, nucleotides, they would stitch together to form chains, or "polymers" of the nucleic acid RNA (Rajamani et al. 2008). Along with his earlier discovery of membranous materials coming from ancient meteorites, Dave worked out that if these meteoritic organics were deposited into a hot spring pool, dried down with nucleotides present, they could self-assemble to form RNA -filled "protocells" the starting units which could be the earliest ancestors of living cells.

Dosing Up

This is where the science stood in 2013, four years after Dave and I first started sharing tea together. Protocells, each containing random sequences of RNA glowed with a fluorescent dye under our microscopes. This was compelling but was only a first step toward life. It was time for another thought experiment, this time reaching out into a truly yawning chasm of complexity. The question was: how could a starting population of trillions of protocells, each one different, acquire the molecular machinery in just the right sequence to give rise to the first living, reproducing cells? I intuitively felt that a visionary flash of extraordinary proportions would have to materialize to move us to the next step. What came next amounted to dosing up with a high-octane fuel able to boost my staid station wagon of a mind into a neurological drag racer.

In late 1998 I hosted Terence McKenna and his son Finn, together with Ralph Abraham on a visit to my property in the Santa Cruz Mountains. Terence's interest was that I was then a "maven" of the medium of multi-user avatar virtual worlds. I sat Terence and his compadres down in front of a computer connected to the Internet by creepingly slow modem and toured them into vivid 3D landscapes, conversing with users inhabiting these worlds and building their dream structures. Terence was sufficiently enthralled to purchase a new PC and plan to host *in-world* fan gatherings from his new house in Hawaii. We set a date to meet there in February, 1999 and I then mentioned to Terence that I was the grand old age of 36, yet "inexperienced" in psychedelic realms. He kindly offered to help open a doorway for me into his own version of very vivid psychedelic virtual worlds. Before traveling to Hawaii, I experienced my first psychedelic trip on a high dose of mushrooms at a remote location in the southern Sierra Nevada in California. Arriving on the Big Island and sitting with our smokes in his library, Terence and I compared notes, contrasting the weird tryptamine worlds of the be-mushroomed psyche with the crude but surprisingly immersive 3D landscapes of the early "metaverse" (Damer, 1999). Terence offered after we concluded the "Virtual AllChemical Powwow" with forty of his fans touring tryptamine-inflected worlds that these experiences were "not unlike DMT". Our late-night discussions seeded his ideas of "novelty" and the "cosmic giggle" into my future work to sprout into mathematics of the EvoGrid as the "cosmic wiggle" and into chemistry as a testable scenario for the origin of life.

Over the next decade I continued to explore the full range of "classic" psychedelics, settling on a regular practice with the jungle medicine ayahuasca. Journeying to take my first "dieta" in a remote location north of Pucallpa, Peru in late 2011 I was inducted into what became the most healing, and intellectually productive period of my life. Over the next five years I partook in three dozen sessions, each building on the previous ones, and refining my relationship with the medicine. Surprisingly perhaps, I began to take ever lower doses. On a return to Peru in October, 2013 I undertook a major personal goal, which was to heal a "hard knot" of pain which I associated with a major life event: being given up at birth for adoption. A growing body of research indicates that the risk of adoptees experiencing psychiatric disorders is in some cases approximately twice as high as that of non-adoptees. Elevated risks of disorders included: attention-deficit/hyperactivity, anxiety, depression, substance use, and psychoses (Behle and Pinquart, 2016). I would have certainly been diagnosed on the autism spectrum had pediatric psychiatrists been looking for that in the 1960s! I was therefore burdened (or blessed) with a lifelong state of heightened self-awareness and external sensitivity, but sometimes converting into states of anxiety. I coped with some of the less pleasant aspects of my reality by focusing on multiple, diverse projects. In other words, I was neurotypical of the personality type we now call "nerds".

First the Healing, then the Revealing

Resolution of my presumed birth trauma came one night toward the end of our group's time in the jungle. I finally felt ready to face fundamental insights about how I was conceived. In an intense tryptamine-driven stream of events, I experienced the journey of my personal sperm to its destined egg and my moment of creation and embryonic growth in my birth mother's belly. Perhaps most important for my healing resolution was that I felt for the first and only time, a love connection with my birth mother. Emerging, I experienced a peace and clarity that had never been present in my life, an unbroken line stretching from my innards to my crown. I was now ready to follow Einstein's example, to chase my own beam of light: the spark that lit up the living world. Perhaps in this work what must come first is *the healing*, then what becomes possible is a full opening to *the revealing*.

Our group leader called for a ten minute "no hustling, no bustling" period of silence and I realized that a unique opportunity had arrived. I closed my eyes and pulled a mental lever which triggered the running of a previously encoded endo-trip in which I visualized the sperm of my father which had created me traveling in reverse. That sperm re-merged with his body which in turn was created by the sperm of my grandfather, itself swimming backwards to his father and so on. I pulled the lever harder, traveling through genus *Homo*, through our ape precursors, then all the land animals, fishes, simple multicellular forms, and then passing into the great ancestral cloud of single-celled organisms. A breathtaking number of join points were presented and I transited them in a blur as I checked my forehead for elevated brain temperature. Too hot and this would signify I was way into the red in terms of neuronal activity and should pull the rip-cord on the scientific endo-trip I was running supercharged within the framework and chemical milieu of an ayahuasca exo-trip. A cool head prevailed and I passed through the cloud, emerging into a vision of the beige skies of the Hadean Earth, over four billion years ago. In my high-speed chase through the ancestor's tales, I had run a mental reenactment of life in reverse to just before its beginning. Beneath my soaring viewpoint now lay a volcanic island with smoke and ash rising from erupting cones. The much fainter young sun radiated as a soft orange ball and meteorites and dust particles crashed and flashed through the hazy atmosphere. Like a gigantic version of Saturn's rings, the brilliant disc of accretion material orbiting the sun was visible in full daylight stretching from horizon to horizon. Within it was a rich flow of interstellar organics ready to impregnate new born worlds with the building blocks of life. I pivoted my observer self into a free fall aiming for the place on the island I knew I had to reach to address my question: how did the first protocells cross the enormous chasm of molecular evolution to become living microbes?

A steaming field of pools, periodically filled by pulses from hot geysers, appeared on the flanks of a volcano below my flight path. This was a best guess of an "urable" locality, a place where the spectacular act of abiogenesis could happen. In scientific terms, it was a zone where away-from-equilibrium chemistry could form the first populations of protocells and run them through untold numbers of cycles to become living cells (Deamer et al. 2022). An instant later my observer was immersed in one such pool, surrounded by silvery objects, the protocells Dave and I had witnessed so many times down the barrel of our microscope. Peering into them much more closely than I could under a 400x lens, I noted that they contained stringy forms, glowing like neon: the polymers. Glancing from protocell to protocell I noticed one which hosted a much more complex interacting mesh of polymers than the others. I parked my observer next to it and entered into a state of emptiness, asking into the ether for the next step, evidently assuming there was *some thing* there to reply. From wherever the reply came, the instruction was simple: "become it, become it now."

I took this to mean *become that protocell*. But I asked myself, how do you become a protocell? The scene then began to fade to black and I felt I was losing consciousness. "What is happening?" I thought, and the reply, was "you must die to experience your own birth." An unknown

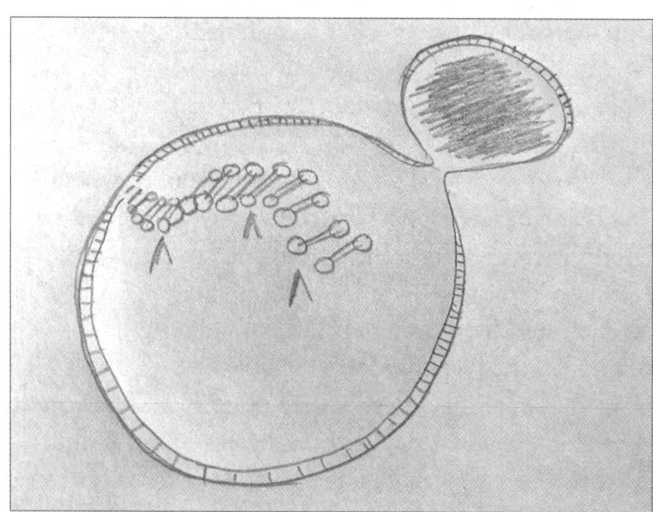

Fig. 2 Simplified sketch of the author's October 2013 flash of insight of a protocell in the process of budding.

duration of time passed and I breached back into consciousness in a "scream" which lit up a new scene. I was now immersed in the illuminated interior of the protocell, my body had now become a pulsating membrane-bounded sack. All around and within me surged a molecular-energetic storm. The scream centered my attention on a tearing action, a ripping of the membrane some distance from my observing center. As I glanced toward that point my observing camera passed by an undulating string of polymers (Fig. 2). Turning to focus on this, I noticed points of motion signifying some sort of action within its chain-links. It was as if the keys of a piano were being played by an unseen hand. My attention was grabbed again by the ripping action, a compartment was budding off, of "me", my body was fissioning! The compartment was small, and within its volume were no illuminated polymers, just blackness. As the compartment blebbed, separated and drifted off, seemingly totally inert, the membrane that defined my boundary closed up, I suddenly felt *more alive*. What did this all mean? There were more questions than answers. Our leader clapped his hands and the ten minute break was up.

I rocked back on my haunches in amazement and stunned happiness. The entire session had been manifested on an exogenous micro-dose of ayahuasca potentiating a presumably more powerful macro-dose of "endo," my home grown endogenous visionary practice. I had finally learned how to merge the two in a type of alchemical symbiosis I came to call "winding the vine." Returning to my little tin-roofed tambo hut in the rainforest I lay for hours replaying the scene. A completely novel class of technical questions and scenarios were now roiling in my brain. These questions contained clues and a logical chain of reasoning slowly emerged: "the action of the polymer was somehow connected to the budding off of the compartment, it was controlling it" but "the results were not viable, the budded protocell was not yet living, it was stillborn." I entered a deeper inquiry: "how can a protocell 'learn' to divide into two viable daughter cells?" and concluded that "the protocell must try and try again until the encoded polymer instructions successfully carry out the duplication and division.". In other words, it seems that "death writes the code of life" even at its very beginning. But how could a relatively simple protocell, floating on its own in a pool, carry out complicated attempts to divide itself? Surely this would be too risky, and not even plausible! This act would be akin to you or me jumping into a swimming pool and slitting oneself from head to stern hoping to birth a pair of twins. One misstep could lead to the dissolution of the entire protocell and loss of all that had evolved and accumulated to that point. It just did not make sense.

Landing a Solution

Three months later, on December 30, 2013 I was at a family relation's house on a hilltop overlooking Los Angeles engaged in a morning set of stretches and a practice of breathwork. I often find that breathwork opens me to a flow state in which inspiring thoughts appear more easily so I was not surprised by what came next. Months of cogitation around the mystery posed by the vision in the jungle had prepared the way. That morning the trigger thought for the download began with me posing a new question: "how can we best construct a laboratory chamber to simulate real hot spring pools, complete with a mineral basin, injectors, and a rocker system to subject the mineral basin's edge to wet-dry cycles?"

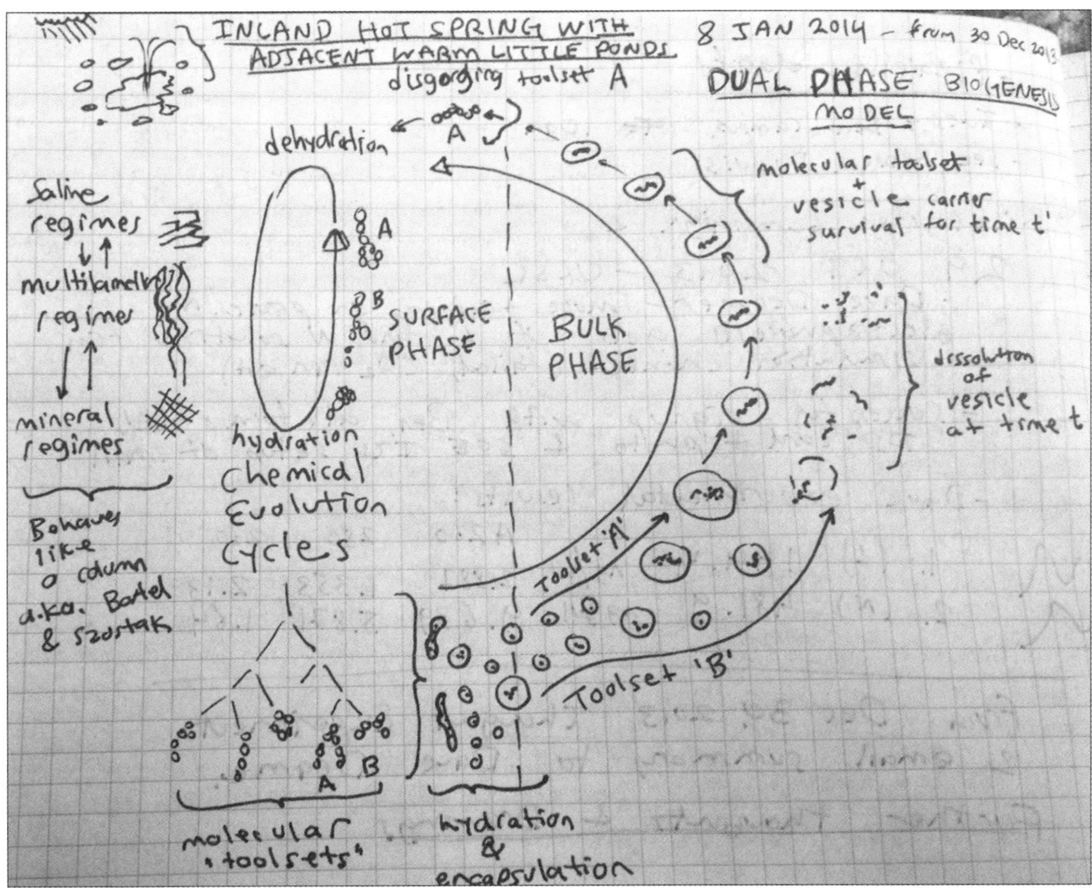

Fig. 3 Sketch of the author's conception of the "coupled phases scenario" envisioned in December 2013 which became the basis of a novel proposal for life's origins on Earth.

Suddenly, I felt the oncoming takeover of my particular brand of thought experiment, and a full-on endo-trip unfolded as I fell headlong into this design for a laboratory hot spring. There I witnessed, without the aid of psychotropic substances, protocells forming in their trillions by budding off from the dry layers of lipid into a refilling pool, each protocell containing complex mixtures of polymers. The protocells floated freely into the bulk of the water, some popping and losing their contents, some staying stably in one piece. The pool began to dry down and the surviving protocells with their polymer cargoes aggregated together at the pool bottom, forming a gelatinous mass. The protocells dried down further and their membranous compartments began to fuse together. As each fusion event happened, a flush of polymers flowed, mixing together with those of adjacent protocells. Protocells fused and fused, forming vast layered lipid sheets. Between the sheets seething populations of polymers and innumerable other molecules moved like the busy automata from Conway's early bio-inspired computer program "the Game of Life" (Gardner, 1970). Complex interactions occurred, sunlight and sources of chemical energy were captured, polymers competed for building blocks, broke up, and grew longer in a nod to Darwin, undergoing "still more complex changes". A flush of water again raised the pond level, and dried films of membrane were submerged, budding off trillions more protocells, each carrying new cargoes of now more complex polymers. The polymers were "coupling" between dry, wet and an intermediate moist phase. They were circulating within the "glassware" of semi-permeable membranes and able to undergo selective changes away from thermodynamic equilibrium. What was emerging was truly novel in the brief history of the young Earth, and perhaps in the entire universe.

I took another breath, as the endo-trip was continuing to roll forward. An untold number of cycles poured protocells into the pool, with colonies forming and growing along different shores and bays. Each colony grew as organics accumulated, membranes formed, and were stabilized by initially random polymers. Gradually each separate colony assumed a distinct character. There was something emerging in each that differentiated it from the others. The protocells seemed to be taking on different colors. Looking closely at these rainbow colonies there were sets of specific polymers engaged in tasks. Some colonies were stagnant or decreasing in size until rafts of protocells from other colonies reached them, merged in with a new color and then the combined colony grew with increased vigor. The circuits of life were lighting up: first, passive pores formed through membranes, allowing nutrients in and other molecules out. Catalysts picked up the nutrients at the entry point of the pores and cycled to produce more catalysts and other products into existence. Those products diffused and joined into other chemical circuits. Amidst it all, little undulating segments of polymers were templated, read and rewritten, beginning to exert control over the circuits. Those information-carrying polymers clumped together into sets, along with other molecular origamis. Budding protocells picked up bigger toolsets of polymers on each round and began to retain them indefinitely through subsequent cycles. Then, one day, after thousands, or millions of years of cycling across a whole landscape of interconnected pools, a protocell executed the instruction to bud off a smaller compartment, and then another, and another. This could only happen while protocells were surrounded by the protective and supportive matrix of other protocells as they aggregated together as the pool was drying down. Protocell division attempts could happen again and again, and even if they failed, all the precious molecular cargoes would be conserved and recycled into the communal matrix. So, this is how protocells would be safeguarded from their own dissolution even as they were driven to attempt their own fission. A chemical economy of mutual support, division of labor, and resource sharing enabled this final step to life. The amorphous, sharing community of protocells had lifted some of their members into singular identity as living cells and birthed billions of years of future lines of descendants.

I sat back, as the download was done. Mulling it over, what I had witnessed I later realized was the "progenote" predicted by the great microbiologist Carl Woese (Woese and Fox, 1977) and which I then later developed in my first sole author publication (Damer, 2016). This was the proposed environment which could support that final reproductive step to cellular life, and every other step leading up to it. The progenote is the deepest ancestor of microbial communities and booted up within the substrate we now term the "progenitor," a veritable womb enabling fragile inanimate protocells to traverse the combinatorial chasm to life (Deamer et al. 2024). Indeed, *death did write the code of life*, but perhaps more fundamentally is perhaps that life began in a very different way than the Victorian notion of the strict competitive regime of "survival of the fittest." Through this discovery in this era of the Internet, we might be able to re-cast life's beginnings and subsequent evolution in the terms of networked emergence powered by cooperation sustained by sharing relationships, yet till driven by innovation-compelling competition and selection. This refiguring could instigate an important philosophical and societal revisioning of life, and our place in it. What a morning reverie! I immediately sketched the scenario (Fig. 3) while it was still fresh in my mind and wrote several pages of notes to my colleague David Deamer. I knew, however, that the concept was still very much in the "hand waving" territory, until it was developed into a scientific proposal which included testable predictions.

Publish and Test, and Test Again

This process took just over a year for the vision to be landed in the scientific language of a hypothesis, an article to be drafted, proceeding through peer review, and first appearing in print in (Damer and Deamer, 2015).

For the next several years, Dave and I presented the scenario to colleagues around the world who had been unsatisfied with the longstanding hypothesis that life must have begun in the oceans at hydrothermal vents. We also began to take our science from the lab to the field, performing prebiotic chemistry at hot springs on three continents which were analogs for volcanic hydrothermal fields on the early Earth. With additional evidence accumulating, the conjecture morphed into a matured hypothesis which began to be tested by multiple laboratories. Dave and I then derived a more extensive scenario, broadened our testable predictions, and made a new case for the third, moist phase, in which we believe the first metabolic circuits might arise. Colleagues from multiple disciplines contributed to a "composite figure" (Fig. 4, left) which formed the explanatory core of our next publication: The Hot Spring Hypothesis for an Origin of Life (Damer and Deamer, 2020). This article was supported by a very nice cover image in the April 2020 issue of the journal *Astrobiology* depicting protocells cycling in a hot spring on a Hadean landscape, four billion years ago (Fig 4. right).

There is no substitute, and no other route to land the hypothetical products of visionary conceptions in science than patient hard work in close collaboration with specialists, and being

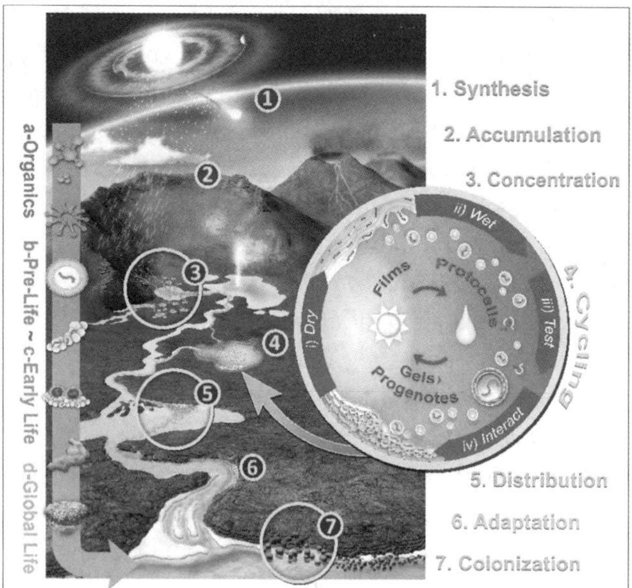

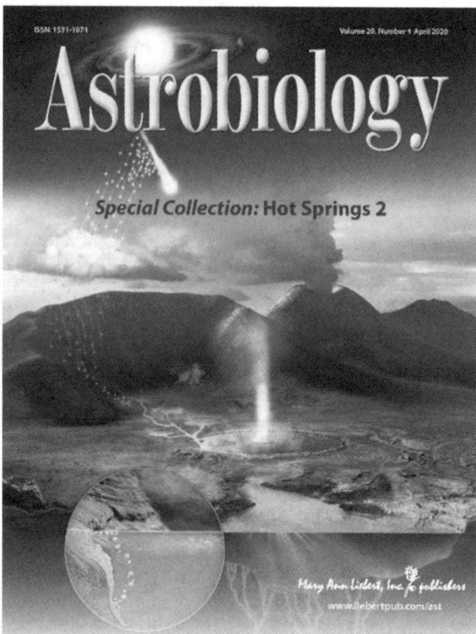

Fig. 4 Final rendition of the composite figure describing the "hot spring hypothesis" for an origin of life (left); Scenario depicted on the cover of the journal Astrobiology (right) which published the full hypothesis article in April, 2020. *Images courtesy Bruce Damer and Ryan Norkus, Mary Ann Liebert Inc. Publisher*

ever ready to receive criticism and respond to potential falsification from the data. Since 2020, increasing numbers of teams around the world have adopted the wet-dry cycling method pioneered by Dave Deamer and our group. Other stages of our end-to-end scenario have also begun to be tested. One of these is the recent confirmation that organics recovered from two sample return missions to asteroids did contain some of the organic compounds that would have been falling into our ancient hot little cycling pools (Yada et al. 2022). We have continued our field work as well and (Fig. 5 left) shows me performing cycling experiments at Fly Geyser in Nevada, USA with visual confirmation of films of silica, lipids and nucleotides drying down on our slides (right). When analyzed, samples like this show long strands of RNA, and even DNA which can become encapsulated in protocells (Hassenkam and Deamer, 2022).

From my first "endo trip" thought experiment at the age of fourteen, through a long string of visionary downloads over half a lifetime, followed by two decades of psychedelic experimentation as an admixture for the creative process, I am convinced that a well-crafted "endo & exo" creative practice can work wonders for problems in science, engineering and even the complex challenges faced by leadership.

TAKEAWAYS FROM A SCIENCE HIGH

Distilling decades of the pursuit of creative solutions, I feel some confidence to offer the following anecdotal extract of the practices that have worked in my case. None of this is yet grounded in neuroscience or models of cognition, yet they might be informative to formalize a future, better-defined practice. Seven distinct methodologies around *set, setting and setup* come to mind:

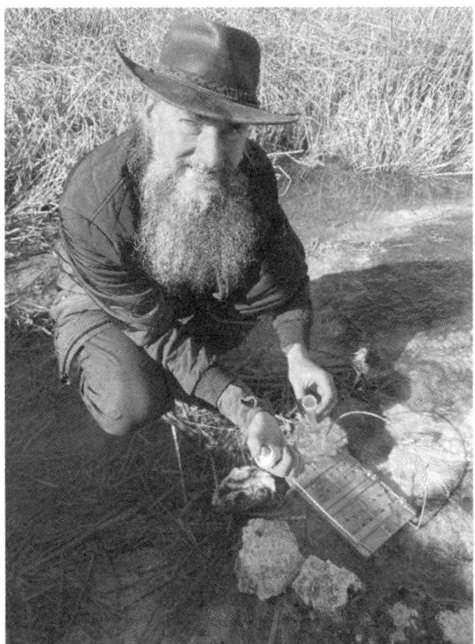

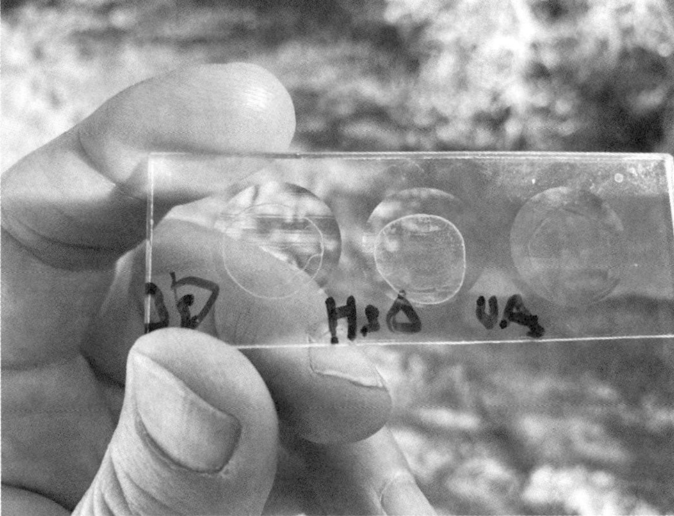

Fig. 5 Testing the hypothesis at Fly Geyser, Nevada, USA in December 2021 (left); Slide showing dry-down films of silica, lipids and nucleotides from Fly Geyser experiments (right).
Images courtesy Kathryn Lukas and Bruce Damer

1. *Holding the Kernel of Commitment*

Key to the start of my creative journey was a kernel storing my commitment and abiding passion for the pursuit of the problem. This kernel lives in a part of my psyche where has been held for forty years almost as a sacred trust. Even in times when the dream of working on the problem seemed very remote, I held to the question, patiently waiting for the right for the problem to be tackled.

2. *Paying Attention, Picking up Probabilistic Marbles and Taking Action*

At periods throughout my life, proverbial *probabilistic marbles of opportunity* would roll my way. Paying attention to their arrival, picking them up, and taking the actions they proscribed was always the right move to push my creative agenda forward. For example, in the late 1980s I was writing code to create a document design environment. One day, a Scientific American issue arrived on my doorstep with a special issue titled "artificial life" (A-Life). I picked up the code from one article and, as I had on my desk an early computer with a bit-mapped display, I could program that environment to run in high resolution. For months I studied fields of mobile, pixelated herbivores devouring virtual plants. I picked up the A-Life thread again in the late 1990s when I founded a working group called *Biota.org* and hosted a conference at the famous Burgess Shale fossil deposit in the Canadian Rockies. A speaker at that meeting, ecologist Tom Ray, demonstrated his *Tierra* A-Life environment. This interest and connection led to a meeting with renowned evolutionary biologist Richard Dawkins who was also working with A-Life. This in turn led to my PhD work on the EvoGrid and meetings with physicist Freeman Dyson, some of whose suggestions resulted in a stronger theoretical underpinning for the work with David

Deamer on the hot spring hypothesis. Failing to notice or pick up each of these and hundreds of other such lovely marbles would have likely irrevocably altered my course on this quest.

3. Embracing Youthful Endo-trips and Nurturing them into Adulthood

In my experience, endo-trips and their "downloads" can arrive spontaneously without an engaged practice or exogenously ingested substance. During childhood and my early teen years these downloads, along with a great deal of daydreaming, were part of my mental media landscape. With the social and intellectual challenges of middle and high school stacked up with hormonal changes, the frequency of such reveries became reduced. From my first endo-trips as a very internal, probably *Asperger* spectrum kid, I determined to keep this "secret inner landscape" alive. Starting to draw at age 12 was one technique paired with imagining entire worlds while walking in my neighborhood. After thousands of full color renderings of these worlds, I felt that I could visualize the moving parts of complex environments, including a board game I designed and ran in my head before fabricating the whole thing out of cardboard and glazed clay pieces. This was a form of self-training that became the foundation of all my adult career, from software development to science. Thus, the core practice of endo-tripping became baked into my creative practice and was well online before I added a psychedelic overlay in my late 30s. In fact, I believe that a non-psychedelic "endo" core dwells at the center and synthesizes my best insights in the free-association storm of a psychedelic melee.

4. Techniques to Pre-load, Run, and Shut Down Endo-trips

Endo-trips are not something new-fangled. I suggested earlier that they are well-chronicled in all manner of creative individuals and that Albert Einstein's thought experiments are perhaps their most famous example in science. I believe they are different from imaginative rumination, nighttime dreams, or lucid dreaming states. They have been described to me by others as wide-awake takeovers of conscious awareness; in most cases, the recipient being swept away into another world. They can come on after months, or years of pondering a problem, having preloaded one's mind with questions, clues, designs, data and notions. The better the quality and extent of pre-loading the more likely the endo-trip will produce a viable product. I find that for endo-trips to wend their way into my waking consciousness, I must be undisturbed, and unconcerned. Whether it be walking in the forest, mowing a lawn, engaging in breathwork or yoga, or lying in bed, a neutral and quiet state sets the stage. These trips take on a softer character than a full-blown psychedelic exo-journey, but can reach an impressive attention-grabbing intensity that for me can last from a few minutes to up to an hour. Their run rate seems to travel on an arc and when the endo-trip is running out of juice, I find it is best to gracefully let it go, shut down the process, and not yield to the temptation to let imagination grab hold and try to stretch it out.

5. A Cautionary Tale of Mixing Endo and Exo

From an early age, and possibly from my status as an adoptee, a kid on the spectrum and my particular arrangement of psychic parts, I was perhaps pre-adapted to enter and navigate the world of endo-trips. Having encountered paranoid schizophrenia in my family (and in my wife's family) I can offer caution around the fine line between constructive endo-tripping and harmful delusional or psychotic ideation. Perhaps endo-tripping is not possible for everyone and may require a specific neurotype and a home environment to nurture it. Waiting until I was in my late 30s before adding the overlay of psychedelics was an indication of my sense of the fragility and possible destabilization of my cognitive system. For the first few years of experimentation with psilocybin, MDMA, LSD, and other substances, I took what I felt to be a mental housekeeping step of "setting up a firewall" to protect my purported endo-tripping neuronal machinery. This may be a completely made-up notion on my part but I felt that even during high-dose experiences I should and could safeguard and shut down my so-called "envisionary consciousness." I recall the moment in 2013 in Peru on a low exo-dose of ayahuasca when I first "powered up" the endo-system within a psychedelic surround. That moment of merging these two modalities was significant for me as I could run an A/B comparison of how *endo* and *exo* manifested behind closed eyes. At the time I was attempting to obtain confirmation that endo-tripping was made possible by a flush of endogenous DMT by comparing the visual effects with an introduced low-dose of exogenously-sourced plant DMT (and other compounds). The decision to enable endo-tripping within the framework of a low-dose ayahuasca trip was instrumental in the healing and scientific breakthroughs described earlier. I would like to caution, however, that this interweaving of endo and exo practice may not be for everyone, and that my predilection for this may be unusual. However, it might be that psychedelics can augment ordinary waking consciousness in the absence of a capacity for endogenous reveries. This is grist for the mill of future research, which might start with the collection of experience reports to build a historical anecdotal understanding of *what is going on out there*?

6. Operating the Endo Observer, Recorder Camera, and Questioner

Given that you self-identify as experiencing productive endo-trips, or that you have entered into a creative visionary state on a psychedelically enabled exo-trip, or some combination of the two, what is the best way to operate your mental control panel during the download phase? From an early age, when an endo-trip took control of my cognitive stick-shift, I decided to both fully immerse in the ride, but maintain my own, separate observer which would neutrally watch and record the journey. I have later learned that the holding of an observer is widely promoted in Buddhism, especially in meditation and other practices. This observer view is especially important in healing practices such as IFS (Internal Family Systems) therapy. One of the jobs of the observer is to provide a safe platform so that the trip does not completely take over the view of self, of time, and of the world. If awareness joins with the parts of oneself and falls into the trip, the tripper might begin to believe that this is their only reality and enter into a state of panic or despair. Another job for the observer is to operate what I called a *high-speed visoneering camera* to record the entire "endo-movie". In some intense hourlong experiences my observer has made it possible for me to "pause" the trip itself, open a notebook, draw and take notes. Closing my eyes again I found that the movie of the trip had advanced into a new scene but I was still able to dive back in. Lastly, the observer can listen to conversation, and mediate questions into the space of the endo-trip. For instance, I could pose questions like: "why are we in colder, darker water, what is happening here?" and the endo-machinery would visually deliver an answer, in that particular case showing stable protocells merging, illustrating a possible early chemical form of sexual recombination.

7. Rendering and Post-processing Endo Deliveries

As the storm of an endo-trip recedes, I let it go gracefully, keeping the mind empty and in many cases reaching for a notebook and pencils to draw some of the visions, often capturing their cinematic nature frame-by-frame. A few scribbled points can scaffold a longer essay where in a stream of words the experience is laid down like a studio track. I strive to not embellish the memory, but to capture the images and feelings as faithfully as possible, even if there are bizarre or incomplete elements. If the vision came with a psycho-spiritual personal insight, I often "re-trip" the experience from still-fresh memory by making an audio recording, voicing the emotional content to its fullness. These practices serve not only to transcribe the experience but also to re-render it such that subsequently, even years later, the endo-trip can be recalled and re-run. I have found that building up a remembered library of "trip-takes" provides something extraordinary: the ability to engage in multi-stage problem solving. By appending experiences together like chapters in a book, and re-tripping them later as a single-story stream as I did with my time-reversal journey through life's ancestry, the next chapter has a much higher probability of emerging. This method works for multi-stage problems or ones containing subsumed detail that must be revealed like the peeling of an onion. Complex scientific solutions like the standard model of particle physics, or a plausible scenario for an origin of life require such a multi-stage, multi-layered approach. The class of highly challenging problems facing Humanity from climate change, viral pandemics and the complications of our psyches might just fit the bill for this approach. I hope that the practices I have tested and reported here might be adapted by others to tackle these existentially important challenges.

Dusting off my drawings and notes a decade after they were first sketched, I am struck by how fresh they all still appear. By not embellishing or drifting from these visions, instead keeping them preserved like insects in amber, they can continue to be a source for new directions, and new science. For example, in the ayahuasca vision, my attention was grabbed by the mysterious budding, dark vesicle and I only briefly focused on the motion of an undulating polymer. This year, a new student joined our group at UC Santa Cruz and the BIOTA Institute and is returning to the question posed by that polymer, taking up the first steps of testing templating of RNA instructions from DNA in hot spring conditions. I will take a new trip to visit that part of the original protocell division experience to see if there are clues for our next laboratory approaches to uncovering mechanisms leading to the origin of genes.

AN AGENDA FOR PSY-SOLUTIONING?

I hope that the above anecdotal sharing of my own experiences might provide some input for future colleagues who could truly formalize hypotheses and approaches around the role of psychedelics in high states of creative problem solving. Moving forward with an agenda and some next steps, perhaps we could first adopt a stand-in term for this endeavor, perhaps "psy-solutioning?"

Harman and Fadiman (1970) summarized their 1966 pilot study with a follow-up review "Selective Enhancement of Specific Capacities Through Psychedelic Training" providing three key questions which might move a psy-solutioning agenda forward in the 2020s:

1. Can the psychedelic experience enhance creative problem-solving ability, and if so, what is the evidence of enhancement?
2. Can this result in enhanced production of concrete, valid, and feasible psy-solutions assessable by the pragmatic criteria of modern industry and positivistic science?
3. Working with a non-clinical population and with a non-therapy orientation, would there nevertheless result demonstrable long-term personality changes indicative of continued increased creativity and self-actualization?

At the ESPD55 meeting I took the liberty of suggesting the following for the anatomy of a psy-solutioning session. This straw-person protocol is based upon my own experience and should only be taken as a starting point.

Prepare the mind, pose the question, engage in extensive reading in the subject area, but also off-axis into other fields which might have a bearing. Take up other activities with nothing to do with the problem, adopt a problem-tackling approach like the one put forward in Zen & the Art of Motorcycle Maintenance (Pirsig, 1999).

Patiently await the right moment as an endo-trip may spontaneously occur after some months, or solutions may arise during an endo-exo experience. Also important is the "digestion and rest time", which cannot be rushed.

Practices during the trip (post-peak intensity of an ingested substance):

- Surrender, quieten the mind, pay attention.
- Allow endo to meet exo in a free association storm.
- Anneal the insight, receive, record, re-trip and draw, write or otherwise render a record of the downloaded vision.

Translate the download into the language of science, engineering, or leadership and then share with peers for a quality critique.

Develop a serious proposal, collaborate, publish, and then test the proposed hypotheses, product designs or organizational methodologies in the real world.

Iterate and wait, propose, publish and iterate again.

If this is not the end of the story, or the fullest exploration of the hypothesis, return to the question, re-trip previous endo-experiences, consider a new carefully planned session with the intention of adding new chapters and develop a next stage for testing.

Be prepared for an ever-deepening level of exploration. Sometimes these inquiries can touch on the infinite.

This article called for the opening of a "fourth path" in psychedelic research and practice in: *altering states for creative breakthroughs in technical fields*. Given that the first three paths could be understood as: indigenous and cultural use; personal growth and expression; and therapeutic applications, how can a community be catalyzed around this next path?

I might suggest that we have some idea of who the "clients" or "practitioners" might be but who would be the overall stakeholders? Does the constituency for psy-solutioning include a wide swath of society or a narrow one? Could this research be broadly carried out amongst scientists and technologists in labs and startup companies, Fortune 500 firms, students and professors at colleges and universities, and also within government agencies? The "psy-curious" abound in these worlds, together with a strong need for creative, out-of-the-box thinking. Would psy-solutioning clinical trials such as those carried out by Harman, Mason, and by future workers fall inside or outside of existing psychedelic therapeutic research into treatments for trauma, anxiety, PTSD, and other conditions? Would an objective be to eventually staff "psy-solutioning clinics or retreats?" To get started, could psy-solutioning sessions be added as a module in the latter stages of government sanctioned psychedelic-assisted psychotherapy? Who would regulate this space and what would constitute legal and normative practices? And last, but not least, who would the financial backers be?

Next Steps?

Might we best begin this initiative by sponsoring an open and anonymous survey to invite psy-solutioning practitioners to file their own experience reports and establish a body of historical data for the practices, and the eventual science?

I'd like to conclude by calling for collaboration and the formation of a working group of advisors, commentators, experts, students and those with practical experience to take the next steps toward *validation* and *valorization* of psy-solutioning as a worthwhile endeavor in society.

RECKONING WITH THE EXTREME ENDS OF GENIUS

We are all familiar with the productive contributions of genius to society throughout our history. However, some of the behaviors of highly creative persons can veer into the territory of psychopathology. The popular idea that "madness and genius are often close bedfellows" is borne out by studies in which "creative people and people suffering from mental disorders appear to share some common personality and cognitive traits" (Fink et al. 2012). Two extreme ends of genius in society are worth noting as more proposals to engage in clinical studies and promote the use of psychedelics in highly creative, yet possibly problematic individuals.

Genius Lost

We are all familiar with impassioned and bright solo individuals proposing their own "theory of everything." We find them isolated and quiet or perhaps more public, transforming themselves into storytellers or even gurus of a sort. They may have pounded on the doors of the Academy to then be somehow rejected, or never sought education beyond a few years at college, or lacked a mentor or collaborator to help shape their thinking. Without the "hazing" of defending one's PhD thesis to a tough review committee, the brutal knocks of grant writing and rejection, the discipline and grit of pulling long hours at the bench or breaking rocks in harsh locations, the hopeful dreamer cannot be transformed into a productive scientist. With no peer review, and no testable experiments proposed, their life's work is destined to be ignored and lost, or worse, converted into a form of quasi-religious system, similar to those chronicled in Manly P. Hall's epic encyclopedia *The Secret Teachings of All Ages* (1973).

Physicist Sabine Hossenfelder, a research fellow at the Frankfurt Institute for Advanced Studies, encountered such individuals first hand. For a time, she hung out a shingle as "as a hired consultant to autodidact physicists" (Hossenfelder, 2016). Dozens of self-taught individuals contacted her for consulting sessions. They were uniformly lacking in the tools of the trade (especially mathematics), understanding of current science, and put forth proposals emerging from isolated ideation, often expressed as elaborate colored drawings with a smattering of equations. The demarcation between real science, scientists and serious work, and these pseudoscience proposals was quite stark. This was not a formal study and none of Hossenfelder's clients were reported to have derived their visions using psychedelics. It might well be that the increasing use of psychedelics in the general population will produce new harvests of pseudoscience and their close cousins, conspiracy theories.

Regardless of the source of any insight about the workings of reality, it must run the gauntlet of formal training and testable hypotheses and vetting within a scientific community of peers. Without structure, mentorship and other guidance, institutional support, translation of their insights into serious proposals for funding, and follow-through (and in some cases, mental health support) many potential "genius level" producers are lost to society, and often to themselves. Even within academic environments, potential genius can be snuffed out through politics or misunderstanding. It is likely that perhaps only a few percent (or less) of those capable of major technical or scientific breakthroughs are ever able to express their potential gifts. In this time of major challenges to Human civilization, of complexity beyond the capacity of day-to-day coping strategies, of planetary ecosystems entering into convulsions, can we afford to waste any potential genius in our ranks? Perhaps these individuals should be sought out, resourced, and if appropriate, given access to the healing, and the revealing powers of psychedelics.

Evil Genius

As the 1960s wound down, so wilted the rose of a psychedelically fueled *Eleusinian return* so colorfully described by the chronicler Patrick Lundborg (2012). An archetypal dark figure from this time was Charles Manson who, through his followers, effected a half dozen grisly murders in Los Angeles in 1969. Recent revisiting of case files and new extant evidence established a link between Manson's use of LSD and these events, possibly provided through a program supported by the US Government (O'Neill, 2019). LSD researcher David Smith reported that the change in Manson's personality "was the most abrupt [another researcher] Roger Smith had observed in his entire professional career" (Smith, 1971). Subsequently Manson began preaching a philosophy surrounding a coming race war based on a conspiratorial mashup of the science fiction novel Stranger in a Strange Land, the Bible, Scientology, Dale Carnegie, and the Beatles (Guinn, 2013). This garnered him the cult following that would later execute the widely publicized murders.

Psychologists Paulhus and Williams (2002) have proposed a "dark triad" of personality traits "three conceptually distinct but empirically overlapping personality variables... Machiavellianism, narcissism and subclinical psychopathy [which] often show differential correlates but share a common core of callous-manipulation" (Furnham et al. 2013). Perhaps this dark triad is a likely marker for potential "evil" practitioners who pluck poisoned fruits from the verdant tree of psychedelic inspiration. Charles Manson may be an exemplar and a warning of what can happen when the dark triad meets the ego-amplification and delusion-enhancing capacity of psychedelics.

Before psychedelics hit the local pharmacy, we might ask: "can we afford to vastly expand the population of evil geniuses walking the streets, running companies and leading countries?" Personality maps and pre-session screening as well as introspective training are already being developed within protocols for MDMA-assisted psychotherapy. Methodologies such as IFS have been selected (Whitfield, 2021) to permit patients a deeper introspection on what Michael Mithoefer (2013) calls the "multiplicity of the psyche." It seems our minds are not unitary but made up of "parts," also referred to in psychiatry as "dissociation," "sub-personalities," "selves," and "complexes." At the extreme manifestations of multiplicity, we find dissociative identity disorders and other pathologies. When deeply suppressed parts do emerge, a state ensues that healers and shamans throughout history have named a "possession" by demons, angels, or animal spirits.

Perhaps IFS and other preparatory practices can cushion the full shock to the system of "what shows up" for the psychedelically naïve and guide even those carrying the burdens of the dark triad to navigate toward positive outcomes. The recent implementation of several school-based anti-bullying programs (Ferguson et al. 2007) have valorized the norm that it might just be OK to "screen and intervene" for those capable of future grave misdeeds within society. From vast human casualties caused by strongmen demagogues to school shooters, untreated psychopathy and traumas call to us from the headlines to consider psychedelics as critical tool for such intervention. Our very survival as a civilization and species may depend upon their widespread therapeutic use especially among those who, through innate traits of personality, might be destined to become our future leadership.

RE-IGNITION

The psychedelic renaissance is considered by many to be something very newborn, of and for our time. Yet the use of psychoactive substances likely suffused of all human history and has underpinned much of our spiritual, and intellectual development even well before antiquity. Perhaps it is we who are myopic to its presence all around us, despite the absence of these practices for a half millennium in the West and other parts of the world. The forces that led to the end of ancient mystery schools, shamanic practices, and the healing arts of women, temporarily scrubbed our memories of the pivotal role of trance states and their attendant potions. Brian Muraresku (2020) built on the earlier works of Wasson, Hoffman and Ruck (1978, 2008) reporting on new evidence that the great mystery school at Eleusis in Greece provided psychedelic visionary rites to many who went on to fashion civilization in the Mediterranean. If this is the case, along with Plato and other initiants present in the Telesterion temple sat the engineers who conceived of grand aqueducts, the geometers who calculated the diameter of the Earth, and the political architects who created the first representative governments of the Greek and Roman worlds.

In concluding this exploration, one of the most remarkable subject reports from the Harman study came from an architect and is worth repeating here to understand the indisputable potential of these tools. Sometime following his peak experience and after taking up his psychedelic creativity session, he reported:

> *"I looked at the paper I was to draw on. I was completely blank. I knew that I would work with a property 300 ft. square. I drew the property lines .... Suddenly I saw the finished project. I did some quick calculations .... it would fit on the property and not only that . . . it would meet the cost and income requirements . . . it would park enough cars.., it met all the requirements. I visualized the result I wanted and subsequently brought the variables into play which could bring that result about. I had great visual (mental) perceptibility; I could imagine what was wanted, needed, or not possible with almost no effort. In what seemed like ten minutes I had completed the problem . . . I was amazed at my idealism, my visual perception, and the rapidity with which I could operate."*

Harman and colleagues then offered this reflection (with my **emphasis**):

> *"Bertrand Russell once remarked that in the discovery of the theory of relativity, Einstein began with a* ***kind of mystical or poetical insight into the*** *truth which took the form of* ***visualizing the totality of the law in all its ramifications****. The* ***Gestalt view*** *conceives creativity as an action which produces* ***a new idea or "insight" full-formed****; it comes to the individual* ***in a flash****. Similarly, the* ***illuminating flash of insight*** *in which the completed solution is grasped in its entirety constitutes the most distinctive feature of Rugg's '****transliminal*** *experience' and Maslow's '****peak*** *experience.'"*

As the psychedelic community reignites this inquiry so wrongly and forcibly abandoned a half century ago, we will mine rich veins of philosophy, forge a theory of mind fully baked with a novel modern mysticism, and speak again in the poetry of transcendental states. Perhaps through new initiatives that might be undertaken by you, dear readers, we can ignite a psychedelic culture in which the **medicines of healing** can also serve as the **elixirs of discovery.**

EPILOGUE: LEST WE FORGET!

In my experience, and perhaps yours as well, the pragmatic products of visionary reverie must cross a liminal boundary from majestic whole-cloth realization to become transmuted into a more plain and oftentimes pedantic form. The transcendent beauty of an equation that defines the structure of the universe, or a chemical cycle that has the power to initiate life must land in the proscribed, bland language of peer-reviewed journal articles and testable hypotheses. To reify the products of genius in our world, their original grand conception is destined to be whittled down and reinterpreted into the language of science, engineering, and business. Yet, if we hold in our minds a carefully preserved record of the original vision of their conception, we can retain a connection to the source of their being. This is precious as it provides water for the long trek across the desert of implementation, and at the end of that long road, gives us buttoned-down technocrats our own private feast of spiritual sustenance. I find that as I revisit carefully stashed reveries, they provide a ready supply of unexplored avenues for my ongoing scientific work. In other words, a careful and faithfully filed visionary entry into our mental media library can remit a long-term annuity.

This is the path some of us choose, to take a ride on the mystical side and manifest its magic into working widgets in our day-to-day reality. Perhaps many more of us can become liminal surfers on the wave between the fully witnessed essence of the psychedelic light and the brilliant incarnations of science and technology. For me, there is no irreconcilable gap between these two great magisteria. We encounter their pure forms in visionary experience, each flowing into the other with equanimity. Perhaps then, one day the "mystic scientist" will gaze into a mirror, give a wink to the "scientific mystic" peering back, and go on to fearlessly and lovingly remake the world.

All of this said, there is an ineffable elephant patiently drumming his trunk in our psychedelic drawing room: the extraordinarily otherworldly reality of the full-blown psychedelic peak state, which Sasha and Ann Shulgin referred to as a "Plus 4" experience (Shulgin and Shulgin, 1995). Often, these peak states cannot be "Englished" in the words of psychedelic raconteur Terence McKenna (who may nonetheless have successfully "Irished" them). After we experience Terence's "death by astonishment" we draw a breath and slide off the peak, oftentimes hardly remembering that we had just merged with some version of the totality of the universe. The products of endo-exo visionary renderings may nonetheless join us on the downslope off the peak, or later as we come to rest in the far hills of integration. The products are gifts of, but in no way can fairly represent the enormity of that place from whence they emerged. So perhaps, we should take a moment honor the elephant, lest we forget its presence. It may provide the gravitas and the mind manifesting dissolution we need to return as humbled yet hopeful children of the cosmos, seeking to do something in our short lives to return the favor of our remarkable existence.

The elephant has been touched by innumerable blind men and women who offer their own description of what it actually is, but this tribute by George Andrews, excerpted from his full poem *Annihilating Illumination* from the Psychedelic Reader (1965), hints at the true ineffable depths and scale of its genius (and ours):

"I am alive within the living God
I throb unique among the infinite variations
and so what if all the evolution of consciousness only leads to the knowledge
that I am a germ in the guts of a greater being
I am older than creation, older than all beings
the stars revolve within me
I voyage through the inner space between my atoms
I take space ships to the different parts of my body
each organ becomes a constellation as I spread across the sky
wheeling through the zodiac, weaving the fate of future races
I conceive a cosmos where life does not need to kill to live
create a system free from pain

And in the spawn and seethe of the primeval ocean
out of chaos I pass the current
immortal diamonds shimmering on the foam of the instant now"

AFTERWORD

This chapter and the ESPD55 talk on which it is based became catalysts for the formation of a new non-profit research organization, the Center for MINDS (Multidisciplinary Investigation into Novel Discoveries and Solutions) established in September 2023 in Austin, Texas. Modeled partly on MAPS and with support and guidance from many in the psychedelic community, MINDS has taken its first baby steps, funding a study at the University of Texas on psilocybin's impact on memory fluency, hosting a workshop for UK researchers at Broughton Sanctuary, presenting many conference talks and podcasts, and developing a roster of upcoming scientific meetings and programs. Manesh Girn, an author cited here, joined MINDS as Scientific Director and is developing a white paper to help platform and catalyze the newly emerging field of psychedelically-catalyzed insight and creative problem solving. I would like to thank Dennis McKenna who joined MINDS as an early advisor and look forward to providing updates on this emerging science at future ESPD meetings. More information on MINDS including a substantial database of personal stories, news items, documentaries, studies, and events can be found at centerforminds.org.

ACKNOWLEDGEMENTS

The author would like to thank Dennis McKenna and the entire McKenna Academy for their kind invitation to participate in the ESPD55 meeting and my wife, Kathryn Lukas-Damer for her support in this very personal telling of my story. Additional thanks go to Rebecca Lazarou for her kind hand in helping to edit this novel synthesis.

BIBLIOGRAPHY

Abraham, Ralph. 2008. "Mathematics and the psychedelic revolution." MAPS 18, no. 1:6-8.

Andreasen, N. C. 2005. The creating brain: The neuroscience of genius. Dana Press.

Baggott, Matthew J. 2015. "Psychedelics and creativity: a review of the quantitative literature." PeerJ PrePrints 3: e1202v1.

Barron, F. 1962. Creativity and psychological health. Princeton: Van Nostrand, 1963. Bruner, J.S. *On knowing*. Cambridge, Mass.: Harvard Univ. Press.

Barron, F. 1965. The creative process and the psychedelic experience. *Explorations Magazine*, 4(2), 48-51.

Behle, Anika E., and Martin Pinquart. 2016. "Psychiatric disorders and treatment in adoptees: A meta-analytic comparison with non-adoptees." Adoption Quarterly 19, no. 4: 284-306.

Bornemann, Joel. 2020. "The viability of microdosing psychedelics as a strategy to enhance cognition and well-being—an early review." Journal of Psychoactive Drugs 52, no. 4: 300-308.

Carhart-Harris, Robin L., and Karl J. Friston. 2010. "The default-mode, ego-functions and free-energy: a neurobiological account of Freudian ideas." Brain 133, no. 4: 1265-1283.

Carhart-Harris, Robin L., David Erritzoe, Tim Williams, James M. Stone, Laurence J. Reed, Alessandro Colasanti, Robin J. Tyacke et al. 2012. "Neural correlates of the psychedelic state as determined by fMRI studies with psilocybin." Proceedings of the National Academy of Sciences 109, no. 6: 2138-2143.

Carhart-Harris, R., R. Leech, and E. Tagliazucchi. 2014. "How do hallucinogens work on the brain." Journal of Psychophysiology 71, no. 1: 2-8.

Carhart-Harris, Robin L., and KJ Friston. 2019. "REBUS and the anarchic brain: toward a unified model of the brain action of psychedelics." Pharmacological reviews 71, no. 3: 316-344.

Christoff, Kalina, Zachary C. Irving, Kieran CR Fox, R. Nathan Spreng, and Jessica R. Andrews-Hanna. 2016. "Mind-wandering as spontaneous thought: a dynamic framework." Nature Reviews Neuroscience 17, no. 11: 718-731.

Damer, B. 1999. "The Virtual AllChemical Powwow" Available online: https://digitalspace.com/damer.com/projects/fan-terencem/index.html (accessed 23 October 2022).

Damer, B. 2011. "TIMELINES The DigiBarn computer museum: a personal passion for personal computing." Interactions 18, no. 3: 72-74.

Damer, B. 2011. Curator note from a catalogue of the Timothy Leary extant archives.

Damer, Bruce Frederick. 2011. "The EVOGRID: An Approach to Computational Origins of Life Endevours." PhD diss., University College Dublin.

Damer, Bruce, Peter Newman, Ryan Norkus, John Graham, Richard Gordon, and Tom Barbalet. 2012. "Cyberbiogenesis and the EvoGrid: A twenty-first century grand challenge." In *Genesis-In The Beginning*, pp. 267-288. Springer, Dordrecht.

Damer, Bruce, and David Deamer. 2015. "Coupled phases and combinatorial selection in fluctuating hydrothermal pools: A scenario to guide experimental approaches to the origin of cellular life." Life 5, no. 1: 872-887.

Damer, Bruce. 2016. "A field trip to the Archaean in search of Darwin's warm little pond." Life 6, no. 2: 21.

Damer, B. 2019. "David Deamer: Five Decades of Research on the Question of How Life Can Begin." Life 9, no. 2: 36.

Damer, Bruce, and David Deamer. 2020. "The hot spring hypothesis for an origin of life." Astrobiology 20, no. 4: 429-452.

Darwin C. 1871. Darwin Correspondence Project, "Letter No. 7471". Available online: http://www.darwinproject.ac.uk/DCP-LETT-7471 (accessed 23 October 2022).

Deamer, David W. 1985. "Boundary structures are formed by organic components of the Murchison carbonaceous chondrite." Nature 317, no. 6040: 792-794.

Deamer, David, Bruce Damer, and Vladimir Kompanichenko. 2019. "Hydrothermal chemistry and the origin of cellular life." Astrobiology 19, no. 12: 1523-1537.

Deamer, David, Francesca Cary, and Bruce Damer. 2022. "Urability: A Property of Planetary Bodies That Can Support an Origin of Life." Astrobiology.

Deamer, David, Simonis, Povilas, and Damer, Bruce. 2024. Assembly of membranous compartments: An essential step in the emergence and function of protocellular systems in V.Kolb (ed.). *Guidebook for Systems Applications in Astrobiology*. Forthcoming. CRC Press.

Einstein, A. 1920. Volume 7: The Berlin Years: Writings, 1918-1921 (English translation supplement) P. 136. Accessed 10-23-2022 from the Collected Papers of Albert Einstein: https://einsteinpapers.press.princeton.edu/

Eisner, B. 1997. Set, setting, and matrix. Journal of Psychoactive Drugs, 29(2), 213-216.

Fadiman, J. 2011. The psychedelic explorer's guide: Safe, therapeutic, and sacred journeys. Simon and Schuster.

Fadiman, James, and Sophia Korb. 2019. "Microdosing psychedelics." Advances in Psychedelic Medicine: State-of-the-Art Therapeutic Applications 318.

Ferguson, Christopher J., Claudia San Miguel, John C. Kilburn Jr, and Patricia Sanchez. 2007. "The effectiveness of school-based anti-bullying programs: A meta-analytic review." Criminal Justice Review 32, no. 4: 401-414.

Fink, Andreas, Mirjam Slamar-Halbedl, Human F. Unterrainer, and Elisabeth M. Weiss. 2012. "Creativity: Genius, madness, or a combination of both?." Psychology of Aesthetics, Creativity, and the Arts 6, no. 1: 11.

Friston, Karl. 2010. "The free-energy principle: a unified brain theory?." Nature reviews neuroscience 11, no. 2: 127-138.

Furnham, Adrian, Steven C. Richards, and Delroy L. Paulhus. 2013. "The Dark Triad of personality: A 10 year review." Social and personality psychology compass 7, no. 3: 199-216.

Gardner, Howard, and Thomas Hatch. 1989. "Educational implications of the theory of multiple intelligences." Educational researcher 18, no. 8: 4-10.

Gardner, Howard E. 2011. Frames of mind: The theory of multiple intelligences. Basic books.

Gardner, Martin. 1970. " The fantastic combinations of John Conway's new solitaire game 'life'" Sc. Am. 223: 20-123.

Girn, Manesh, Caitlin Mills, Leor Roseman, Robin L. Carhart-Harris, and Kalina Christoff. 2020. "Updating the dynamic framework of thought: Creativity and psychedelics." Neuroimage 213: 116726.

Guinn, Jeff. 2013. Manson: The Life and Times of Charles Manson. Simon & Schuster. P. 95

Harman WW, McKim RH, Mogar RE, Fadiman J, Stolaroff, MJ. 1966. Psychedelic agents in creative problem-solving: a pilot study. *Psychol Rep.*;19(1):211-27. doi: 10.2466/pr0.1966.19.1.211. PMID: 5942087.

Harman, W., and Fadiman J. 1970. "Selective enhancement of specific capacities through psychedelic training." from PSYCHEDELICS, The Uses and Implications of Hallucinogenic Drugs. Bernard Aaronson and Humphrey Osmond, editors, Doubleday & Company.

Hassenkam, Tue, and David Deamer. 2022 "Visualizing RNA polymers produced by hot wet-dry cycling."

Heard, G. in Weil, Gunther M., Ralph Metzner, and Timothy Leary, eds. 1965. *The psychedelic reader.* University Books.

Hodges, James A. 2019. "Comparing born-digital artefacts using bibliographical archeology: a survey of Timothy Leary's published software (1985–1996)".

Hossenfelder, S. 2016. "What I learned as a hired consultant to autodidact physicists. Aeon.".
Huxley, A. 1954. The Doors of Perception New York. Harpers.
Isaacson, W. 2011. Steve Jobs. Simon & Schuster.
Hall, Manly P. 1973. The secret teachings of all ages. Lulu.com.
Kuypers, K. P. C. 2018. "Out of the box: A psychedelic model to study the creative mind." Medical Hypotheses 115: 13-16.
Letheby, Chris. 2016. "The epistemic innocence of psychedelic states." Consciousness and cognition 39: 28-37.
Lundborg, Patrick. 2012. Psychedelia: An ancient culture, a modern way of life. Lysergia.
Markoff, John. 2005. What the dormouse said: How the sixties counterculture shaped the personal computer industry. Penguin.
Mason, N. L., K. P. C. Kuypers, J. T. Reckweg, F. Müller, D. H. Y. Tse, B. Da Rios, S. W. Toennes, P. Stiers, A. Feilding, and J. G. Ramaekers. 2021. "Spontaneous and deliberate creative cognition during and after psilocybin exposure." *Translational psychiatry 11*, no. 1: 1-13.
McKenna, T. 1998. From a talk "Dreaming Awake at the End of Time".San Francisco, December 13, 1998. Text sourced online from: https://www.organism.earth/library/document/dreaming-awake-at-the-end-of-time. (accessed 8 June 2023).
Mithoefer, Michael. 2013. "MDMA-assisted psychotherapy: How different is it from other psychotherapy." Manifesting minds: A review of psychedelics in science, medicine, sex, and spirituality 125.
Mullis KB 2000 Dancing Naked in the Mind Field. New York: Vintage Books.
Muraresku, Brian C. 2020 The Immortality Key: The Secret History of the Religion with No Name. St. Martin's Press.
Norton, J.D. 2013. "Chasing the Light: Einstein's Most Famous Thought Experiment" in Frappier, Mélanie, Letitia Meynell, and James Robert Brown, eds. *Thought experiments in philosophy, science, and the arts*. Vol. 11. Routledge.
Nichols, David E. 2016. "Psychedelics." Pharmacological reviews 68, no. 2: 264-355.
O'Neill, Tom. 2019. Chaos: Charles Manson, the CIA, and the Secret History of the Sixties. Hachette UK.
Palhano-Fontes, Fernanda, Katia C. Andrade, Luis F. Tofoli, Antonio C. Santos, Jose Alexandre S. Crippa, Jaime EC Hallak, Sidarta Ribeiro, and Draulio B. de Araujo. 2015. "The psychedelic state induced by ayahuasca modulates the activity and connectivity of the default mode network." PloS one 10, no. 2: e0118143.
Paulhus, Delroy L., and Kevin M. Williams. 2002 "The dark triad of personality: Narcissism, Machiavellianism, and psychopathy." Journal of research in personality 36, no. 6: 556-563.
Pirsig, Robert M. 1999 Zen and the art of motorcycle maintenance: An inquiry into values. Random House.
Pollan, M. 2018. How to change your mind: What the new science of psychedelics teaches us about consciousness, dying, addiction, depression, and transcendence. Penguin.
Rajamani S., Vlassov A., Benner S., Coombs A., Olasagasti F., Deamer D.W. 2008. Lipid-assisted synthesis of RNA-like polymers from mononucleotides. *Orig. Life Evol. Biosph.* 38:57-74.
Runco, Mark A. 2019. "Creativity as a dynamic, personal, parsimonious process." In Dynamic perspectives on creativity, pp. 181-188. Springer, Cham.
Sessa, Ben. "Is it time to revisit the role of psychedelic drugs in enhancing human creativity?." Journal of Psychopharmacology 22, no. 8 2008: 821-827.
Shulgin, A.T. and Shulgin, A., 1995. PIHKAL: a chemical love story (p. 978). Berkeley: Transform Press.
Shulgin, A. T., T. Manning, and P. F. Daley. 2011. "The Shulgin Index: Volume One.".
Simonton, D. K. 1999. Origins of genius: Darwinian perspectives on creativity. Oxford University Press.
Simonton, Dean Keith. 2004. Creativity in science: Chance, logic, genius, and zeitgeist. Cambridge University Press.
Smith, David E; Luce, John 1971. Love Needs Care: A History of San Francisco's Haight-Ashbury Free Medical Clinic and Its Pioneer Role Treating Drug-abuse Problems. Boston, Little, Brown. Retrieved April 30, 2021. p. 257
Wasson, G., A. Hoffman, and C. Ruck. 1978. The Road to Eleusis. New York: Harcourt Brace Jovanovich, Inc.
Wasson, R. Gordon, Albert Hofmann, and Carl AP Ruck. (2008) The road to Eleusis: Unveiling the secret of the mysteries. North Atlantic Books.
Weil, A., Rosen, W. 1993, From Chocolate To Morphine: Everything You Need To Know About Mind-Altering Drugs. New York, Houghton Mifflin Company. p. 93.
Wießner, I., Falchi, M., Maia, L. O., Daldegan-Bueno, D., Palhano-Fontes, F., Mason, N. L., ... & Tófoli, L. F. 2022. LSD and creativity: Increased novelty and symbolic thinking, decreased utility and convergent thinking. Journal of Psychopharmacology, 36(3), 348-359.
Whitfield, Henry J. 2021. "A Spectrum of Selves reinforced in multilevel coherence: A Contextual Behavioural response to the challenges of psychedelic-assisted therapy development." Frontiers in psychiatry: 2095.
Woese, Carl R., and George E. Fox. 1977. "Phylogenetic structure of the prokaryotic domain: the primary kingdoms." Proceedings of the National Academy of Sciences 74, no. 11: 5088-5090.
Yada, Toru, Masanao Abe, Tatsuaki Okada, Aiko Nakato, Kasumi Yogata, Akiko Miyazaki, Kentaro Hatakeda et al. 2022. "Preliminary analysis of the Hayabusa2 samples returned from C-type asteroid Ryugu." Nature Astronomy 6, no. 2: 214-220.

Beyond the Doors of Perception: What Else Can William Blake Tell Us about How Psychedelics Work?

David Nutt, PhD

Professor of Neuropsychopharmacology and Head of the Centre for Psychedelic Research, Division of Psychiatry, Imperial College London

"Our recent neuroimaging studies of depressed patients recovering after psilocybin treatment reveals that the increased connectivity seen during the trip persists for weeks afterwards and is associated with increased flexibility of brain function, an outcome not seen with traditional antidepressant treatments." —David Nutt

David Nutt shares with us how psychedelics work both in the brain and clinically. He also shares a fascinating perspective on how artist, poet and thought leader William Blake from England in the 1700's is connected to the psychedelics movement.

Many people are aware that Aldous Huxley used a famous phrase from William Blake as the title of his first book on the psychedelic experience—*The Doors of Perception*. The title of his later book on psychedelics, "Heaven and Hell," was also taken from one of Blake's works "The Marriage of Heaven and Hell." Clearly Blake had a major impact on Huxley's understanding of the impact of psychedelics on his mind. As a child Huxley had had ambitions to become a scientist like many of his family (his half-brother Andrew Huxley later won the Nobel Prize for medicine and physiology), but eye problems precluded this possibility, so he turned to the study of literature whilst keeping close to science.

Like Huxley I encountered Blake before psychedelics, in my case via his "Songs of Innocence and Experience" that were being studied at the time (1968) by my then girlfriend Jan. When I went up to Cambridge in 1969, she and I visited an exhibition of his paintings at the Fitzwilliam Museum where I discovered Blake was also an artist. But it wasn't until I started reading the works of Aldous Huxley that the importance of Blake's writings for him became apparent and I began to reflect further on Blake's insights and philosophy of the mind. More recently as my own research on psychedelics has developed, they have helped me make sense of the effects of psychedelic drugs on the workings of the human mind.

In this chapter I review how modern neuroscience studies on psychedelics have revealed Blake's insights to have been extraordinarily prescient. I then explore some of the other writings and art of Blake that further help us understand the human mind and how psychedelics may work to change these, ending with the tension between science and feelings that underpinned Blake's disagreements with Newton.

THE NEUROSCIENCE OF PSYCHEDELICS

The last ten years have provided a revolution in the science of psychedelics. One of the prime movers of this has been a series of brain imaging studies, mostly fMRI but also EEG/MEG, that have revealed an unexpected disorganisation of brain rhythms during the psychedelic experience. This state has been called the entropic brain and helps explain many of the features of the psychedelic trip. The entropic state is produced by psychedelics activating the serotonin 5-HT_{2A} receptors on a group of neurons that are located in the deeper layers of the cerebral cortex—the layer 5 pyramidal neurons. These neurons are critical for the ability of the brain to connect its vast range of different activities; they provide cross-cortical information transfer that allows the brain to construct the range of images, sounds, feelings, thoughts and ideas of which it is capable. When the function of these neurons is disrupted, the brain cannot perform its normal integrative processes and so a state of altered consciousness is produced.*

To understand these effects, we have first to understand some basic aspects of how the brain works. A description of this for the visual system is provided in Figure 1. The brain is not a camera, it does not take millions of pictures of the world day after day. This would be extremely energy inefficient and would use up the memory capacity of the brain very quickly. The way the brain allows us to "see" is by creating a hypothesis of the outside world based on the electrical signals that reach it from the retina. This process is explained in Figure 1.

When we look at anything, photons of light from the outside image enter the retina and activate photoreceptors (rods and cones) in the eye. This photoreceptor activation then changes the firing of neurons in the retina which begin to organise and collate inputs from many receptors, and then send their own outputs as electrical impulses to the brain via the optic nerve. Different retinal outputs go to different regions of the visual cortex system which are located at the back of the brain. Different regions of the visual cortex are responsible for receiving and then decoding specific elements of the retinal outputs—e.g. colour, shape, movement. Then these different analyses are pulled together to create an estimate of what is outside—i.e. what has generated the retinal signals. In other words, the visual cortex creates a hypothesis of the outside world based on analysing the light entering the eye.

Often the brain then tests this hypothesis—e.g. when we see something that looks like an appetising piece of food we might move to eat it. If it isn't food but maybe a piece of coloured paper, we rapidly learn this. The hypothesis is then re-framed and we don't repeat the mistake the next time we see the coloured paper. Such learning processes occur very early in life as babies begin to explore the world, and continue till death. Similar inferential processes apply to all different forms of sensory inputs—all sensations are brain constructs that are then tested out and either validated or re-made. In the words of one of the founders of modern neurosci-

* For an overview see Nutt, Erritzoe, and Carhart-Harris (2020).

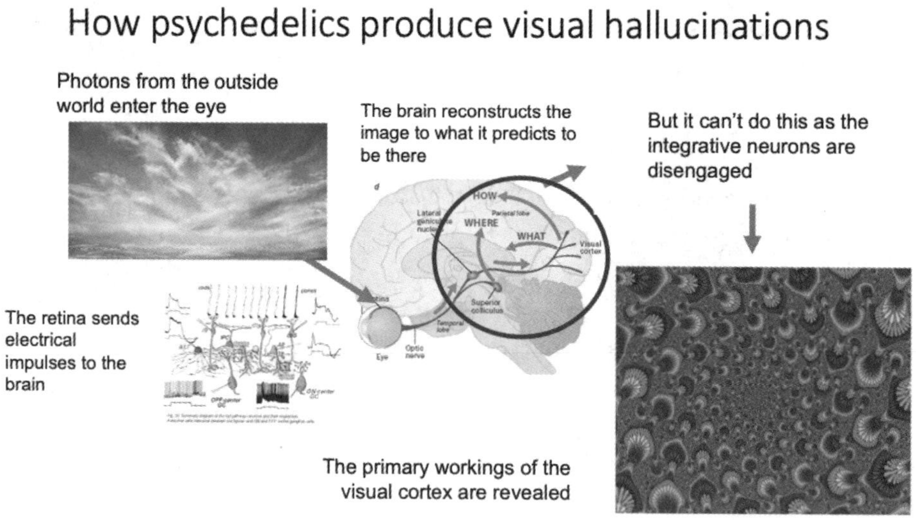

How psychedelics produce visual hallucinations

Photons from the outside world enter the eye

The brain reconstructs the image to what it predicts to be there

But it can't do this as the integrative neurons are disengaged

The retina sends electrical impulses to the brain

The primary workings of the visual cortex are revealed

Fig.1 How psychedelics affect vision. Images sourced from (Orpwood 2013).

ence Helmholtz "the brain is an inference-making machine". This explains why the brain is so much more energy efficient than any computer. Its software is analytical and iterative. The brain continually upgrades the estimates it makes. Modern AI computing programmes use a similar approach to learn and improve their decision-making as it repeats its assessments.

As mentioned earlier serotonin-receptor acting psychedelics such as psilocybin and LSD powerfully disrupt these predictive processes. This is because the neurons responsible for the integration of the activity of different parts of the brain (the layer 5 neurons of the cortex) have a very dense expression of the 5-HT_{2A} receptors that psychedelics bind to. When psychedelics bind to these receptors this activates and dramatically increases the firing of these neurons. This disrupts their ability to integrate activity across different regions—so this critically important function of the brain breaks down.

So, for example in the visual cortex this means that a normal hypothesis (the "picture" that the brain produces) of the outside world cannot be generated because the different parts of the cortex that need to work together to produce this "picture" are not optimally integrated. Therefore, they cannot produce their usual best estimates of what is out there producing the retinal inputs. The sensory inputs from the retina are still present and can be experienced, but not computed into a full image. The pretty coloured simple (elemental) visual hallucinations (often described as like Christmas tree lights) so common with psychedelics I think can be explained as the person experiencing the early workings of the primary visual cortex.

We know from work in other animals such as frogs the first stage of a brain creating images from retinal inputs is to create simple shapes, that are then coalesced into more complex images. These simple geometric images are normally not seen because they are immediately fused into a whole completed image which the person perceives as the outside world. So, one remarkable aspect of the psychedelic state is that it allows people to experience this early-stage primary level function of the visual system. This is a special experience that probably only previously happens in the very early weeks of a baby's life before the visual system's cortical networks become fully developed and functionally integrated.

Another much rarer example of this disrupting phenomenon of visual reconstruction was shared with me by a magic mushroom user who in a memorable (maybe unforgettable?) trip had a period when the world was upside-down. To understand how this could occur we have to remember that the lens of the eye inverts the light form the outside world, so the image of the outside world on the retina is upside down. Our brain learns from a very early age to adjust for this this, to flip the images to the same plane as we are, so we can function in our usual upright mode. I think the experience of the upside-down world was because under psilocybin this process was interrupted: for the upside-down period the person saw what the retina sees all the time, an upside-down image of the world.

Sometimes psychedelics especially *Amanita Muscaria* can produce alterations in the perceived size of objects—think of Alice in Wonderland and the growing and shrinking potions. The perception of the size of objects in the outside world is a special feature of the visual system that is particularly affected by the active ingredient in *Amanita Muscaria*– muscimol. This stimulates GABA receptors that are highly expressed in the visual cortex and so alters function in that part of the visual cortex that predicts the perceived size of objects.

Another profound experience produced by psychedelics is the sense of body disorganisation or dissolution. People often describe a sense of changing body form and position, sometimes moving into another place or different dimension. Other times they experience a sense of atomisation with their body dispersing into atoms. These experiences occur because the psychedelic disrupts a part of the brain called the posterior cingulate cortex, where our sense of self is generated. If this self-generation process is interrupted, we can feel our body as being very different and possibly somewhere else. Electrical stimulation of this part of the brain performed during brain surgery can produce similar "out of body" experiences.

The initial hypotheses (inferences) the brain generates and then tests are called "priors". These exist in relation to both the external world of the senses e.g., what we expect to see in a particular place, and to the internal world of all brain processes such as language, cognition, emotions etc. Of course, these are harder for the brain to evaluate than those predicting sensory inputs because they are harder to test. That requires introspection, self-awareness and perhaps communication with others of our species. In this way the brain orchestrates and defines the content of its productions and activity in relation to both the outside and inside worlds. This then becomes the content of the mind—the brain determines the content and hence the focus of the mind.

I now believe that conditions such as depression and addiction come to dominate a person's behavior because their brain develops false assumptions and then fails to correct them. These incorrect ways of thinking (priors) are wrong or maladaptive but become more and more dominant because the evaluation system has broken down. Worse—in some cases rather than reappraising the priors they become reinforced; more on this later.

As well as altering perception psychedelics also open the mind. This is graphically illustrated in the image below in which different brain regions are positions around the edge of the circle and the connectivity between as the size of the black lines. The left-hand image shows the connectivity of the brain after placebo and the right-hand image that after psilocybin. Each image has the same number of connections but in the normal (placebo) brain state these are mostly around the edge—local connectivity within specific brain circuits e.g., within the visual network or auditory networks. This is called the "small-world" brain. It is developed in all of us by years of generating and testing inferences about the inner and outer worlds that started as babies and is reinforced by schooling and other forms of education. These connections are very efficient in allowing normal daily life functions. Although this form of brain functionality is very efficient in terms of energy use and explains why the brain is ten times more efficient than any known computer, it comes at a cost—inflexibility and loss of creativity. And if the efficient connections are maladaptive then mental illness can result.

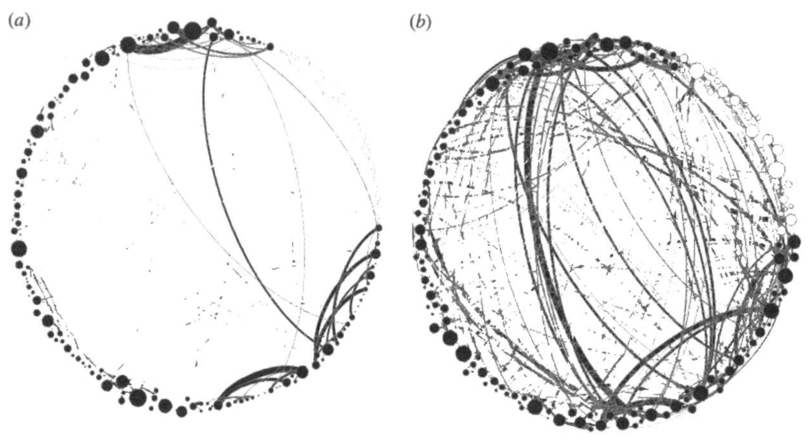

Fig.2 Graphic illustrations that show different brain regions connectivity after placebo (a) and after psilocybin (b) (Petri et al, 2014).

Under psilocybin there is a massive increase in connectivity because the control centres of the brain are disrupted. This allows areas that have been functionally disconnected since childhood to reconnect during the trip. We believe that this enhanced connectivity explains why psychedelic trips allow people to think differently about their past and remember events that have been supressed. It also allows new ways of thinking about how they might deal with these memories and also gives new insights into how they might deal with the future providing new solutions to old problems. Moreover, the enhanced neuroplasticity that psychedelics also produce can help these new ideas and plans embed in the brain and so endure well beyond the trip. This explains the long-lasting clinical outcomes of psychedelic therapy which we cover in the next section.

The psychedelic opening of the mind, allowing it to return to a more child-like state is a remarkable finding. We have already mentioned how Huxley utilised Blake's concept of "the doors of perception" to explain his psychedelic experience and will talk more about that later. But another of Blake's great creations were his poems for children, the Songs of Innocence and Experience. Here is one that sums up that transition from the innocent open mind of a child where all things are possible and pleasurable to the adult experience of loss and depression.

The Garden of Love

I went to the Garden of Love,
And saw what I never had seen:
A Chapel was built in the midst,
Where I used to play on the green.
And the gates of this Chapel were shut,
And Thou shalt not. writ over the door;
So I turn'd to the Garden of Love,
That so many sweet flowers bore.
And I saw it was filled with graves,
And tomb-stones where flowers should be:
And Priests in black gowns, were walking their rounds,
And binding with briars, my joys & desires.

CLINICAL RESEARCH WITH PSYCHEDELICS

Psychedelic drugs such a psilocybin LSD and DMT/ayahuasca offer remarkable insights into how the brain works. They also change user's minds, an experience established by many who have taken them and perhaps best encapsulated in the recent book by Michael Pollan, "How to change your mind".

In a way psychedelics have also changed my mind. When I started out using neuroimaging to explore the effects of these drugs on the brain, I had no inkling that I would soon be writing grants to study psilocybin as a treatment for depression. My neuroimaging work was undertaken to explore the nature of the psychedelic experience and to gain insights into the role of the serotonin 5-HT_{2A} receptors that these drugs stimulate. At the start of this research, I was clueless to the fact that it would explode into the revolution in neuroscience and psychiatry it is today: I saw them initially as tools to explore brain function.

The fact that they are now the most significant innovation in psychiatry treatments in the past 50 years tells us several things. One is that psychiatric medicine hasn't made much progress over the past 50 years. All the drugs we use today are derivatives of drugs discovered by serendipity in the 1950s. True their molecular structures have been refined so they are safer especially in overdose, but there has been no equivalent improvement in efficacy. Treatment innovation hasn't developed as predicted in parallel with the massive rise in neuroscience knowledge that has occurred in the past 30 years.

The second is that basic research into brain mechanisms can be relevant to treatment innovation. We had no idea that the brain images we obtained from our first psilocybin MRI studies would uncover a new more powerful route to treat depression, especially those which had failed to respond to conventional antidepressant and psychotherapy treatments. Our transition from imaging psychedelic effects on the brain to treating depression is a remarkable example of translational medicine. Our brain imaging revealed psilocybin to have an impact on the brain circuits that underpin depression in a manner similar to that seen with other treatments of depression such as antidepressant drugs, electroconvulsive therapy (ECT) and even Cognitive Behavioural Therapy (CBT). Like all these other successful treatments psilocybin decreased activity in a part of the brain that is known to drive depressive thinking, the (sub-genual) pre-frontal cortex. This led us to argue a trial in depression was warranted, the UK Medical Research Council agreed, and the results were remarkable.

We treated 20 people whose depression had not responded to at least two antidepressant medicines (some had tried over ten) and all had not responded to CBT. These patients were very much treatment resistant. We found a single psychedelic (25mg) dose of psilocybin produced more powerful antidepressant effects than any previously reported antidepressant treatment in treatment-resistant patients before. It halved the depression scores within a week (usually the effect was seen the very next day) and in a few of these patients the depression has stayed at bay for over 8 years. Sadly, in the majority of the patients the depression began to creep back over the next 6 months and some eventually returning to as bad a state as they were in before (Carhart-Harris et al, 2016).

How can we make sense of these phenomena? How does depression get set in the brain to an extent it doesn't respond to traditional antidepressant medicines or to psychotherapy? A key feature of depression is rumination, repetitive thought loops with negative valence, often of low self-worth or guilt. Even when the person realises that these are plainly wrong or at least out of proportion to what they have done the thoughts can be very hard to stop. And eventually they can become so ingrained that the person doesn't even challenge them, they become "true". The biological basis of this ingraining—sometimes called thought canalisation—is discussed in depth in this recent review (Carhart-Harris et al, 2022).

This is not a new idea, and can be seen in the concept of Buddhist "formations", as described by Andy Olendzki, a Buddhist scholar (Germer and Siegel 2012):

> *'An image is offered in the Pali texts of early Buddhism to help us understand what formations are, and I think it is an image remarkably adaptable to our current understanding of the brain and its architecture. Picture a chariot driving across a dusty plain. The chariot may presumably be steered wherever its driver wishes to go, within the constraints of the terrain. It might have to dodge around some rocks or stay away from the swampy areas, but it is under the driver's volitional control. This image captures the first sense of formations: the intention or executive function in the mind that makes moment-to-moment decisions.*
>
> *Then, as the chariot actually traverses one path or another, it makes an imprint of the wheel upon the earth. This imprint represents the actual carrying out of an action or activity. In Buddhist thought every moment entails some sort of action, by body, speech, or mind, and all such activity is called karma, a word that basically just means "action." The second meaning of "formations" has to do with the fact that volitional activity leaves traces—the tracks of the chariot are embedded in the dust on the plain for all to see. One can gaze out over that plain and have a very good idea of where the chariot has been because it leaves a. clear record of its activity carved in the ground. Moreover, if it takes the same route many times over, a path (or even a rut) gets constructed, so the entire history of that chariot's activities is recorded in the patterns it has laid down on the plain".*

We can use the analogy of the ruts to explain how depressive thinking gets more and more ingrained in the brain. The more we go over the same thought the deeper the rut it produces, so escaping from it gets harder and harder, its less and less under volitional control.

The reasons for the return of the depression are at present unclear. It seems that the longer the depression has been present the more likely it will be to come back. We presume the more times the person has gone over a negative thought the more ingrained it and the depression becomes, so the harder it is to eliminate fully. Though psychedelics can disrupt ongoing depressive thinking the underlying brain processes might remain dormant and later resurface if not fully dealt with.

How best to prevent relapse is one of the biggest questions facing the field at present with a number of possible options. One is more intensive or enduring integration psychotherapy such as the new ACER approach developed by the lead therapist on our trials, Dr Rosalind Watts.* An alternative would be to use another "top-up" dose of psychedelic when the depression creeps back. A third option would be to reinstate one of the antidepressants that had previously proved ineffective, since it might now work in a prophylactic fashion in the new improved brain state: perhaps even a mood stabiliser against depression such as lamotrigine might work?

Subsequent trials by us and other groups at Johns Hopkins university and the new pharmaceutical company COMPASSPathways have confirmed the antidepressant effects of psilocybin (Goodwin et al, 2022). Moreover, our comparative study of psilocybin versus the gold standard selective serotonin reuptake inhibitor (SSRI) escitalopram (Carhart-Harris et al, 2021) confirmed our hypothesis that psilocybin worked in quite a different way to the SSRI's (Carhart-Harris and Nutt, 2017). Again, using fMRI neuroimaging we found that psilocybin increased connectivity and flexibility in the brain whereas escitalopram did not (see later). However as predicted escitalopram reduced activity in the emotional circuit of the brain—especially the amygdala—whereas psilocybin had no impact there.

These findings mirror the reported experiences of patients. Those who recovered on psilocybin report increased flexibility of thinking with greater connectedness to other people, to nature and to the world. They often use computer analogies to explain this feeling. Some say it's like when you reformat or de-frag the hard drive of a computer to clear away the bugs or background programmes that are interfering with its normal running. Others talk about cleaning out a virus that impedes fluent running. Most say that their minds are much freer- they have escaped from the internal loops of negative thinking that are the cardinal feature of depressive thought processes. These experiences probably explain why wellbeing is so markedly improved after psilocybin treatment (Watts et al, 2017).

In contrast escitalopram lifts mood by protecting the emotional circuits of the brain from stress. These regions become super-sensitive in depression and so perpetuate the low mood and other disturbances such as loss of appetite and insomnia. Escitalopram in common with all SSRI's and other traditional antidepressant medicine dampens stress-reactivity in this circuit, and so allows that part of the brain to heal. This process takes many weeks, which is why SSRI's do not reveal their full therapeutic effect for 6-10 weeks. But one drawback of the suppression of activity in this brain circuit is that the responses to all emotions are supressed, and many

* For more information on this see https://acerintegration.com.

patients on SSRI's complain of an unwanted dampening of positive emotions that accompanies the (desired) dampening of their sensitivity to stress.

As a result of this and many other supporting studies from other research labs we can now be pretty certain that psychedelics offer a new and unique was of lifting depression, quite different from that of traditional antidepressants. This is exciting for researchers and pleasing for patients—they now know if one treatment fails, they have another totally different one to try—once psychedelics become approved medicines.

THE MIND OF WILLIAM BLAKE

As a child Blake was moted for seeing visions of religious figures, for example at a garden party he claimed to see the Prophet Elijah under a tree. This ability to "see" things that were not there, or at least that others could not see, is common in great artists, performers and visionaries. Blake knew he was different from most others. In a letter written in 1799 he said "*I know that This World Is a World of Imagination & Vision; I see Everything I paint In This World, but Everybody does not see alike. (...) Some See Nature all Ridicule & Deformity & by these I shall not regulate my proportions, & Some Scarce see Nature at all. But to the Eyes of the Man of Imagination Nature is Imagination itself. As a man is So he Sees.*"

Seeing things that others can't is reminiscent of the impact of psychedelics on perception, particularly the tendency for believers to experience religious content or contact with meaningful others such as entities. It is thought that this power of Blake's to see things very differently to others underpinned the very novel and "unworldly" nature of much of his art. And of course, he was aware that others couldn't see in the same way as he could—being limited in their vision by social norms, education and ignorance. It was this insight that led to the quote *"If the doors of perception were cleansed everything would appear to man as it is, infinite. For man has closed himself up, till he sees all things thro' narrow chinks of his cavern"*. Many users of psychedelics would confirm that only in the trip can the human mind really appreciate the infinite.

This quote was used by Huxley for *The Doors of Perception* because Huxley realized that mescaline had opened the chinks in his mind's cavern, allowing him to see things very differently. He then made the logical inference that if mescaline had opened his mind something must have been closing it. The most likely explanation for Huxley was that that something was the brain and so he theorized that "*the brain is an instrument for focusing the mind*". This hypothesis of Huxley's was conceived in 1953 and has been substantiated over the subsequent decades by sophisticated neuroscience research from many pre-clinical labs. The final proof that this is true for humans I believe came from the current neuroimaging studies of psychedelics. As described above psychedelics alter brain function in a way that disrupts the long-practiced predictive ongoing processing of external inputs and internal constructs. This disruption changes consciousness usually in a direction that is mind-opening. Hence Huxley was correct—psychedelics change brain function and so allow the mind to open.

But Blake's quote meant more than just open your eyes, he understood that all aspects of human consciousness were limited in the same way, in all aspects of life most of us fail to see the bigger picture. What is less well known is that more of Blake's insights and visions are also relevant to other aspects of psychedelics and psychedelic therapy.

The paintings of Blake such as his image of God, other biblical characters and the scientist Newton are some of the most recognised works of English art. Though ignored and actively opposed in his own time for his liberal philosophies he is now universally recognised, which is why he is considered by Jonathan Jones the 21st-century art critic to be *"far and away the greatest artist Britain has ever produced"*. Blake was also very religious but from a personal spiritual perspective, and so conflicted with the Church of England and other organised religions. The poem already quoted—The Garden of Love—clearly expresses his view of the established religion of the time.

Blake was a supporter of the ideas of the French and American revolutions and the philosophy of Thomas Paine who in his treatise on the Rights of Man said *""Whatever is my right as a man is also the right of another; and it becomes my duty to guarantee as well as to possess."*
Blake's poem "The little black boy" shows his support for racial equality:

My mother bore me in the southern wild,
And I am black, but O! my soul is white;
White as an angel is the English child:
But I am black as if bereav'd of light.

And thus I say to little English boy.
When I from black and he from white cloud free,
And round the tent of God like lambs we joy:
I'll shade him from the heat till he can bear,
To lean in joy upon our fathers' knee.
And then I'll stand and stroke his silver hair,
And be like him and he will then love me.

Blake was also a committed rationalist building on the social aspirations of the Enlightenment. He was vocally anti-war and anti-slavery and in favour of female equality, three traits that made him a threat to the establishment of the time. This fear was rekindled in the 1960s by the rising use of LSD in freethinkers who too wanted to change society to one that was more just and equal and, especially in the 1960s, not engaged in warfare, particularly with Vietnam.

He was once tried in court for his views. This originated in a war of words with a soldier called Skofeld that led Blake to being accused of treason and taken to court. Though acquitted, this episode led him to write in his most famous work, *Jerusalem,* how soldiers were controlled and made to fight because society had made them tie themselves up with their "*mind forged manacles*'. After this episode Blake produces the print shown on the next page.

There is little doubt that after the *"doors of perception"* Blake's most well-known phrase is *"mind forged manacles"*. Though he first applied it to soldiers it had more general applicability e.g. to those workers choosing to leave the countryside and go to work in the "*dark satanic mills*" of the northern industrial towns. The theme of the Jerusalem book is this enslavement of the people, their complicity in this process because of their manacled thinking, and how insights such as the "*arrows of desire*" could be used to help them escape from these manacles.

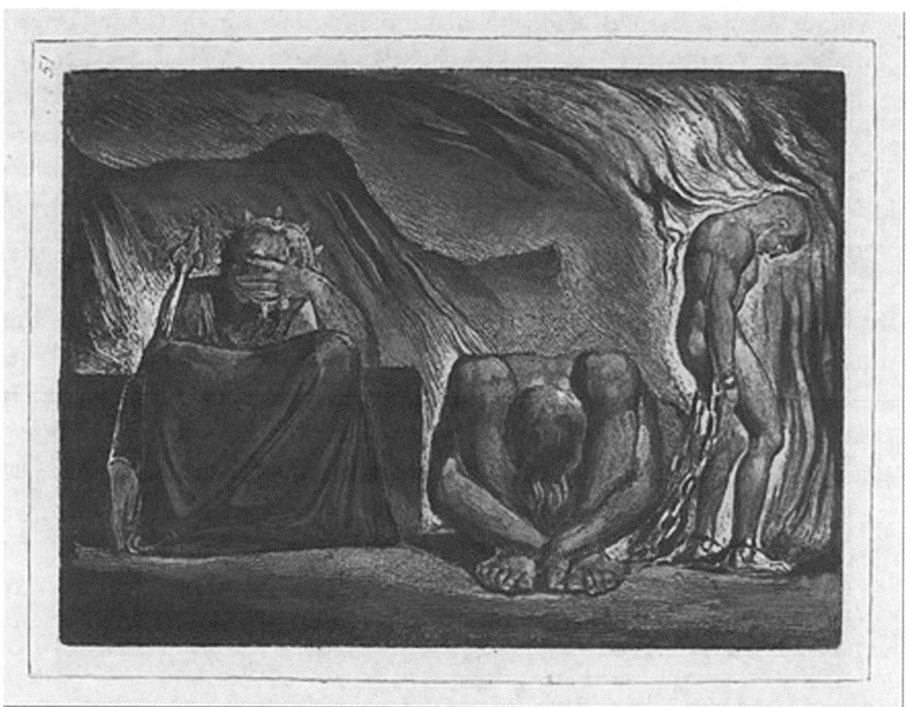

Fig.3 The Emanation of the Giant Albion Plate 51. Here Skofeld' is wearing "mind forged manacles" in Jerusalem.

"Mind forged manacles" is a powerful analogy for how the brain controls behavior. This is now a central aspect of my neuroscientific view of how the brain is involved in conditions such as depression and addiction and helps offer new ways to think about how psychedelic treatments work. Earlier we discussed how the brain creates inferences about the outside world—so called priors—and then tests them through trial and error. In the same way the brain also creates the internal constructs we call thoughts, plans, memories, imaginations etc.

For most of us these internal constructs are positive—happy memories, positive plans for the future etcetera. But for some people for example those with depression, OCD, anorexia or substance/behavioral dependences, these contracts are negative thoughts or damaging and ultimately self-destructive behaviors. Many such individuals know that that their thoughts and desires are not what they want but they can't stop them. It is as if they become habitual rather than volitional. What might start off in the case of addiction as a desire with pleasurable outcomes, over time ends up becoming a curse. Many people dependent on alcohol and other drugs continue to use them despite getting no pleasure from them, and they do not just use them to deal with withdrawal symptoms. Substance use, which started as a mind-made decision ends up becoming a sub-conscious reflex behavior or habit that has escaped from conscious override- it has become manacled to action. The mind that started the behavior is no longer able to unshackle it because the behavior it is now embedded in brain systems below conscious control. As described above thinking loops become deeply rutted or canalised.

In the case of OCD most people know that their compulsive thoughts or rituals are pointless, but they can't stop them. OCD was the first mental illness to have its brain circuits characterised: an overactivity of the orbitofrontal cortex to caudate nucleus pathway was discovered. Further neuroimaging research showed that over time both pharmacological and psychotherapy interventions dampened down this over-activity. Many depressed people feel the same about their negative thoughts but can't stop this rumination. In this case we know that this thinking process is driven by overactivity of parts of the frontal cortex.

Brain imaging studies mentioned above show a profound disruption of normal ongoing brain activity following psilocybin. So, could this disrupt the thinking processes underpinning depression? And what are these anyway? Here again Blake has a profound insight with his quote *"For man has closed himself up, till he sees all things thro' narrow chinks of his cavern"*. For most of us though our view through the chinks is limited the content of our vision is generally positive—blue skies white clouds etc. But people with mental illness see things differently. Depressed people see a bleak dark grey miserable landscape, people with OCD see threats, germ-containing objects etc. Addicts see their love objects, for example a vodka bottle, a hypodermic syringe, a white powder or a roulette wheel.

Figure 4 below helps to explain the neural processes of cognitive biases that underpin these mental illnesses again using the visual system as the exemplar. The mind begins the process but over time the brain takes over and determines the cognitive and thinking processes. The ill person becomes trapped by their brain in their thinking and behavior processes. In one way Blake was wrong, these are not "mind forged manacles" but brain-forged ones.

Psychedelics by disrupting the brain processes of entrapment can free people from their illness. The rutted loops of thinking from which they have not been able to escape are flattened so they can think differently. For some this may be temporary, but at least during the trip they can understand (in colloquial terms "see") that there is the possibility of escape from them (recovery): whereas for some lucky ones the escape can be permanent.

Our most recent research helps throw a light on the brain mechanisms underpinning the more enduring effects of psychedelics (Daws et al, 2022). This is shown schematically in figure 4.

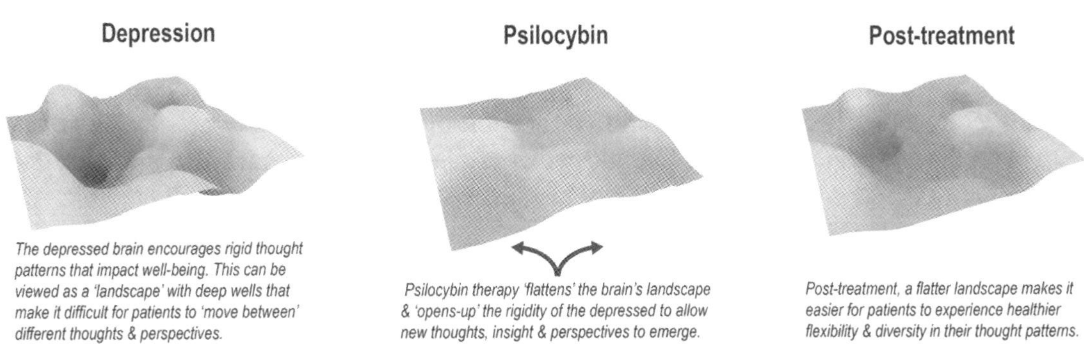

Fig 4. The energy landscape of the brain in different states

Colour Vision

Blakes pictures are some of the most unique and recognised pieces of printed art in the world, for both their design and colour. His use of white to express innocence and closeness to God—a colour experience commonly encountered during trips that take people to heaven, holy places and even God. This aspect of the psychedelic experience is like that reported in near death experiences and probably reflects similar physiological changes in visual processing areas. Black of course represented death and the dark reality and psychology of human life especially in the industrial cities—"*those dark satanic mills.*" One advantage of Blakes special copper-plate printing process was that he could experiment with different colours in progressive prints, evolving and exploring the impact of altered shades and colours.

But colour was at times a challenge to Blake as he explained innovation an 1804 letter to William Hayley: "*Suddenly, on the day after visiting the Truchsessian Gallery of pictures, I was again enlightened with the light I enjoyed in my youth, and which has for exactly twenty years been closed from me as by a door and by window-shutters*". Why this transformation occurred is not known but the gallery comprised over 900 pictures, the greatest selection in one place ever assembled and the sheer scale and content seemed to jolt Blake back into an interest in both colour and form.

Psychedelics can also do this. Most are familiar with the wonder-filled descriptions of Hofmann and Huxley on how psychedelics made colours more vivid, more discrete, and more awesome. Similar experiences are commonly reported by many less well-known users; in fact this is one of the more generally reported phenomena of the psychedelic experience. Perhaps paradoxically improvements in colour perception are also reported by people with colour-blindness, enabling them to see colours better. One such person spontaneously emailed me some years ago saying "*all my life I suffered from red-dichromacy/ protanopia.* One day during a magic mushroom trip my brother showed me a screen image of Monet's San Giorgio Maggiore at Dusk. A painting which I had previously seen as a dull mass of brown and blue. All of the colours I was previously unable to see were there on the screen, and the emotion that I felt made me unable to speak for about half an hour.*" This report started us asking our volunteers in previous psychedelic imaging studies if they had colour blindness and we discovered that several had, and many of these reported improved colour perception during and after the trip.

Because of this intriguing feedback we then put a special short questionnaire into the Global Drug Survey addressing this specific point. We asked colour-blind respondents to comment on the impact that psychedelic use had on their colour vision. Of the 47 colour-blind people who responded nearly half (23) stated that their colour vision had improved during the use of a psychedelic with many reporting this effect lasted for weeks or months (Anthony et al, 2020).

How can we explain this? It seems unlikely that psychedelics can normalise a genetic change in the photoreceptor protein. There are 5-HT_{2A} receptors on cells in the retina so it might be that stimulating these somehow enhances the gain from the photoreceptors into the neurons transmitting colour signals to the brain. More likely I think is that psychedelics release a degree of suppression of colour perception that is commonly present in the "small world" brain described

---

* Protanopia is a hereditary type of colour blindness that comes from insensitivity to red light, which causes confusion of reds, greens and yellows.

earlier. For most of us (artists excepted) colour is a useful but not essential aspect of visual life. This whole chapter has gotten by without it! The function rather than the colour of objects tends to dominate our interactions with them: knowing a door is in front of you is more important than knowing its colour. I suspect colour perception becomes diminished in importance in the brain as we mature through childhood, perhaps even actively supressed. Psychedelics release this minimisation of the value of colour by the brain and so allow it to resume its previous place as a vital aspect of vision. In the next section you will discover just how Blake had foreseen this.

Blake And Newton: Two Different Visions Of Vision?

Although the lives of these two great pillars of British intellectual thought did not overlap (Blake lived 1757-1827 and Newton 1642-1726) Newton clearly had a great influence on Blake as he did on most other thinkers that followed him. Blake's print of Newton scaling the world is one of his most famous and is thought to reflect Blake's opposition to a simple scientific view of the world. He was particularly opposed to Newton's view that reason and logic (scientific materialism) could explain everything. In Jerusalem Blake states *"I will not Reason & Compare: my business is to Create"*.

Where Blake most opposed Newton was in relation to colour perception. One of Newton's great discoveries was, from the use of the prism, that white light was composed of lights of different colours—as we see in a rainbow. But Blake thought the physics of optics were inadequate to explain humans' appreciation of colour. He argued there were two aspects to vision, the simple "vegetive eye" that does the seeing, and the spiritual appreciation of that vision. Eventually Blake developed a four level explanation of visual experience which directly challenged the "single vision" of Newton, whose "natural religion" he characterized as like being asleep.

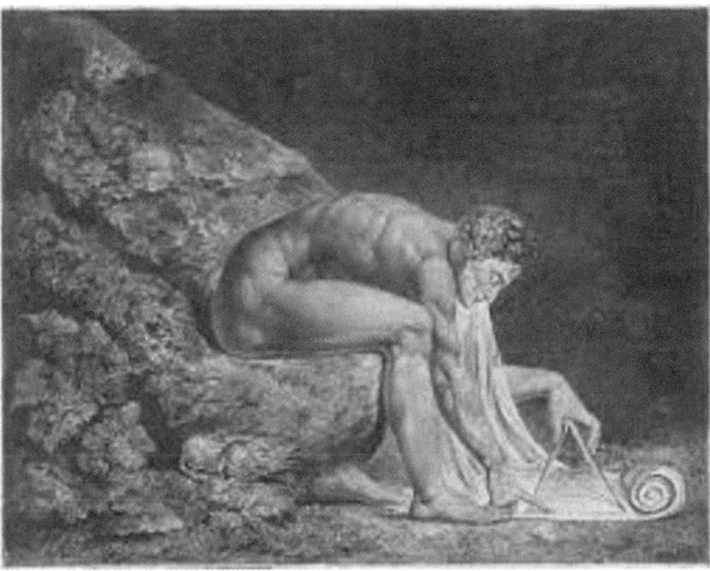

Fig 5. William Blake painting of Newton scaling the world 1795-c.1805. *Tate, 2018*

"Now I a fourfold vision see
And a fourfold vision is given to me
Tis fourfold in my supreme delight
And three fold in soft Beulah's night
And twofold Always. May God us keep
From Single vision & Newton's sleep"
—Excerpt from a letter from William Blake to Thomas Butts*

The fourfold vision is a state of ecstatic or mystical bliss. Threefold vision arises naturally from Beulah, which, in Blake's mythology, is the place of poetic inspiration and dreams, "*where Contrarieties are equally True*". Twofold vision is seeing not only with the eye, but through it, seeing contexts, associations, emotional meanings, connections. Single vision is the literal, rational, scientific or Newtonian view of the world: for the artist the least important. One can argue that psychedelics support Blake's theories by opening the doors to the higher stages of vision.

This early challenge to science that Blake's visionary experiences produce has been much more eloquently discussed by Aldous Huxley in his book "Heaven and Hell". Many users of psychedelics would undoubtedly side with Blake in the idea that there are different (possibly higher) levels of consciousness that psychedelics reveal to them. They pose a major, maybe the greatest challenge to modern neuroscience: can they be explained in the context of current theories of brain activity? Blake would likely say we don't need to. I would say that if we could, then this would be an advance equivalent to that made for physics by the Theory of Relativity. Whatever the outcome the question will stand, and Blake will remain as one of the leading thinkers in this field.

BIBLIOGRAPHY

Anthony, Jec, Adam R. Winstock, Jason Ferris, and David J. Nutt. 2020. "Improved Colour Blindness Symptoms Associated with Recreational Psychedelic Use: Results from the Global Drug Survey 2017." *Drug Science, Policy and Law* 6 (November): 205032452094234. https://doi.org/10.1177/2050324520942345.

Daws, Richard E., Christopher Timmermann, Bruna Giribaldi, James Sexton, Matthew B. Wall, David Erritzoe, Leor Roseman, David J. Nutt, and Robin L. Carhart-Harris. 2022. "Increased Global Integration in the Brain after Psilocybin Therapy for Depression." *Nature Medicine* 28 (4): 844–51. https://doi.org/10.1038/s41591-022-01744-z.

Carhart-Harris, Robin L., Mark Bolstridge, James Rucker, Camilla M. Day, David Erritzoe, Mendel Kaelen, Michael a P Bloomfield, et al. 2016. "Psilocybin with Psychological Support for Treatment-Resistant Depression: An Open-Label Feasibility Study." *The Lancet Psychiatry* 3 (7): 619–27. https://doi.org/10.1016/s2215-0366(16)30065-7.

Carhart-Harris, Robin L., and David J. Nutt. 2017. "Serotonin and Brain Function: A Tale of Two Receptors." *Journal of Psychopharmacology* 31 (9): 1091–1120. https://doi.org/10.1177/0269881117725915.

Carhart-Harris, Robin L., Bruna Giribaldi, Rosalind Watts, Michelle Baker-Jones, Ashleigh Murphy-Beiner, Roberta Murphy, Jonny Martell, Allan Blemings, David Erritzoe, and David J. Nutt. 2021. "Trial of Psilocybin versus Escitalopram for Depression." *The New England Journal of Medicine* 384 (15): 1402–11. https://doi.org/10.1056/nejmoa2032994.

Carhart-Harris, Robin L., S Chandaria, David Erritzoe, Adam Gazzaley, Manesh Girn, Hannes Kettner, P a M

* You can read more about William Blake archives and letters (The William Blake Archive, 1977)

Mediano, et al. 2022. "Canalization and Plasticity in Psychopathology." *Neuropharmacology* 226 (December): 109398. https://doi.org/10.1016/j.neuropharm.2022.109398.

Germer, Christopher K., and Ronald A. Siegel. 2012. "Wisdom and Compassion in Psychotherapy: Deepening Mindfulness in Clinical Practice." *American Psychological Association*, January. https://psycnet.apa.org/record/2012-13277-000.

Goodwin, Guy M., Scott T. Aaronson, Oscar Alvarez, Peter C Arden, Annie Lilian Baker, James C. Bennett, Catherine Bird, et al. 2022. "Single-Dose Psilocybin for a Treatment-Resistant Episode of Major Depression." *The New England Journal of Medicine* 387 (18): 1637–48. https://doi.org/10.1056/nejmoa2206443.

Nutt, David J., David Erritzoe, and Robin L. Carhart-Harris. 2020. "Psychedelic Psychiatry's Brave New World." *Cell* 181 (1): 24–28. https://doi.org/10.1016/j.cell.2020.03.020.

Orpwood, Roger. 2013. "Qualia Could Arise from Information Processing in Local Cortical Networks." *Frontiers in Psychology* 4 (March). https://doi.org/10.3389/fpsyg.2013.00121.

Petri, Giovanni, Paul Expert, Federico Turkheimer, Robin L. Carhart-Harris, David J. Nutt, Peter J. Hellyer, and Francesco Vaccarino. 2014. "Homological Scaffolds of Brain Functional Networks." *Journal of the Royal Society Interface* 11 (101): 20140873. https://doi.org/10.1098/rsif.2014.0873.

Tate. 2018. "'Newton', William Blake, 1795–c.1805 | Tate." October 2018. https://www.tate.org.uk/art/artworks/blake-newton-n05058.

The William Blake Archive. 1977. "A Suggested Redating of a Blake Letter to Thomas Butts | E. B. Murray | Blake/An Illustrated Quarterly | Volume 13, Issue 3." Https://Www.Blakearchive.Org/. 1977. https://bq.blakearchive.org/13.3.murray.

Watts, Rosalind, Camilla M. Day, Jacob Krzanowski, David J. Nutt, and Robin L. Carhart-Harris. 2017. "Patients' Accounts of Increased 'Connectedness' and 'Acceptance' After Psilocybin for Treatment-Resistant Depression." *Journal of Humanistic Psychology* 57 (5): 520–64. https://doi.org/10.1177/0022167817709585.

Phytosphere

Teachings from the Psychotropic Plant Kingdom

Are the Fruits Too High or Have We Been Clumsy? A Critical Analysis of Ethnopharmacological Research Techniques

Elaine Elisabetsky, PhD

Ethnopharmacologist, Departamento de Bioquímica, Universidade Federal do Rio Grande do Sul, Porto Alegre, Brazil | WHO Traditional, Complementary and Integrative Medicine advisor

"This presentation investigates possible reasons to explain the meager results of ethnopharmacology-driven leads in the development of psychoactive drugs."

Ethnopharmacology is a diverse discipline with high potential, but much room for improvement. This paper explores how it can be improved and optimized for the betterment of medicine and humanity.

ABSTRACT

Despite the prominent role of natural products in the history of psychopharmacology, and the unquestionable need for more effective drugs for treating mental disorders, new plant-derived psychoactive drugs are lacking. The advantages of natural products over synthetic ones in the interaction with biological targets of therapeutic interest has been documented. A higher hit rate of ethnopharmacology-driven plant collections over those guided by biodiversity and/or chemotaxonomy is acknowledged in retrospective analysis of medium to large drug discovery bioactivity evaluation programs. Scientific journals focusing on the biological evaluation of plant species used in traditional medical systems often conclude that the data is coherent with the reported use. Therefore, why is it that there are no new psychoactive drugs are in the market? This manuscript discusses possible reasons that may contribute to the meager results of ethnopharmacology-driven leads in the development of psychoactive drugs. Ethnopharmacology studies, including the plants *Ptychopetalum olacoides* and *Psychotria colorata*, and the botanical isolates linalool (a monoterpene), and alstonine (an indole alkaloid) are used to illustrate methodological issues relevant to the question in place. The collection of relevant clinical data in the field, the discipline mainstream *modus operandis* (or though style) for phytochemical and pharmacological investigations, the scarcity of accumulated knowledge on promising species, and the issues of reproducibility and translational values of experimental models are discussed. The identification and potential solutions for bottlenecks, as well as the development of adequate conservation and benefit sharing policies, will be instrumental to foster the discovery of innovative psychoactive drugs from traditional knowledge.

INTRODUCTION

Ethnopharmacology is a multidisciplinary subject that includes disciplines from social and biomedical sciences and is an approach to understand various aspects of traditional systems of medicine. The ethnopharmacology approach can be used to document history, change and subsidize health policies, work with traditional communities in a culturally sensitive manner, and produce improved (or branded) herbals, among others. The focus here is on its use for the discovery and development of psychoactive drugs.

The International Society of Ethnopharmacology (ISE) was founded in 1990 at a conference in Strasbourg, France, organized by the toxicologist Prof. Laurent Rivier. It has met biannually ever since, with additional regional meetings, in various Asian, European and Latin American countries (see www.ethnopharmacology.org). The Journal of Ethnopharmacology has been in print since 1979 and was adopted in 1997 as the official journal for the society. Along with other journals devoted to natural products research (such as Journal of Natural Products, Planta Medica, Phytochemistry, Journal of Herbal Medicine, Pharmaceutical biology, among others) or traditional medicine (such as Phytomedicine, Fitomedicina, Evidence Based Complementary and Alternative Medicine, J. Alternative and Complementary Medicine), a significant amount of research has been put forward and documented by a sizable community of researchers from various fields who believe that there are therapeutic agents to be discovered and developed from plants traditionally used for medical purposes in different cultural settings. Yet, in the last decades, the successful development of plant-based medicines that were subjected to the rigors of modern pharmaceutical formulation and clinical trials have been meagre,* and, to the best of my knowledge, none have been approved for mental disorders. Of note, clinical trials have been performed on numerous phytomedicines and supplements (such as those based on *Gingko biloba*, St John's Wort, Saw Palmetto, among numerous others) and important plant derived compounds (such as taxol, vinblastine, vincristine, artemisinin, resveratrol, and cannabidiol, to name a few) have been successfully developed as medical products. This paucity of regulatory agency (e.g. FDA) approved plant-based prescription drugs by no means implies that plant medicines have been of meagre service to mankind. On the contrary, the majority of the global population rely primarily on traditional medicines or Indigenous medicines for primary healthcare (World Health Organization, International Union for Conservation of Nature and Natural Resources, and World Wide Fund for Nature 1993/4), as there is an indisputable place for herbals in the service of global health, either in natural unprocessed form, as phytomedicines or as traditional remedies (Willcox et al. 2011; Seck et al. 2018; Graz et al. 2015).

Despite the prominent role of plants and/or plant derived molecules in healthcare, only about 200 of the 10,000–15,000 higher plants with reported medicinal properties are meaningfully incorporated in Western medicine (Birari and Bhutani 2007; McChesney, Venkataraman, and Henri

* Basically comprising of: Acheflan®, an anti-inflammatory ointment based of *Cordia verbenacea* developed in Brazil by the Aché laboratories; Mytesi™, an antidiarrheic agent based on polymeric proanthocyanidins from *Croton lechleri* developed in the USA by Shaman/Napo Pharmaceuticals (Nee et al. 2019; Greene et al. 2021), and Veregen®, a topical treatment for external genital and perianal warts, based on sinecatechins from *Camelia sinensis*) (Scheinfeld 2013).

2007). While the herbal market is established, newly approved botanical drugs are rare (Wu et al. 2020). Although ethnopharmacological data has been found to be more effective than chemotaxonomy-driven or random plant collection strategies in the search for biologically active extracts/compounds (Gyllenhaal et al. 2012), it is often considered as a second-class scientific approach.

It does not seem likely that the problem lies in the lack of interesting bioactive compounds of natural origin. On the contrary, natural products present advantages over synthetic molecules for drug discovery as recently reviewed (Harvey, Edrada-Ebel, and Quinn 2015; Skirycz et al. 2016). It is noteworthy that 34% of the new medicines approved by the US Food and Drug Administration (FDA) between 1981 and 2010 were based on natural products and/or their direct derivatives, and the vast majority of all drugs have a close match to natural-products (Harvey, Edrada-Ebel, and Quinn 2015). The chemical and analytical methods used for identifying active compounds have progressed significantly, and are instrumental in overcoming the snags in compound isolation and identification that marked the field in the past (Harvey, Edrada-Ebel, and Quinn 2015; Skirycz et al. 2016). Yet, only 5–15% of higher plants have been systematically examined as sources of compounds with medicinal properties (McChesney, Venkataraman, and Henri 2007), the 200,000 plant metabolites already identified have not been evaluated for biological effects, and neither have tens of thousands of plant and fungi based homemade remedies used daily for therapeutic purposes by a majority of mankind.

Given the proven record in the identification of bioactive formulas/extracts/compounds uncovered by ethnopharmacological studies, why have these efforts not reflected the development rate of therapeutic drugs from these leads? What are the bottlenecks? There appears to be not a single answer, but a multiplicity of problems. The issues include supply chain problems, the low yield and often complex nature of the chemical structure of compounds (Skirycz et al. 2016), leading to challenges in commercial scale-up production; the sociopolitical nature of drug development (especially for bioprospection initiatives); intellectual property rights (IPR) and benefit sharing issues (established by the 1992 Biological Convention) viewed as up-front hurdles driving the pharmaceutical industry's interest away (Elisabetsky 1991; Wynberg and Laird 2022). In 1984, Professor Norman Farnsworth (University of Illinois at Chicago) posed the same question in his article "How can the well be dry when it is filled with water?" (Farnsworth 1984). In the nearly 40 years since the publication of this article, advances in phytochemistry discovery and complex molecule synthesis methods can largely overcome the complications of commercial supply/resupply issues that were faced at that time. Where does the problem lie today? The purpose of this paper is to contemplate how we can improve tapping this well.*

THE TRUNCATED DIALOG BETWEEN MEDICAL SYSTEMS

Ethnopharmacology has undergone several definitions over time. Of interest to this discussion is Daniel Moerman's: "Essentially ethnopharmacology is the examination of non-Western (not mine) medicinal plant use in terms of Western (mine) plant use" (Heinrich 2015). As an old version of the "bed to bench strategy," ethnopharmacology records therapeutic practices reported

* Some of the ideas discussed in this paper have been previously published (Elisabetsky 2021).

by users as the basis to articulate a working hypothesis to drive subsequent chemical/pharmacological investigation of home-made remedies. In agreeance with Moerman's definition, studies in this field often conclude on the "validation" (or lack of) of a traditional used remedy; a positive validation is reached when the *in vitro* or *in vivo* effect observed for the extract/fraction/compound under study was as expected, or made sense, in relation to the original therapeutic claim (Verpoorte 2012). Though Moerman's definition is perfectly accurate to describe most of the published papers in journals of this field, I argue that this understanding and the *modus operandis* that follows is counterproductive to identify potential drugs with truly innovative mechanisms of action. Fleck explains how a "thought style" may limit thinking and experimentation to the expected results according to the dominant understanding of a given scientific question (Fleck 1981, 39). Therefore, if we explore a different medical tradition in biomedical western terms, we may well fail to explore truly innovative medical practices, medication included. Considering the high rate of drop-outs when translating pre-clinical data to successful clinical outcome, the report of a specific therapeutic outcome (and adverse reactions) from plant-based formulas ingested orally by people is an advantage for drug development that cannot be underestimated (Mullane, Winquist, and Williams 2014).

The seemingly simple idea to use traditional medical systems as sources of relevant information for drug development contrasts with the realities that there are difficulties in translating traditional medical practices to the to the now dominant evidence based Western biomedical paradigm. Firstly, traditional (Indigenous) and modern (Western biomedical) medical systems evolved from distinct sociohistorical contexts, relate to singular belief systems, and accordingly, are based on different models of disease causality, diagnosis, and treatment (Etkin 2001). Secondly, traditional medical systems and practices are inevitably shaped by and immersed in culture, regardless of which medical system one looks at. In spite of such profound differences, people worldwide make use of concepts and practices from various medical systems in order to maintain or re-establish health (Ceuterick and Vandebroek 2017; Crandon 1986; Freymann et al. 2006). An informed multidisciplinary research team can extract from the description of signs, symptomatology, disease and treatment courses reported by healers and/or users key information to formulate a sound working hypothesis to drive the desired laboratory examination (Elisabetsky 2007). Sadly, though, less than 10% of the Journal of Ethnopharmacology's papers are multidisciplinary in nature (Etkin and Elisabetsky 2005; Vandebroek and Moerman 2015).

Traditional medical practices are not easily integrated into the contemporary Western medicine paradigm because they differ in fundamental meanings of health, disease, aetiology, and cure (Wang 2012; Etkin, Ross, and Muazzamu 1990; Moerman 2002). If this difficulty is applicable in most areas of medicine, not only the understanding, but the very description of psychiatric symptomatology may vary from culture to culture (Gadit 2003; Shepard 1998; Weisman et al. 2000). Nonetheless, descriptions of symptoms and the natural course of the disease can be effectively used to bridge emic and Western disease categories. Valuable information can be obtained on the clinical outcome of therapies, when and how amelioration and/or resolution is perceived and adverse effects, among others. Unfortunately, much of this relevant information is lost or distorted because a significant (if not major) part of ethnopharmacology is based on secondhand information and/or field data collected (and interpreted) by personnel with no biomedical training/knowledge. As a result, often literature searches and cultural-driven libraries might be built upon misleading information. Despite cultural beliefs that don't align with the Western paradigm, informed clinical data collected in the field is highly instrumental for constructing a sound working hypothesis to drive laboratory and/or clinical studies (Graz 2013). In fact, observational studies and/or retrospective treatment outcomes have been proposed as initial steps to optimize the choice of plant species to be evaluated/studied, to format research designs, and/or to develop improved phytomedicines (Akubue and Mittal 1982; Graz 2013; Willcox et al. 2011).

Being often narrow in view and scope, interest in traditional medical systems for drug development is usually limited to the assumption that plants (admittedly a rich source of chemical diversity), used as traditional medicines may have a higher probability of containing bioactive compounds of interest for drug development. Nevertheless, by not truly considering traditional medicines as medicines, the research designs rarely (if ever, in industrial settings) embrace basic pharmacological hallmarks, such as formulation and posology, which are certainly relevant to the outcome. As Etkin put it "ethnopharmacologists of all backgrounds can enhance their work by projecting pharmacologic data against a backdrop of medical ethnography" (Etkin 2001). With the following examples, I hope to illustrate that if the field of ethnopharmacology is to be helpful for drug discovery and development, ethnopharmacological research approaches and methods must be optimized.

THE TEACHINGS OF TRADITIONAL PHARMACOTECHNIQUES

In the course of biomedical investigation, more often than not, the lack of respect for traditional knowledge results in a "one size fit all" approach in which the plant-based medicine research/development material/product is prepared/formulated into one (or a series of) extracts obtained according to a pre-defined laboratory protocol regardless of how the traditional remedy is made. Traditional pharmacotechniques reflect the best way to extract the compounds of interest with the limited available resources. As it is likely that only a fraction of the number of chemical compounds present in a plant species will be present in the traditional remedy, a phytochemical profiling of of an extract/formulation prepared as originaly used should indicate which compound(s) are actually ingested by the patient. However, the chemical study of such a preparation that is useful to generate hypothesis driven investigation is rarely performed. If such a customized analysis is not feasible for screening large libraries of extracts, there is no obvious reason to understand why it is often overlooked at academic settings. It should be obvious that it is simply counterproductive to initiate preclinical experiments with extracts bearing little resemblance to the original formulation, given that traditional modes of preparation may concentrate the active compounds of interest.

By narrowing the possibilities of active compounds, and thus decreasing the workload, traditional pharmacotechniques also bring insights into the best choices for extraction and isolation procedures. For instance, one can expect components of volatile aromatic components of essential oils to be the active compounds in aromatic teas (where the plant is added to hot water for a few minutes, often with a cover lid), while thermal sensitive compounds can be excluded from non-aromatic teas (where the plant is boiled in water for minutes). In the case of psychoactive drugs one must be attentive to the presence of alkaloids (as free bases, glycosides, salts of primary, secondary, tertiary amines, or quaternary ammonium salts), and explore 9:1 or 1:1 water:ethanol extracts for bottled remedies (*garrafadas* in Brazil) prepared in wine or distilled spirit (Nunes 1996). The analysis of a traditional formula used for epilepsy in the Brazilian Amazon illustrates the point: the remedy (used for *Mal de Guta and/or convoluções*) is prepared by mashing fresh leaves of *Aeollhantus suaveolens*, *Ruta graveolens*, and *Cissus sycioides* together with black sesame seeds; and the resulting mixture is filtered through a clean cloth, and ingested orally. Whereas this exact formula only delayed pentylenetetrazol-induced convulsions in mice (i.p. treated), linalool (the major component of *A. suaveolens* essential oil) was found to possess a clear and broad anticonvulsant profile (Elisabetsky and Brum 2003). With an unusual mechanism of action, linalool acts by inhibiting glutamate release with no apparent direct interaction with GABAa receptors (Elisabetsky, Brum, and Souza 1999; Silva Brum et al. 2001). The sesame seeds are likely to facilitate the extraction of the essential oils and it was the marked aroma of the active fractions of the crude extract that gave the hint to investigate the essential oil components from *A. suaveolens*. A standard fractionation/isolation protocol could well have de-fatted the sample, thus losing or modifying the active component, and would have led to a more extensive and convoluted path to identify linalool.

As is the case with allopathic drugs, traditional remedies are to be used according to a set of instructions (how much, how often, for how long, etc). It is expected that long term use may have effects significantly different than acute (single administration) or sub-chronic (a few administrations) challenges to any molecular target. Nevertheless, for planning drug development programs the traditional posology is rarely taken into consideration. Understandably, the correspondence between traditional use and its laboratory investigation collide with practical matters, such as the need for higher amounts of compounds/extracts/fraction for *in vivo*, orally administered and/or repeated administration. Be that as it may, the answer to the research hypothesis of a given biological activity based on users' claims cannot be conclusive before a fair assessment of the traditional medicine, including its posology, is accomplished. Regarding CNS active drugs this issue is of upmost importance since the long-term effects on initial targets is often required to achieve a new functional state (Hyman and Nestler 1996). Importantly, *in vitro* methodologies are unfortunately more often than not inadequate for the purposes of checking the clinical value of bioactivity (Houghton et al. 2007). The use of single administration experimental model's with good predictive validity are suitable to initiate the investigation. That is if these initial results are positive, and especially if they show dose dependent and sizable effects, in which case a more elaborate phase using models with translational value and attention for the original posology can be put in place for further investigation.

The study of alstonine shows how a traditional formulation and posology that was truer to real life use can be informative. A working hypothesis of antipsychotic properties was raised for the plant-based medicine used by Dr. Chidi Osondu, a Nigerian traditional psychiatrist. The study led to the identification of the indole alkaloid alstonine as the active compound, with a clear antipsychotic profile (positive, negative and cognitive symptoms in mice models), and a unique mechanism of action (Linck et al. 2015). Alstonine proved to be active in mice models at 0.5-2.0 mg/kg dose range, far lower than the usual 20-200mg/kg used in most studies, but compatible with the alkaloid yield in the traditional preparation recorded at field work (Costa-Campos et al. 1998). After the negative results obtained with 10 and 20 mg/kg, the entire line of research would have been abandoned, if it was not for the original preparation being considered leading us to investigate doses way lower than what is usually employed in such studies.

MULTIFACTORIAL DISEASE TARGETS VERSUS THE MAGIC BULLET

Traditional remedies are often composed of a mixture of plants, and even a single plant-based remedy may contain dozens of secondary metabolic compounds. Plants of relevance in the herb market such as Gingko (Liu et al. 2018; Tian, Liu, and Chen 2017), Gingseng (Murthy et al. 2018), and Kava Kava (Celentano et al. 2019) are examples of bioactivity resulting from an aggregate of active compounds, where activity is lost or diminished when any one is separately assessed. Synergistic interaction may be expected from different ingredients in complex formulas, as in Japanese Kampö (Satoh 2013), and Traditional Chinese Medicine (TCM) (Hong et al. 2017). Nevertheless, the majority of ethnopharmacological studies still aim to identify "the" active component, which may be only part of what is of research interest.

The use of *Psychotria colorata* based remedies in the Brazilian Amazon is a clear case which illustrates the point. Caboclos (a population also referred as "Ribeirinhos") at the Pará state in the Brazilian Amazon use *Psychotria colorata* to prepare an analgesic remedy to manage earache: a handful of cut-up fresh flowers are mashed in milk (preferably "mother's milk"), packed in banana leaves and left for a few minutes over warm ashes; the resulting mixture is filtered through a piece of cloth and drops applied into the ear; it is said that abdominal pain also responds to the species, but for that purpose roots and fruits are mixed with water, left to boil and the decoction taken orally (Elisabetsky and Castilhos 1990). Pharmacological studies of *P. colorata* flower extracts showed marked analgesic activity in various pain models in mice (Elisabetsky et al. 1995) and they contained pyrrolidino indoline alkaloids which were identified as the major active components. One of these alkaloids, hodgkinsine, possess a dual mechanism of action acting as an opioid agonist (Amador et al. 2000) and a glutamate N-methyl-D-aspartate receptor (NMDAR) antagonist. Another alkaloid constituent, psychotridine, acts as a glutamate NMDAR antagonist (Amador et al. 2001). The potent analgesic effects resulting from this cooperative mechanism of action, is equivalent to that of combining morphine and dizocilpine. Dual mechanisms of action was also identified for Kanna (*Sceletium tortuosum*) used by the Namaquas, among other peoples in the Cape area, from which selective serotonin reuptake inhibitor (SSRI) alkaloids mesembrine and mesembrenone were isolated and characterized (Gericke, 2018). Further, mesembrenone was also found to also be a specific phosphodiesterase 4 inhibitor (Harvey et al. 2011).

Results such as these call attention to the advantage of starting with *in vivo* animal model analysis, given that active compounds and/or mechanisms of action can be lost if a pre-defined target drives the research approach, which ultimately diminishes the chance to unveil innovative unforeseen mechanisms of action. Unfortunately though, even with the changes in mainstream pharmacology with regard to multiple mechanisms of action and network pharmacology (Hopkins 2008; 2007), a significant part of medicinal plant research continues to pursue *the* active compound.

ORIGINAL VERSUS AGGREGATE KNOWLEDGE

The analysis of meetings annals or journal volumes shows that the fields of natural products pharmacology and ethnopharmacology-driven biological evaluation, are marked by a pattern of limited data for a given species and/or compound, instead of a body of complementary knowledge regarding one species or formula. Typically, a congress will show limited data for a great diversity of plant species, scattered over dozens of plant families. This pattern contrasts with the extensive investigation of different aspects of new drug candidates.

For example, let us examine the study of essential oils (EO), an example of complex mixtures of compounds extensively used in traditional systems of medicines. The effects of EO inhalation in anxiety and depression has been documented in clinical settings (Aponso, Patti, and Bennett 2020; Malcolm and Tallian 2017), and they are often shown to often interact with more than one CNS target (Wang and Heinbockel 2018). A review was performed to build EO psychoactive profiles to understand the underlying mechanism(s) of actions. Because experiments performed with essential oils as such are difficult to reproduce due to their characteristically complex chemical composition (a core feature for their uniqueness), and marked quantitative and qualitative variability among EO samples, the review focused only on single compounds isolated from essential oils.

A Web of Science™ survey with the key words "essential oil" and "hypnotic/anxiolytic/anticonvulsant/antidepressant and/or neuroprotector" properties revealed 785 abstracts, from which 300 studies were selected on the basis of the scientific quality of the reports. Sixty-one (61) compounds were thus identified as being psychoactive. The Web of Science survey was repeated using the compound name and the same keywords. After dismissing reports with scientifically frail data, the sample size was reduced to 34 compounds, which were subjected to a final thorough analysis/evaluation. Of these compounds, 25 were reported to have anxiolytic, 9 hypnotic, 18 anticonvulsant, 9 antidepressant and 10 neuroprotective activity/profile, based on at least one behavioral and/or *in vivo* electrophysiology assay.

Of the 34 compounds or soanalyzed, a substantial body of data is only available for linalool, α-asarone, and thymoquinone, for which studies were replicated by different research groups suggesting a reliable psychoactive antiepileptic/anticonvulsant profile. For most compounds only one study was reported or has only been studied, which limits the data reliability (Ioannidis 2018). Among the compounds claimed to act as neuroprotectors, data is scattered over compounds and models, except for the antioxidant activity assessed in all but one compound. More often than not, only one experimental model is used, whereas a battery of models would yield a more reliable picture, and will likely rule out false positives. Another potential limitation is that the mechanism of action is often inferred from the antagonist effect performed with single dose experiments, as pointed out by Zhu and colleagues (Zhu et al. 2014) in their review of anticonvulsant compounds isolated from medicinal plants. Although this search model for potential pharmacologically active lead compounds may be acceptable in exploratory research (Kenakin et al. 2014), these compounds are unlikely to be selected for drug development until a far more rigorous analysis has taken place (Kimmelman, Mogil, and Dirnagl 2014).

Unfortunately, this pattern of a single or small set of studies on a wide range of species is dominating the field, perhaps because the idea of original research is translated into studying a species for which data is lacking. As a result, a limited set of results obtained during a Master or PhD study is left where it was, with the new student focusing on a different less studied species. Be that as it may be, the lack of accumulated data, including a battery of *in vivo* and *in vitro* tests, phytochemistry and toxicology, certainly does not help to make any given species a compelling case for drug development.

THE POWER OF "THOUGHT STYLE"

The history of pharmacology in general, and psychopharmacology in particular, is full of examples of drugs introduced to medical practice long before the mechanism of action was properly elucidated. A plant-based product example is Saint John's Wort (*Hypericum perforatum*), which was widely used for decades in the management of mild depression in various countries and continents (Linde, Berner, and Kriston 2008; Ng, Venkatanarayanan, and Ho 2017), even though its active compounds and/or mechanisms of action were, and still are, not fully clarified (Barnes, Anderson, and Phillipson 2001). This is perhaps not surprising in a field of medicine, in which the disorder's pathophysiology is often elusive. In his seminal book "Genesis and Development of a Scientific Fact" Ludwik Fleck states that "Cognition is the most socially-conditioned activity of man, and knowledge is the paramount social creation" (Fleck 1981, 42). Fleck calls attention to the point that the prevailing understanding of any topic is a basic factor of all new knowledge, as it impacts the relationship of a scientist and his/her object of study. I argue that the often-employed research design in ethnopharmacology that starts with *in vitro* tests based on known mechanisms of action may steer us away from finding innovative drugs.

To illustrate the point, let us examine a study on potential antidepressant species from South African traditional medicine. Ethnopharmacology information was used as the basis to select 34 medicinal plant species; 75 extracts were prepared and evaluated for serotonin transporter activity. From the five positive plant species found, two were discarded because they contained tropane alkaloids or cardiac glycosides, which were judged to be inappropriate for long term therapeutic use. The three remaining species were examined and found to exhibit varying degrees of activity in the forced swimming and tail suspension tests. Bio-guided fractionation led to the identification of buphanamine type alkaloids (including lycorine) and the monoterpene lactone, (-)-loliolide (Jäger 2015). It is not simple to translate emic therapeutic indications to potential antidepressant activity; even so, was this workflow appropriate to investigate these 34 selected candidates? For example, were these traditional remedies consumed for long periods of time? Could the two candidate species deemed too toxic for long term use by the investigator(s) be fast acting antidepressants, without the need for long term use, thus avoiding toxic side effects? Were the traditional formulations (emic mode of preparation) examined to verify if significant amounts of the potentially toxic alkaloids were present? Could any of the ruled out candidate plants function in the form of pro-drugs since ingested orally? Finally, would it be possible that some of the candidate plants' pharmacological actions were mediated through an entirely different mechanism of action not involving serotonin?

The failure to take into account detailed traditional knowledge (such as posology, observed therapeutic effects and side effects) when designing experiments for drug discovery research programs based on traditional medical systems resources, the choice of workflow (eg., *in vitro* before *in vivo studies*), and the limited use of pre-clinical animal models with good translational value are to blame for many/most of the misapplied investments in the study of medicinal plants. It is also part of the explanation for the extremely poor record of lead compound yields of high throughput screening programs that were once the hype and hope in the search for drugs/lead compounds from natural product libraries (Fox et al. 2006). Although studies such as the one described above in the search for antidepressants might be seen as the most valuable in academic settings, where students research training is of point, the main stream *modus operandis* adds little to the discovery of innovative therapeutic agents in general, and psychoactive drugs in particular.

A CALL FOR TRANSLATIONAL ETHNOPHARMACOLOGY

Drug development is not an academics pursuit, nor is it their responsibility. Nevertheless, academics working with medicinal plants, or their isolated compounds, do wish for their studies to contribute to the discovery of new drugs, to the development of high quality herbals, or at least for a better-informed use of these health care resources. Among these academic researchers are ethnobotanists, ethnopharmacologists, pharmacognosists/natural products chemists. Of relevance is the argument that the financial resources that fund academic research, often public, require at least an inherent intent to provide a tangible benefit to society (Horrobin 2003). If the justifiable goal of the study is simply to clarify aspects of traditional remedies, the often found concluding remarks, which explain the relevance of the study for drug development should be avoided.

It is a consensus that the full pharmaceutical potential of natural products has yet to be explored (Cragg and Newman 2013). The preference of relying on combinatorial over natural product libraries in the search of drug candidates may have contributed to the small number of new bioactive chemical lead compounds, fueling the pharmaceutical industry's productivity crisis (Ogbourne and Parsons 2014). In reference to the search for psychoactive drugs, only 5% out of 2000 studies that included ethnopharmacology in the title or key words focused on CNS studies (Heinrich 2015). Collaborative efforts in drug development have been put in place where consortia are formed with specific goals such as defining biomarkers or sharing specific data (Patridge et al. 2016; Wehling 2009). Such efforts, perhaps steered by scientific organizations devoted to specific neuronal and mental disorders could combine different academic skills and resources to attain a substantial enough body of knowledge on promising extracts/compounds to attract industrial research.

Starting the evaluation of medicinal plants with methodologies that gauge the effect on experimental models with translational value, rather than checking if it matches a pre-determined mechanism of action, may be especially relevant in the field of mental disorders for which the pathological basis are still elusive (Ledford 2014). A fair assessment of traditional remedies requires hypothesis driven and customized research designs that consider its modes of preparation (types and dose range of components) and posology (single versus repeated doses, time required for effects). With biomedical sciences in general, a more rigorous standard is required to lend credibility and reproducibility to ethnopharmacology studies (Ioannidis 2005), in which the null hypothesis is often accepted or rejected even when plant part, type of extract, dose range and the experimental model bear little resemblance to the traditional use.

The extended interpretation of cause-effect relationships in physics calls for the substitution of "cause" to "determining conditions", where all the conditions of a process or state are equally important. For complex diseases such as mental disorders, where genetic, developmental, and ontogenetic factors are increasingly recognized, the concept of determination fits better than causality (Vineis and Porta 1996). When diseases are understood as processes, where an interplay of multiple factors have to be considered, it becomes attractive to study complex extracts and/or plant formulas that may simultaneously modulate more than one target (Rasoanaivo et al. 2011; Roth, Sheffler, and Kroeze 2004). In order to truly benefit from studying traditional medical systems as such, rather than just medicinal plants as sources of bioactive molecules, ethnopharmacologists, pharmacologists, pharmacognosits and phytochemists need to be unprejudiced and open-minded, adopting an unbiased appreciation of potentially new drug classes or even paradigms. The somewhat new paradigm of network pharmacology (Hopkins 2008) is much in alignment with traditional/Indigenous remedies (e.g., they have more than one active compound, varied/multiple-mechanisms of action) than the now outdated single "silver bullet" drug model. Yet phytomedicine is often seen as messy and untrustworthy by the establishment pharmacologists/medical practitioners. I argue that incorporating ethnopharmacology and applying rigorous, hypothesis-driven laboratory evaluation, while also considering traditional medical concepts and practices, can be a fruitful strategy for developing innovative psychoactive drugs.

CONCLUSION

Ludwik Fleck says that "fundamentally new facts can be discovered only through new thinking" (Fleck 1981, 51). We are supposed to be investigating medical systems that profoundly differ from ours. If we do not recognize this we risk conducting what Fleck calls a self-fulfilling type of investigation, which in ethnopharmacology is "validating" traditional use by looking for data that fits in the boxes we know. In doing so, instead of using ethnopharmacology leads to help discover truly innovative medicines, we will continue to attempt to tap a well that just seems dry due to our shortsighted minds and biased research approaches.

ACKNOWLEDGEMENTS

I wish to thank Dennis McKenna and the McKenna academy for making ESPD55 happen, and for the opportunity to present these ideas to such a unique audience. I want to express my gratitude for the impeccable editing of this manuscript by Professor Harry Fong, with whom I have the continuing pleasure to discuss traditional medicines and natural products in relation to drug discovery and public health.

BIBLIOGRAPHY

Akubue, P. I., and G. C. Mittal. 1982. "Clinical Evaluation of a Traditional Herbal Practice in Nigeria: A Preliminary Report." *Journal of Ethnopharmacology* 6 (3): 355–59. https://doi.org/10.1016/0378-8741(82)90056-3.

Amador, Tania A., L. Verotta, D. S. Nunes, and E. Elisabetsky. 2000. "Antinociceptive Profile of Hodgkinsine." *Planta Medica* 66 (8): 770–72. https://doi.org/10.1055/s-2000-9604.

Amador, Tania.A., L. Verotta, D.S. Nunes, and E. Elisabetsky. 2001. "Involvement of NMDA Receptors in the Analgesic properties of Psychotridine." *Phytomedicine* 8 (3): 202–6. https://doi.org/10.1078/0944-7113-00025.

Aponso, Minoli, Antonio Patti, and Louise E. Bennett. 2020. "Dose-Related Effects of Inhaled Essential Oils on Behavioural Measures of Anxiety and Depression and Biomarkers of Oxidative Stress." *Journal of Ethnopharmacology* 250 (March): 112469. https://doi.org/10.1016/j.jep.2019.112469.

Barnes, J., L. A. Anderson, and J. D. Phillipson. 2001. "St John's Wort (Hypericum Perforatum L.): A Review of Its Chemistry, Pharmacology and Clinical Properties." *The Journal of Pharmacy and Pharmacology* 53 (5): 583–600. https://doi.org/10.1211/0022357011775910.

Birari, Rahul B., and Kamlesh K. Bhutani. 2007. "Pancreatic Lipase Inhibitors from Natural Sources: Unexplored Potential." *Drug Discovery Today* 12 (19): 879–89. https://doi.org/10.1016/j.drudis.2007.07.024.

Celentano, Antonio, Andrew Tran, Claire Testa, Krishen Thayanantha, William Tan-Orders, Stephanie Tan, Mitali Syamal, Michael J. McCullough, and Tami Yap. 2019. "The Protective Effects of Kava (Piper Methysticum) Constituents in Cancers: A Systematic Review." *Journal of Oral Pathology & Medicine* 48 (7): 510–29. https://doi.org/10.1111/jop.12900.

Ceuterick, Melissa, and Ina Vandebroek. 2017. "Identity in a Medicine Cabinet: Discursive Positions of Andean Migrants towards Their Use of Herbal Remedies in the United Kingdom." *Social Science & Medicine* 177 (March): 43–51. https://doi.org/10.1016/j.socscimed.2017.01.026.

Costa-Campos, Luciane, D. R. Lara, D. S. Nunes, and E. Elisabetsky. 1998. "Antipsychotic-like Profile of Alstonine." *Pharmacology, Biochemistry, and Behavior* 60 (1): 133–41. https://doi.org/10.1016/s0091-3057(97)00594-7.

Cragg, Gordon M., and David J. Newman. 2013. "Natural Products: A Continuing Source of Novel Drug Leads." *Biochimica Et Biophysica Acta* 1830 (6): 3670–95. https://doi.org/10.1016/j.bbagen.2013.02.008.

Crandon, Libbet. 1986. "Medical Dialogue and the Political Economy of Medical Pluralism: A Case from Rural Highland Bolivia." *American Ethnologist* 13 (3): 463–76. https://doi.org/10.1525/ae.1986.13.3.02a00040.

Elisabetsky, Elaine. 1991. "Sociopolitical, Economical and Ethical Issues in Medicinal Plant Research." *Journal of Ethnopharmacology*, Special Issue Proceedings of the First International Congress on Ethnopharmacology, 32 (1): 235–39. https://doi.org/10.1016/0378-8741(91)90124-V.

Elisabetsky, Elaine. 2007. "PHYTOTHERAPY AND THE NEW PARADIGM OF DRUGS MODE OF ACTION.Elisabetsky," Scientia et Technica, 33: 459–64.

Elisabetsky, Elaine. 2021. "Ethnopharmacology and the Development of Psychoactive Drug: A Critical Overview." In *NeuroPsychopharmacotherapy*, edited by Peter Riederer, Gerd Laux, Toshiharu Nagatsu, Weidong Le, and Christian Riederer, 1–15. Cham: Springer International Publishing. https://doi.org/10.1007/978-3-319-56015-1_459-1.

Elisabetsky, Elaine, Amador, Albuquerque, Domingos Nunes, and Carvalho. 1995. "Analgesic Activity of Psychotria Colorata (Willd. Ex R. & S.) Muell. Arg. Alkaloids." *Journal of Ethnopharmacology* 48 (2): 77–83. https://doi.org/10.1016/0378-8741(95)01287-N.

Elisabetsky, Elaine and Brum, Lucimar. 2003. "Linalool as Active Component of Traditional Remedies: Anticonvulsant Properties and Mechanisms of Action." *Curare* 26 (January): 45–52.

Elisabetsky, Elaine Brum, and Souza. 1999. "Anticonvulsant Properties of Linalool in Glutamate-Related Seizure Models." *Phytomedicine: International Journal of Phytotherapy and Phytopharmacology* 6 (2): 107–13. https://doi.org/10.1016/s0944-7113(99)80044-0.

Elisabetsky, Elaine and Castilhos, Zuleica. 1990. "Plants Used as Analgesics by Amazonian Caboclos as a Basis for Selecting Plants for Investigation." *International Journal of Crude Drug Research* 28 (4): 309–20. https://doi.org/10.3109/13880209009082838.

Etkin, Nina 2001. "Perspectives in Ethnopharmacology: Forging a Closer Link between Bioscience and Traditional Empirical Knowledge." *Journal of Ethnopharmacology* 76 (2): 177–82. https://doi.org/10.1016/s0378-8741(01)00232-x.

Etkin, Nina and Elisabetsky, Elaine. 2005. "Seeking a Transdisciplinary and Culturally Germane Science: The Future of Ethnopharmacology." *Journal of Ethnopharmacology* 100 (1–2): 23–26. https://doi.org/10.1016/j.jep.2005.05.025.

Etkin, Nina, Ross, and Muazzamu. 1990. "The Indigenization of Pharmaceuticals: Therapeutic Transitions in Rural Hausaland." *Social Science & Medicine* 30 (8): 919–28. https://doi.org/10.1016/0277-9536(90)90220-M.

Farnsworth, Norman R. 1984. "How Can the Well Be Dry When It Is Filled with Water?" *Economic Botany* 38 (1): 4–13. https://doi.org/10.1007/BF02904411.

Fleck, Ludwik. 1981. *Genesis and Development of a Scientific Fact*. Edited by Thaddeus J. Trenn. Translated by Robert King Merton. Chicago: University of Chicago press.

Fox, Sandra, Shauna Farr-Jones, Lynne Sopchak, Amy Boggs, Helen Wang Nicely, Richard Khoury, and Michael Biros. 2006. "High-Throughput Screening: Update on Practices and Success." *Journal of Biomolecular Screening* 11 (7): 864–69. https://doi.org/10.1177/1087057106292473.

Freymann, Heike, Timothy Rennie, Ian Bates, Sabine Nebel, and Michael Heinrich. 2006. "Knowledge and Use of Complementary and Alternative Medicine among British Undergraduate Pharmacy Students." *Pharmacy World & Science* 28 (1): 13–18. https://doi.org/10.1007/s11096-005-2221-z.

Gadit, Amin 2003. "Ethnopsychiatry—a Review" 53 (10): 1–6.

Gericke, Nigel 2018. "The Past, Present and Possible Future of Kanna." In *Ethnopharmacological Search for Psychoactive Drugs.*, 122–50. Synergetic Press,.

Graz, Bertrand. 2013. "What Is 'Clinical Data'? Why and How Can They Be Collected during Field Surveys on Medicinal Plants?" *Journal of Ethnopharmacology* 150 (2): 775–79. https://doi.org/10.1016/j.jep.2013.08.036.

Graz, Bertrand, Merlin Willcox, Diafara Berthé, Denis-Luc Ardiet, Jacques Falquet, Drissa Diallo, and Sergio Giani. 2015. "Home Treatments Alone or Mixed with Modern Treatments for Malaria in Finkolo AC, South Mali: Reported Use, Outcomes and Changes over 10 Years." *Transactions of the Royal Society of Tropical Medicine and Hygiene* 109 (3): 209–13. https://doi.org/10.1093/trstmh/tru181.

Greene, Claire, Brigid Barlesi, Sigrid Tarroza-David, and Terence Friedlander. 2021. "Improved Control of Tyrosine Kinase Inhibitor-Induced Diarrhea with a Novel Chloride Channel Modulator: A Case Report." *Oncology and Therapy* 9 (1): 247–53. https://doi.org/10.1007/s40487-021-00147-3.

Gyllenhaal, Charlotte, M. R. Kadushin, B. Southavong, K. Sydara, S. Bouamanivong, M. Xaiveu, L. T. Xuan, et al. 2012. "Ethnobotanical Approach versus Random Approach in the Search for New Bioactive Compounds: Support of a Hypothesis." *Pharmaceutical Biology* 50 (1): 30–41. https://doi.org/10.3109/13880209.2011.634424.

Harvey, Alan L., RuAngelie Edrada-Ebel, and Ronald J. Quinn. 2015. "The Re-Emergence of Natural Products for Drug Discovery in the Genomics Era." *Nature Reviews Drug Discovery* 14 (2): 111–29. https://doi.org/10.1038/nrd4510.

Harvey, Alan L., Louise C. Young, Alvaro M. Viljoen, and Nigel P. Gericke. 2011. "Pharmacological Actions of the South African Medicinal and Functional Food Plant Sceletium Tortuosum and Its Principal Alkaloids." *Journal of Ethnopharmacology* 137 (3): 1124–29. https://doi.org/10.1016/j.jep.2011.07.035.

Heinrich, Michael 2015. "Ethnopharmacology: A Short History of a Multidisciplinary Field of Reserach." In *Ethnopharmacology*, 1–9. UK: Wiley Blackwell.

Hong, Chunlan, Anja Schüffler, Ulrich Kauhl, Jingming Cao, Ching-Fen Wu, Till Opatz, Eckhard Thines, and Thomas Efferth. 2017. "Identification of NF-⊠B as Determinant of Posttraumatic Stress Disorder and Its Inhibition by the Chinese Herbal Remedy Free and Easy Wanderer." *Frontiers in Pharmacology* 8 (April). https://doi.org/10.3389/fphar.2017.00181.

Hopkins, Andrew L. 2007. "Network Pharmacology." *Nature Biotechnology* 25 (10): 1110–11. https://doi.org/10.1038/nbt1007-1110.

Hopkins, Andrew L. 2008. "Network Pharmacology: The next Paradigm in Drug Discovery." *Nature Chemical Biology* 4 (11): 682–90. https://doi.org/10.1038/nchembio.118.

Horrobin, David F. 2003. "Modern Biomedical Research: An Internally Self-Consistent Universe with Little Contact with Medical Reality?" *Nature Reviews. Drug Discovery* 2 (2): 151–54. https://doi.org/10.1038/nrd1012.

Houghton, Peter J., M.-J. Howes, C. C. Lee, and G. Steventon. 2007. "Uses and Abuses of in Vitro Tests in Ethnopharmacology: Visualizing an Elephant." *Journal of Ethnopharmacology* 110 (3): 391–400. https://doi.org/10.1016/j.jep.2007.01.032.

Hyman, Steven E., and E. J. Nestler. 1996. "Initiation and Adaptation: A Paradigm for Understanding Psychotropic Drug Action." *The American Journal of Psychiatry* 153 (2): 151–62. https://doi.org/10.1176/ajp.153.2.151.

Ioannidis, John P. A. 2005. "Why Most Published Research Findings Are False." *PLoS Medicine* 2 (8): e124. https://doi.org/10.1371/journal.pmed.0020124.

Ioannidis, John P. A. 2018. "Meta-Research: Why Research on Research Matters." *PLoS Biology* 16 (3): e2005468. https://doi.org/10.1371/journal.pbio.2005468.

Jäger, Anna 2015. "Medicinal Plant Research: A Reflection on Translational Tasks." In *Ethnopharmacology*, 11–16.

Kenakin, Terry, David B. Bylund, Myron L. Toews, Kevin Mullane, Raymond J. Winquist, and Michael Williams. 2014. "Replicated, Replicable and Relevant–Target Engagement and Pharmacological Experimentation in the 21st Century." *Biochemical Pharmacology* 87 (1): 64–77. https://doi.org/10.1016/j.bcp.2013.10.024.

Kimmelman, Jonathan, Jeffrey S. Mogil, and Ulrich Dirnagl. 2014. "Distinguishing between Exploratory and Confirmatory Preclinical Research Will Improve Translation." *PLoS Biology* 12 (5): e1001863. https://doi.org/10.1371/journal.pbio.1001863.

Ledford, Heidi. 2014. "Medical Research: If Depression Were Cancer." *Nature* 515 (7526): 182–84. https://doi.org/10.1038/515182a.

Linck, Viviane M., Marcelo Ganzella, Ana P. Herrmann, Christopher O. Okunji, Diogo O. Souza, Marta C. Antonelli, and Elaine Elisabetsky. 2015. "Original Mechanisms of Antipsychotic Action by the Indole Alkaloid Alstonine (Picralima Nitida)." *Phytomedicine: International Journal of Phytotherapy and Phytopharmacology* 22 (1): 52–55. https://doi.org/10.1016/j.phymed.2014.10.010.

Linde, Klaus, Michael M. Berner, and Levente Kriston. 2008. "St John's Wort for Major Depression." *The Cochrane Database of Systematic Reviews*, no. 4 (October): CD000448. https://doi.org/10.1002/14651858.CD000448.pub3.

Liu, Hong, Li-ping Tan, Xin Huang, Yi-qiu Liao, Wei-jian Zhang, Pei-bo Li, Yong-gang Wang, et al. 2018. "Chromatogram-Bioactivity Correlation-Based Discovery and Identification of Three Bioactive Compounds Affecting Endothelial Function in Ginkgo Biloba Extract." *Molecules* 23 (5): 1071. https://doi.org/10.3390/molecules23051071.

Malcolm, Benjamin J., and Kimberly Tallian. 2017. "Essential Oil of Lavender in Anxiety Disorders: Ready for Prime Time?" *The Mental Health Clinician* 7 (4): 147–55. https://doi.org/10.9740/mhc.2017.07.147.

McChesney, James D., Sylesh K. Venkataraman, and John T. Henri. 2007. "Plant Natural Products: Back to the Future or into Extinction?" *Phytochemistry* 68 (14): 2015–22. https://doi.org/10.1016/j.phytochem.2007.04.032.

Moerman, Daniel E. 2002. *Meaning, Medicine, and the "Placebo Effect."* Cambridge Studies in Medical Anthropology 9. Cambridge ; New York: Cambridge University Press.

Mullane, Kevin, Raymond J. Winquist, and Michael Williams. 2014. "Translational Paradigms in Pharmacology and Drug Discovery." *Biochemical Pharmacology* 87 (1): 189–210. https://doi.org/10.1016/j.bcp.2013.10.019.

Murthy, Hosakatte Niranjana, Vijayalaxmi S. Dandin, So-Young Park, and Kee-Yoeup Paek. 2018. "Quality, Safety and Efficacy Profiling of Ginseng Adventitious Roots Produced in Vitro." *Applied Microbiology and Biotechnology* 102 (17): 7309–17. https://doi.org/10.1007/s00253-018-9188-x.

Nee, Judy, Katherine Salley, Andrew G. Ludwig, Thomas Sommers, Sarah Ballou, Eve Takazawa, Sarah Duehren, et al. 2019. "Randomized Clinical Trial: Crofelemer Treatment in Women With Diarrhea-Predominant Irritable Bowel Syndrome." *Clinical and Translational Gastroenterology* 10 (12): e00110. https://doi.org/10.14309/ctg.0000000000000110.

Ng, Qin Xiang, Nandini Venkatanarayanan, and Collin Yih Xian Ho. 2017. "Clinical Use of Hypericum Perforatum (St John's Wort) in Depression: A Meta-Analysis." *Journal of Affective Disorders* 210 (March): 211–21. https://doi.org/10.1016/j.jad.2016.12.048.

Nunes, Domingos S. 1996. "Chemical Approaches to the Study of Ethnomedicines." In *Medical Resources of the Tropical Forest*, 41–47. Columbia University Press.

Ogbourne, Steven M., and Peter G. Parsons. 2014. "The Value of Nature's Natural Product Library for the Discovery of New Chemical Entities: The Discovery of Ingenol Mebutate." *Fitoterapia* 98 (October): 36–44. https://doi.org/10.1016/j.fitote.2014.07.002.

Patridge, Eric, Peter Gareiss, Michael S. Kinch, and Denton Hoyer. 2016. "An Analysis of FDA-Approved Drugs: Natural Products and Their Derivatives." *Drug Discovery Today* 21 (2): 204–7. https://doi.org/10.1016/j.drudis.2015.01.009.

Rasoanaivo, Philippe, Colin W. Wright, Merlin L. Willcox, and Ben Gilbert. 2011. "Whole Plant Extracts versus Single Compounds for the Treatment of Malaria: Synergy and Positive Interactions." *Malaria Journal* 10 Suppl 1 (March): S4. https://doi.org/10.1186/1475-2875-10-S1-S4.

Roth, Bryan L., Douglas J. Sheffler, and Wesley K. Kroeze. 2004. "Magic Shotguns versus Magic Bullets: Selectively Non-Selective Drugs for Mood Disorders and Schizophrenia." *Nature Reviews. Drug Discovery* 3 (4): 353–59. https://doi.org/10.1038/nrd1346.

Satoh, Hiroyasu. 2013. "Pharmacological Characteristics of Kampo Medicine as a Mixture of Constituents and Ingredients." *Journal of Integrative Medicine* 11 (1): 11–16. https://doi.org/10.3736/jintegrmed2013003.

Scheinfeld, Noah. 2013. "Update on the Treatment of Genital Warts." *Dermatology Online Journal* 19 (6): 18559.

Seck, Sidy Mohamed, Dominique Doupa, Diatou Guéye Dia, ElHadji Assane Diop, Denis-Luc Ardiet, Renata Campos Nogueira, Bertrand Graz, and Boucar Diouf. 2018. "Clinical Efficacy of African Traditional Medicines in Hypertension: A Randomized Controlled Trial with Combretum Micranthum and Hibiscus Sabdariffa." *Journal of Human Hypertension* 32 (1): 75–81. https://doi.org/10.1038/s41371-017-0001-6.

Shepard, Glenn H. 1998. "Psychoactive Plants and Ethnopsychiatric Medicines of the Matsigenka." *Journal of Psychoactive Drugs* 30 (4): 321–32. https://doi.org/10.1080/02791072.1998.10399708.

Silva Brum, Lucimar , Souza, and Elisabetsky. 2001. "Effects of Linalool on Glutamate Release and Uptake in Mouse Cortical Synaptosomes." *Neurochemical Research* 26 (3): 191–94. https://doi.org/10.1023/a:1010904214482.

Skirycz, Aleksandra, Sylwia Kierszniowska, Michaël Méret, Lothar Willmitzer, and George Tzotzos. 2016. "Medicinal Bioprospecting of the Amazon Rainforest: A Modern Eldorado?" *Trends in Biotechnology* 34 (10): 781–90. https://doi.org/10.1016/j.tibtech.2016.03.006.

Tian, Jinfan, Yue Liu, and Keji Chen. 2017. "Ginkgo Biloba Extract in Vascular Protection: Molecular Mechanisms and Clinical Applications." *Current Vascular Pharmacology* 15 (6). https://doi.org/10.2174/1570161111566617071 3095545.

Vandebroek, Ina, and Daniel E. Moerman. 2015. "The Anthropology of Ethnopharmacology." In *Ethnopharmacology*, 1st ed., 17–28. John Wilwy & Sons, LTd.

Verpoorte, Robert 2012. "Good Practices: The Basis for Evidence-Based Medicines." *Journal of Ethnopharmacology* 140 (3): 455–57. https://doi.org/10.1016/j.jep.2012.02.033.

Vineis, P., and M. Porta. 1996. "Causal Thinking, Biomarkers, and Mechanisms of Carcinogenesis." *Journal of Clinical Epidemiology* 49 (9): 951–56. https://doi.org/10.1016/0895-4356(96)00118-7.

Wang, Qi 2012. "Individualized Medicine, Health Medicine, and Constitutional Theory in Chinese Medicine." *Frontiers of Medicine* 6 (1): 1–7. https://doi.org/10.1007/s11684-012-0173-y.

Wang, Ze-Jun and Heinbockel. 2018. "Essential Oils and Their Constituents Targeting the GABAergic System and Sodium Channels as Treatment of Neurological Diseases." *Molecules (Basel, Switzerland)* 23 (5). https://doi.org/10.3390/molecules23051061.

Wehling, Martin. 2009. "Assessing the Translatability of Drug Projects: What Needs to Be Scored to Predict Success?" *Nature Reviews. Drug Discovery* 8 (7): 541–46. https://doi.org/10.1038/nrd2898.

Weisman, Amy G., Steven R. López, Joseph Ventura, Keith H. Nuechterlein, Michael J. Goldstein, and Sun Hwang. 2000. "A Comparison of Psychiatric Symptoms Between Anglo-Americans and Mexican-Americans With Schizophrenia." *Schizophrenia Bulletin* 26 (4): 817–24. https://doi.org/10.1093/oxfordjournals.schbul.a033496.

Willcox, Merlin L., Bertrand Graz, Jacques Falquet, Chiaka Diakite, Sergio Giani, and Drissa Diallo. 2011. "A 'Reverse Pharmacology' Approach for Developing an Anti-Malarial Phytomedicine." *Malaria Journal* 10 Suppl 1 (March): S8. https://doi.org/10.1186/1475-2875-10-S1-S8.

World Health Organization, International Union for Conservation of Nature and Natural Resources, and World Wide Fund for Nature, eds. 1993. *Guidelines on the Conservation of Medicinal Plants*. Gland, Switzerland: World Health Organization : World Conservation Union : World Wide Fund for Nature.

Wu, Charles, Su-Lin Lee, Cassandra Taylor, Jing Li, Yen-Ming Chan, Rajiv Agarwal, Robert Temple, Douglas Throckmorton, and Katherine Tyner. 2020. "Scientific and Regulatory Approach to Botanical Drug Development: A U.S. FDA Perspective." *Journal of Natural Products* 83 (2): 552–62. https://doi.org/10.1021/acs.jnatprod.9b00949.

Wynberg, Rachel, and Sarah Laird. 2022. "Access and Benefit Sharing and Biodiversity Conservation." In *Access and Benefit Sharing of Genetic Resources, Information and Traditional Knowledge*, by Charles Lawson, Fran Humphries, and Michelle Rourke, 1st ed., 50–70. London: Routledge. https://doi.org/10.4324/9781003301998-6.

Zhu, Hui-Ling, Jian-Bo Wan, Yi-Tao Wang, Bao-Cai Li, Cheng Xiang, Jing He, and Peng Li. 2014. "Medicinal Compounds with Antiepileptic/Anticonvulsant Activities." *Epilepsia* 55 (1): 3–16. https://doi.org/10.1111/epi.12463.

Kratom (*Mitragyna Speciosa*): Recent Advances in Understanding the Chemistry, Pharmacology, and Human Use

Christopher R. McCurdy, PhD

Department of Medicinal Chemistry, College of Pharmacy, University of Florida | Director of the UF Translational Drug Development Core

"This polypharmacology renders kratom unique from other opioids and to label kratom an opioid is scientifically and factually incorrect." —Chris McCurdy

Kratom is a popular, and commonly misunderstood plant that can support many healthcare issues. Christopher McCurdy shares with us the science and potential behind this traditional medicine.

Originally, I think that this plant found me when I was studying *Salvia divinorum* and I was asked by the National Institute on Drug Abuse to present a talk about naturally occurring analgesics (McCurdy & Scully, 2005). During my research for that talk, I came across this plant (*Mitragyna speciosa*) and it just sort of kept coming back and coming back and coming back. Soon, *Salvia divinorum* faded away from my interest and our teams' research. *Mitragyna speciosa* really percolated to the top and became something that was at first, an effort to isolate alkaloids, as we were determined to create new analgesics from derivatization of these alkaloids.

We were met with a lot of resistance because these compounds had nowhere near the affinities for opioid receptors that the traditional opiate like molecules of morphine and oxycodone and other prescription opiates had. So, study sections at National Institutes of Health basically left us out of consideration. It was interesting, when I was in the shower one day, I was thinking, why? Why is this plant so important? How is it utilized and how does it exist within its native population? Of course, it is used as a tea decocted from the leaves or simply the leaves are chewed. So I said, why are we trying to isolate out every single compound and understand each compound alone? It's a unique symphony orchestra that is existing together, so why take each instrument out? Well, we must take each instrument out from that objective, scientific standpoint to look at what those potential contributions are to the overall orchestra. Since ESPD50, we have learned so much from this approach and about the plant. Our team includes horticulturists and plant biosynthetic chemists and pharmacologists to go a little deeper and further into understanding what this plant is really trying to teach us.

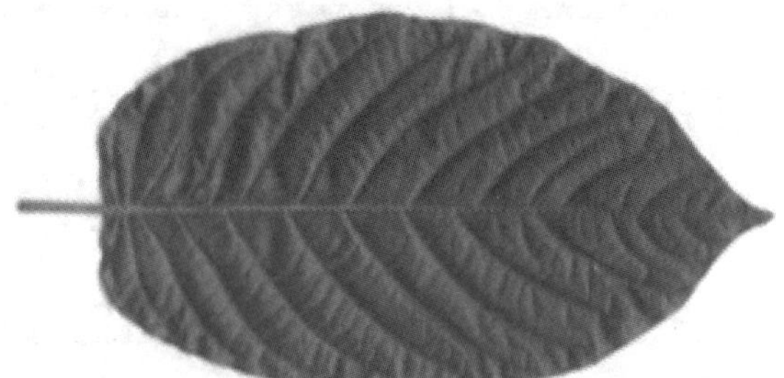

Fig.1 Leaf of *Mitragyna speciosa*

First, for those that do not know about kratom or *Mitragyna speciosa*, let me bring you up to speed. This plant comes from the family Rubiaceae, which is the same family of the coffee plant (Jansen & Prast, 1988). This plant and this genus doesn't seem to contain caffeine in it so, we don't see that similarity that we do with coffee plant. The *Mitragyna* genus was named from the shape of the leaf. If you take the leaf shown in Figure 1 and turn it -90 degrees and stand it sort of straight up, you'll see that it resembles a bishop's hat or a mitre, and that's where the name came from.

This is a tree that is found in tropical Southeast Asia, particularly at the interface of peninsular Malaysia and Thailand. This is the richest area of concentration of these trees. It's since spread probably by human propagation all across Southeast Asia, and most of the material that's coming into the United States and into the Western world is actually coming out of Indonesia now, not from Malaysia or Thailand based on word of mouth from kratom vendors in the USA.

In Thailand, the plant is referred to as kratom (Krat-Tom) and we hear a lot of it in the Western world pronounced "Craytum". Craytum (Kratom) is a pronunciation that was pretty much created in the USA or the Western world. That pronunciation is not recognized in Southeast Asia. So, kratom or craytum or ketum (Key-tum), which it is called in Malaysia, are the known pronunciations.

There are over 40 different alkaloids that have been reported to have been isolated from this plant and nobody has looked at anything else- most of the focus has been on alkaloids (Adkins et al., 2011). Historically, that makes sense because plants that contain alkaloids are thought to have their bioactivity resulting from these compounds. However, there are other perceptive qualities that don't seem to be coming from the alkaloids, and so this is something that is totally untouched right now. There's a whole plethora of other compounds within the plant that researchers haven't really even scratched the surface of yet. So, our team has focused on the alkaloids because that's sort of the low hanging fruit, if you will.

Figure 2 shows the flowering seed pod of this plant that occurs about once a season. It's a beautiful and fragrant flower that contains a number of different alkaloids or a concentration of different alkaloids than do the leaf materials. However, most of the individuals that we've talked with in Malaysia don't tend to use the flower as anything special. They just harvest the leaves freshly and use those.

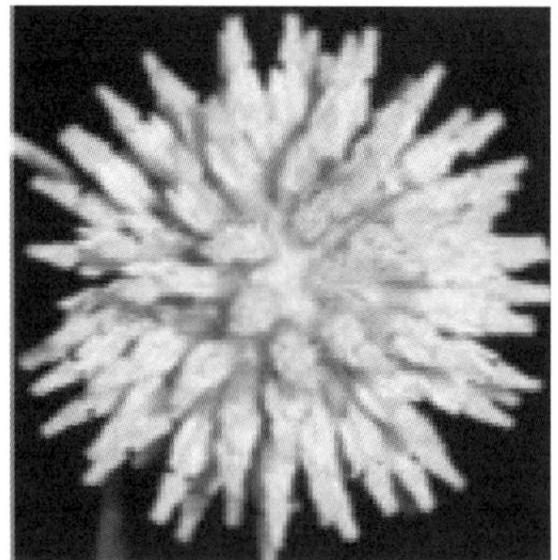

Fig.2 *Mitragyna speciosa* flower/seed pod

What does that look like? The typical use of kratom in Malaysia and Thailand is derived from the leaves of the tree shown in Figure 3.

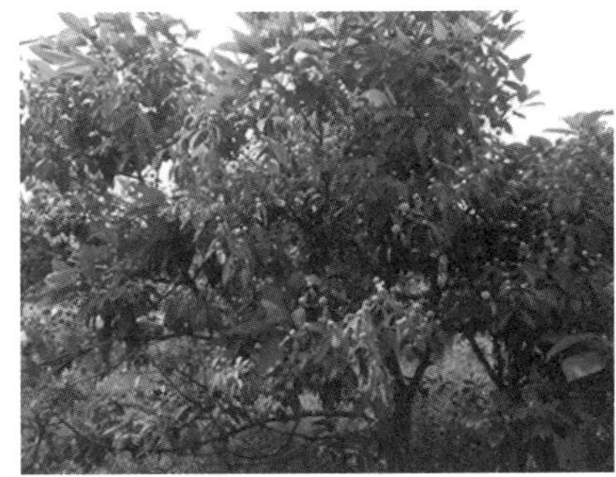

Fig.3 *Mitragyna speciosa* tree in flowering stage

Those trees are really in almost everybody's yard in that region and it's legal to have your own tree and it is legal to have your own production of and use of kratom. It's not legal to sell it in Malaysia, however, you can see in Figure 4A, a roadside stand where you can stop and pick up your beverage of choice.

In this case, the traditional preparation is made from fresh leaves that are plucked, about five kilograms are put into about five liters of water. Those leaves are cut with just regular scissors (or ripped by hand) to expose more of the surface area. They're boiled for about 2 to 3 hours to create the tea (Figure 4B). Then the tea, or juice, as they call it, is consumed at the roadside stand or packaged into baggies to take away (Figure 4C).

Native users in Malaysia will say that after 48 hours, the tea has no more activity. The interesting part of that is all the alkaloids are still intact based on our analyses over time. So, there is something that this plant is again trying to teach us that we seem to be ignoring and something that we are very, very interested in really trying to understand. The brewed juice is utilized about three times a day, morning, afternoon and late afternoon/early evening. They will split this about 1:1 with either ambient or warm water, and then they'll consume those very much like many of us would consume coffee or tea in our normal day of activity. Like coffee, kratom is also something that's titrated to the effect. For example, some mornings I wake up and one cup of coffee is enough for me, whereas some mornings I need maybe two or three. So, it's something that's titrated to the effect and is not a fixed or prescribed dosage. Afterall, it is a natural product and variation exists from batch to batch.

Kratom has been used historically by outdoor laborers to be able to prolong their ability to work in the hot sun climate, also to relieve pain as they work (Singh et al., 2019). It has a para-

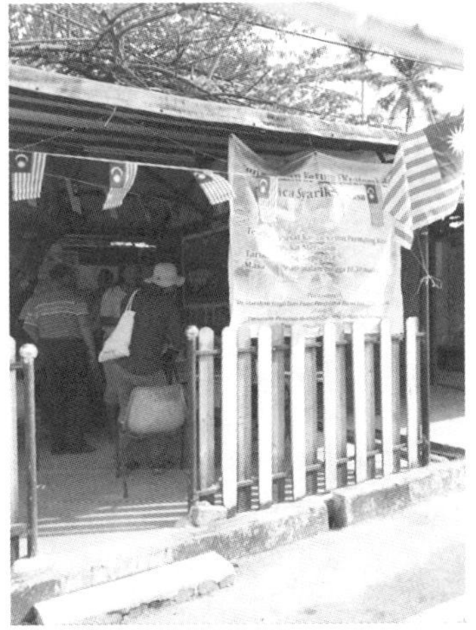

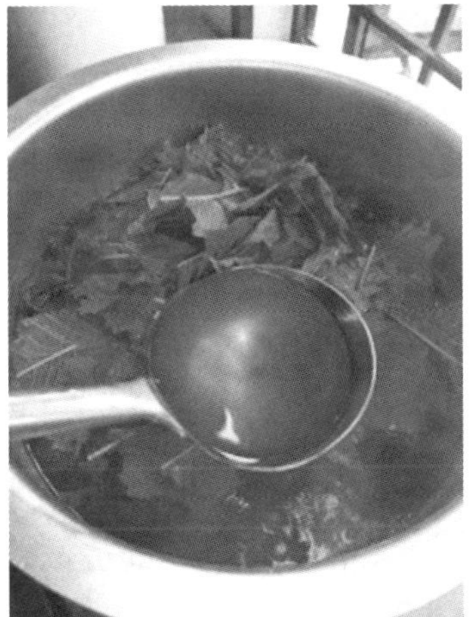

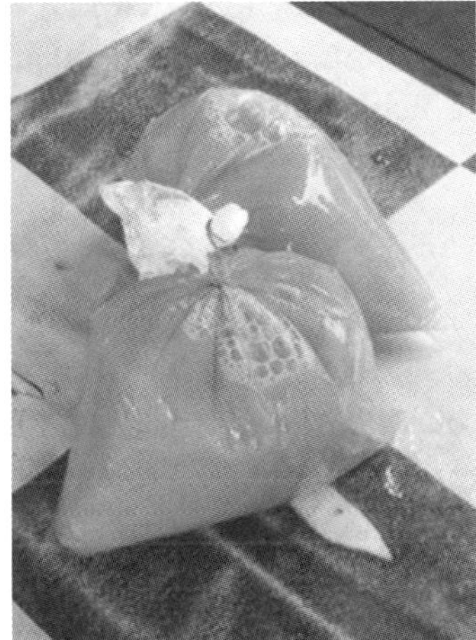

Fig.4 A) Roadside kratom stand in Malaysia. B) Preparation of kratom tea. C) Kratom tea package "to go".

doxical pharmacological approach which I have started to coin as "disruptive pharmacology". I really think of kratom as having disruptive pharmacology and this is because it has a categorical emptiness and is unique. The FDA in the United States categorizes kratom as an unregulated opioid. It's not an opioid. It's fundamentally wrong, in my opinion, to classify it as an opioid. It has been stuck in this box because we want to put things into a box. But it's completely not opioid. It has qualities of opioids; it interacts with opioid receptors but also so many other receptors. One could argue that it is an opioid simply because it interacts with opioid receptors. However, the way we currently classify opioid compounds are those that *only* interact with opioid receptors. Again, kratom is this symphony orchestra of activity that is really fascinating, and it does have stimulant and mood elevating activity as well. Many indigenous farmers and laborers also use traditional opium preparations to this day. When they run out of opium, they claim to increase their consumption of kratom to avoid going into withdrawal (Singh et al., 2019). This use is what really sparked our interest because we have a worldwide, particularly in the United States, opioid crisis. Could kratom be something that could help? Is it possible that nature has providing a remedy to balance or augment what nature has provided us with the opium poppy, and the crisis that has resulted? Personally, I have long believed that nature has solutions to problems or diseases derived from nature as it plays into the balance of the universe.

This really started to crystallize our thought process around where we want to go with our research program, moving away from really looking at analgesic activity (although we're still doing that), and really examining if kratom can be useful in opioid use disorders and helpful to the world in that sense.

We have done a lot of collaborative work with scientists at the Universiti Sains Malaysia (University of Science Malaysia), located in Penang, Malaysia. One of the most recent surveys that conducted with them found that poly drug users, individuals that are using opiates along with methamphetamine, are actually finding that kratom is able to reduce their usage of methamphetamine (Singh et al., 2020). This is interesting from many standpoints, especially since there are no approved treatments for methamphetamine use disorder or stimulant use disorders. We do know that kratom has stimulant like effects and it is not clear if use of kratom is substituting or actually reducing the desire for intake of stimulants. How is kratom supposedly reducing methamphetamine intake? Is there some pharmacokinetic consequence that's causing this or is it working on neurotransmitters to block out that effect? This is something we are also interested in.

The predominant or at least thought to be predominant active alkaloid in kratom is mitragynine, a corynanthe-based indole alkaloid. It is an interesting molecule from many standpoints, and we finally feel like we have an understanding of how it's interacting with different G-protein coupled receptors (GPCRs) in a different fashion than what we thought of originally when we compared it to structures of opioids (Kruegel et al., 2016). I will come back to that as everyone was pointing out it was some sort of opioid, and we're learning that it has many more activities.

Kratom use in the United States, and in the Western world looks very different. Shown in Figure 5 are products that you would see available through the Internet or smoke shops.

In fact, right off our campus at the University of Florida, one can walk to a smoke shop where an entire wall section of kratom products are available. Our team has purchased and ana-

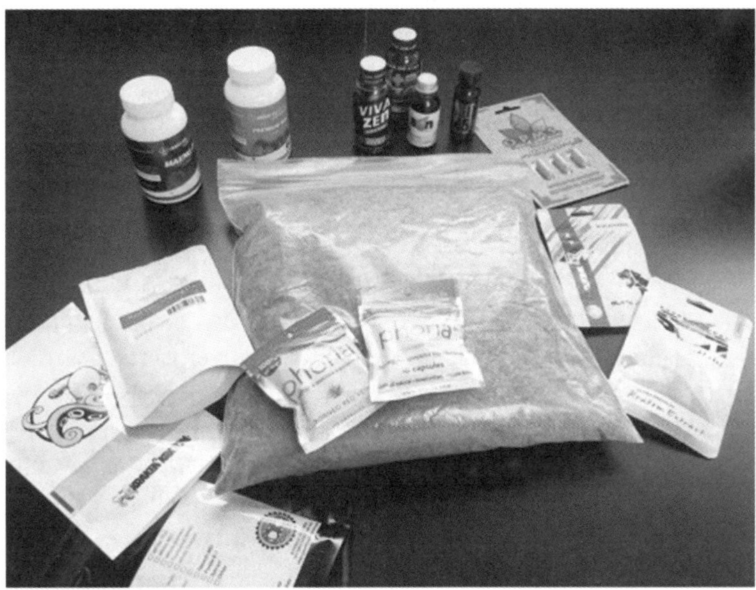

Fig.5 Commercial kratom products available in the USA

lyzed most of these, and interestingly enough, they're alkaloid contents are quite different, which isn't too surprising for a natural product. Thankfully, I would say more than 95% of the products we analyzed over the past decade actually contain what they claim, which is a step in the right direction for herbal products in general. As shown in Figure 5 there are energy shots, pure leaf material that's either been crushed or finely ground into powders, there are tablets and capsules. Some of these are marketed as a herbal product where the label states "Premium Bali" or "Maeng Da—*Mitragyna speciosa*" that is claimed to be the highest quality. Then there are other products marketed, such as "Phoria", which definitely have a different connotation to what you might expect when you purchase and ingest a product like this. And then you also have products like Viva Zen. Viva Zen is one of the energy shots. It's combined with many other herbal products. The name sounds reminiscent of the opioid product, Vicodin.

Just some examples of how this has moved from a traditionally used product to a legitimate use by many, many people across the world to really get off of opioids or to improve their energy versus the very small population that's using this to get high which has turned it into a very controversial product. There's old data, now three years old, that approximately 2000 metric tons is exported to the United States every year, according to the American Kratom Association (American Kratom Association, 2017). And if you look at a typical dose of about 3 to 5 grams that suggest in the United States alone, there are potentially 15 million users. This puts it into a high level of use category within the US, and I think that number is probably greater now. Definitely during COVID, the sales, according to a lot of the vendors of kratom products, has been substantially higher than it was pre-COVID, and these exportation quantities are pre-COVID numbers. Interestingly, with the presumed large increase in users in the past few years there does not appear there is a parallel or accelerated increase in adverse events being reported to poison control centers or emergency departments.

This brings us to the question, is kratom a credible threat or is it therapeutic and how do we determine this? As I mentioned anecdotally, kratom has been used for chronic pain, mood elevation, and opioid use disorders, among others. Our team has reported adulterated and contaminated products into the scientific literature (Lydecker et al., 2016) (Vo et al., 2022). Why individuals would take a very inexpensive natural product and put highly purified, expensive pharmaceuticals into it and then sell it at a very inexpensive price to me seems nefarious. What they're trying to do with that, in that marketplace is to capture a group of people to get return customers, not really contribute to making the world a better place, and that is really sad.

But I will take it a step further and say that our team has seen adulterated products with substances that we cannot identify as well. So, our team has fingerprinted legitimate, pure kratom and we know what alkaloids should be present. This allows us to suspect adulteration when we observe abnormal spikes in the mass spectrometry analysis, and we search databases to try and determine what might be present. Sometimes, there are no matches which could indicate a novel synthetic or something completely harmless. When you have a small amount to analyze, it is like looking for the sort of proverbial needle in a haystack. You really must know what you're looking for in order to identify what the adulterant is. A lot of our thoughts and a lot of the mass range that are in there probably fall into the synthetic cannabinoids, and synthetic fentanyl type derivatives that are around. When we learn of individuals that have consumed too much kratom and that have ultimately passed on, there exist very few reports that have kratom as the sole source of death. On those few reports that appear, we still have the question because they may have been contaminated with other items that we just do not have the ability to detect, because in Southeast Asia there's not been one report of death linked to kratom over centuries of traditional use.

This is a very interesting paradox in the world as there are claims that kratom is severely addictive and deadly. I've been working with a lot of addiction physicians over the years, and interestingly enough, some of them are starting to use kratom in their practice to move serious opioid addicts off of those opioids and onto kratom. Then the question is, where do we go from there? We have begun working on that piece as well because these physicians are also starting to treat individuals that have been extremely heavy users of kratom that are not able to stop their use. The big question is, how do we treat these individuals? Do we give them buprenorphine like we would a normal opioid addict? We have had discussions that maybe this is not the right approach, because if kratom is truly not a pure opioid, why would you put somebody on a pure opioid and now make them opioid dependent on a buprenorphine product? As one can imagine, there is a lot of debate and questions that we do not have answers to. However, if one looks in the medical literature right now, buprenorphine treatment (Brogdon et al., 2022) seems to the standard of care for kratom dependency. So, from a basic science research question, our team is trying to figure out what the best treatment(s) might be to obtain the best outcome for the patient.

The US Food and Drug Administration has driven a lot of action towards regulation around kratom. In fact, when I spoke at the 2017 conference, we had just come off a historical decision by the DEA (Drug Enforcement Agency) that was trying to place kratom in schedule one of the controlled substances act, and for the first time ever backed off of an intention to do so. It's still in that gray area that it could be scheduled at any point in time. To the best of our knowledge, we don't feel that it's headed in that direction any time soon. The US FDA put pressure on to the World Health Organization (WHO) to put an international ban on kratom into place. I was fortunate to be one of the few scientists invited to speak to the WHO Expert Committee on Drug Dependance. This United Nations panel rejected the international kratom ban because of a couple of reasons. One, it's an indigenous medicine that many people are using, or the indigenous product that many people are using in Southeast Asia daily. And two, the emerging science really shows that there is some therapeutic promise here in terms of helping a greater population.

Unfortunately, today, kratom is still illegal in six states in the U.S.; Alabama, Arkansas, Indiana, Rhode Island, Vermont, and Wisconsin. It's illegal in certain counties and cities throughout other states, which only means that individuals need to travel a distance outside of those areas to obtain materials. The United States government and several state legislatures have been working on passing what's called the Kratom Consumer Protection Act (KCPA). That legislation has passed in eight states (as of May 2022) where there will be some regulatory backing behind products that are sold in those states to ensure that they're meeting labor requirements and unadulterated and passed GMP (Good Manufacturing Practices) production. There are some things going in the right direction, but there's still this sort of overall question, is it a threat or is it a therapeutic? There was a story from USA Today, the headline read "U.S. Herbal Drug Kratom linked to almost 100 overdose deaths from the CDC" (Today, 2019). If you read that article in the entirety, the very end of that article says most all the samples were laced with fentanyl!

As I mentioned, few deaths have been attributable to kratom alone. We're questioning if any are. Of course, we do believe the poison is in the dose and if you take enough of any substance, it can have adverse consequences including death. We do know that mitragynine, the major alkaloid in kratom, is a partial mu opioid receptor (MOR) agonist, but that's not all the activity that occurs (more on this later). Mitragynine exerts a 40% maximal activation effect on MOR (Kruegel et al., 2016). So, by definition, it is a partial agonist, which is very similar to what buprenorphine behaves at MOR, also a partial agonist. Buprenorphine is highly selective for opioid receptors over other proteins and is very effective at getting people off of a full MOR agonist. Since buprenorphine is a partial MOR agonist, how do we ultimately transition individuals off buprenorphine? This remains an unanswered question.

One thing that made mitragynine interesting at this time was that it was found to be a biased agonist or what we think of as an agonist that only recruits and activates the G protein of a G protein coupled receptor and does not recruit another protein called beta-arrestin (Kruegel et al., 2016). Beta-arrestin, as the name suggests, would arrest the signaling and arrest the function of the receptor or desensitize it, which is thought to be tied to many of the side effects associated with opioids. For example, respiratory depression, constipation, tolerance, but nothing around the abuse or addictive possibilities. However, these molecules are exciting because with low respiratory depression and low constipation effects, they could offer a better alternative to the opioids that are used in clinic today.

Our team decided to really dive into this and think from a therapeutic potential of how kratom would work. Where could we go? The first and foremost for us was opioid detoxification. What follows is some pharmacology that suggests that kratom alone would be a single concoction that someone could ingest instead of having to take several prescription medications to detox, which would really improve medication adherence and the chances of them completing detoxification. This is because we learned that there is not only opioid activity here, but significant adrenergic and serotonergic activity. This all starts to make sense based on the anecdotal reports of mood elevation and pain relief together. Pure opioids are depressants and do not increase energy or elevate mood. Again, another interesting paradoxical effect of kratom is that it has, by nature, poly-pharmacology.

The other area is medication assisted therapy, which is really what is currently done with the use of methadone and buprenorphine, but instead using kratom to reduce opioid use. We know that this has been reported with the traditional use, but it is also seen anecdotally through surveys in the United States and around the world. Many people are using kratom to move themselves off prescription opioids, and one of the biggest reasons is because they report that they do not go into withdrawal. Also, these users indicate that kratom has a mood enhancing property that helps them re-engage back into society. I get emails all the time from people that say, "before I found Kratom, I was laid out on the couch. My family sort of disowned me. I wasn't paying attention to my children or my pets or my plants or anything. I found kratom and I'm back up, you know, preparing meals for my family, doing whatever it is that I used to do, and my pain is under control and I'm not taking hardcore prescription opioids". There seems to be a lot of promise from the anecdotal side, and really the reports of withdrawal are quite mild.

On the subjective opioid withdrawal scale (SOWS), the overall withdrawal seems to be mild. There are cases and exceptions to the mild withdrawal where individuals will say they cannot stop using kratom without having significant problems. Most of these individuals are using very high amounts of kratom daily maybe because they have developed tolerance and increased consumption. Studies that have been conducted by interviewing users indicate that those using a typical dose (3-5 grams of leaf), maybe two or three times a day, have very little withdrawal. Unfortunately, chronic kratom use has not been scientifically studied (even in animals) to understand long-term use. A major problem in the field is the lack of standardized product to conduct rigorous clinical trials to evaluate any claims associated with the pharmacology and not rely on anecdotal evidence.

One advantage about the being at the University of Florida is we have the Institute for Food and Agricultural Sciences (UF/IFAS) and all the health care sciences together under one umbrella. This is not typical for universities in the United States. This university structure allowed for interactions with horticulturists! Dr. Brian Pearson, who is an assistant professor at the University of Florida reached out to me with an interest in learning how to grow this plant and understand the environmental needs for it to be cultivated, perhaps as a commercial crop. We now have our own kratom farm at the University of Florida. There are approximately 100 trees in the ground (Figure 6) and around 300 or so trees in the greenhouses. What it has allowed us to do is start to really study what are the plants requirements for nutrients, what are the plants requirements for sunlight, basically all the environmental needs for production (Zhang et al., 2020, 2022) (Zhang et al., 2022). This affords the study of alkaloid biosynthesis and factors that can influence the ratio of alkaloids that make up this complex symphony! (Schotte et al., 2023) (Laforest et al., 2023).

Why is this of interest particularly in Florida? Well, the University of Florida has been a strong supporter of this cross-collaborative research project between the UF Health Center and

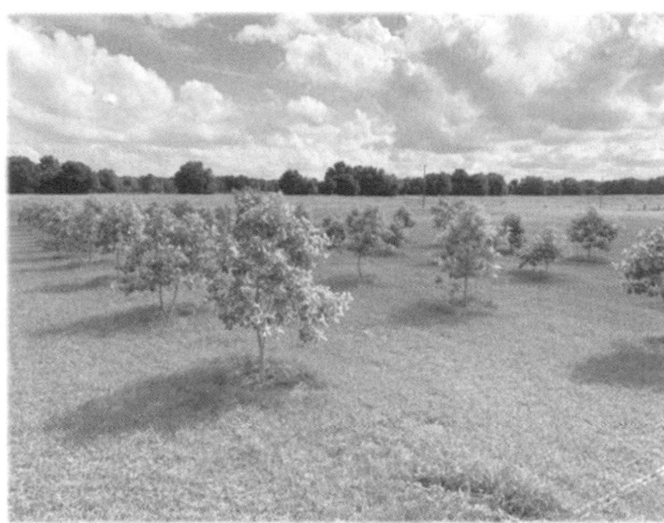

Fig.6 *Mitragyna speciosa* growing at the University of Florida

the Agricultural school. This has turned into a huge project where we are working on understanding how we can potentially improve the economy of the state of Florida. If you are not familiar, Florida is very famous for citrus. The citrus farms are in in great danger right now because of citrus greening, one of the most devastating citrus plant infections for which there is no cure. What Dr. Pearson has been able to do is figure out that *Mitragyna speciosa* could serve as a replacement of citrus trees. Interestingly, the trees can be planted with the same spacing, utilize the same irrigation equipment, the same farming equipment and potentially "rescue" these farms. It will become a matter of educating the farmers on how to grow these trees properly. So, if this becomes a viable option, we believe that this will help the economy of Florida by transferring the citrus industry into hopefully some sort of beneficial herbal and botanical drug product industry.

During these studies with the trees, it has been determined that there are at least two, potentially three different chemotypes of *Mitragyna speciosa*. This immediately brought to mind *Cannabis* where the plants dramatically vary in the production of the cannabinoids. The same could be the case with *Mitragyna speciosa* where there are trees that produce high levels of mitragynine and others that produce very low amounts.

The interesting part of that story is all these trees were donated to us by individuals from around the state of Florida that have been using them as personal fresh material, instead of going and buying dried material. Every single one of them said that they gave them the exact same experience as the dried materials that they have bought. Dry materials are really sold in the marketplace based on the percent of mitragynine they contain. So again, we're starting to think that the big spotlight has been on mitragynine for all these years because it is the most abundant alkaloid in some trees, and it would seem logical to be the most pharmacologically active. In the products that are available in the United States, mitragynine is absolutely the most abundant because that's how those products are selected for sale in the US. Because mitragynine is at high levels in leaf material that researchers have access to, it is easier to extract and purify mitragynine for studies. Almost all the studies that are in the literature have been conducted with mitragynine alone, not with the whole leaf kratom itself. So, it is a big difference when you when you start to really look at those. As a scientific community, mitragynine has become the poster child of kratom and because of this, many extrapolate the findings with mitragynine (a single isolated instrument) to what the entire leaf (complex symphony orchestra) actions are. This is also fundamentally wrong!

Recently, enough material was available from the low mitragynine producing trees to have a harvest large enough to prepare tea in the traditional way with fresh leaves. We just finished freeze drying all of that and I jokingly call it astronaut kratom. Now animal studies are being planned to determine if this material that essentially lacks mitragynine are going to be as beneficial as those that are commercially available with the main ingredient of mitragynine.

Taking a closer look at the various alkaloids shown in Figure 7, mitragynine has always been touted as the major one. It is reported to make up 66% of the total alkaloid content (Shellard et al., 1978). Interestingly, that number came from a sampling of three trees and has become dogma in the field/industry. Now sampling from individual trees, either that we have been growing or from farms in Malaysia, and samples that have been purchased in the marketplace show that mitragynine accounts for 0.7% to 38.7% of total alkaloid content, so much less than what was initially thought of and initially reported. This could also be due to the fact that 4 isomers exist naturally in the plant and we can separate these with current analytical techniques. Next, 7-hydroxymitragynine (7HMG) is also one of the more studied metabolites of mitragynine and it was thought to be produced in the plant and make up about 2% of the total alkaloid content. We now believe that 7HMG is most likely a post-harvest artifact. Two independent collaborators cannot find any biological enzyme within the plant material that will convert mitragynine into 7HMG leading us to believe that it is possibly formed once the leaf is separated from the tree and dried. Our team has been looking into the post-harvest hypothesis as to how it could be formed as well, perhaps by heat, light, air-drying, or all these things. What we find in almost every sample and thankfully in many of the products that our lab has been testing in the marketplace is that the 7HMG content is less than 0.01% of the total alkaloid content. This becomes important when we start talking about the pharmacology associated with these.

Another observation from the chemical structures of the alkaloids is that every one of these molecules has a similar appendage at the bottom of the molecule or the southern part of the molecule. This chemical group is called a beta-methoxyacrylate and why would the plant decorate every single one of these unique alkaloids with that same chemical feature became of interest. Again, what is the plant trying to tell us about what is going on here? These are chemical groups that are found in a class of natural products called strobilurins, which are naturally occurring antifungals or fungicides and are used in agricultural practice (Bartlett et al., 2002). We started to wonder, do these have antifungal properties because the natural environment where *Mitragyna speciosa* grows is swampy? In fact, they can grow in standing water and seem perfectly happy in standing water. In that environment, one must think that the pressure from fungus is going to be tremendous and interestingly enough, we have found that the genes for all alkaloid production are within the root system, but we do not find many alkaloids in the roots, which is interesting. So, I think they're being synthesized there and quickly distributed, whether it's into the environment around them, which we haven't explored yet, but they are quickly sent through the tree into the leaves. There's very little alkaloid in the bark, there's very little in the stem, but there's high concentrations in the leaf material and we believe probably in the in the surrounding ground area. Those thoughts pushed us to investigating the antifungal properties. Interestingly, we do not see anti-fungal activity on human fungal pathogens, but we have seen a nice broad spectrum of activity against plant pathogenic fungus. This is another scientific area that we are fortunate to be collaborating with our colleagues in the agricultural school.

Again, shown in Figure 7 are just some of the alkaloids that our team has isolated and studied out of that symphony orchestra. We have "listened" to every single one of these alkaloids on full blast, ignoring their actual ratio to others, or role in the full plant material context. Doing this is a totally different story compared to looking at the full plant material in the complex mixture it exists. We always remind ourselves what we are doing in this situation and the effects of each individual alkaloid must be looked at in that context. We were the first group to profile mitragynine against 82 different central nervous system drug targets. The results or "hits" are shown in Table 1 where we screened human receptors at a 10 micromolar (10,000 nM) concentration. A 10 micromolar concentration is basically bathing these protein targets in this molecule. And what was found is that there is some serotonergic activity, some alpha adrenergic, dopaminergic,

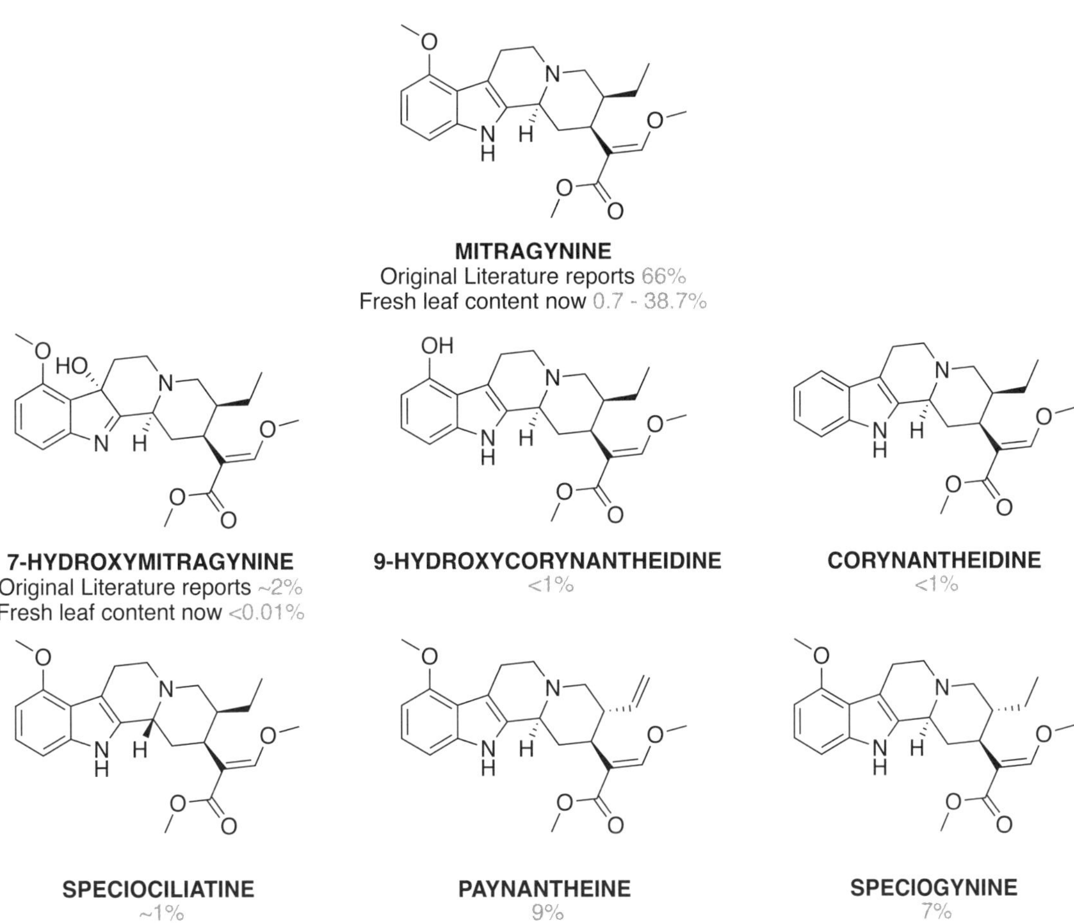

Fig 7. Some isolated kratom alkaloids with their percentage of total alkaloid content.

Assay	100 nM (1.0E-07 M)	10000 nM (1.0E-05 M)
5-HT$_{1A}$*(h)* (agonist radioligand)		x
5-HT$_{2B}$*(h)* (agonist radioligand)		x
α_{1A}*(h)* (antagonist radioligand)		x
α_{1D}*(h)* (antagonist radioligand)		x
β_2*(h)* (antagonist radioligand)		x
D$_1$*(h)* (antagonist radioligand)		x
D$_{2S}$*(h)* (agonist radioligand)		x
D$_3$*(h)* (antagonist radioligand)		x
κ (KOP) (agonist radioligand)		x
μ (MOP) *(h)* (agonist radioligand)		x
Na$^+$ channel (site 2) (antagonist radioligand)		x
Potassium Channel hERG (human)- [3H] Dofetilide		x

Table 1. Eurofins screening panel over 82 CNS drug targets. Mitragynine was screened at two concentrations. First screen was conducted at 10,000 nM and if radioligand was displaced at >50% a second screen at 100 nM was conducted to determine if the target was a hit for further study (again if 50% of radioligand was displaced) and no targets met the criteria at this level.

and opioid activity all from the single alkaloid. We take these hits at this high concentration and then interrogate those receptors at a concentration of 100 nanomolar, which is a level that we would expect to see pharmacological activity. When the concentration of mitragynine was dropped down to 100 nanomolar, there were no hits. This is where one starts to question where the pharmacological activity is really coming from in kratom? Yes, mitragynine has opioid affinity and it also has affinity at all these other proteins too, so how physiologically relevant is any of this or all of it? To determine this, we performed precise affinity measurements at each of these targets.

One of the targets of most interest was the alpha-adrenergic receptor activity. This is because when opioid use disorder patients are treated, they are given methadone or buprenorphine, and as they are going into withdrawal, they are oftentimes given clonidine or lofexidine, which are alpha-two receptor adrenergic agonists. What we found, interestingly, and many of the kratom alkaloids, is that they have this partial mu-opioid receptor activity, plus this alpha-adrenergic activity, which would make them suitable as single agent treatments for opioid withdrawal syndrome.

We have been conducting studies along this avenue (opioid withdrawal) as well with isolated mitragynine, but also with whole plant material in those same paradigms. We found that of course this is a mu-opioid partial agonist that interacts with kappa-opioid receptors, and it does interact with alpha adrenergic receptors to degrees that are physiologically relevant (Obeng et al., 2020). We can observe these behavioral activities in animals, particularly animals that have been genetically modified to not contain opioid receptors, what are referred to as knock-out animals. The adrenergic activity is real.

Poison control centers across the United States provided us another key indicator here that kratom overdoses resemble stimulant overdoses, not opioid overdoses. You get agitated delirium, you get seizures or convulsions, but you do not see very often respiratory depression. This was another indicator that tells us other things are going on within this plant. So, we wanted to look at just the hot plate assessment of mitragynine (Figure 8). This work was carried out by my col-

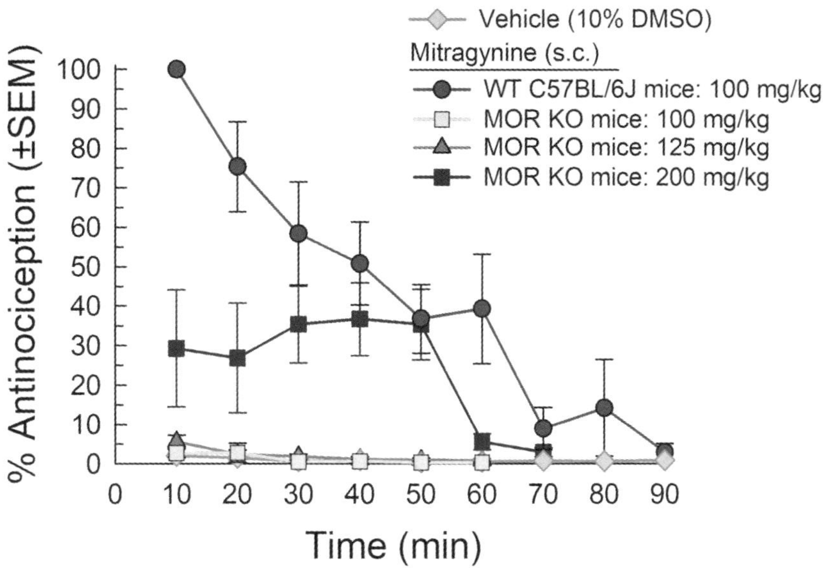

Fig.8 Antinociceptive activity of mitragynine in wild-type (WT C57BL/6J) and mu-opioid receptor knockout (MOR KO) mice. *Data generated in collaboration with Dr. Jay McLaughlin at the University of Florida*

league at the University of Florida, Dr. Jay McLaughlin. The hot plate assay can be though of just as if a human is walking barefoot out on the pavement in the summertime, the first couple of steps are okay and then all of a sudden you want to get to the grass as quickly as possible because your feet are burning. We do that with these animals, we put them on for a limited period of time and as we increase doses, you can get to a point where you achieve 100% antinociception (or pain relief). They stay on that apparatus the full amount of time, then we take them off of the apparatus because of we do not want to damage their skin, we don't want to harm the animal in any way, but we can get to 100% analgesia. That is in the wild-type mouse represented by the brown colored circles (WT C57BL/6J). Then we took the genetically modified mu-opioid receptor knockout mouse (MOR KO).

We took that same dose of 100 milligrams per kilogram and you can see there's absolutely no analgesic activity, which really, if you stop the experiment there you can conclude it's mu-opioid receptor mediated analgesia. We pushed the dose in those knockout mice a little higher and then a little higher and what you can see at 200 milligrams per kilogram was actually about 40% analgesic response. We could see some of those other receptor mechanisms are kicking in at the higher doses, and we wanted to really push that and see what was happening. Since we hypothesized this was alpha-adrenergic activity we used yohimbine, an alpha-adrenergic antagonist, to try and block the analgesia. As shown in figure 9, we pretreated those mu-opioid receptor knockout animals with yohimbine and what we were able to do is pretty much completely block that analgesic efficacy that was seen in those animals. This shows there is an adrenergic component of analgesia to mitragynine and by extension then to kratom as a whole, which is very exciting.

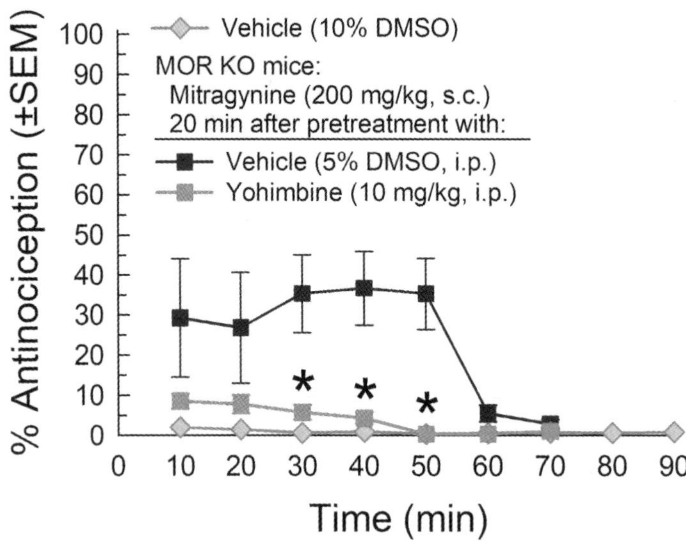

Fig.9 Reversal of antinociception in MOR KO mice with the alpha-adrenergic antagonist yohimbine. *Data generated in collaboration with Dr. Jay McLaughlin at the University of Florida*

I think one of the most striking pieces of data that we've collected so far is a neuropathic pain model and looking at mitragynine with our collaborators Jenny Wilkerson and Lance McMahon. We took rats and created what is called a chronic constriction injury where we surgically open their thigh and ligate their sciatic nerve on one leg while leaving the other leg normal. Those animals heal for about three or four weeks. Then they are subjected to grams of pressure through apparatus called Von Frey, where a monofilament is inserted through a mesh floor and pokes them in the paw. An advantage of this assay is one can use the same animal as its own control because one leg has not been damaged, the other leg is damaged, and we can look at the contralateral and ipsilateral paws in the same animal. What we found was that mitragynine is effective in reversing this type of neuropathic pain and interestingly, it is not fully blocked by the opioid antagonist naloxone, indicating other pain mechanisms are at play. We have not yet published this data so no figures can be shown here. This is really encouraging because this means that the treatment of chronic pain in many, many individuals that are using kratom are saying it's great for their chronic neuropathic pain. It appears not to be opioid related mechanisms, and so we're really digging into this now to understand this in more detail.

So, what about 7HMG, which again was the other controversial compound in the plant, which we found out is not really in the plant. It's a metabolite probably made through oxidation. Now that we have enough trees growing of the true chemotype or what we think of as the high mitragynine chemotype, we are starting to conduct postharvest studies on our own to see what causes the production of 7HMG and possibly understand the high levels we saw in samples that were examined from the US marketplace almost a decade ago. The 7HMG molecule is probably the most selective opioid I have ever seen over the quarter century I have been working in opioid chemistry, and most of the opiates will start to pick up other receptor activity at high concentrations. This molecule at that high 10 micromolar concentration does not interact with anything other than opioid receptors, and when you drop the concentration down to the 100 nanomolar level, it exclusively interacts with the mu-opioid receptor. After a full profiling of 7HMG, it is clear that it's a very high affinity opioid receptor agonist. Then it brought up the question as to several things. One is this the abuse component within the full plant mixture? Is this an addictive component of the mixture? Should we try to figure out how to "de7-hydroxymitragynine" kratom mixtures like decaffeinated coffee? Is this the problem?

Following this line of questions, the first study that we did was with a colleague, Scott Hemby, at High Point University (Hemby et al., 2019). Scott is an expert in animal models of drug self-administration so we wanted to study mitragynine and 7HMG in this model. This paradigm is the gold standard and if it shows that a compound can be self-administered, then it most likely has abuse potential. Scott was able to train rats to self-administer morphine, and what you generally observe in this case is the rats are pressing a lever and after so many times they will get an injection of drug and then there is a timeout period where no drug is available. Then they are able to get access to the drug at a higher dose the next time, then they will continue to self-administer and feel good until they get to a dose that is so high that they do not need to administer as often. Some refer to this are the "drunk or intoxicated phase" where the observation appears the rats are pressing less often and the dose-response curve goes in the opposite direction, you get this inverted U-shaped pharmacological curve. Once you have an animal trained on how to self-administer morphine, you can swap out that bottle of morphine for any other drug and see if they will self-administer that compound or not. We did this with mitragynine first and the result was no substitution over a large range of increasing doses. It never really was self-administered in those animals and was comparable to saline. As a conclusion, we do not think mitragynine alone has abuse potential or abuse liability. On the other hand, 7HMG produces that typical inverted U-shaped curve and readily substitutes for morphine in the self-administration assay, indicating it has high abuse potential.

Another similar study was published by a longtime collaborator of mine, Jonathan Katz at the National Institute on Drug Abuse (Yue et al., 2018). He called me up and asked me for mitragyine, and I said we were already doing the studies with Scott Hemby so I cannot give you any mitragynine but directed him to a place where he could to buy it for research purposes. He bought it and performed an elegant study showing that pretreatment with mitragynine, dose-dependently, decreases and completely blocks heroin self-administration. This is another nice piece of evidence that shows that this molecule again, not the whole plant material, may have potential in this area of treating those with opioid use disorder.

There was some evidence in a 1972 publication by Macko, et al.,[21] from SmithKline and French that when mitragynine was given orally, it was more potent than when it was given by any other route. We found this to be interesting. So, we did a quick comparison in a warm water withdrawal test. Shown in Figure 10 is morphine in blue where increasing doses have increasing anti-nociception, 7HMG (in green) is much more potent than morphine. Not surprisingly, mitragynine (in yellow) was much less potent than morphine.

These were given subcutaneously, and when you give a mitragynine orally shown in the yellow triangles there in Figure 11, it is almost equivalent to morphine. There is a definite difference

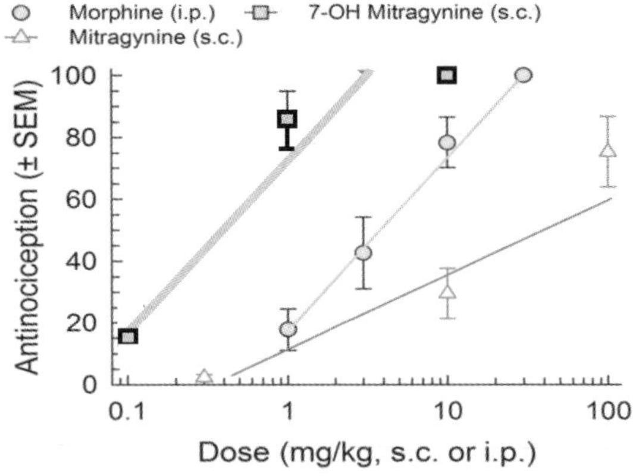

Fig.10 Antinociception of morphine (i.p.).

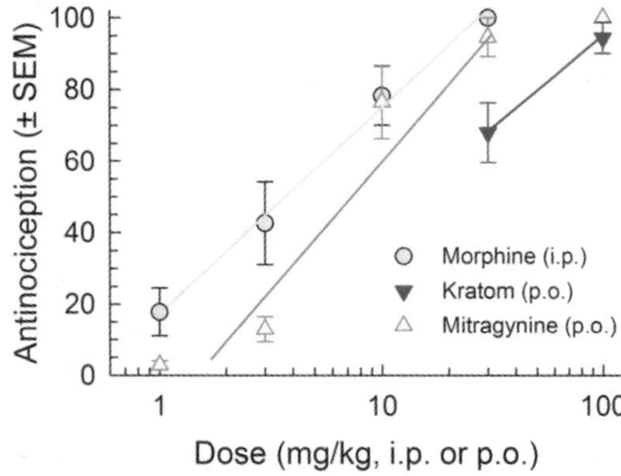

Fig. 11 Antinociception of morphine (i.p.), mitragynine (p.o.), and kratom (p.o.) in mice. *Data generated in collaboration with Dr. Jay McLaughlin at the University of Florida*

between oral delivery, which is the way that humans are ingesting kratom, versus an injectable. Figure 11 also shows two doses of orally administered kratom. It takes much higher doses of the whole plant material to get to the efficacy, but good analgesic efficacy is still achieved by ingesting the full plant material orally.

What this made us think was obviously there's some sort of intestinal or first-pass liver metabolism that is taking place. We went through and looked at rat liver microsomes and rat intestinal microsomes, and we incubated those with pure mitragynine and we monitored for the disappearance of mitragynine and the subsequent metabolic formation of 7HMG. As shown in Figure 12, as mitragynine concentrations decrease, concentrations of 7MG start to increase. It seems that this alone would explain the increased analgesia seen when mitragynine is administered orally.

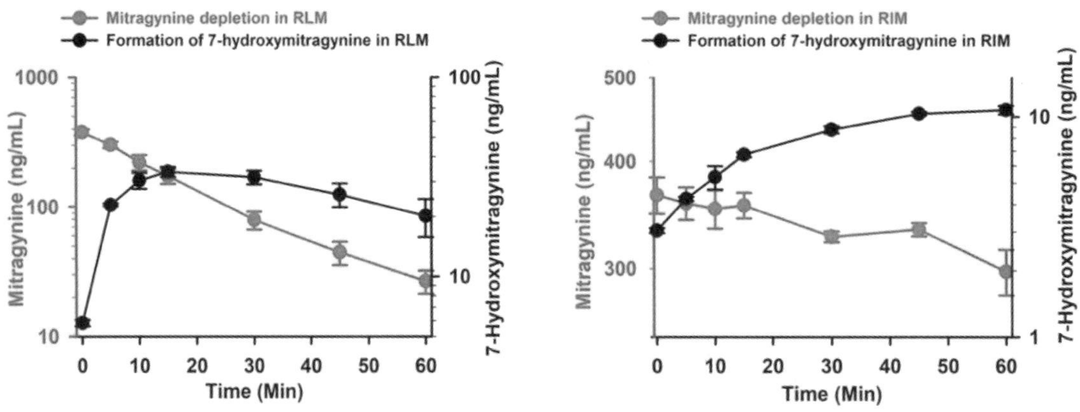

Fig.12 Mitragynine metabolism in rat liver microsomes (left) and rat intestinal microsomes (right) over time and the formation of the metabolite 7HMG over time. *Data generated in collaboration with Dr. Abhisheak Sharma at the University of Florida*

We wanted to know if this slight production of 7HMG is pharmacologically relevant? Is the generated 7HMG metabolite responsible for the overall analgesic effects from the parent compound? So, we took mitragynine and dosed mice and examined this hot plate assay on them as well. This was as very sophisticated pharmacokinetics and pharmacodynamic study where we looked at the amount of compound that was getting into the brain versus the amount of compound that was present in the plasma (Berthold et al., 2021). Then with those amounts we also looked at the hot plate assay, and we were able to figure out what brain concentration was relevant to the pharmacological activity. What we found was the maximum 7HMG levels that could be produced in those studies fell far below any of the actual pharmacodynamic effect that we found with 7HMG alone. It is not possible to achieve the analgesia from just the metabolite alone, and that is a sort of popular myth that has grown in the literature. We have been arguing this, but hopefully this study will really help to underline there is no relevance of the small amount of 7HMG generated as a metabolite from mitragynine, at least in mice and in these single dose studies.

During this process we discovered a unique metabolite in human plasma, as we were doing plasma stability studies with 7HMG we observed another compound appearing with the exact molecular weight and mass transitions. This resulted in a scale up of the plasma study to be able to obtain enough of the unknown compound to perform structure elucidation (Kamble et al., 2020). We went through NMR and mass spectrometry analysis to determine it was a known compound, mitragynine pseudoindoxyl (Figure 13).

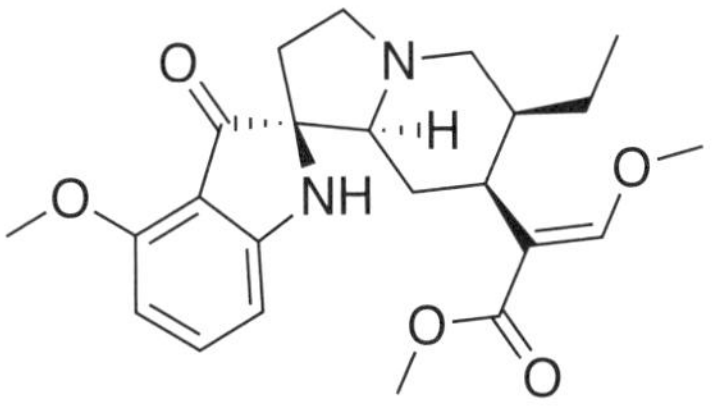

MITRAGYNINE PSEUDOINDOXYL

Fig.13 structure of mitragynine pseudoindoxyl.

This compound was previously reported in the literature decades ago from a study that fed mitragynine to a fungus to see what metabolites would be produced (Zarembo et al., 1974). The fungus spit out mitragynine pseudoindoxyl which is an even more potent mu-opioid receptor agonist than 7HMG. We embarked on several studies only to learn it has very poor brain penetration and since it is a minor metabolite from the 7HMG metabolite we believe that there is no functional consequence of this metabolite in humans. We were able to find this in all preclinical species that we've been studying mouse, rat, dog, and monkey but it seems to be more common in humans.

We then wanted to interrogate which cytochrome P450 enzymes were involved because this is important when you start looking at herb-drug interactions and fortunately or unfortunately, whichever way you want to look at it, two of the most important CNS drug metabolizing cytochrome P450s are involved here (Kamble, Sharma, et al., 2020). CYP3A4, which is one of the major drug metabolizing cytochrome P450s is the major pathway for the metabolism of mitragynine, and then CYP2D6, which is one of the major cytochrome P450s that metabolizes drugs like antidepressants and antipsychotics is also a pathway here.

What we really wanted to know is, is this a problem when people are taking kratom? Because what we did was go through the FDA's Adverse Event Reporting System (FAERS) database and searched for drug interactions have been reported to the FDA. Most of the drugs that have caused adverse events with kratom are CNS active drugs, antipsychotics, antidepressants, and anti-anxiety agents. We really wanted to understand is there some pharmacokinetic issue that is happening with the co-ingestion of those substances? We examined many of the alkaloids that we isolated, particularly those that we know reach plasma concentrations after kratom is ingested. We looked for the inhibition of the major cytochrome P450s. Mitragynine and corynantheidine, two of the compounds that are relevant when ingesting the whole plant do that have moderate inhibition of CYP2D6, the one that is responsible for all those CNS drugs as well as many prescription drugs. There could be some caution needed if co-ingesting anti-depressants and antipsychotics along with kratom, which sadly is many of the population that is using these because they're using kratom for the mood elevation/mood enhancement property. It is something that we need to be aware of.

The take home message about mitragynine is it is not, in any way, a typical opioid and does have additional non-opioid pharmacology-what I call disruptive pharmacology. It shares some effects as an opioid agonist in that it has a low potency and low efficacy. I did not go into all of the studies we have conducted but mitragynine has less tolerance than morphine and less dependance. It also has a very different discriminative stimulus effect than morphine. Essentially, we can teach rats to be connoisseurs of morphine and then we can switch out morphine with any other substance and see if they consume it like morphine. When you do that with mitragynine they don't think it's like morphine at all. In contrast, 7HMG they consume just as if it were morphine. Mitragynine also shows less tolerance, abuse, and dependance liability. Again, this is mitragynine alone and not the whole kratom leaf material, but mitragynine does have the desired characteristics for a candidate for opioid addiction and withdrawal.

The take home message around 7HMG is that it should be considered a constituent with high abuse potential. It may increase the intake of other opiates. I didn't show that, but in the collaborative work with Scott Hemby, we did show that 7HMG in its purified form, can act to sort of kindle the use of other opioids in that it increased the intake of morphine after animals were exposed to it (Hemby et al., 2019). We don't think that the extent that 7HMG is metabolically converted from mitragynine is physiologically relevant in the actions of kratom.

This brings us back to kratom itself? We performed much of our work with lyophilized kratom, what I call the astronaut kratom, because it is as close the traditional use of a brewed tea, albeit with the dried leaf material that is available in the US market. We basically look at it in comparison to morphine, either orally or intraperitoneally (in the abdomen) when dosing the lyophilized kratom tea (Figure 14) (Wilson et al., 2020). With this preparation, there is a ceiling effect on the analgesia and so whether we give one gram,

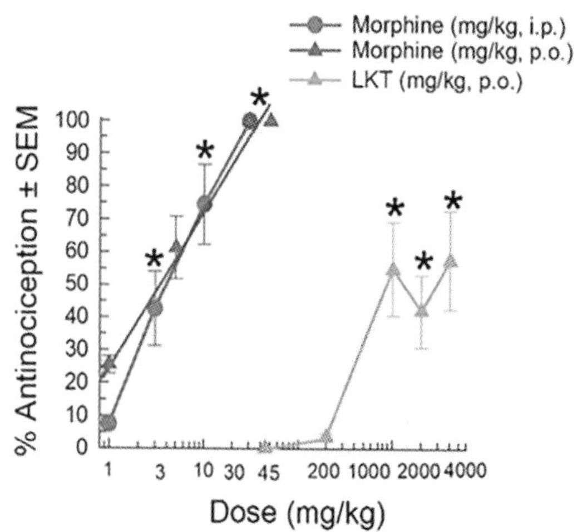

Fig.14 Antinociception of lyophilized kratom tea (LKT) orally in mice. *Wilson et al., 2020*

two grams, four grams per kilogram of this lyophilized kratom tea and we don't get any higher than 40% maximal analgesic efficacy. That is first and foremost.

One thing that is interesting is it doesn't seem that you could push the opioid system over the top. There are other mechanisms and other pharmacology's within this plant that are balancing and counterbalancing effects that are going on. We do know that at those high doses it will last as long in terms of its length of action. The effect lasts as long as a typical five mg per kilogram dose of morphine. So interestingly, it can be probably a legitimate analgesic substitute although maybe not as fully effective. We do know that the analgesia appears to be mediated through opioid receptors when you look at kratom as a whole, and so this backs up some of the claims that the FDA is making. But I still think that it needs to be put in the proper context and corrected as there is so much more pharmacology going on here.

Another way we investigate abuse potential is through the Conditioned Place Preference assay. Place preference is a drug seeking paradigm, animals will seek out a drug and we have observed that, even at high doses of lyophilized kratom tea, there is no desire to seek it out. They are not interested in really trying to find kratom as they would be with morphine (Wilson et al., 2020). We also investigated some of the liabilities, particularly sedation. We don't see kratom tea causing sedation, which makes sense because one of the things that is always reported is the stimulant-like activity (Wilson et al., 2020). The other thing that we investigated was respiratory depression, as this is a key issue with opioids. In this study, as expected, morphine caused respiratory depression. There was a slight drop in respirations in the in the first 5 minutes with the lyophilized kratom tea but overall, that rebounds quickly and there appears to be no issue in terms of respiratory depression (Wilson et al., 2020). We also looked at precipitated naloxone withdrawal in several animal groups on different treatment mixtures of morphine and kratom or kratom alone. One of the key side effects from precipitated opioid withdrawal in mice is jumping, which is not something that a mouse does normally. When mice are in withdrawal they do what is called popcorn jumping and they really move all over the container they are in. We can attenuate this with kratom nicely, and another effect that can be attenuated with kratom is teeth chattering which is another withdrawal symptom (Wilson et al., 2020). So what is going on when we give the whole product? What is happening? If we look at the pharmacokinetics and plasma levels of exposure, mitragynine is clearly the most exposed alkaloid. After that we see speciociliatine, which will be detailed below, as the second highest exposure. The 7HMG, which was not detectable in the tea we made and dosed the animals with is in the plasma as a result of metabolism from mitragynine. There are two other alkaloids, speciogynine (another isomer of mitragynine) and paynantheine (a precursor to speciogynine) which show up in the plasma during the first hour but are quickly metabolized. Their metabolites have similar activity and are longer lasting. We are just learning about these metabolites and starting to study them.

So, what is this second highest exposure alkaloid? Speciociliatine, an isomer of mitragynine with the only difference being the configuration of the three-position hydrogen (Kamble et al., 2021). In speciociliatine that hydrogen is in the beta configuration instead of the alpha configuration as it is in mitragynine. That small change effects the entire 3D structure of the molecule from something that is sort of flat to something that is bent. Because of this conformational change, a higher affinity and potency at opioid receptors is realized. This does have more potent partial mu-opioid agonist effects as well, and it may be the key alkaloid that has been overlooked in the plant. It is more active than mitragynine and it is almost as abundant as mitragynine, even though older reports indicated it only made up about 1% of the total alkaloid content. More work has been completed with this compound and we will have more details published soon. Unfortunately, there is not enough information to share yet.

Another alkaloid, corynantheidine, was profiled through the 82 CNS target screen and interacted with several targets at 10 micromolar. When it was screened at 100 nanomolar, we got a hit at the alpha-adrenergic receptor. Upon further study, we determined that it has a 40 nanomolar affinity for the alpha-1D adrenergic receptor and a 75 nanomolar affinity for the mu-opioid receptor. The only difference between corynantheidine and mitragynine is the 9-methoxy group on the indole ring position of the molecule. This is very interesting that when that is removed from mitragynine, the resulting alkaloid has high affinity for alpha-adrenergic receptors. From a medicinal chemistry standpoint of view, I mentioned paynantheine and speciogynine, and these are two other compounds that we found that are in high concentration in the plant that also have high affinity for 5HT1A and 5HT2B receptors (León et al., 2021). They are both around 30 nanomolar at these targets. These are some of the highest affinity compounds at any target in the plant, yet the focus remains on opioid receptors!

This activity at the 5HT1A receptor is of high interest since agonists at this receptor are reported to reverse or reduce opioid-induced respiratory depression. That is within the plant's whole symphony orchestra that we have something to counteract respiratory depression. 5HT2B is known to be an anti-drug target, as agonists are involved in cardiac valvulopathy. These alkaloids are antagonists at that receptor, so we do not have an issue or concern. These alkaloids are also weak agonists at the mu opioid receptor. The only difference between speciogynine and paynantheine is the reduction of one exocyclic double bond. Speciogynine is also an isomer of mitragynine, this time the difference is found in the exocyclic ethyl group where it is in the alpha configuration instead of the beta configuration (as it is in mitragynine). That small change completely flip flops the pharmacology to high affinity serotonin activity. Interesting stuff. In this context, we have shown that serotonin activation results in analgesic effects that can be blocked with a selective serotonin antagonist, WAY-100635 (León et al., 2021).

I will not go into this into much detail other than to say clinical pharmacokinetics was published in a 2015 Thai study (Trakulsrichai et al., 2015) where they showed the maximal plasma concentrations of mitragynine in regular kratom users reached about 120 nanograms per milliliter. Two of the individuals that passed in the United States from reported kratom overdose did not have 120 nanograms per milliliter, instead they had mitragynine levels at 1,800 and 3,500 nanograms per milliliter in their blood supply (Speciosa.org, 2017). Any substance in excess can be a little too much. In these two cases, mitragynine was found at 17 to 189 times higher plasma concentrations than traditional users of kratom.

I wish to finish with the first clinical pharmacokinetic study that was published in the United States on March 11th of 2022, not from our team, but from Professor Mary Paine's group at Washington State University (Tanna et al., 2022). In this study, a 2 gram dose of dried kratom leaf powder was administered to volunteers in the form of a tea or solution. Two grams is a very low dose. They had eight patients that they signed up to participate, two patients had nausea and vomiting when they started and they were excluded from the trial, so six were included in the final data analysis. This work showed for the first time, the exposure profile of kratom alkaloids in humans, not just mitragynine. This provides a really good foundation for more clinical research to take place. There are some other planned human trials, and there's an FDA contract that's been awarded to Alta Sciences and planning is underway for safety and subsequent human abuse potential studies. Then Nutrasource, a company in Canada has carrying out a study as well, looking at safety and effectiveness as well as cognitive performance with three different kratom products. That study has over 250 human volunteers enrolled. We are all anxious to see the results of that work.

Again, there long safe history of use in Southeast Asia but lots of adverse events have been reported in the Western world. But I really want to throw this disruptive pharmacology term out there and say that we we've got something *really* important here. We just don't want to throw it away and ignore what the plant is trying to teach us.

BIBLIOGRAPHY

Adkins, J. Y., Boyer, E. W., & McCurdy, C. R. (2011). *Mitragyna speciosa*, A Psychoactive Tree from Southeast Asia with Opioid Activity. *Current Topics in Medicinal Chemistry*, *11*(9), 1165–1175. https://doi.org/10.2174/156802611795371305

American Kratom Association. (2017, June). The increase in consumer use of kratom in the United States. *https://www.americankratom.org/*. Retrieved May 30, 2023, from https://assets.website-files.com/61858fcec654303987617512/619dd9d68bd48315873c4952_Kratom_Population_2019.pdf

Bartlett, D., Clough, J. D., Godwin, J. R., Hall, A. K., Hamer, M., & Parr-Dobrzanski, B. (2002). The strobilurin fungicides. *Pest Management Science*, *58*(7), 649–662. https://doi.org/10.1002/ps.520

Berthold, E. C., Kamble, S. H., Raju, K. S. R., Kuntz, M., Senetra, A. S., Mottinelli, M., León, F., Restrepo, L. F., Patel, A., Ho, N., Hiranita, T., Sharma, A., & McCurdy, C. R. (2021). The Lack of Contribution of 7-Hydroxymitragynine to the Antinociceptive Effects of Mitragynine in Mice: A Pharmacokinetic and Pharmacodynamic Study. *Drug Metabolism and Disposition*, *50*(2), 158–167. https://doi.org/10.1124/dmd.121.000640

Brogdon, H. D., McPhee, M. M., Paine, M. F., Cox, E. R., & Burns, A. (2022). A Case of Potential Pharmacokinetic Kratom-drug Interactions Resulting in Toxicity and Subsequent Treatment of Kratom Use Disorder With Buprenorphine/Naloxone. *Journal of Addiction Medicine*, *16*(5), 606–609. https://doi.org/10.1097/adm.0000000000000968

Hemby, S. E., McIntosh, S., León, F., Cutler, S. J., & McCurdy, C. R. (2019). Abuse liability and therapeutic potential of the *Mitragyna speciosa* (kratom) alkaloids mitragynine and 7-hydroxymitragynine. *Addiction Biology*, *24*(5), 874–885. https://doi.org/10.1111/adb.12639

Jansen, K., & Prast, C. J. (1988). Ethnopharmacology of kratom and the Mitragyna alkaloids. *Journal of Ethnopharmacology*, *23*(1), 115–119. https://doi.org/10.1016/0378-8741(88)90121-3

Kamble, S. H., León, F., King, T. I., Berthold, E. C., Lopera-Londoño, C., Raju, K. S. R., Hampson, A. J., Sharma, A., Avery, B. A., McMahon, L. R., & McCurdy, C. R. (2020). Metabolism of a Kratom Alkaloid Metabolite in Human Plasma Increases Its Opioid Potency and Efficacy. *ACS Pharmacology & Translational Science*, *3*(6), 1063–1068. https://doi.org/10.1021/acsptsci.0c00075

Kamble, S. H., Berthold, E. C., King, T., Kanumuri, S. R. R., Popa, R. A., Herting, J. R., León, F., Sharma, A., Avery, B. A., & McCurdy, C. R. (2021). Pharmacokinetics of Eleven Kratom Alkaloids Following an Oral Dose of Either Traditional or Commercial Kratom Products in Rats. *Journal of Natural Products*, *84*(4), 1104–1112. https://doi.org/10.1021/acs.jnatprod.0c01163

Kamble, S. H., Sharma, A., King, T. I., Berthold, E. C., León, F., Meyer, P. K. L., Kanumuri, S. R. R., McMahon, L. R., McCurdy, C. R., & Avery, B. A. (2020). Exploration of cytochrome P450 inhibition mediated drug-drug interaction potential of kratom alkaloids. *Toxicology Letters*, *319*, 148–154. https://doi.org/10.1016/j.toxlet.2019.11.005

Kruegel, A. C., Wulf, M. G., Kapoor, A., Váradi, A., Majumdar, S., Filizola, M., Javitch, J. A., & Sames, D. (2016).

Synthetic and Receptor Signaling Explorations of the *Mitragyna* Alkaloids: Mitragynine as an Atypical Molecular Framework for Opioid Receptor Modulators. *Journal of the American Chemical Society*, *138*(21), 6754–6764. https://doi.org/10.1021/jacs.6b00360

Laforest, L. C., Kuntz, M. A., Kanumuri, R. S., Mukhopadhyay, S., Sharma, A., O'Connor, S. E., McCurdy, C. R., & Nadakuduti, S. S. (2023). Metabolite and Molecular Characterization of *Mitragyna speciosa* Identifies Developmental and Genotypic Effects on Monoterpene Indole and Oxindole Alkaloid Composition. *Journal of Natural Products*, *86*(4), 1042–1052. https://doi.org/10.1021/acs.jnatprod.3c00092

León, F., Obeng, S., Mottinelli, M., Chen, Y., King, T., Berthold, E. C., Kamble, S. H., Restrepo, L. F., Patel, A., Gamez-Jimenez, L. R., Lopera-Londoño, C., Hiranita, T., Sharma, A., Hampson, A. J., Canal, C. E., & McCurdy, C. R. (2021). Activity of *Mitragyna speciosa* ("Kratom") Alkaloids at Serotonin Receptors. *Journal of Medicinal Chemistry*, *64*(18), 13510–13523. https://doi.org/10.1021/acs.jmedchem.1c00726

Lydecker, A. G., Sharma, A., McCurdy, C. R., Avery, B. A., Babu, K. M., & Boyer, E. W. (2016). Suspected Adulteration of Commercial Kratom Products with 7-Hydroxymitragynine. *Journal of Medical Toxicology*, *12*(4), 341–349. https://doi.org/10.1007/s13181-016-0588-y

Macko, E., Weisbach, J. A., & Douglas, B. (1972). Some observations on the pharmacology of mitragynine. *PubMed*, *198*(1), 145–161. https://pubmed.ncbi.nlm.nih.gov/4626477

McCurdy, C. R., & Scully, S. (2005). Analgesic substances derived from natural products (natureceuticals). *Life Sciences*, *78*(5), 476–484. https://doi.org/10.1016/j.lfs.2005.09.006

Obeng, S., Kamble, S. H., Reeves, M. E., Restrepo, L. F., Patel, A., Behnke, M., Chear, N. J., Ramanathan, S., Sharma, A., León, F., Hiranita, T., Avery, B. A., & McCurdy, C. R. (2020). Investigation of the Adrenergic and Opioid Binding Affinities, Metabolic Stability, Plasma Protein Binding Properties, and Functional Effects of Selected Indole-Based Kratom Alkaloids. *Journal of Medicinal Chemistry*, *63*(1), 433–439. https://doi.org/10.1021/acs.jmedchem.9b01465

Schotte, C., Jiang, Y., Grzech, D., Dang, T. T., Laforest, L. C., León, F., Mottinelli, M., Nadakuduti, S. S., McCurdy, C. R., & O'Connor, S. E. (2023). Directed Biosynthesis of Mitragynine Stereoisomers. *Journal of the American Chemical Society*, *145*(9), 4957–4963. https://doi.org/10.1021/jacs.2c13644

Shellard, E. J., Houghton, P. J., & Resha, M. (1978). The Mitragyna Species of Asia. *Planta Medica*, *34*(07), 253–263. https://doi.org/10.1055/s-0028-1097448

Singh, D., Narayanan, S., Müller, C. P., Swogger, M. T., Chear, N. J., Dzulkapli, E. B., Yusoff, N. I. M., Ramachandram, D. S., León, F., McCurdy, C. R., & Vicknasingam, B. (2019). Motives for using Kratom (*Mitragyna speciosa* Korth.) among regular users in Malaysia. *Journal of Ethnopharmacology*, *233*, 34–40. https://doi.org/10.1016/j.jep.2018.12.038

Singh, D., Chear, N. J., Narayanan, S., León, F., Sharma, A., McCurdy, C. R., Avery, B. A., & Balasingam, V. (2020). Patterns and reasons for kratom (*Mitragyna speciosa*) use among current and former opioid poly-drug users. *Journal of Ethnopharmacology*, *249*, 112462. https://doi.org/10.1016/j.jep.2019.112462

Speciosa.org. (2017, October 12). *Analysis of Two Deaths Reportedly Associated with Kratom*. http://speciosa.org/analysis-of-two-deaths-reportedly-associated-with-kratom/

Tanna, R. S., Nguyen, J., Hadi, D. L., Manwill, P. K., Flores-Bocanegra, L., Layton, M. E., White, J. H., Cech, N. B., Oberlies, N. H., Rettie, A. E., Thummel, K. E., & Paine, M. F. (2022). Clinical Pharmacokinetic Assessment of Kratom (*Mitragyna speciosa*), a Botanical Product with Opioid-like Effects, in Healthy Adult Participants. *Pharmaceutics*, *14*(3), 620. https://doi.org/10.3390/pharmaceutics14030620

Today, R. W. M. U. (2019, April 12). Herbal drug kratom linked to almost 100 overdose deaths, CDC says. *USA TODAY*. https://eu.usatoday.com/story/news/health/2019/04/11/kratom-herbal-drug-linked-overdose-deaths-cdc-says/3441560002/

Trakulsrichai, S., Sathirakul, K., Auparakkitanon, S., Krongvorakul, J., Sueajai, J., Noumjad, N., Sukasem, C., & Wananukul, W. (2015). Pharmacokinetics of mitragynine in man. *Drug Design Development and Therapy*, 2421. https://doi.org/10.2147/dddt.s79658

Vo, K. T., Yin, S., Sharma, A., Avery, B. A., McCurdy, C. R., & Waksman, J. C. (2022). Acute Renal Insufficiency Associated With Consumption of Hydrocodone- and Morphine-Adulterated Kratom (*Mitragyna Speciosa*). *Journal of Emergency Medicine*, *63*(1), e28–e30. https://doi.org/10.1016/j.jemermed.2022.02.004

Wilson, L. M., Harris, H., Eans, S. O., Brice-Tutt, A. C., Cirino, T. J., Stacy, H. M., Simons, C. A., León, F., Sharma, A., Boyer, E. W., Avery, B. A., McLaughlin, J. P., & McCurdy, C. R. (2020). Lyophilized Kratom Tea as a

Therapeutic Option for Opioid Dependence. *Drug and Alcohol Dependence*, *216*, 108310. https://doi.org/10.1016/j.drugalcdep.2020.108310

Yue, K., Kopajtic, T. A., & Katz, J. (2018). Abuse liability of mitragynine assessed with a self-administration procedure in rats. *Psychopharmacology*, *235*(10), 2823–2829. https://doi.org/10.1007/s00213-018-4974-9

Zhang, M., Sharma, A., León, F., Avery, B. A., Kjelgren, R., McCurdy, C. R., & Pearson, B. J. (2020). Effects of Nutrient Fertility on Growth and Alkaloidal Content in *Mitragyna speciosa* (Kratom). *Frontiers in Plant Science*, *11*. https://doi.org/10.3389/fpls.2020.597696

Zhang, M., Sharma, A., León, F., Avery, B. A., Kjelgren, R., McCurdy, C. R., & Pearson, B. J. (2022). Plant growth and phytoactive alkaloid synthesis in kratom [*Mitragyna speciosa* (Korth.)] in response to varying radiance. *PLOS ONE*, *17*(4), e0259326. https://doi.org/10.1371/journal.pone.0259326

Zarembo, J., Douglas, B., Valenta, J. R., & Weisbach, J. A. (1974). Metabolites of Mitragynine. *Journal of Pharmaceutical Sciences*, *63*(9), 1407–1415. https://doi.org/10.1002/jps.2600630916

Leshoma, Southern Africa's Visionary Plant and Arrow Poison

Nigel Gericke, MBBCh

Medical Doctor | Ethnobotanist | Ethnopharmacologist |
Founding member of the Association for African Medicinal Plants Standards

The African continent is full of diverse plants and fungi which have psychoactive effects and have been traditionally used. In this paper Nigel Gericke shares the case of leshoma, a plant native to South Africa.

INTRODUCTION

The African continent, and especially southern Africa, has been considered to have relatively few psychoactive plants of cultural importance compared to the rich utilization of psychoactive plants in the New World (Schultes & Hofmann 1979, de Smet 1996). The purpose of this paper is to introduce southern Africa's leading visionary plant *Boophone disticha*, leshoma, to a wider audience, to recognize the traditional healers who committed important new information to the public domain, to highlight the therapeutic potential of the plant, to encourage further research on isolated compounds from the plant, and to draw attention to the cultural and spiritual dimensions of the use of the plant. The inherent toxicity of the plant, illustrated with case histories, safely managed through preparation and dosage by experienced traditional healers, presents a grave danger to the dilettante.

Boophone disticha, leshoma, was familiar to me as a young botany student through the magnificent tome, Medicinal and Poisonous Plants of Southern and Eastern Africa (Watt & Breyer-Brandwijk 1962), and my fascination with this plant began in earnest in 1994 when I was establishing the Traditional Medicines Programme (TRAMED), a collaboration between researchers and traditional healers, at the Pharmacology Department of the University of Cape Town. I was introduced to Bani Mayeng, a Tswana-speaking South African who was not only a practicing traditional healer, but had also graduated with a BSc degree in medicinal chemistry from the University of Buffalo in New York. At the time Bani was working in the Department of Organic Chemistry, and I asked if he would like to work with me in TRAMED. Since this would involve research on traditional medicines Bani first needed to ask his traditional mentor for permission to join the project. We set off together on a 1300 km drive from Cape Town to Puthaditjhaba (meaning 'meeting place of the tribes'), to meet Bani's traditional mentor, John Molefi Sekaja. Shortly after our arrival at the modest rural dwelling, and after introductions and pleasantries had been exchanged, I noticed the unmistakable fan-like leaves of a fine specimen of *Boophone*

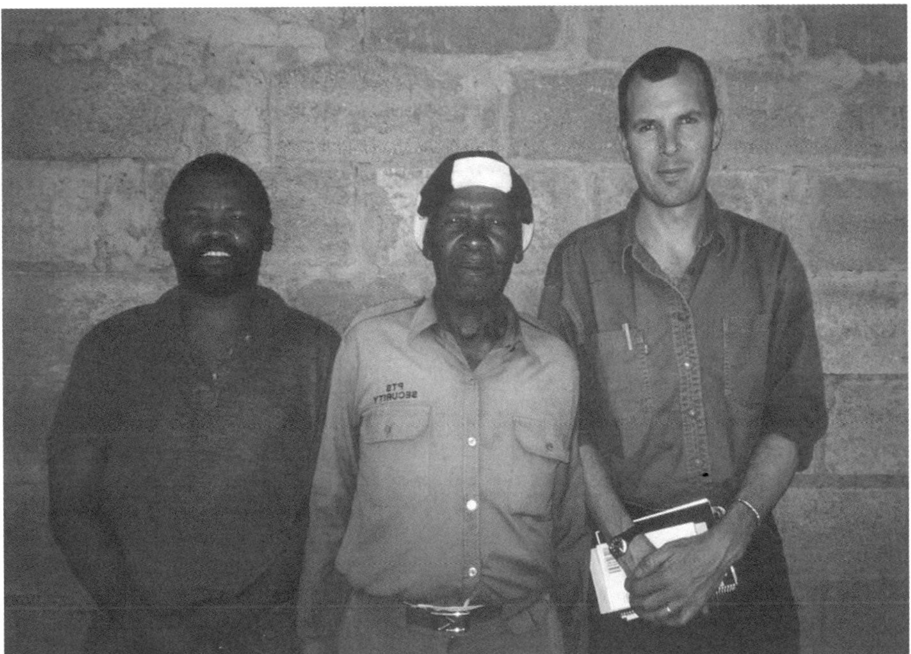

Fig. 1 Bani Mayeng, John Molefi Sekaja, Nigel Gericke in Puthadjithaba, 1994.

disticha growing in the yard. Pointing to the plant, I asked John Molefi Sekaja what he used leshoma for and was told he primarily used decoctions of the plant to sedate violent psychotic patients, and that dose was important as too much could cause visions and was dangerous. He explained that there was variability in the effect of wild plants from different areas so he had transplanted this specimen from the wild for all his treatments with the plant.

I asked if he would be willing to give me the dose of leshoma that would typically be administered to a psychotic patient so that I could experience the effect. At dawn the following morning I was instructed not to eat, and John Molefi Sekaja removed what looked like only two dry papery outer scales from the bulb, and boiled them in about a liter of water on the wood-fired stove. When the pot had cooled, I was given an enamel mug of the clear decoction to drink and told to go and rest. After about twenty minutes he came to check on me, saying "now we must get the poison out of you", which should have been alarming, but I was feeling pretty relaxed and had confidence in his knowledge. I was told to drink about a liter of warm water and then self-induce vomiting (traditionally called *phalaza*) into a plastic basin. The contents of the basin were examined, and I was told that "not all the poison is out", so I had to drink another liter of warm water and repeat the *phalaza*. This time the clear watery content of the basin was given a nod of approval and I was allowed to go off on my own in the bright morning sunshine and enjoy a state of deep calm, relaxation and contemplation which lasted some four to five hours, the calming effect tapering imperceptibly. John Molefi Sekaja, the maestro, had given me a gentle initiation into the therapeutic potential of leshoma, and a lesson on the finesse used in the preparation and safe dosing of this enigmatic plant.

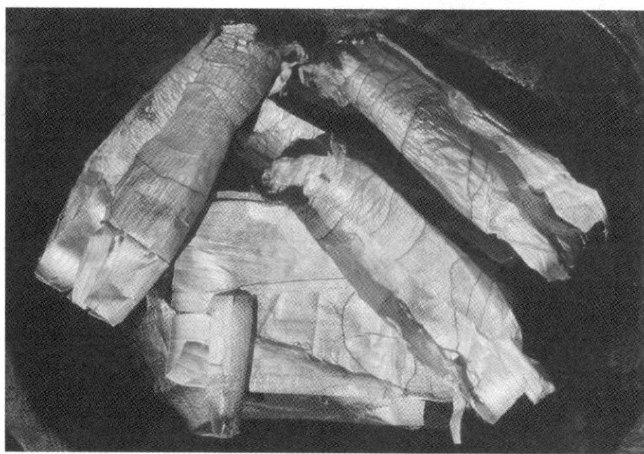

Fig. 2 Dry bulb scales of leshoma, *Boophone disticha*.

BOTANY

Boophone disticha (L.f.) Herb. is a member of the family Amaryllidaceae, and is a perennial herbaceous plant with a prominent bulb. A fan of grey-green opposite leaves in a characteristic single plane are produced annually. After the leaves have been shed in winter, an umbel of dense red flowers is produced annually. The fruits are borne terminally on elongated pedicels, and are disseminated as the characteristic tumbleweed of the dry inforescence, up to 60 cm in diameter, is blown along the ground by the wind. The bulb can be up to 20 cm long, invested in a thick layer of fire-resistant papery brown bulb scales. The name *Boophone* is derived from the Greek *bous* = ox, and *phone* = death, referring to the poisonous properties of the bulb which have caused death in cattle browsing on the plants. The species name *disticha* refers to the erect fan shape of the leaves.

Sixteen synonyms are recognized in Plants of the World Online:

Homotypic synonyms

Amaryllis disticha L.f., Suppl. Pl.: 195 (1782)
Amaryllis toxicaria (L.f. ex Aiton) D.Dietr., Syn. Plant. 2: 1181 (1840)
Boophone toxicaria (L.f. ex Aiton) Herb., Appendix: 18 (1821)
Brunsvigia disticha (L.f.) Sweet, Hort. Brit.: 404 (1826)
Brunsvigia toxicaria (L.f. ex Aiton) Ker Gawl., Bot. Reg. 7: t. 567 (1822)
Haemanthus distichus (L.f.) L.f. ex Savage, Herbertia 4: 97 (1937)
Haemanthus toxicarius L.f. ex Aiton, Hort. Kew. 1: 405 (1789), nom. superfl.

Heterotypic Synonyms

Boophone intermedia M.Roem., Fam. Nat. Syn. Monogr. 4: 59 (1847)
Boophone longipedicellata Pax, Bot. Jahrb. Syst. 10: 4 (1888)
Boophone toxicaria var. *obtusifolia* Herb., Appendix: 18 (1821)
Brunsvigia ciliaris (L.) Ker Gawl., Bot. Reg. 3: t. 192, 193 (1817)

Brunsvigia rautanenii Baker, Bull. Herb. Boissier, sér. 2, 3: 667 (1903)
Haemanthus ciliaris L., Sp. Pl. ed. 2.: 413 (1762)
Haemanthus lemairei De Wild., Contr. Fl. Katanga: 33 (1921)
Haemanthus robustus Pax, Bot. Jahrb. Syst. 15: 140 (1892)
Haemanthus sinuatus Schult. & Schult.f., J.J.Roemer & J.A.Schultes, Syst. Veg. ed. 15bis. 7: 892 (1830), nom. nud.

FOLK NAMES

Namibia

n/ara (Thaddeus Chedau pers. comm. 1 August 2022)	Khwe
/a'ana (Gibson, 2018)	Ju/'hoansi
||hou ||hou (Bleek & Lloyd archive)	!Kun

South Africa

century plant, *Cape poison bulb*, *candelabra flower*	English
gifbol (poison bulb), *malgif* (mad poison), perdespook (startles horses), *seeroogblom* (sore-eyes flower)	Afrikaans
leshoma, *lesoma*, *motlatsia*	South Sotho
kgutsanayanaha	Sotho
ibhade, *inkotha*	Zulu
incumbe, *siphahluka*	Swati
inkoto	Ndebele
incotha	Pondo
incotho, *iswadi*, *inkwadi*	Xhosa
leshona, *kgutsana ya naha*	Tswana

Zaire

lunteunteu	Tabwa
luteoto	Luba
mba dia tseke	Jaka

Zimbabwe

muwandwe, *mumhandwe*, *munzepete*	Shona
ingkoto	Ndebele

DISTRIBUTION AND HABITAT

Country plant collection records of *Boophone disticha* are from Angola, Botswana, Burundi, Kenya, Lesotho, Malawi, Mozambique, Namibia, Rwanda, South Africa, Sudan, Swaziland,

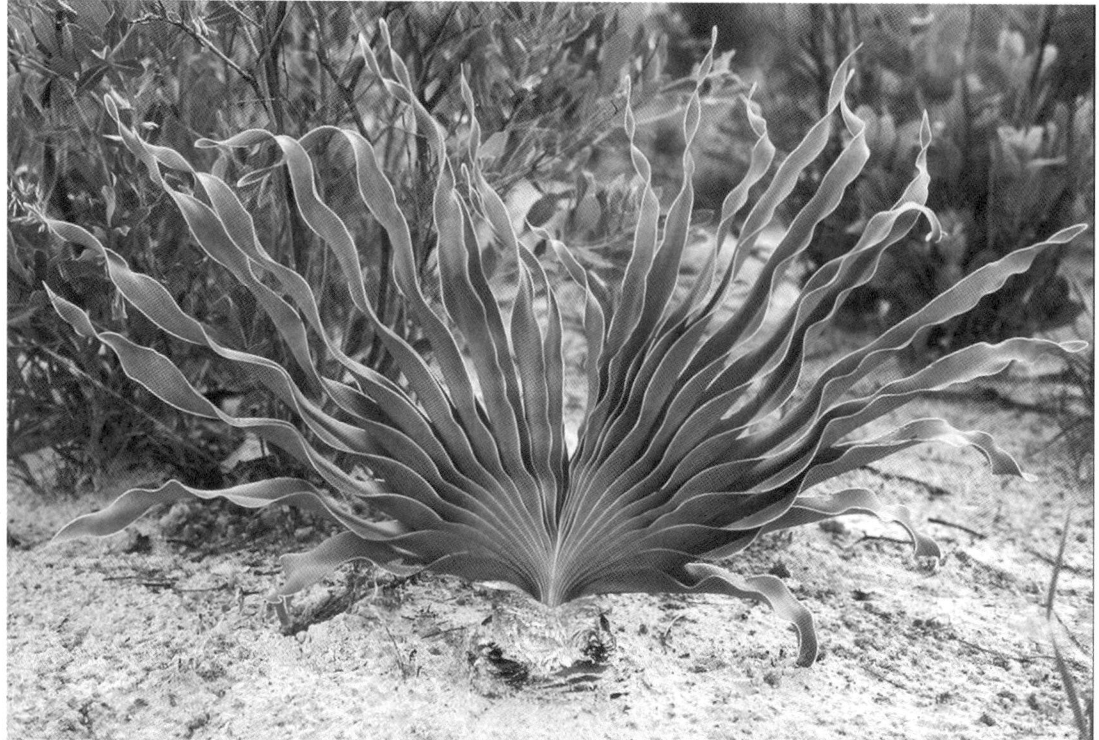

Fig. 3 *Boophone disticha* showing the characteristic fan-like leaves growing in a single plane.

Tanzania, Uganda, Zambia, Zaïre and Zimbabwe (POWO). The plant grows in temperate and tropical sandy or rocky grassland and bushland, up to an altitude of 2450 m (Neuwinger 1994).

PSYCHOACTIVE USES OF LESHOMA

In April 1999 a remarkable archaeological find was made in the Kouga Mountains in the Langkloof region of the Eastern Cape Province of South Africa. The well-preserved mummified remains of a San hunter-gatherer were found in a shallow grave against the back wall of a rock shelter. The grave had been marked by a large flat stone with San paintings, and beneath the stone were two layers of sticks, leaves and branches. The body was that of an adult male, 50–55 years old who had been buried in a traditional flexed position, lying on the left side facing East. Most of the body was covered in a thick layer of leaves of leshoma, *B. disticha,* (Binneman 1999, Steyn et al., 2007). The Kouga mummy has been dated to almost 2000 years old (1930 +/- 20 years BP) (Steyn et al., 2007). While there is no direct evidence from this site of leshoma having a spiritual significance, its use to invest the body attests to the San peoples' intimate familiarity with the plant for at least two millennia. The leaves may have been used simply to preserve the body as the plant does have antimicrobial properties, but they may have been used symbolically.

It is widely known that San shamans entered into altered states of consciousness for healing in trance dances. In her paper titled "Enigma of drug-induced altered states of consciousness

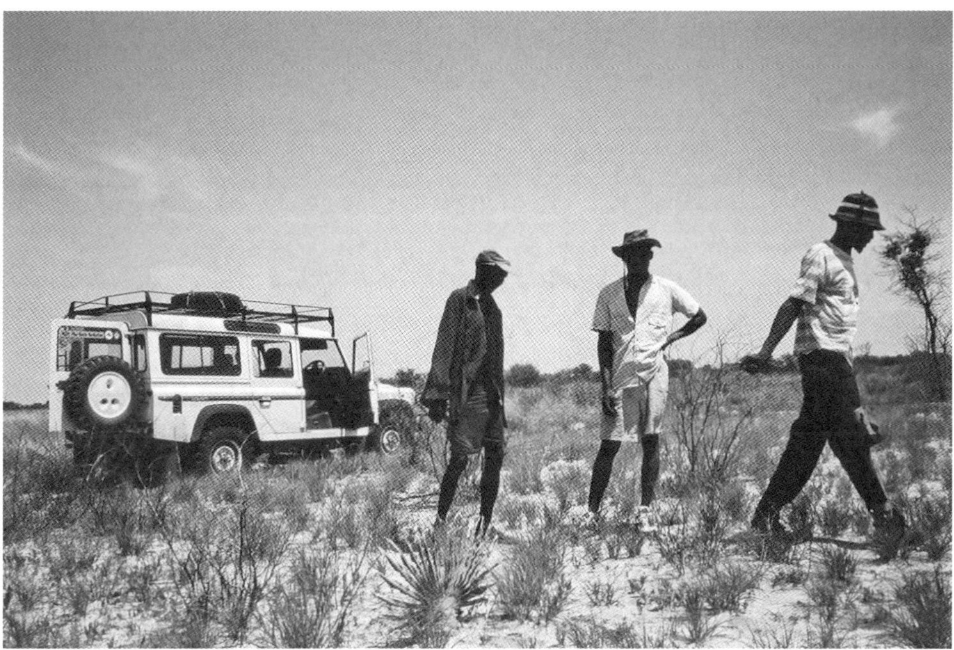

Fig.4 San people keeping their distance from *Boophane disticha* in the Kalahari, Botswana.

among the !Kung bushmen of the Kalahari desert", De Rios explained that the enigma in this title refers to the unknown influence that psychoactive plants may have had on the trance phenomenon and on the healing beliefs of the Kalahari Bushmen (de Rios 1986). Kalahari plants which have been suspected of inducing the San trance state known as *kia* include a *Pancratium* species, Amaryllidaceae, known to the San of the Dobe area in Botswana as *kashi*; the bulb is cut and rubbed into scarifications on the head to induce hallucinations (Schultes, 1970), and *Ferraria glutinosa,* Iridaceae, known to the !Kung as *!gaishe noru noru* (Dobkin de Rios 1986). While the alkaloidal composition of *Pancratium* species suggests they may have entheogenic potential, the use of *Ferraria glutinosa* as an entheogen is unlikely. On coming across a corm of a *Ferraria* species in January 1998 in the settlement of Molapo, Central Kalahari, Botswana, the local Ju/'hoansi people still called the plant *!gaishe*, but told me it had no use and that children simply played with the corms as toys. *Ferraria* species are known to be eaten as *veldkos* (wild food) in southern Africa: *Ferraria glutinosa* has been recorded as a wild food (Welcome & van Wyk 2019), while on the West Coast of the Cape in South Africa the corms of *Ferraria crispa* were baked on hot coals and eaten as a pleasant tasting starch-rich food (Dawid Bester personal communication 1995), and *Ferraria divaricata* is also eaten as a food (Welcome & van Wyk 2019).

In Molapo in January 1998, Ju/'hoansi people seemed very wary—or very respectful of—a specimen of *Boophane disticha* we came across in the field. They gave it a wide berth, and stated they did not use the plant. One evening while watching the community dancing the healing Gemsbok Dance, I spoke to a young San man who acknowledged that certain plants (names were not mentioned) were sometimes used by some of the elders to aid in the trance state during healing dances, and I wondered if *B. disticha* may have been one of these plants. The first documented evidence that *Boophone disticha* is indeed used to induce trance by the Ju/'hoansi San was reported by Gibson, 2018:

> *"In 2008 in Namibia, /Kunta Kashe, an aged n/umkxao (the owner of n/um healing power), told me that his uncle Dam Toma, also a n/umkxao, had sometimes used malgif (Boophone disticha) to induce a trance and to heal"*
>
> *"He explained: If you take the malgif (|a'ana) for himself, in a respectful relationship (/ xoa kòàqà khòè), not being afraid of each other: then he can help you. The bulb is poisonous. If you use it correctly, his nature/ being (tca´to'à hè ku´|xoa), he is owner of power (kgwe xau), he becomes medicine([n/om) or to help you to heal other people. The plant, plants are living beings with the knowledge/knowing (!'hàn ka) of nature (tci !u), the land (kxàlhò). You must take/ approach the plant for himself, from kgwe (power) and the knowledge/knowing of nature. Through that bulb, if you can warm its medicine/healing power (tzi n/om), you use it for the [trance] dance, then you see what the problem is and also the spirits (//gauwasi), but only if all are together/in relation (||káe´)."*

In the note accompanying this report, Gibson explained "the Ju/'hoansi who participated in the study understood Afrikaans well but preferred to speak their own language. I spoke Afrikaans and a certified guide and native Ju/'hoan speaker translated for me. Because the healers understood me as well as the translation, they interrupted the translator when they did not agree with his translation. I also often asked for more clarity on words and meanings. We would then all engage in a discussion about the most appropriate translation from the Ju/'hoan language into Afrikaans or vice versa. There are a number of words which cannot be directly translated into Afrikaans or English. In such cases I use more than one word to try to provide an approximation of the meaning. I also asked the translator to write words down for me and subsequently checked these against a Ju/'hoan English Dictionary as I translated the interviews from Afrikaans to English for the purpose of this article" (Gibson 2018).

The renowned Zulu *sangoma* (diviner and healer), traditional historian and mystic Vusamazulu Credo Mutwa related to me the use of leshoma when Nehanda of Dande died in 1973 (Vusamazulu Credo Mutwa, personal communication 2001). Nehanda is the name of a female spirit venerated in traditional Shona religion in Zimbabwe, and it is also the name given to the human medium that invokes the spirit of Nehanda. At the end of the nineteenth century, the Shona medium Charwe Nyakasikana, who embodied the spirit of Nehanda, inspired the first uprisings against the authorities and settlers in British-occupied Southern Rhodesia in 1896-97, known as the first *chimurenga* (meaning fight or struggle). Nehanda was arrested and prosecuted by the colonial authorities, and hanged in 1898. Just before she died, she is said to have prophesised "My bones shall rise again." During the second *chimurenga*, the Zimbabwean war of independence from the 1960's to 1980, the freedom fighters invoked the history and mythology of Nehanda through stories and songs, and considered themselves her followers (Bertho 2017), and a second spirit medium of Nehanda did indeed appear once more, known as the Nehanda of Dande (Dande is an area in northern Zimbabwe). Because of her importance to the liberation struggle, the elderly Nehanda of Dande was taken to safety to guerrilla camps in Mozambique by fighters of the Zimbabwe African National Liberation Army (ZANLA), and her presence continued to inspire the fighters until she died in 1973. According to Vusamazulu Credo Mutwa, the body of the Nehanda of Dande was wrapped in the bulb scales of leshoma before her burial in Mozambique, and after independence her body was brought back to Zimbabwe for burial.

The association of leshoma with death and with the world of the ancestors continues to this day. The Northern Sotho of South Africa consider the plant sacred and pray next to the plant to communicate with their ancestors, together with offerings of sorghum and tobacco (Bani Mayeng, personal communication 1 November 2022).

Two African traditional healers independently gave similar information on the use of leshoma by the Basotho during the initiation into manhood (Laydevant 1932):

> "The bulb is very poisonous; and when mixed with the food of the initiates at the circumcision lodge, it must first be carefully measured. The taste is not bitter, and the boys do not object to its flavour. In this instance, the *buphane* [*Boophone*] is not used alone, but mixed with several ingredients of other plants and remedies"

> "The initiates are taught that such a remedy will imbue them with the qualities of their ancestors and will tend to make men of them. When the signs of intoxication produced by the mixture are apparent, they are accepted as a token that the spirit of manhood has entered the youth's body."

> "This remedy is also considered as a cup or draught of inspiration for the initiates at the circumcision lodge. During the initiation period, every boy has to compose a piece of poetry or praises, which he will recite publicly when he is liberated and the medicine which is given to them is supposed to communicate the gifts of poetry and eloquence."

After circumcision Basotho initiates were given a large bowl of medicine (Pasquali 2021, quoting Ashton 1952):

> "roasted anhydrous butterfat mixed with a potent narcotic made from the bulb of leshoma. Everyone eats a handful and within minutes falls into a deep stupor that lasts for a day or more and soothes all the pain".

The first documented cases of the recreational use of *Boophone disticha* for its hallucinogenic activity was reported in 1979 by Dr. R.O. Laing, the Government Medical Officer at Fort Victoria, Zimbabwe. According to the three boys presenting at the hospital, aged from 15 to 18 years of age, the hallucinatory effect of the bulb was well known in the Gutu district of Zimbabwe. Two of the three boys had to be hospitalised after ingesting a decoction of the bulb. Dr. Laing's clinical case notes from the boys' misadventure are instructive, and included in full under the paragraph titled Toxicity. He concluded: "Cases such as these may become more common as young rural dwellers seek to join the 'drug culture' with locally available herbs" (Laing 1979).

In 1995 a visitor arrived unannounced at the TRAMED Programme at University of Cape Town. He was a traditional healer named David Matthe, who had heard about TRAMED in Johannesburg and had caught a train to Cape Town to meet Bani Mayeng and myself to find out more about the programme's objectives and to explore a potential cooperation. Smartly dressed in a suit and carrying a briefcase, David Matthe exemplified the modern urban traditional healer, and announced with pride that he had published his first paper titled 'Ethnomedical science and African medical practice' (Matthe 1988). We discussed the use of leshoma, and David Matthe shared with us the first information that we were aware of that traditional healers in Johannesburg administered decoctions of the bulb orally or by enema to patients specifically to induce visual hallucinations. He informed us this phenomenon is called "bioscope" in Johannesburg (a South African colloquial for cinema) when the patient is seated in front of a white cloth fixed to a wall to await the onset of visions, or "the mirror", when the patient is seated in front of a mirror. The visions are interpreted by the healer to represent events from the person's past, or of future events that are yet to come to pass (David Matthe, personal communication 1995). The Zulu term *bhayiskhobho* is also used to describe divination through leshoma-induced visions (Sobiecki 2008), derived from the English word bioscope, and called *lispëel* in Zulu, derived from the Afrikaans word *spieël* for mirror, and *tshivhone* in Venda, meaning "mirror" or "vision" (Thornton, 2017).

Divination aimed at identifying a person responsible for the suspected bewitching of another is prohibited by law in South Africa, but bogus healers are known to use leshoma to induce hallucinations which they then claim to be evidence that their client was bewitched (Bani Mayeng, personal communication 1 November 2022), requiring treatment for a fee.

In Zimbabwe, botanical drugs are not typically required by the *n'anga* (traditional healer) to initiate spirit possession or communication with ancestral spirits. *B. disticha* is used, however,

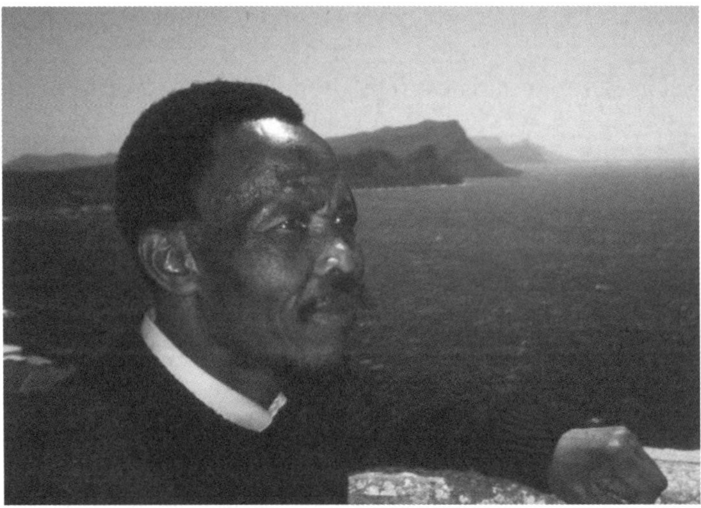

Fig.5 Traditional healer David Matthe, Cape Town 1995.

when the traditional healers believe that their own spirit is unable to communicate with the patients' spirit. In such cases the bulb of the plant is crushed into water and boiled together with an unidentified plant called *mukundagona*, and a single teaspoon of the decoction is given to the patient (Gelfand et al., 1985).

Amafufunyana is a culture-bound syndrome recognised by local communities and traditional healers throughout South Africa. The term is used to describe a syndrome of disordered thought and behavior traditionally believed to have a number of possible causes including neglecting duties honouring the ancestors, possession by a malevolent spirit, or ignoring a calling by the ancestors to undergo training as a traditional healer. There is some overlap between the presentation of *amafufunyana* and conversion syndrome and schizophrenia (Niehaus et al., 2004). South African doctors working in rural or township areas are familiar with patients presenting with *amafufunyana* and acute treatment may be benzodiazepine anxiolytics. In rural areas traditional healers first divine the cause of the condition and may use healing rituals and traditional sedative and anxiolytic remedies. *Boophone* has been reported as a treatment for *amafufunyana* (Watt & Breyer-Brandwijk 1962).

In the Karoo area of South Africa near Touws River it was believed by local people of European extraction that stuffing mattresses and pillows with the dry bulb scales of *B. disticha* will calm hysteria and treat insomnia (Watt 1967). Preparations of the bulb are used to treat anxiety in Zimbabwe, and hallucinations and psychosis have been reported as side-effects (Nyazema 1986).

Low doses of decoctions of the bulb scales of *B. disticha* are administered to sedate violent psychotic patients (John Molefi Sekaja, personal communication 1994).

Rastafarians in the Western cape Province of South Africa recommend one leaf of *B. disticha*, [likely taken as an infusion or decoction] to be taken orally to abstain from drinking alcohol (Philander 2011).

TOXICITY

Fatalities from overdose of *B. disticha* are well-known, and preparations administered rectally and vaginally have been used to commit suicide (Juritz 1914, Watt & Breyer-Brandwijk 1962). The characteristic signs of *Boophone disticha* poisoning in non-fatal cases are the rapid development of ataxia, dizziness, impaired vision, talkativeness or quietness, and depression, stupor and coma. A case of non-fatal poisoning in Zimbabwe has been described as follows (Gelfand and Mitchel 1952):

> "A 24 year old patient was told by a traditional healer to drink juice of the bulb of *B. disticha* if he felt weak or developed abdominal pain. After experiencing such discomfort the patient cut off the root of the bulb, allowing a few drops from the bulb to collect on a plate. He mixed this with some porridge, eating only two spoons of the porridge mixture. His mouth immediately became painful and he experienced burning pain down to his epigastrium. Within minutes he became dizzy and fell to the ground, regaining consciousness in hospital twenty hours later. He was

> irrational, talkative, restless and had intense photophobia. Pupils were dilated but reacted to light. The following morning he was still irrational, talkative and resisting examination. By five in the afternoon he regained [full] consciousness and made an uneventful recovery."

Case notes on three teenage boys aged 15 to 18 presenting at hospital with signs and symptoms of acute poisoning following ingestion of a decoction of *Boophane disticha* for recreational visionary use have been reported by Dr. Laing, the Government Medical Officer at Fort Victoria, Zimbabwe. Aspirate of stomach contents and remnants of the actual bulbs were sent to the Government Analyst and the National Herbarium, and it was confirmed that the bulbs were from *Boophane disticha* (Laing 1979):

> Case 1.
> "The eldest, 18 years, was deeply unconscious, with widely dilated pupils which reacted sluggishly, a tachycardia (110—120 beats per minute), raised blood pressure 150/110 mm Hg, a slight temperature (37,4- 37,6 °C) and laboured respiration. He remained in this state for 24 hours and then gradually recovered and was discharged after 72 hours with a normal pulse, BP and temperature."
>
> Case 2.
> "The younger relative of Case 1. presented as an acute psychotic episode and appeared to be having violent hallucinations. The physical signs were similar to those in Case 1. but less marked. He was treated with intravenous chlorpromazine to sedate him and after 36 hours had recovered. He was allowed home after 48 hours."
>
> Case 3.
> "This young man, who was not admitted to hospital, claimed that ·he had taken the decoction with the other two and had spent the night feeling drunk and seeing visions and felt perfectly well the following morning. On examination the only abnormal sign was slightly dilated pupils."

A homicidal psychotic reaction to a dose of leshoma has been reported from South Africa. A traditional healer gave a patient who claimed to be bewitched 150 ml of a decoction of *B. disticha.* Soon after ingestion the patient became paranoid, and imagining he was being attacked drew a pistol and fired shots randomly, killing one person and wounding several others. A sample of the decoction was analyzed by the South African Police Forensic Service, confirming the presence of alkaloids from *B. disticha* (du Plooy et al., 2001).

NON-PSYCHOACTIVE USES

The papery dried outer bulb scales of leshoma are still widely used in southern Africa as a dressing to cuts, wounds, burns, abscesses and boils, and to relieve urticaria. They are also applied to

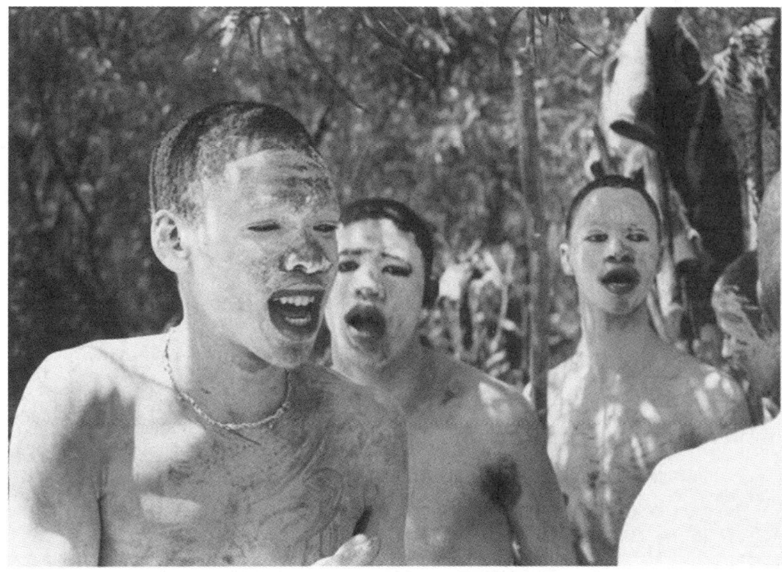

Fig. 6 Abakweta—Xhosa circumcision initiates—Western Cape in 1991.

contusions and to painful joints. The treatment is reputed to draw pus from abscesses, and to relieve pain. Bulb extracts are administered for headache, chest pain and abdominal pain. Pillows stuffed with the dry bulb scales are used to provide relief from asthma (Neuwinger 1994). In Zimbabwe the plant is used to treat general body pains, vertigo, edema of the legs, constipation, burns, wounds and skin rashes (Gelfand et al., 1985).

The dry bulb scales of leshoma are used to this day as an antiseptic and analgesic dressing for the wound after traditional circumcision.

In January 1998 on an ethnobotanical expedition to Molapo village in Central Kalahari Game Reserve, Botswana we were approached one evening by an elderly !Kung-speaking San couple who asked for help. The woman had been stung on the hand by a scorpion about a week earlier and was in great pain. Her hand was extremely swollen and tender, and she was running a high fever. The hand had become secondary infected, and the clinical presentation was that of severe cellulitis requiring antibiotics, or a hand abscess which would need surgery to drain the pus together with a course of antibiotics. Since we had no suitable medicine's we planned on driving the patient to a clinic in the small town of Ghanzi the following morning. Earlier that day we had photographed a specimen of *Boophone disticha* growing not far from our campsite, and we went back to collect the dry bulb scales, much to the surprise of the local San people who appeared wary of the plant. As a first aid measure I applied aqueous cream to the skin of the swollen hand and wrapped the hand in a thick layer of the *Boophane* bulb scales which were held in place by a firm crépe bandage. The woman was instructed to keep the hand elevated during the night and to return at dawn. We were anticipating that we would have to abandon the ethnobotany expedition and take her to the town of Ghanzi for treatment. When the woman returned at dawn, her temperature was back to normal, the pain was much reduced, and the swelling of her hand had reduced by about a third. I resolved to continue with the daily dressings of the bulb scales, and by the third day her hand was back to normal. Clinically, the *Boophone* bulb scale treatment exhibited significant analgesic, anti-inflammatory and antimicrobial activities.

A popular weekly South African agricultural magazine reported the case of a retired engineer from the rural town of Prins Albert, who suffered from a chronic non-healing sore on his leg that doctors had been unable to heal. After another ineffective visit to doctors in Cape Town, his domestic worker presented him with a whole bulb of *B. disticha* and recommended daily dressings with the outer bulb scales. According to the article, by the end of two weeks of daily dressings with the plant the wound healed completely (Landbouweekblad 1995).

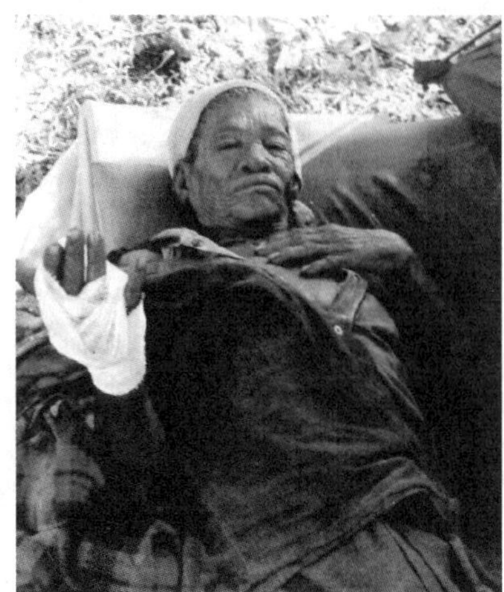

Fig.7 San woman resting with swollen septic hand dressed with *Boophone disticha* bulb scales, Molapo, Central Kalahari, 1998.

HUNTING POISON

Boophone disticha has been well documented as an arrow poison. Thunberg and Masson appear to have been the first Europeans to report on the use as an arrow poison in 1774 (Smith 1966). *B. disticha* was the main source of hunting poison in southern Africa among the San hunter-gatherers and Khoi khoi pastoralists (Paterson 1778, Lichtenstein 1806).

Alexander, 1838:

> "The *Buphane disticha* or *Haemanthus toxicaria*—the 'giftbol' of the old Colonist—was used chiefly by the tribes of Bushmanland and Little Namaqualand. The bulbs were taken at just about the time they are putting out their leaves and cut transversely; the thick fluid which was then extracted was kept in the sun till it was the consistency of gum, and in that form was smeared on the arrows and allowed to dry. This poison was employed chiefly for the purpose of killing animals which were intended for food, such as antelope and other small quadrupeds."

David Livingstone, 1857, noted that *B. disticha* was widely used as an arrow poison, often added to *Euphorbia* latex, by local people in the vicinity of Victoria Falls, and also by the San of northern Botswana. Wellman, 1907, reported on the use of *B. disticha* bulbs as an arrow poison in south Angola. Dornan, 1916, witnessed the use of *B. disticha* bulbs as an additive to other poisons by San people in Zimbabwe (formerly Rhodesia).

The online digital Bleek and Lloyd archive of the Centre for Curating the Archive of the University of Cape Town includes collections of drawings and watercolours made by four !Kun boys who lived in the Mowbray, Cape Town household of Llucy Lloyd. !nanni was the oldest of the four boys, and had been abducted from his home area in north east Damaraland (in what is now Namibia) by Makoba people. He was then possibly exchanged or bartered and brought to Cape Town by a Mr. Eriksson and arrived in Mowbray, Cape Town on the 1st of September 1879. He was placed (along with a younger !Kun boy called Tamme) at the Lloyd household. !nanni's people were known as |kam-ssin !ku or 'Sun' Bushmen (page 9175v). !nanni was able to provide Lucy Lloyd with a number of stories of the !Kun in his region, as well as many drawings depicting local fauna and flora and folklore. He was repatriated to Damaraland in the care of Mr. Eriksson on the 28th March 1882. A watercolour painting of a plant by !nanni dated 8 July 1881, with the !Kun name transcribed by Lucy Lloyd as ||*hó* ||*kó*, looks strikingly like *Boophone disticha* (Bleek & Lloyd 2022[a]).

A simple pencil drawing of a plant by !nanni with a very similar !Kun name transcribed as ||*hou* ||*hou*, is described as a leafy plant, the juice of the root is boiled and used to poison arrows (Bleek & Lloyd 2022b).*

In 2022 older former hunter-gatherers now settled in the Kavango area of Namibia recognised *B. disticha* when shown photographs of the plant, and called it *n/aro*. They had used it as an arrow poison in their younger days when living in Botswana and had also used it to poison the tips of the long lances used to impale springhares in their holes (Thaddeus Chedau, personal communication 1 August 2022).

ALKALOID CHEMISTRY

Eleven alkaloids were identified from the bulb of *B. disticha* , and of the total the major alkaloids were buphanidrine (19.4%), undulatine (18.6%), buphanisine (16.9%) buphanamine (14.1%) and nerbowdine (11.1%). Minor alkaloids were crinine, crinamidine, lycorine, distichamine, 3-O-acetylnerbowdine and buphacetine (Hauth and Stauffacher, 1961), and 3-O-methylcrinamidine and acetyl-3-nerbowdine (Dictionary of Natural Products 2008), and a new alkaloid, 1-O-acetylbuphanamine (van Rensburg et al., 2017).

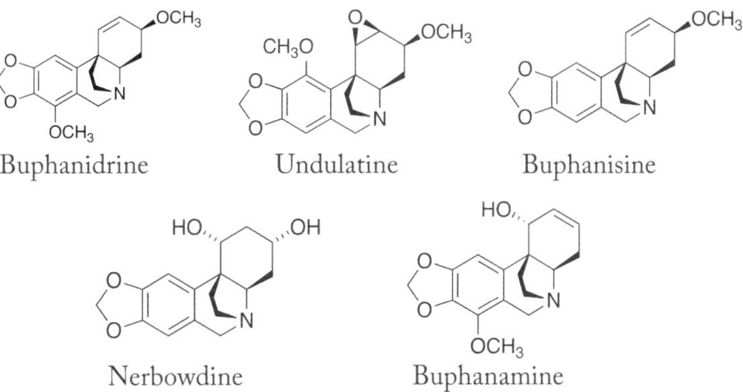

Fig. 8 Major alkaloids in *Boophone disticha*.

* To see these image's go to http://lloydbleekcollection.cs.uct.ac.za/drawings/NLLB_D_!n078.html

CENTRAL NERVOUS SYSTEM PHARMACOLOGY

In-vitro

Methanol extracts from two specimens of *B. disticha* gave 37.2 % and 50.5% inhibition respectively of actelycholinesterase (Sibanyoni et al., 2020). Two alkaloids isolated from *B. disticha*, buphanadrine and buphanamine were tested in-vitro for affinity to the serotonin transporter (SERT) in a binding assay using [^{3}H]-citalopram as ligand. The IC50 values of buphanidrine and buphanamine were 274 μM (*K*i = 132 μM) and 1799 μM (*K*i = 868 μM), respectively. The two alkaloids showed weak affinity to the 5HT1A receptor, and were not tested on 5HT2A receptors (Sandagar et al., 2005). An ethanol extract of *B. disticha* was tested in-vitro and found to inhibit SERT with IC50 = 423 μg/ml, inhibit the dopamine transporter (DAT) with IC50 = 93 μg/ml and the noradrenalin transporter with IC50 = 77 μg/ml (Pederson 2008). The four isolated compounds from *B. disticha*, buphanamine, buphanidrine, buphanisine and distichamine, were tested for affinity to SERT and had IC50 values of 55 μM, 62 μM, 199 μM and 65 μM respectively (Neergard et al., 2009).

In-vivo

In a mice forced swim model of depressive behavior, an ethanol extract of *B. disticha* showed antidepressant-like activity at the high doses of 250 mg/kg and 500 mg/kg, and in rats at a dose of 250 mg/kg (Pederson et al., 2008).

Aqueous-ethanolic extract of *B. disticha* bulb in mice showed long term antihypertensive activity, and like the positive control diazepam gave increased heart rate variability, indicative of the anxiolytic potential of the extract (Pote et al., 2014).

Aqueous-ethanolic extract of *B. disticha* bulb was tested for anxiolytic activity in the Souk test (ST) elevated plus maze (EPM) and open field tests (OF) in mice. The 25 mg/kg *B. disticha* dose group exhibited highest anxiolytic-like activity in both the ST and OF, while the 10 mg/kg was most active in the EPM. It was concluded that the extract of *B. disticha* exerted good anxiolytic-like activity in both the ST and OF at medium dose (25 mg/kg), while the low dose (10 mg/kg) showed prominent anxiolytic-like activity in the EPM (Pote et al., 2018).

The antidepressant effects of *Boophone distic*ha was studied in mice exposed to the five-day repeated forced swim stress, and the extracts of *B. disticha* were compared to distilled water control and fluoxetine. The *B. disticha* treatment (10 mg/kg/p.o for 3 weeks) significantly attenuated the depressive-like behavioral abnormalities induced by the repeated forced swims test and the elevated serum corticosterone levels observed in stressed mice. Additionally, repeated forced swim exposure significantly decreased the number of neuroblasts in the hippocampus and BDNF levels in the brain of the mice, while both fluoxetine and *B. disticha* treatment attenuated these changes. The antidepressant effects of *B. disticha* were comparable to those of fluoxetine, but unlike fluoxetine, did not show any anxiogenic effects, suggesting it may be better tolerated. This study demonstrated that the *B. disticha* extract exerted antidepressant-like effects which were mediated in part by normalizing brain corticosterone and BDNF levels (Xhakaza et al., 2022).

TOXICOLOGY

A freeze dried hydro-ethanolic plant extract of the bulb of *B. disticha* was tested in thirty-three adult rats. The oral LD50 of this plant extract was between 120 and 240 mg/kg. Signs of toxicity began approximately 10 minutes after gavage, and the most prominent initial signs were head tremors (at 50 mg/kg) and body tremors, and severe body tremors (>360 mg/kg) followed by convulsions. Symptoms of toxicity lasted approximately 2 hours for doses of 240 mg/kg and less, and 3 hours for doses over 240 mg/kg for animals that survived. The results indicate rapid gastrointestinal absorption of the active principles in the plant extract. The most prominent neurotoxicological effects were limb paralysis. Tachypnoea was noted at low doses, while higher doses produced laboured breathing. Retropulsion (the tendency to walk backwards) was observed with higher doses supporting the hallucinogenic potential of the plant extract (Gadaga et al., 2011).

Pre-treatment of mice with the serotonin antagonist cyproheptadine led to a dose-dependent decrease in mortality, from 80% mortality in the group not pre-treated with cyproheptadine, to 30% mortality in the 15 and 20 mg/kg cyproheptadine pre-treated groups. There was also a dose-dependent increase in median survival times amongst the groups. Pre-treatment with cyproheptadine also resulted in a decrease of other toxic symptoms associated with *Boophone disticha*, indicating that excess serotonin signalling plays a role in the toxicity of the plant (Mutseura et al., 2013).

Neurobehavioral toxicity of an extract of *B. disticha* was studied in rats in a 28-days sub-acute test. Rats were allocated to four treatment groups (n=6); control and three experimental group (100, 200 and 400 mg/kg p.o. *Boophone* extract). Functional Observational Battery (FOB) and motor activity testing were carried on day 1, 14 and 28 of the study. Signs of toxicity included stupor followed by tremor affecting the whole body. In more severe cases the rat would progress to tremors at rest with the head sloping to one side. These responses were most pronounced at higher doses. Retropulsion was observed in some rats after repeated dosing. The observed toxic responses lasted approximately 30 minutes. At low single doses, however, it appeared that *Boophone disticha* had stimulant properties (Ganga et al., 2017).

TRADE AND CONSERVATION STATUS

In spite of its potential toxicity wild-harvested leshoma is commonly sold on medicinal plant street markets and in *muthi* (traditional medicine) shops in South Africa (Moeng 2010). In the Eastern Cape Province of South Africa leshoma was the 23rd most frequently traded medicinal plant out of 60 plants with more than 1.6 tonnes estimated to be sold annually in this province alone (Dold and Cocks 2002). Leshoma was found in 56% of the Witwatersrand *muthi* shops in 1994, and it was sold by 11% of the traders in the Faraday Street *muthi* market in Johannesburg in 2001. *Boophone disticha* is a popular medicinal plant with approximately 60% of traditional medicines traders stocking a quantity equivalent to least three medium-sized shopping bags per trader (Williams et al., 2020).

Boophone disticha is widespread and long-lived but has been assessed as Declining by the Red List of South African Plants. Wild plants are over-harvested and sold in large quantities at traditional medicine markets, causing the wild population to decrease, particularly in the provinces of

KwaZulu-Natal and Gauteng. Over-harvesting and habitat destruction are impacting wild plant populations (Williams et al., 2020).

CONCLUSIONS

Leshoma, *Boophone disticha*, is the main visionary plant of southern Africa (Pasquali 2021, Samorini 2022). Direct evidence from the Kouga mummy indicates that the plant has been known by San people for at least two millennia (Binneman 1999, Steyn et al., 2007), and it has recently been confirmed to have been used by the San to induce trance states for healing (Gibson 2018). The plant is still commonly used by traditional healers and local people in southern Africa to facilitate communication with the patient's spirit and with the ancestors (Bani Mayeng, personal communication 1 November 2022), to induce visual hallucinations in patients for diagnostic and divinatory purposes (David Matthe personal communication 1995, Sobiecki 2008, Thornton 2017), and it has been deliberately used as a hallucinogen by teenagers in rural Zimbabwe (Laing 1979).

Leshoma has been used as a major tranquillizer or antipsychotic to treat violent psychotic patients (John Molefi Sekaja, personal communication 1994), and to treat a culture bound mental health syndrome known as *amafufenyana* (Watt & Breyer-Brandwijk 1962), to treat anxiety (Nyazema 1986), and to treat alcoholism (Philander 2011). There is a well-recognized dose-response and a narrow therapeutic index, with toxicity manifesting with acute psychosis, visual hallucinations, coma, and death (Laing, 1979, du Plooy 2001, Nyazma 1986, Watt & Breyer-Brandwijk 1962). Toxicity manifests with signs and symptoms similar to those of poisoning with *Datura* alkaloids, with initial excitation or sedation, frank psychosis, hallucinations, mydriasis, rapid pulse, raised blood pressure, raised temperature, and ultimately coma and death (Laing 1979, du Plooy 2001).

To date none of the key alkaloids of the plant have been studied on a wide range of central nervous system targets, including on neurotransmitter receptors and receptor subtypes, neurotransmitter transporters and enzymes that metabolize neurotransmitters and ion channels. In-vivo behavioral studies on extracts of the plant have demonstrated promising anxiolytic and antidepressant potential, supporting traditional uses (Pederson et al., 2008, Pote et al., 2014, Pote et al., 2018, and Xhakaza et al., 2022). There are no human clinical studies on extracts of leshoma. Preparations of leshoma have been administered orally, rectally, vaginally, topically, and by inhalation of smoke, but the actual doses of *Boophone* alkaloids useds in traditional preparations have not yet been quantified.

While it is clear that the plant needs thorough traditional training and considerable experience for correct preparation and careful dosing, the surprisingly large volumes of the plant sold annually in the informal traditional medicines trade, and the popularity of the plant on traditional medicine markets (Dold & Cocks 2002, Williams et al., 2020) suggest that the morbidity and mortality from toxic doses of the plant may not be as common as one would expect.

It should be appreciated that in rural southern Africa the traditional use of a psychoactive plant like leshoma to treat psychosis is only one part of the overall traditional management of the patient. For example, in the village of Sagole in Venda in the Limpopo Province of South Africa, when a psychotic patient was brought to the traditional healer by relatives, the patient would first be sedated by traditional herbal medicines, and then restrained to prevent self-harm and harm to others. As the patient's mental state improved they would be closely accompanied by two local men to prevent the patient from absconding, and to see to it that the patient begins to help with familiar daily tasks like collecting firewood and weeding crops. As the patient's mental state and behavior improved, they were invited to become part of the healers' household for a time, helping with the gradual re-integration to normal life, before he was finally allowed to return home. At the outset, the original cause of the psychosis was divined and given an explanation within the cultural paradigm, understandable and acceptable to the patient (Joseph Tshikovha, personal communication 1988). The use of leshoma was the entry point for the overall traditional management of the patient. The final part of the healing process would typically be a ceremony, usually with drumming, which served to announced to the local community, and to the patient, that the patient was now a fully healed person with no remaining stigma (Ncindani Maswanganyi, personal communication 1988).

Writing this overview of leshoma, I am conscious how my own relationship to plants has changed over the years. As a young doctor working in rural and township hospitals in South Africa thirty-five years ago, I found that many of my patients were consulting traditional healers in addition to using the public health system, and I endeavoured to learn as much as I could about African traditional medicine and the traditional *materia medica*. At the time, I was most interested in understanding the uses of medicinal plants from a purely biomedical perspective on the basis of the plant's chemistry and pharmacology. I hoped to one day develop an evidence-based botanical extract that could contribute to human health and well-being. I was eventually fortunate to realize this dream with a successfully researched and commercialized extract of kanna, *Sceletium tortuosum* (Gericke 2018). Now, as I enter my later years and draw closer to the realm of the ancestors, I find myself capable of transcending my rational scientific mind, embracing additional dimensions of the plant. In this state, leshoma transcends its identity as a subject of scientific enquiry, a psychoactive medicine, or even as a visionary sacrament. I have learned to try to contemplate the plant in the wild as a sacred presence connected to all Nature and to the realm of the ancestors, and to appreciate humankinds' place as inextricably part of Nature.

ACKNOWLEDGEMENTS

The authors of excellent reviews on *Boophane disticha* are thanked for their valuable publications that informed aspects of this paper and guided me to key primary literature (Neuwinger 1994, Nair & van Staden 2014, Pasquali 2021 and Samorini, accessed 5 November 2022). I am grateful to Bani Mayeng for many years of friendship, collaboration and discussions on African traditional medicine and medicinal plants. I am grateful to the late John Molefi Sekaja, Bani Mayeng's traditional mentor, for introducing me to the dosing and use of leshoma, and to David Matthe, the late Vusamazulu Credo Mutwa, and to Thaddeus Chedau for sharing information on traditional uses of leshoma. I am grateful to my first traditional mentor Ncindani Maswanganyi, for introducing me to Tsonga traditional medicine at Mbokota village, and to Joseph Tshikovha for introducing me to Venda approaches to managing mental health in the village of Sagole. Professor

Manuel Lopéz-Romero is thanked for kindly providing structural diagrams of *Boophone disticha* alkaloids.

BIBLIOGRAPHY

Alexander, J. E. 1838. Expedition of Discovery into the Interior of Africa, Henry Colburn, London.

Bertho, E., 2017. Reworkings of a Literary Myth and Historical Construction: Nehanda (Zimbabwe). In *Literary Location and Dislocation of Myth in the Post/Colonial Anglophone World*(pp. 103-119). Brill.

Binneman, J.N.F. 1999. Mummified human remains from the Kouga Mountains, Eastern Cape. *The Digging Stick* 16: 1-2.

Bleek & Lloyd Archive, 2022[a] http://lloydbleekcollection.cs.uct.ac.za/drawings/Iziko_SAMLB_!nBook4_019.html accessed 13 November 2022)

Bleek & Lloyd Archive, 2022[b]

http://lloydbleekcollection.cs.uct.ac.za/drawings/Iziko_SAMLB_!nBook4_019.html

accessed 13 November 2022.

De Rios, M.D., 1986. Enigma of drug-induced altered states of consciousness among the! Kung Bushmen of the Kalahari desert. *Journal of ethnopharmacology*, *15*(3), pp.297-304.

De Smet, P.A., 1996. Some ethnopharmacological notes on African hallucinogens. *Journal of Ethnopharmacology*, *50*(3), pp.141-146.

Dold, A.P. and Cocks, M.L., 2002. The trade in medicinal plants in the Eastern Cape Province, South Africa. *South African Journal of Science*, *98*(11), pp.589-597.

Dornan, S.S. 1916. Some notes on Rhodesian native poisons. S.A. Association for the Advances of Science, 356-361.

Du Plooy, W.J., Swart, L. and Van Huysteen, G.W., 2001. Poisoning with Boophane disticha: a forensic case. *Human & experimental toxicology*, *20*(5), pp.277-278.

Gadaga, L.L., Tagwireyi, D., Dzangare, J. and Nhachi, C.F., 2011. Acute oral toxicity and neurobehavioral toxicological effects of hydroethanolic extract of *Boophone disticha* in rats. *Human & experimental toxicology*, *30*(8), pp.972-980.

Ganga, T., Gadaga, L.L. and Tagwireyi, D., 2017. Neurobehavioral Toxicity Study of a Hydro-Ethanolic Extract of *Boophone disticha* in Sprague Dawley Rats. In Drug Discovery From Herbs: Approaches and Applications (pp. 277-290). Publisher: Daya Publishing House.

Gelfand, M. and Mitchel, C.S. 1952. Buphanine poisoning in man. *South African Medical Journal* 26, 573-4.

Gelfand, M., Mavi, S. Drummond, R.B., Ndemera, B. 1985. The Traditional Medical Practitioner in Zimbabwe. Mambo Press, Zimbabwe.

Gericke, N. Kabbo's !Kwaiń: The Past, Present and Possible Future of Kanna, in McKenna, D. et al., . (Eds.) 2018. The Ethnopharmacologic Search for Psychoactive Drugs. Synergetic Press, Santa Fe. ISBN-13: 978-0907791683

Gibson, D. 2018. Rethinking medicinal plants and plant medicines, *Anthropology Southern Africa*, 41:1, 1-14, DOI: 10.1080/23323256.2017.1415154

Hauth, H., Stauffacher, D., 1961. Die alkaloide von Buphane disticha (L.f.) Herb. *Helvetica Chimica Acta* 44, 491–502.

Juritz, C.F. 1914. South African plant poisons and their investigation. *South African Journal of Science* 11:109-145.

Laing, R.O., 1979. Three cases of poisoning by Boophane disticha. *Central African Journal of Medicine*, *25*(12), pp.265-266.

Landbouweekblad, 17 February 1995. Gifbol genees man se been.

Laydevant, F. 1932. Religious or sacred plants of Basotholand. *Bantu Studies* 6, 65-66.

Lichtenstein, H. 1812. Reisen im südlichen Afrika 1803-1806. Teil, Berlin.

Livingstone, D. 1857. Missionary travels and researches in South Africa. John Murray, London.

Matthe, D.S., 1988. Ethnomedical science and African medical practice. *Med. & L.*, 7, p.517.

Moeng, T.E., 2010. *An investigation into the trade of medicinal plants by muthi shops and street vendors in the Limpopo province, South Africa* (Doctoral dissertation, Department of Biodiversity School of Molecular and Life Sciences Faculty of Science and Agriculture, University of Limpopo).

Mutseura, M., Tagwireyi, D. and Gadaga, L.L., 2013. Pre-treatment of BALB/c mice with a centrally acting serotonin antagonist (cyproheptadine) reduces mortality from *Boophone disticha* poisoning. *Clinical Toxicology*, *51*(1), pp.16-22.

Nair, J.J. and Van Staden, J., 2014. Traditional usage, phytochemistry and pharmacology of the South African medicinal plant *Boophone disticha* (Lf) Herb.(Amaryllidaceae). *Journal of Ethnopharmacology*, *151*(1), pp.12-26.

Neergaard, J.S., Andersen, J., Pedersen, M.E., Stafford, G.I., Van Staden, J. and Jäger, A.K., 2009. Alkaloids from *Boophone disticha* with affinity to the serotonin transporter. *South African Journal of Botany*, *75*(2), pp.371-374.

Neuwinger, H.D. 1994. African Ethnobotany. Poisons and Drugs. Chapman and Hall, Weinheim.

Niehaus, D.J.H., Oosthuizen, P., Lochner, C., Emsley, R.A., Jordaan, E., Mbanga, N.I., Keyter, N., Laurent, C., Deleuze, J.F. and Stein, D.J., 2004. A culture-bound syndrome 'amafufunyana' and a culture-specific event 'ukuthwasa': differentiated by a family history of schizophrenia and other psychiatric disorders. *Psychopathology*, *37*(2), 59-63.

Nyazema, N.Z., 1986. Herbal toxicity in Zimbabwe. *Transactions of the Royal Society of Tropical Medicine and Hygiene*, *80*(3), 448-450.

Pasquali, L., 2021. Leshoma, the visionary plant of southern Africa. *Antrocom: Online Journal of Anthropology*, *17*(1), 5-20.

Paterson, W. 1789. A Narrative of Four Journeys into the Country of the Hottentots And Caffraria. J. Johnson, London.

Pedersen, M.E., Szewczyk, B., Stachowicz, K., Wieronska, J., Andersen, J., Stafford, G.I., van Staden, J., Pilc, A. and Jäger, A.K., 2008. Effects of South African traditional medicine in animal models for depression. *Journal of Ethnopharmacology*, *119*(3), pp.542-548.

Philander, L.A., 2011. An ethnobotany of Western Cape Rasta bush medicine. *Journal of ethnopharmacology*, *138*(2), pp.578-594.

Plants of the World Online (POWO), Royal Botanic Gardens, Kew. https://powo.science.kew.org/taxon/60455694-2 accessed 1st November 2022.

Pote, W., Tagwireyi, D., Chinyanga, H.M., Musara, C., Pfukenyi, D.M., Nkomozepi, P., Gadaga, L.L., Nyandoro, G. and Chifamba, J., 2014. Long-term cardiovascular autonomic responses to aqueous ethanolic extract of *Boophone disticha* bulb in early maternally separated BALB/c mice. *South African Journal of Botany*, *94*, pp.33-39.

Pote, W., Musarira, S., Chuma, D., Gadaga, L.L., Mwandiringana, E. and Tagwireyi, D., 2018. Effects of a hydroethanolic extract of *Boophone disticha* bulb on anxiety-related behavior in naive BALB/c mice. *Journal of Ethnopharmacology*, *214*, pp.218-224.

Samorini, G. Il leshoma de Sud Africa. Leshoma, the visionary plant of Africa. https://samorini.it/antropologia/africa/leshoma-pianta-visionaria-sud-africa/ accessed 5 November 2022

Sandager, M., Nielsen, N.D., Stafford, G.I., Van Staden, J., Jäger, A.K., 2005. Alkaloids from *Boophane distica* with affinity to the serotonin transporter in rat brain. Journal of Ethnopharmacology 98, 367–370.

Schultes, R.E. 1970. *Bull. Narcotics*, 22 (1): 25-53.

Schultes, R. E. & Hofmann, A. 1979. Plants of the gods: origins of hallucinogenic use. Hutchinson, London.

Sibanyoni, M.N., Chaudhary, S.K., Chen, W., Adhami, H.R., Combrinck, S., Maharaj, V., Schuster, D. and Viljoen, A., 2020. Isolation, in vitro evaluation and molecular docking of acetylcholinesterase inhibitors from South African Amaryllidaceae. *Fitoterapia*, *146*, p.104650.

Smith, C.A. 1966. Common Names of South African Plants. Botanical Survey Memoir No. 35. Government Printer, Pretoria.

Sobiecki, J.F. 2008. A review of plants used in divination in southern Africa and their psychoactive effects. *Southern African Humanities* 20(1): 333-351.

Steyn, M., Binneman, J. and Loots, M., 2007. The Kouga mummified human remains. *South African Archaeological Bulletin*, *62*(185), pp.3-8.

Thornton, R. 2017. *Healing the Exposed Being: The Ngoma healing tradition in South Africa*. Wits University Press, Johannesburg.

van Rensburg, E., Zietsman, P.C., Bonnet, S.L. and Wilhelm, A., 2017. Alkaloids from the Bulbs of *Boophone disticha*. *Natural Product Communications*, *12*(9): 1431-1433.

Watt, J.M. 1967. African plants potentially useful in mental health. *Lloydia* 30:1-22.

Watt, J.M & Breyer-Brandwijk, M.G. 1962. The Medicinal and Poisonous Plants of Southern and Eastern Africa. 2nd edition. E & S Livingstone, Edinburgh and London.

Welcome, A.K. and Van Wyk, B.E., 2019. An inventory and analysis of the food plants of southern Africa. *South African Journal of Botany*, *122*, pp.136-179.

Wellman, C. 1907. *Über Pfeilgifte in Westafrika und besonders eine Käferlarva als Pfeilgift in Angola. Dtsche. Ent. Zeitschrift*, 17.

Williams, V.L., Raimondo, D., Brueton, V.J., Crouch, N.R., Cunningham, A.B., Scott-Shaw, C.R., Lötter, M. & Ngwenya, A.M. 2016. *Boophone disticha* (L.f.) Herb. National Assessment: Red List of South African Plants version 2020.1. Accessed on 2022/11/03

Xhakaza NK, Nkomozepi P, Mbajiorgu EF. *Boophone disticha* attenuates five day repeated forced swim-induced stress and adult hippocampal neurogenesis impairment in male Balb/c mice. Anat Cell Biol. 2022 Oct 21. doi: 10.5115/acb.22.120. Epub ahead of print. PMID: 36267006.

The Ayahuasca Survey Project

Barrett McBride, MSc

Ethnobotanist | Phytochemist

> *"The aim of our project is to understand how the ayahuasca plants Psychotria viridis and Banisteriopsis caapi have evolved across time and place."* —Barrett McBride

A PhD proposal by Barrett McBride in collaboration with University of Reading Biological Sciences and the McKenna Academy of Natural Philosophy.

INTRODUCTION AND BACKGROUND

Recent years have seen the global expansion of ayahuasca. The Amazonian ethnomedicine has spread both in and outside of its traditional setting. The popularity has further surged as recent studies have shown the hallucinogenic brew to be beneficial in the treatment of a range of mental health issues. This trend has the potential to be of great benefit to the collective human condition (Domínguez-Clavé et al., 2016; Coe and McKenna, 2017). However, popularization and commercialization of a medicinal plant can have a substantial impact on the species, its ecosystem and the cultures that carry their knowledge. Two of the greatest challenges that plants with rapidly growing medicinal use face are pressure on harvest volume and the potential for adulteration or substitution of the material itself (WHO, 2005).

AIMS AND OBJECTIVES

With the above in mind, the question that frames our project is— what can be done to help preserve the cultural knowledge and biodiversity of ayahuasca? From our perspective the answer starts with a study to document ayahuasca as it currently is today.

Therefore, the primary aim of this proposed project is to conduct an ethnobotanical and phytochemical survey of ayahuasca brews and to document ayahuasca in its current state. The project will consider if an increased demand for the brew is affecting its composition and quality. It will examine if demand affects use-pressure of the admixture plants, their availability and selection. It will also consider what effect future widespread pharmacological applications might add to the plants.

The project's main objective is to analyze a set of collected ayahuasca samples in order to document their various preparations and admixture plants. The project will seek to authenticate their known ingredients and to better understand their chemical composition and quality. Part of the purpose of this project is to understand the chemical variation found in different ayahuasca preparations and how their ingredients differ. This project aims to unravel some of the mysteries surrounding what admixture plants are used and what the final product's chemical fingerprint looks like after collection, storage and brewing of the plant materials.

RESEARCH QUESTIONS

In short, the present study will investigate what kind of botanical variation exists in ayahuasca preparations and amongst the plant species themselves. Specifically, the project will ask:

- What plant species are in ayahuasca?
- How were they sourced and prepared?
- What is the chemical result?
- Are there unique pharmacological implications to different brews?

ETHICS

In general, this project approaches the scientific study of ayahuasca with the goals of bettering the well-being of humanity and to inform contemporary medicine. With this in mind, we also want to approach it in such a way that betters the plants and the communities that hold them.

At this stage we have assembled principles to guide our ethics process and are prepared to use our resources to follow them.

Principles:

- Maintain ongoing conversations with the communities in which we work
- Work towards the goals and desired outcomes of participating communities
- As outlined by Chacruna's Indigenous Reciprocity Initiative, we will seek to preserve "plant medicines in the environments and communities where they originate" (Mays, 2022)
- Ensure any published data exists in a way that protects cultural information
- Reciprocity through benefit and knowledge sharing

LITERATURE

The following table shows an overview of previous studies that have conducted ethnobotanical surveys of ayahuasca and Yagé. **Figure 1** shows what types of source plants and brews were collected and what analytic techniques were used.

While these studies represent an enormous foundation of both field and lab work, we think there is an opportunity in the present study to update and expand the knowledge of the ever-evolving ayahuasca brew. It is interesting to note that the majority of studies investigated plant specimens and very few to date have investigated the actual brews. In addition to increasing scale, we believe our study will be the first of its kind to use DNA metabarcoding along with the other classic investigation techniques to investigate samples of ayahuasca at all stages: plants, brews and bricks.

STUDY DETAILS				SAMPLES ANALYZED			METHODS		
DATE	AUTHOR	TITLE	LOCATION	PLANTS	BREWS	Preparation	ETHNOGRAPHY	PHYTOCHEMICAL	DNA
2020	Santos	*Biodiversity of β-Carboline Profile of Banisteriopsis caapi and Ayahuasca, a Plant and a Brew with Neuropharmacological Potential.*	Brazil	176 lianas total 159 of B. caapi and 17 others	33	Traditional	Yes	LC-MS/MS	-
2019	Souza	*Validation of an analytical method for the determination of the main ayahuasca active compounds and application to real ayahuasca samples from Brazil*	São Paulo (State), Brazil	-	38	Traditional	-	LC-MS/MS	-
2010	Wang	*Composition, standardization and chemical profiling of Banisteriopsis caapi, a plant for the treatment of neurodegenerative disorders relevant to Parkinson's disease. Journal of Ethnopharmacology*	Hawaii (Cultivars)	6 B. caapi	0	Lab	-	HPLC	-
2009	Mcilhenny	*Direct analysis of psychoactive tryptamine and harmala alkaloids in the Amazonian botanical medicine ayahuasca by liquid chromatography-electrospray ionization-tandem mass spectrometry*	Hawaii (Cultivars)	-	6	Lab	-	LC-ESI-MS/MS	-
2005	Callaway	*Phytochemical analyses of Banisteriopsis caapi and Psychotria viridis*	Brazil	-	29	Traditional	Yes	HPLC	-
1984	McKenna	*Monoamine oxidase inhibitors in South American hallucinogenic plants: Tryptamine and β-carboline constituents of Ayahuasca,*	Peru- Iquitos, Pucallpa and Tarapoto.	6 B. caapi 4 Psychotria 1 Diplopterys 4 other admixture	8	Traditional	Yes	TLC, HPLC, GC/MS	-
1977	Shultes	*DE PLANTIS TOXICARIIS E MUNDO NOVO TROPICALE COMMENTATIONES III: PHYTOCHEMICAL EXAMINATION OF SPRUCE'S ORIGINAL COLLECTION OF BANISTERIOPSIS CAAPI*	Rio Uaupés Brazil	material from voucher specimen "Stems of Banisteria sp. used with the roots and leaves [120] of	-	-	Yes	GC/MS	-
1972	Rivier & Lindgren	*"Ayahuasca," the South American hallucinogenic drink: An ethnobotanical and chemical investigation*	River Purús Peru	17 B caapi 7 Psychotria spp	various	Traditional	Yes	GCMS	-

Fig.1 Previous studies that have conducted ethnobotanical surveys of ayahuasca.
Santos et al. 2020; Souza et al., 2019; Wang et al., 2010; McIlhenny et al., 2009; Callaway, Brito, and Neves 2005; McKenna, Towers, and Abbott 1984; Rivier and Lindgren 1972; Richard Evans, Holmstedt, and Lindgren 1969

METHODS AND PROCESS

By using DNA barcoding and phytochemical techniques, we hope to better understand the current composition and chemistry of ayahuasca. As previously mentioned, this study is a survey to collect and document samples from the field. The primary fieldwork location is Peru, specifically the areas around Pucallpa and Iquitos. However, we would also like to collect samples from other locations, with the goal to learn more about how the composition of ayahuasca and Yagé might have changed as they have spread cross-culturally. The goal is to collect a variety of samples from different traditional and neo-shamanic sources, with the target number of collections being 100. Samples are defined as source plants, brews and condensed brews, also known as bricks.

The study will identify plants visually and prepare voucher specimens to deposit in the Herbarium Amazonense at the Universidad Nacional de Amazonica Peruana (UNAP) in Iquitos. Where possible the study will also deposit living cuttings at a UNAP facility or another local site.

After documenting the collected samples, we will begin the analysis portion, which takes two forms: DNA metabarcoding and chromatography.

First, DNA metabarcoding will be used to identify the list of plant materials in our brew samples as well as identify the species of collected plant specimens. It is our goal to use DNA metabarcoding to look for the presence of specific DNA in a complex mixture. In this way the project aims to produce lists of plant materials from the brews, and to potentially understand if there are different varieties of *Banisteriopsis caapi*, *Psychotria viridis* or other admixture plants being used.

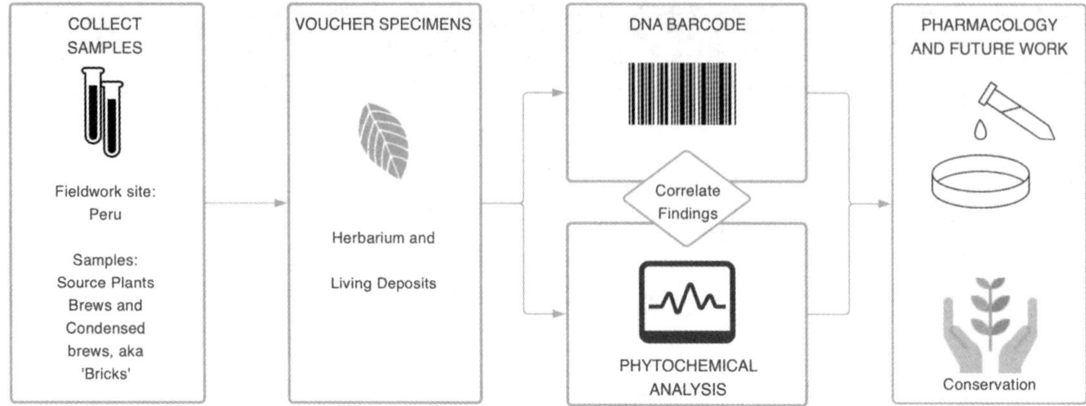

Fig.2 Flow diagram of methods and process.

Proposed DNA Metabarcoding Process:

1. Isolate DNA from the matrix (brewed ayahuasca)
2. Prepare DNA metabarcoding libraries for the target taxonomic groups of plants. (We will construct this library at the outset by sequencing vouchered plants)
3. Sequence the DNA metabarcoding libraries
4. Analyze the data from step 3 to obtain the taxonomic composition of the samples.

It is important to note that we acknowledge the potential limits of attempting to sequence DNA from complex mixtures that have been exposed to high temperatures (boiled) and thus potentially containing a degraded quality of DNA. In the case that we are unable to sequence DNA from the mixtures (brews), we will use the same technique to identify the species of the collected plant specimens prior to preparation.

In addition, chromatography techniques such as HPLC or LC-MS will be used to identify what active compounds our samples contain and in what concentrations. This process can be used on all sample types including plants, bricks and brews and is not sensitive to thermally degraded samples.

SUPPORTING WORK

Two examples from the literature demonstrate how DNA metabarcoding and chromatography can be used in our proposed study.

In 2021, a team from the University of Milan used metabarcoding to identify lists of plant ingredients in herbal tea samples. Using this method, the authors were able to determine the relative abundances of the varying species in each sample tested. The output of this was a published list of detected ingredients, or plant species, they found in each tea (Frigerio et al, 2021).

With regards to phytochemistry, a team of researchers in Brazil used Chromatography–Electrospray Ionization-Tandem Mass Spectrometry (LC-MS/MS) to identify chemical compounds and concentrations in the samples of collected ayahuasca brews. Their project used chromatography techniques to produce chemical fingerprints of both brews and their source plants. With this process the authors were able to produce lists of alkaloids and their associated concentrations found in each sample (Santos et al, 2020).

OUTCOMES

It is our hope that this project will help shed light on the age-old questions surrounding the identity of the admixture plants of ayahuasca. The project could potentially reveal new botanical information regarding the varieties of ayahuasca vine that can be readily identified by some indigenous people yet not by western botanical methods (Schultes, 1986; Sheldrake, 2020).

A specific outcome of this project is to create a database of brew samples with lists of ingredients and associated alkaloids. The goal is that this data could be used in future research, especially if ethnobotanical data, such as cultivation, harvest and production practices are documented with each sample. As noted in the ethics section, we want to ensure our data exists in a way that protects cultural information. As such, any sensitive published data entries would have anonymous identifiers and location data redacted to protect local knowledge.

In regards to ayahuasca in contemporary medicine, we are planning pharmacology work at the University of Reading to investigate if laboratory evidence can be established for the reported therapeutic effects of the brews and if any behavioral correlations can be seen between the brews prepared by different healers. In short, we intend to investigate if different brews have different therapeutic effects and could thus potentially imply unique applications in contemporary medicine.

CONCLUSION

We believe our findings will have the potential to yield higher taxonomic resolution of the admixture plants and produce data that serves as a platform to inform future work in medicine, preservation of biocultural knowledge, biodiversity and highlight any potential threats to individual species. Our intention is that this study will be a contribution to the body of existing scientific knowledge and one that is done respectfully and in conversation with local communities and the plants themselves.

BIBLIOGRAPHY

Callaway, J C, Glacus S Brito, and Edison S Neves. 2005. "Phytochemical Analyses of Banisteriopsis Caapi and *Psychotria Viridis*." *Journal of Psychoactive Drugs* 37 (2): 145–50. https://doi.org/10.1080/02791072.2005.10399795.

Coe, Michael A., and Dennis J. McKenna. 2017. "The Therapeutic Potential of Ayahuasca." In *Evidence-Based Herbal and Nutritional Treatments for Anxiety in Psychiatric Disorders*, edited by David Camfield, Erica McIntyre, and Jerome Sarris, 123–37. Cham: Springer International Publishing. https://doi.org/10.1007/978-3-319-42307-4_7.

Domínguez-Clavé, Elisabet, Joaquim Soler, Matilde Elices, Juan C Pascual, Enrique Álvarez, Mario de la Fuente Revenga, Pablo Friedlander, Amanda Feilding, and Jordi Riba. 2016. "Ayahuasca: Pharmacology, Neuroscience and Therapeutic Potential." *Brain Research Bulletin* 126 (Pt 1): 89–101. https://doi.org/10.1016/j.brainresbull.2016.03.002.

Frigerio, Jessica, Giulia Agostinetto, Valerio Mezzasalma, Fabrizio De Mattia, Massimo Labra, and Antonia Bruno.

2021. "DNA-Based Herbal Teas' Authentication: An ITS2 and PsbA-TrnH Multi-Marker DNA Metabarcoding Approach." *Plants* 10 (10). https://doi.org/10.3390/plants10102120.

Mays, Joseph. 2022. "Indigenous Reciprocity Initiative of the Americas: A Respectful Path Forward for the Psychedelic Movement—Chacruna." Indigenous Reciprocity Initiative of the Americas: A Respectful Path Forward for the Psychedelic Movement. April 28, 2022. https://chacruna.net/psychedelics_indigenous_reciprocity/.

McIlhenny, Ethan H, Kelly E Pipkin, Leanna J Standish, Hope A Wechkin, Rick Strassman, and Steven A Barker. 2009. "Direct Analysis of Psychoactive Tryptamine and Harmala Alkaloids in the Amazonian Botanical Medicine Ayahuasca by Liquid Chromatography-Electrospray Ionization-Tandem Mass Spectrometry." *Journal of Chromatography. A* 1216 (51): 8960–68. https://doi.org/10.1016/j.chroma.2009.10.088.

McKenna, D J, G H Towers, and F Abbott. 1984. "Monoamine Oxidase Inhibitors in South American Hallucinogenic Plants: Tryptamine and Beta-Carboline Constituents of Ayahuasca." *Journal of Ethnopharmacology* 10 (2): 195–223.

Richard Evans, Schultes, Bo Holmstedt, and Jan-Erik Lindgren. 1969. "De Plantis Toxicariis e Mundo Novo Tropicale Commentationes Iii: Phytochemical Examination of Spruce's Original Collection of *Banisteriopsis Caapi*." *Botanical Museum Leaflets, Harvard University* Botanical Museum Leaflets, Harvard University (22, 4): 121–32.

Rivier, Laurent, and Jan-Erik Lindgren. 1972. "'Ayahuasca,' the South American Hallucinogenic Drink: An Ethnobotanical and Chemical Investigation." *Economic Botany* 26 (2): 101–29. https://doi.org/10.1007/BF02860772.

Santos, Beatriz Werneck Lopes, Regina Célia de Oliveira, Julia Sonsin-Oliveira, Christopher William Fagg, José Beethoven Figueiredo Barbosa, and Eloisa Dutra Caldas. 2020. "Biodiversity of β-Carboline Profile of *Banisteriopsis Caapi* and Ayahuasca, a Plant and a Brew with Neuropharmacological Potential." *Plants* 9 (7). https://doi.org/10.3390/plants9070870.

Schultes, Richard Evans. 1986. "RECOGNITION OF VARIABILITY IN WILD PLANTS BY INDIANS OF THE NORTHWEST AMAZON: AN ENIGMA." *Environmental Science*, January.

Sheldrake, Merlin. 2020. "The 'enigma' of Richard Schultes, Amazonian Hallucinogenic Plants, and the Limits of Ethnobotany." *Social Studies of Science* 50 (3): 345–76. https://doi.org/10.1177/0306312720920362.

Souza, Rita C Z, Flávia S Zandonadi, Donizete P Freitas, Luís F F Tófoli, and Alessandra Sussulini. 2019. "Validation of an Analytical Method for the Determination of the Main Ayahuasca Active Compounds and Application to Real Ayahuasca Samples from Brazil." *Journal of Chromatography. B, Analytical Technologies in the Biomedical and Life Sciences* 1124 (August): 197–203. https://doi.org/10.1016/j.jchromb.2019.06.014.

Wang, Yan-Hong, Volodymyr Samoylenko, Babu L Tekwani, Ikhlas A Khan, Loren S Miller, Narayan D Chaurasiya, Md Mostafizur Rahman, et al. 2010. "Composition, Standardization and Chemical Profiling of *Banisteriopsis Caapi*, a Plant for the Treatment of Neurodegenerative Disorders Relevant to Parkinson's Disease." *Journal of Ethnopharmacology* 128 (3): 662–71. https://doi.org/10.1016/j.jep.2010.02.013.

WHO. 2005. "National Policy on Traditional Medicine and Regulation of Herbal Medicines: Report of a WHO Global Survey." *World Health Organization, Geneva, Switzerland.*

Toward a Road Map for Sustainable Ayahuasca Production Using Integral Projection Models

Michael A. Coe, PhD, and Orou G. Gaoue, PhD

Assistant Professor Tarleton State University | Ethnobiologist | Applied Ecologist

Associate Professor University of Tennessee | Ethnobiologist | Applied Ecologist

> *"We must not let this precious opportunity to learn how to respectfully manage ayahuasca production slip through our fingertips for there is much at stake beyond the revenue streams of commercialization, subsistence, and local livelihoods. We must honor the wisdom of the ages and learn from the symbiotic relationships of the natural world to ensure that the diversity of ways of being and ways of knowing inspired by the interconnection between the human experience and ayahuasca teacher plants remain and continue their dialog in reverence. Therefore, it is critical that we develop a deeper understanding of the ecology and demography of these plants and how they respond to increasing harvest pressures and environmental variablility over time."* —MICHAEL COE

Ayahuasca sustainability is of pivotal importance, however sadly it is under threat. This article shares a methodology for the protection and sustainable harvest of Banisteriopsis caapi (Spruce ex. Griseb.) C.V. Morton.

INTRODUCTION

One of the greatest advantages and challenges of ethnobiological research is the diversity of methods available to better understand the interactions between human societies and the natural world (Gaoue et al., 2021, 2017; Hoffman and Gallaher, 2007; Hurrell and Albuquerque, 2012; Albuquerque et al., 2014). Legendary ethnobiologist, explorer and Harvard Professor, Richard Evans Schultes (1915-2001) is known widely for his pioneering methodological work based on his incredible journeys in the Northwest Amazon where he documented the use of sacred plant medicines among Indigenous Amazonian peoples like the Kofàn, Makuna, Kamsá, Yukuna, Ingano and Witoto (Davis 1996, 2004). In following in the footsteps of his childhood hero Richard Spruce, while traveling approximately half-million square miles across Northwest Amazon from Bogota to the Sibundoy Valley, the cloud-soaked forests of the Andes and the sacred headwaters of the Putumayo River, Schultes' methodological accomplishments were both remarkable and captivating (Davis 1996, 2004). Beyond the insurmountable botanical collections of medicinal plants he made (many of which are single-handedly responsible for advancing our scientific understanding of the biological diversity in the Amazon that has long been useful to Indigenous peoples for subsistence, healing, divination, and connecting with the ancestors), Schultes was arguably the first ethnobiologist who used *participant observation*, a method now commonly employed to gain a glimpse into the emic perspective or worldview of particular culture and their relationship with plants (Davis 1996, 2004; Albuquerque et al. 2014; Alexiades and Sheldon 1996). In using this methodology, Schultes lived with Indigenous Amazonian communities, tasted the bitter leaves of plants they used for healing, and participated in daily subsistence activities which allowed him to develop an in-depth understanding of their unique and diverse of ways of being, ways of knowing and relating to the natural world that were far different from his own (Davis 1996, 2004). Beyond this, Schultes's work contributed to accelerating the development of *utilitarian ethnobotany*, a sub-discipline of ethnobiology that gained momentum during the first half of the 20th century and since then has primarily focused on documenting medicinal plants and their uses with practical implications for drug discovery (Albuquerque et al. 2017). Much of Schultes' work, which he articulated in more than 400 publications throughout his lifetime, provides a glimpse into the remnants of an ancestral past of plant use among the Indigenous peoples of the Northwest Amazon that lay in the wake of the Spanish conquest.

EVOLUTION OF A DISCIPLINE

Since Schultes's foundational contributions to contemporary ethnobiological research, ethnobiology has continued to evolve to include numerous sub-disciplines each with their own methodological approaches to investigate the interactions between people, organisms, and culture (Alexiades and Sheldon 1996; Albuquerque et al. 2017). Because of the interdisciplinary nature of ethnobiology, most contemporary ethnobiologists to date are either trained biologists who are comfortable conducting interviews and asking questions about plants, animals, or environmental use; or they are trained anthropologists who are interested in learning about, identifying and cataloging plant or animal species. As such, contemporary ethnobiologists often have expertise or backgrounds in other disciplines such as anthropology, botany, archaeology, pharmacology, sociology, linguistics and other related fields (Alexiades and Sheldon 1996; Gaoue et al. 2021). Given such a multifaceted set of backgrounds consistent with the diverse methodological culture of the discipline, ethnobiologists today have been exposed to a variety of analytical methods of inquiry that combine the intuitions, skills, methods and biases of researchers from all of these areas (Gaoue et al. 2021, 2017; Albuquerque et al. 2014). Because of this sheer methodological complexity, academics have criticized ethnobiology or its sub-discipline ethnobotany for lacking consistent methodological rigor (Alexiades and Sheldon 1996; Gaoue et al. 2017; Albuquerque and Hanazaki 2009; Phillips and Gentry 1993). While this may be considered a challenge as the discipline continues to evolve, it is hardly a limitation and will indeed prove to be the contrary.

Diverse methodologies are becoming necessary to understand the complexity surrounding the drivers of some of the world's current cultural and ecological crises (Vandebroek et al. 2020; Gaoue et al. 2017; Fernández-llamazares et al. 2022; Berkes, Colding, and Folke 2000). Thus, it is essential to consider how ethnobiologists, including those with expertise in ethnobiology's sister-disciplines (e.g. anthropology, botany, ecology, archaeology, pharmacology, sociology, linguistics, etc.), might use their range of expertise collectively using advanced methods spanning across disciplines as an advantage to ensure that the solutions to various traditional and emerging environmental crises are culturally appropriate while aligning with the needs of Indigenous peoples and local communities (Fernández-llamazares et al. 2022). This is critically important now more than ever, especially given the numerous compounding threats to the biological, linguistic and cultural diversity of the planet (Maffi 2005, 2002; Pretty et al. 2009; Fernández-llamazares et al. 2022; Gorenflo et al. 2012). Therefore, it is likely that providing practical solutions to address environmental and cultural challenges that currently threaten the stability of social and ecological systems are going to require creative and collaborative efforts that transcend the boundaries of academic disciplines, individuality, colonial epistemologies embedded within research, social inequalities and notions of academic superiority. Perhaps in this context, ethnobiology as a discipline of diverse methodologies, can provide an essential platform to highlight a range of expertise and essential skill sets that hold the keys to developing a sustainable future and collaborative partnerships aimed at providing creative solutions to address current ecological and cultural conservation challenges.

THE SUSTAINABILITY OF AYAHUASCA USE OVER TIME

The plight of local and Indigenous peoples of the Amazon Basin includes the devastating forces that pose compounding threats to the biological and cultural webs of life that are responsible for the persistence of much of the chemical, linguistic, cultural, and biological diversity of the planet. It is undeniable and warrants considerable conservation efforts; however a current biocultural conservation challenge and sustainability concern of the Amazon Basin that has yet to thoroughly captivate widespread attention, and urgently needs collaborative efforts to address, is the potential overexploitation of ayahuasca. Specifically, its source plants *Banisteriopsis caapi* (Spruce ex. Griseb.) C.V. Morton, *Psychotria viridis* Ruiz & Pav. and *Diplopterys cabrerana* (Cuatrec.) B. Gates (yagé). The effects of the increased harvest pressures of ayahuasca source plants have only begun to be realized in the Amazon Basin. *B. caapi* shortages have been reported in and around major cities like Pucallpa and Iquitos where ayahuasca production has grown exponentially over the last decade to provide the brew for the estimated 100-200 centers in these areas and for the exportation of the concentrated brew to various ayahuasca communities and practitioners around the world (Coe and Gaoue 2023, unpublished data). Conservative estimates indicate that approximately five and a half million servings of ayahuasca were consumed by nearly 820,000 people worldwide in 2019 (Suárez Álvarez & Mazarrasa, 2023). To date, it is unclear exactly how many ayahuasca source plants remain in the wild and we can only estimate how many tons of biomass from these plants are harvested annually to meet exponentially growing supply and demand chains. Although there have been considerable efforts towards sustainability where growers and harvesters, syncretic religions like the União do Vegetal and Santo Daime, and various stakeholders continue to plant more ayahuasca source plants in and around the Amazon Basin and in other parts of the world (see for example Thevenin and Sambuichi 2020; Tupper 2009), it is unclear whether or not these efforts will be enough to provide ayahuasca for the foreseeable future. While increased harvest pressure and intensity does not always result in a decline of culturally important plants such as *B. caapi*, *P. viridis*, or *D. cabrerana* over time (Ticktin

2004; Schmidt, Figueiredo, and Ticktin 2015; Sampaio and Santos 2015), as these plants become increasingly exploited while the ayahuasca brew continues to be commercialized, it is critical to take the necessary steps to evaluate sustainability concerns (Tupper 2009). This brings us to ask, "what is known about ayahuasca sustainability and the effect of increased harvest pressures on ayahuasca source plants?" This set of questions go beyond the unique case of ayahuasca source plants and are important to consider for species that are harvested for non-timber forest products in general, most of which are the basis of local livelihoods and international trade. Answering these questions require methodological tools that are beyond what is commonly used in ethnobiology and this is consistent with the interdisciplinary nature of the discipline.

ADDRESSING KNOWLEDGE GAPS

It is clear there has been much focus and time spent by social and natural scientists studying ayahuasca from both the pharmacological and sociocultural perspectives. Incredible advancements have been made in understanding the brew's chemistry and pharmacology. To date, there is considerable evidence to suggest that ayahuasca consumption can enhance creativity, reduce anxiety, exhibit anti-depressant and anti-addictive effects, improve psychological well-being, quality of life, enhance cognition and more recently there is evidence to suggest that alkaloids present in ayahuasca facilitate the formation of new neurons which indicates that ayahuasca acts at multiple levels of neural complexity (McKenna 2004; Grob et al. 1996; Kuypers et al. 2016; de Osório et al. 2015; Morales-García et al. 2017). All of which point to the great therapeutic potential of ayahuasca in contemporary medicine. It is also undeniable that the use of ayahuasca is deeply-rooted in social organization and world views of numerous cultural communities throughout the Amazon Basin where many lineages of *vegetalistas*, *maestros*, *médicos*, *paies*, *taitas* and other religious and shamanic practitioners are experts in navigating the inner domains of consciousness, the inner paths to outer space, or the realms of the spirits and ancestors invoked by the ayahuasca-induced visionary experience (Luna 1984b; Luna and White 2017; Reichel-Dolmatoff 1971; Narby and Chanchari Pizuri 2021; Brabec de Mori 2012a). While substantial research has led to a greater understanding of ayahuasca's therapeutic potential, traditional applications in ethnomedicine, its cultural importance and array uses among Amerindian societies and syncretic religious organizations, there remains significant knowledge gaps on how ayahuasca responds to harvest from an ecological perspective. Further, collaborative partnerships involving synergistic efforts worldwide— a global ayahuasca project— focused on sustainability so that ayahuasca will remain for future generations, has yet to be developed and are likely needed. Therefore, it is essential to develop a mechanistic understanding of how ayahuasca source plants respond to increasing harvest pressures and environmental variability over time by gaining a deeper understanding of the ecology and demography of these plants. This is a necessary step towards sustainable ayahuasca production. In addition, it is essential to study, thoroughly understand and value local and Indigenous people's knowledge of their environment and how they are actively managing ayahuasca source plants. This greater understanding along with collaborative efforts are essential for developing creative and practical solutions for sustainability. Fortunately, the opportunity to embrace the contribution that interdisciplinary methods of ethnobiology can make in this context may prove invaluable in developing methodological approaches towards sustainable ayahuasca production.

ASSESSING THE SUSTAINABILITY OF AYAHUASCA

To facilitate an in-depth understanding on how ayahuasca lianas [*Banisteriopsis caapi* (Spruce ex. Griseb.) C. V. Morton] respond to varying harvest intensities and provide a means to assess sustainability concerns, here we introduce integral projection models (IPMs) in ethnobiological contexts. IPMs are a more contemporary quantitative method for ethnobiology and its sub-discipline ethnoecology that holds the keys to understanding how we can develop a sustainable future for ayahuasca production. By definition, IPMs are time-discrete population models that have been developed in population ecology over the last several decades and gained momentum for their use to project the population dynamics of a given species in response to various anthropogenic and environmental factors (e.g. climate change and harvesting intensities) (Easterling, Ellner, and Dixon 2000; Rees and Ellner 2009; Ellner and Rees 2006). In this context, IPMs describe how a given population structured by an individual-state variable or continuous trait (e.g. size) changes in discrete time. They do so by allowing the characterization of the complete life cycle of an organism as a function of size. This is one of the advantages of IPMs compared to other population models because IPMs avoid any biological assumptions linked to artificial or synthetic division of life stages across the life history of a given species (Ellner and Rees 2006; Easterling, Ellner, and Dixon 2000).

In this paper we highlight the application IPMs, an interdisciplinary method in ethnobiology that has proven useful in developing a preliminary understanding of how several *B. caapi* populations may be doing ecologically from a conservation standpoint. Although, we primarily focus on *B. caapi* for this study, this same methodology can be applied to understand the population dynamics of other *teacher plants* (e.g. *P. viridis* , *D. cabrerana)* and shamanic medicines (e.g. *L. williamsii, T. macrogonus var. pachanoi*) in response to harvest. In this context, an IPM is a powerful tool because it can be used to quantify measures of fitness of individual ayahuasca vines over their life history and make robust predictions on population-level patterns which can provide a mechanistic understanding how a given population of ayahuasca lianas respond to increased harvest pressures over time. Additionally, we also provide a preliminary contextual framework for the sustainable development of ayahuasca involving relevant stakeholders within four key domains including ecological, cultural, social, and economic to serve as a catalyst for future research, discussion and collaborations among stakeholders.

METHODS

To encourage a deeper understanding of IPMs and to facilitate reproducible science in ethnobiology, we first break it down into several functions mathematically while highlighting some of the basic statistics used to build them. We also provide examples of data collection and analyses from the first known demographic study on ayahuasca to help to facilitate a practical application of IPMs and additional computational tools (e.g. elasticity analyses, LTRE, etc.) in ethnobiological contexts (see Coe and Gaoue 2023).

In examining the IPM mathematically, this integral equation is composed of several size-dependent functions as follows:

$$n(y, t+1) = \int_{\Omega} K(y, x) n(x, t) dx \qquad \text{equation 1}$$

The left side of the equation (eqn 1), is the expected population state, $n(y, t+1)$, where n is the number of individuals in a given plant population, y is their size at $t+1$, a given time interval in the future. On the right hand side of the equation, there is the core of the IPM, $K(y,x)$, known as the *Kernel*. The Kernel is composed of several size-dependent functions that describe how the current size of an individual at an initial time dictates its size and that of its offspring at some future time. In other words, the kernel describes how the current size distribution of individuals in a population changes over one time step. To project the expected population state at some time in the future (left side of the equation), the Kernel is multiplied by the *current population state* $n(x, t)$ where n is the number of individuals of a given size x at time t. Because the operation of integration (right-hand side of equation) here is linear, the current population state at the initial time t can be iterated to give the expected population state at subsequent times in the future (over several years) (Ellner and Rees 2006; Easterling, Ellner, and Dixon 2000). This characteristic equation can be broken down further (eqn 2) for clarity where the kernel is composed of the survival-growth function and the fertility function:

$$n(y, t+1) = \int_{\Omega} [p(y, x) + f(x,y) + c(y, x)] n(x, t) dx \qquad \text{equation 2}$$

The *survival-growth function* $p(y,x)$ describes the probability that an individual plant survives the census interval, and if so, the probability distribution for the size it might become. Mathematically, it consists of the probability $p(y,x)$ that an individual will survive and grow to stage y if it were size x the year prior (eqn 2). The fertility function $f(y,x)$ describes the number of offspring produced by reproductive individuals during the census interval, and the size distribution of those new offspring. The fertility function can also be expanded and is generally composed of several variables based on regression models that estimate the reproductive capacity of an individual in the population and the size-class distribution of new offspring (eqn 3). Mathematically, it consists of the probability that an individual will survive $s(x)$, the probability of fruiting $f_f(x)$ or producing clonal $c_f(x)$, the number of new fruits $f_n(x)$ or clonal offspring $c_n(x)$ produced by reproductive individuals, the probability of seedling germination p_g, the probability that a given germinated offspring will become established p_e and the the size distribution of the new seedlings $f_d(y)$ or clonal offspring $c_d(y)$ in a given population. It is important to mention here that IPMs are flexible and can wide range of life histories such as clonality as a continuous size by partitioning the kernel and fertility function into additional vital rate functions. We illustrate this with the additional vital rate function $c(y,x)$ for clonality in the following equation (eqn 4):

$$f(y, x) = s(x) f_f(x) f_n(x) p_g p_e f_d(y) \qquad \text{equation 3}$$

$$c(y, x) = s(x) c_f(x) c_n(x) c_d(y) \qquad \text{equation 4}$$

To build an IPM for practical applications and to test the effect of harvest on demographic responses of ayahuasca, *B. caapi*, we applied this population model to the entire life cycle of ayahuasca lianas in several localized populations in a previous study (see Coe and Gaoue 2023) where data gathered from censusing the vines were used to estimate each liana's vital rates such as growth, survival, and fertility from one year to the next. Data on vital rates were then used to develop the backbone of the IPM consisting of regression models that relate the size of each individual liana to its vital rates. In other words, the regressions were used to link demographic observations to biological inference. Now beyond the effect of size, we also included the effect of harvest as an additional abiotic covariate (e.g. harvest intensity) in these regressions to help explain variation in vital rates beyond the effect of individual size. Our approach in building an IPM to understand the demographic responses to harvest for ayahuasca (*B. caapi*) is described below.

Study System

Banisteriopsis caapi (Spruce ex. Griseb.) C.V. Morton is a woody jungle liana in the Malpighiaceae family (Figure 1). It is botanically described as a liana with brown bark and dark green ovate to lanceolate leaves up to about 7 in. in length, 2-3 in. wide; inflorescences are axillary with many small 5 petal flowers that are pink or rose-colored; Fruit is a samaroid schizocarp composed of 2 to 3 samaras connected at the torus; each samara has dorsal wings about 1.38 in. long (Figure 1). Flowering generally occurs between December —August with samara production between March—August (Gates 1982; Schultes, Hofmann, and Rätsch. 2001). It can also reproduce asexually or colonially where new ramets are generally formed when either mature shoots take root following to host tree falls or anthropogenic harvests of mother plants and out-planting of cut stems (Coe and Gaoue 2023, unpublished data).

In applying IPM's in ethnobotanical contexts, we conducted the first demographic study of ayahuasca from 2017-2018 in a remote region of Loreto, Peru that has more recently become a central location for ayahuasca harvest that currently supplies the harvested liana for Iquitos, Pucallpa and surrounding areas (Coe and Gaoue 2023, unpublished data). The climate in the area is tropical rainforest with a mean annual temperature of 26.4°C and annual rainfall of approximately 1600mm (Casimiro et al. 2013). We collected data on vital rates for two populations of *B. caapi* consisting of approximately 300 plants in total where each population included three 4-ha

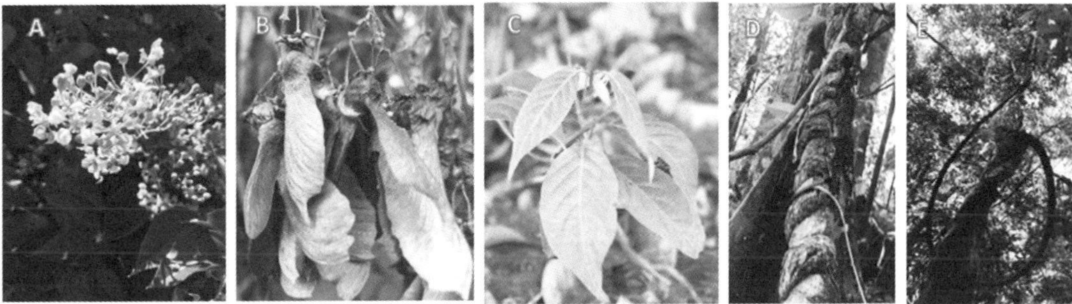

Fig. 1 (A-E). *Banisteriopsis caapi* (Spruce ex. Griseb.) C.V. Morton. (a) Axillary inflorescence, (b) Samaroid schizocarps, (c) vegetative biomass and leaves, (d) mature stem often harvested for the production of ayahuasca, and (e) mature liana growing into the canopy.

plots experiencing differing levels of stem harvest intensity over a 2 year period (July 2017-2018) during the census interval. Differences in harvesting intensity between the two populations were classified based on several criteria including the accessibility of each site to harvesters and the total number of harvested lianas noted during the census interval. Data collection and differences in harvesting intensity between the two populations were estimated and defined as follows:

> Treatment 1 was classified as an ayahuasca population consisting of 3 plots that were less accessible to harvesters and experienced less harvest pressure whereas, treatment 2 was classified as an ayahuasca liana population consisting of 3 plots that were more easily accessible to harvesters and initially experienced increased harvest pressure. There was a total of 41 harvested lianas between the populations at the beginning of the census period whereas, a total of 28 lianas were harvested during the census at *t+1* resulting in an 31% total decrease in harvest over the census period. This significantly reduced the difference in harvest pressure between the treatments with an initial difference of 9 harvested lianas between the populations at time *t* and a difference of 4 lianas at *t+1*. Data for each individual liana were collected to estimate vital rates including growth, survival, fertility to build an IPM where size for each mature liana was measured with precision calipers at DBH and basal diameter for seedlings and clonal ramets following Schnitzer et al. (2008) to estimate growth. Clonal ramets were defined as functionally independent ramets not connected to a mother. New seedlings were characteristic and upright without branching. Mothers were defined as the closest mature vine to a given seedling or clonal ramet. Each point of measurement was marked to ensure precise estimates for individual size from one year to the next. Individual lianas were tagged, and GPS coordinates were taken to ensure a high probability of re-monitoring the population. GPS coordinates were used to locate the stump or root system of harvested lianas under circumstances where tags were removed due to anthropogenic harvest. Survival for each individual was measured from July 2017-2018. We measured reproducing individuals in two parts as (1) the number of seedlings produced nearest to a reproducing adult and (2) the number of ramets in genets produced by a given adult. We estimated fertility in two parts as (1) the proportion of the total number of seedlings produced by a reproducing individual and (2) the proportion of the total number of clones produced by clonally reproducing individuals.

Data analysis for building IPM

Data for vital rates collected during the census interval were used for regression analyses and subsequently used to build the IPM backbone where the survival-growth function was estimated in two parts. For survival, we modeled the probability that each ayahuasca liana will survive at the expected population state under the condition that it survived the year prior. This is done by modeling the probability of survival as a logistic function of size at time *t* following a binomial error structure. We also included the level of harvest at each site as an abiotic covariate. For growth, we modeled the probability that each ayahuasca vine will grow to size x at the expected population state under the condition that it survived the year prior using a linear regression with log-transformed sizes at time t and t+1. We also included size-dependent variance in our models. The linear regression describes the expected size of individuals at the next census, while the log-normal distribution describes the range of possible sizes for each individual at this time interval.

We adapted the fertility function it to include clonality (see equation 4) where fertility was estimated under the condition that plants of size x survived to reproduce. We modeled the probability of seedling and clonal reproduction for each ayahuasca liana at t+1 using a logistic regression following a binomial error structure. The number of clones (ramets) in genets produced is count data, therefore we modeled them using a generalized linear model using a Poisson error structure. We did not have data for the direct average number of fruits produced per reproductive individual. Therefore, based on the known reproductive ecology of *Banisteriopsis muricata* (Cav.) Cuatrec, a closely related species in the same botanical genus (Gates 1982), we estimated an average liana fruit production of 71 fruits produced by flowering individuals given that each fruit produces 2- 3 samaras. As such, each reproductive plant was expected to produce 219 samaras following Zapata & Kalin Arroyo (1978). We used this conservative estimate of size-independent fruit production for individuals that reach reproductive size which is directly accounted for by the probability of fruiting. We then developed a conservative scenario of size-dependent fruit production between harvest treatments by varying the slope for 0.1 (increased harvest pressure, treatment 2) to 0.6 (less harvest pressure, treatment 1). The probability of germination and establishment for seedlings were modeled as constants based on the ratio of new seedlings from field data and fruit production based on conservative estimates.

IPM Regression-model Backbone

To directly assess the effects of harvest on vital rates of *B. caapi*, we developed an IPM (Easterling et al., 2000; Ellner and Rees, 2006; Rees and Ellner, 2009) using functions for growth, survival, and fertility where vital rates were modeled as a function of size. To do so, we first used generalized linear mixed effect models (*glmm*) in *R* 3-4-3 (R Development Core Team 2019) using the *lme4* package (Bates et al., 2015) to assess the effect of harvest and other covariates on vital rates (growth, survival, clonal and sexual reproduction). Random effects included plot number. Fixed-effect explanatory variables included the effect of harvest and size of *B. caapi* individuals. *B. caapi* size measurements were log-transformed to meet normality and homogeneity of variance assumptions. Generalized linear models (*glm*) were also used to assess the effects of harvest and size on the number of seedlings and clones produced. The response variables for our *glmm* models were measurement data for growth, and binary data for survival and the probability of clonal and sexual reproduction. Our response variables for our *glm* models were count data. Therefore, we used *glmm* or *glm* with normal, binomial, and Poisson error structures (Crawley 2013). An information-theoretic approach following Gaoue et al. (2011) was used to select the best fitting models that had greater explanatory power, where, for each response variable we estimated the Akaike information criterion (AIC) for each model, the difference in the AIC between each model, and the model with the lowest Δ AIC. Models with the lowest Δ AIC< 2 were then selected as best model candidates (Gaoue et al., 2011).

We then used these regressions for the survival-growth and fertility functions (see eqn 1; 2) and combined them according to the life-history of the ayahuasca liana (*B. caapi*) to develop the IPM kernel using the *popbio* package (Stubben and Milligan, 2007) in R (R Development Core Team 2019). The kernel was then used to project the size distribution of the population in time following the main equation (eqn 1). To do, so we specified the limits of integration which discretizes the kernel to generate a large population matrix where the boundaries between matrix elements are based on the range of sizes of the lianas in the population (mid-point rule). We then used basic matrix algebra to estimate the eigen values, eigen vectors and for elasticity analysis (Ellner and Rees 2006).

Eigenvalues, eigenvectors and damping ratio

From our IPM, we estimated eigen values, eigen vectors and damping ratio (ρ) for both ayahuasca populations under differing harvest treatments in R (R Development Core Team 2019) to understand population-level patterns of ayahuasca lianas in response to harvest. The largest dominant eigen value lambda (λ) is the long-term population growth rate whereas the largest sub-dominant eigenvalue (λ1) is short-term population growth rate. When $\lambda < 1$, the population is projected to decline, if $\lambda = 1$, then the population is expected to be at equilibrium, and if $\lambda > 1$ the population is expected to increase over time (Ellner and Rees 2006). The right eigenvector of the large population matrix known as the stable size distribution (SSD) and left eigenvector which is the reproductive value (RV) of size-classes in the population. When a population reaches SSD, the proportion of individuals in each size remains constant over time and the population exhibit stable dynamics (Haridas and Tuljapurkar 2007). This is when the population is expected to be at equilibrium. However, populations exhibiting stable dynamics at SSD are not typically seen in nature. For example, ayahuasca lianas of a given size class may respond differentially to environmental cues given the numerous stochastic processes acting in natural systems. As such, populations are in flux and often moved away from SSD. Therefore, understanding SSD dynamics, particularly the rate at which the population is approaching SSD provides an estimate of the projected stability of the population and how the distance away from SSD influences model projections (Haridas and Tuljapurkar 2007). The RV describes the reproductive capacity of individuals in the population and is an important parameter for estimating elasticity analysis (Easterling, Ellner, and Dixon 2000). Damping ratio (ρ) is the rate at which the population is approaching SSD and describes how quickly the population approaches equilibrium. This is mathematically defined as the absolute value of the subdominant eigenvalue (λ1) divided by the dominant eigenvalue (λ). In general, if $\rho < 1$, the population is moved away from equilibrium whereas if $\rho = 1$ the population is closer to equilibrium or structure is at SSD (Haridas and Tuljapurkar 2007).

Elasticity analysis and Life table response experiment (LTRE)

Assessing the demographic responses of ayahuasca to anthropogenic bark harvest requires further analyses beyond estimating population growth rates (Schmidt et al., 2011). It is important also to consider that ayahuasca harvest results in the loss of plant biomass which often leads to changes in vital rates and population structure. These effects of harvest, can also move a given ayahuasca population away from the stable size distribution (Haridas and Tuljapurkar 2007; Stott, Townley, and Hodgson 2011). Therefore, complementary analyses such as elasticity analysis and Life Table Response Experiments (LTRE) can be used to understand prospective and retrospective changes in ayahuasca population dynamics in response to harvest (see Caswell, 2000; Gaoue, 2016; Gaoue, Horvitz, & Ticktin, 2011; Pinard, 1993) which can used to inform sustainable harvest plans. Elasticity analyses are prospective analyses that explore the functional dependence of λ on the vital rates forward in time. Given that λ is a function of the vital rates and this relationship is a property of species' life history which is independent of any actual variation vital rates (Easterling, Ellner, and Dixon 2000), elasticity analyses have become an important and widely used management tool to predict the changes in λ that result from proportional changes in the vital rates (De Kroon, Van Groenendael, and Ehrlén 2000). Life table response experiments (LTRE) are a useful retrospective analysis that assesses the expressed variation of λ as a function variation in vital rates observed backward in time (Easterling, Ellner, and Dixon 2000). As such, LTRE reveal unique population-level patterns that resulted from temporal variation of λ as a function of past variation of vital rates.

In our study on the demographic responses of ayahuasca (*B. caapi*) to harvest, we estimated elasticity values for our IPM using the following equation:

$$\mathrm{e}(x,y) = \frac{\mathrm{k}\,(x,y)}{(\lambda)} \times \frac{v(x)w(y)}{(w,v)}$$

equation 5

where v and w are the left and right eigenvectors of λ and and *K(x,y)* represents the kernel derived from IPM. Given elasticity analysis project the consequences of future changes in the vital rates, we were interested in helping to identify potential management targets for ayahuasca populations because changes in vital rates with high elasticity values will produce large changes in λ. Because we were interested in understanding which demographic processes were responsible for differences in λ between the ayahuasca populations observed backward in time, we carried out life table response experiments (LTRE's) (Caswell, 2000) to identify which vital rates contributed most to differences in population growth rates of B. caapi experiencing less (treatment 1) vs. increased harvest pressure (treatment 2) using the following equation:

$$\lambda^{t} - \lambda^{c} = \sum (K^{t} - K^{c})(\partial\lambda/\partial K)|K^{m}$$

equation 6

where K^t is the kernel element in our treatment matrix, K^c is the kernel element in our reference matrix, $(\partial\lambda/\partial K)$ is the sensitivity of λ to the mean kernel element evaluated by the midway kernel K^m. It is important to mention that because LTRE compare λ between populations, one population kernel must be designated as a treatment and the other as a control (reference kernel) (Caswell 2000). As such, we designated the ayahuasca population kernel for lianas experiencing less harvest pressure (treatment 1) as the reference matrix (λ^c) we obtained from the numerical integration of the IPM so that positive contributions from our LTRE represented differences in vital rates that contributed to the higher population growth rates of ayahuasca populations experiencing increased harvest pressure (treatment 2). Both elasticity analyses and LTRE were conducted using the popbio package (Stubben and Milligan, 2007) in R (R Development Core Team 2019).

RESULTS

Regressions: Effect of Harvest on Survival-Growth and Fertility

There was a linear relationship between ayahuasca lianas of a given size at time t (July 2017) and the following year t+1 (July 2018) indicating the as size of individual lianas increased so did the growth of individuals in the population (Figure 2a). There was no significant effect of harvest on the growth for *B. caapi*. Overall, the probability of survival of individuals increased with size (Figure 2b). Annual changes in plant size from t to t+1 (2017-2018) were independent of harvest and plot as supported by our model (β= 0.908 ± 0.033, t = 27.78, p < 0.0001). The ayahuasca population experiencing treatment 2 (greater harvest pressure) had a lower survival rate than the population experiencing treatment 1. There was a significant interactive effect of harvest and plant size on survival of *B. caapi* (β= 0.876 ± 0.319, z=2.741, p = 0.006) indicating survival of smaller individuals is greater in the population experiencing treatment 2 than the population experiencing treatment 1. The size of individual liana's had a significant effect on survival (β= 0.436± 0.204,

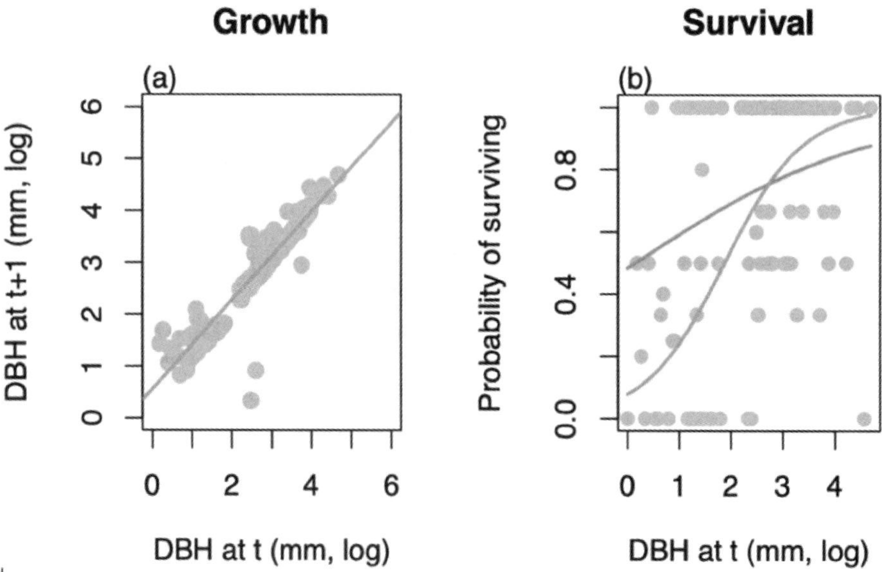

Fig. 2 Demographic functions (vital rates) for *B. caapi*. (a) growth (log scale) as a function of size (measured in mm) July 2017–July 2018, (b) the probability of survival to July 2018 as a function of size (log scale, previously measured in mm) in July 2017. The red dashed line represents the regression coefficient for high harvest whereas the blue dashed line represents the regression coefficient for lower-to-medium harvest intensity.

z=2.132, p=0.033) suggesting the probability of survival was size-dependent. Large individuals 0.5 inches (2.8mm, log) diameter and greater were more likely to experience mortality in the population experiencing greater harvest (treatment 2) (Figure 2b). For such a long-lived species, life history theory suggests that survival of mature ayahuasca lianas are most likely to drive the long-term population dynamics (Silvertown et al. 1993; Enright, Franco, and Silvertown 1995). The reduced survival of large lianas in harvested sites suggests that the level of harvest of large individuals may result in reduced in overall population growth rate between the sites.

Harvest did not have a significant effect on the probability of fruiting and clonality (Figure 3a; Figure 3b). These probabilities were dependent on size where ayahuasca lianas of larger size classes (1.3 inches ≥) produced the greatest number of seedlings (b=1.680 ± 0.755, z= 2.226, p= 0.0026; Figure 3a) and clones (β=1.025 ± 0.4288, z= 2.390, p= 0.0168; Figure 3b). Beyond the effect of size, harvest also had a significant effect on the number of clones produced (β= 0.9153 ± 0.428, z=2.138, p=0.032).

Population growth rate, λ

In our study, the ayahuasca populations experiencing less harvest pressure (treatment 1) were projected to increase at 3.2% per year (λ = 1.032) whereas the ayahuasca population experiencing increased harvest pressure (treatment 2) was projected to decline (λ = 0.987) by 1.3% per year. While these long-term projections are important, they should be understood and interpreted with caution because the short-term population growth rate (λ1) indicated that both ayahuasca populations included in our study are initially projected to decline λ < 1 where the population

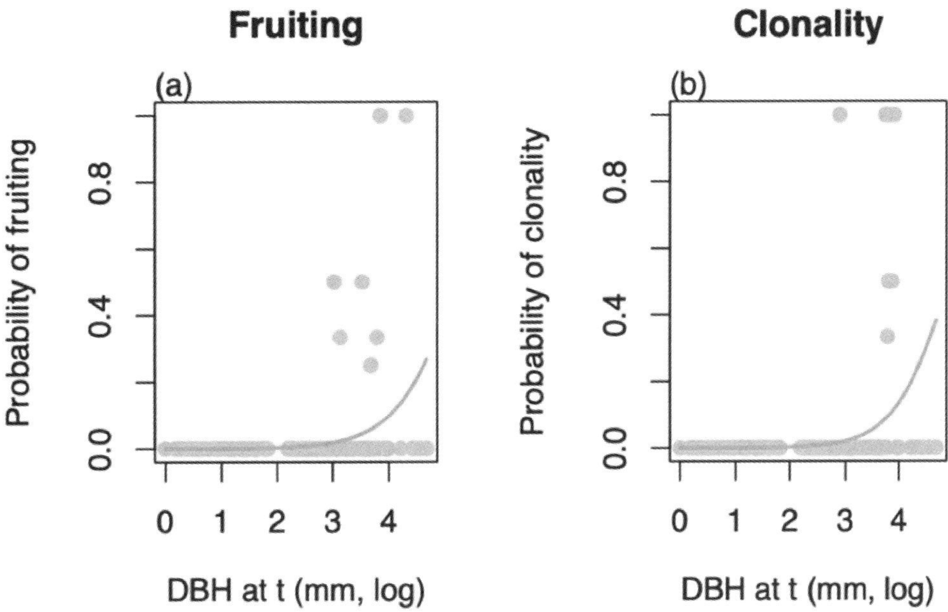

Fig. 3 Demographic functions (vital rates) for *B. caapi*. (a) the number of seedlings produced as a function of size (log scale, previously measured in mm) in 2017. (b) the number of clones produced as a function of size (log scale, previously measured in mm) in 2017.

experiencing treatment 2 was expected to decline faster at a rate of 26% per year (λ1 = 0.74) compared to the population experiencing treatment 1 (less harvest pressure) (λ1 = 0.796). While conservation strategies have historically been informed by long-term projections, it is becoming increasingly clear that short-term and long-term population dynamics differ and are often driven by variability in abiotic and biotic factors (e.g. climate change, plant-herbivore interactions, harvest, etc.) (Bialic-Murphy, Gaoue, and Kawelo 2017; Gaoue 2016; Bialic-Murphy et al. 2022). Consistent with previous studies, these findings support the growing number of studies that have demonstrated the importance of short-term or transient projections in informing sustainable harvest and species management plans which are often designed in the short-term (Gaoue 2016; Stott, Townley, and Hodgson 2011; Koons et al. 2005; Wong and Ticktin 2015; Fox and Gurevitch 2000; Bialic-Murphy et al. 2022).

Damping ratio ρ and SSD

Ayahuasca populations included in our study had a ρ < 1 indicating these populations are away from equilibrium. The ayahuasca population under treatment 1 approached equilibrium at a greater rate (ρ = 0.772) than the population experiencing greater harvest pressure (treatment 2) (ρ = 0.740). This was expected given that the ayahuasca population under treatment 2 experienced greater harvest pressure which likely influenced population structure and subsequently SSD dynamics (Haridas and Tuljapurkar 2007; Stott, Townley, and Hodgson 2011) moving it farther away from equilibrium.

Ayahuasca elasticity values

Elasticity patterns for *B. caapi* indicated that survival of long-lived mature individuals under both harvest treatments had the greatest influence on the short-term λ and long-term population dynamics. (Figure 4a; Figure 4b). Thus, the best approach to improve the short-term population growth rate is to ensure the high survival of large individuals with size greater than 3.5 inches (4.5 mm, log) (Figure 4a; Figure 4b) diameter. This contrasts with previous studies suggesting that survival of young individuals contribute most to the short-term population dynamics of long-lived species (Enright, Franco, and Silvertown 1995; Koons et al. 2005). Such differences could be explained by low seedling recruitment in the ayahuasca liana populations and subsequent lack of change in the number of young individuals over time. Given both populations are projected to decline in the short-term, management targets could focus on the proportional contributions of survival of larger size classes to fitness because of their high elasticity values (Figure 4a; Figure 4b).

Analyzing differences in λ using LTRE

Life table response experiments showed the greater relative contribution of survival of larger size lianas (3.5mm, log ≥; 1.3 ≥ inches), including sexually reproductive individuals, to the ayahuasca population experiencing treatment 1 indicating there was greater survival-growth these size-classes in the population (Figure 5). Consequently, increased harvesting reduced the

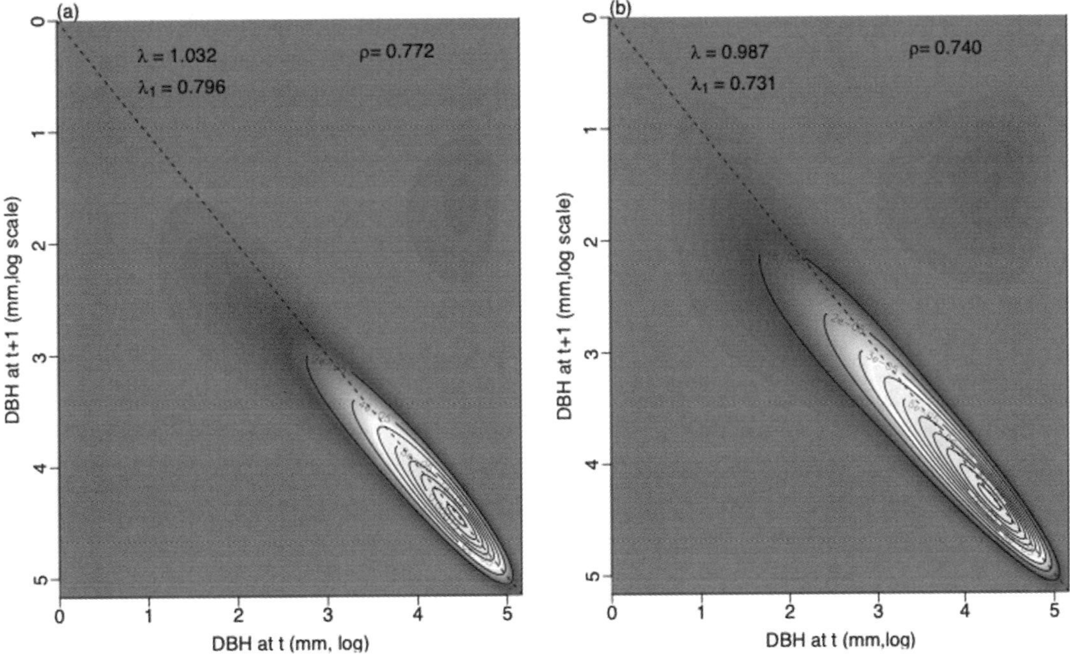

Fig. 4 Elasticity contour plot for the ayahuasca (*B. caapi*) kernel. Elasticity patterns of the short-term population growth rate are represented as follows where (a) elasticity patterns of *B. cappi* under less harvest pressure (treatment 1) and (b) elasticity patterns of *B. caapi* under increased harvest pressure (treatment 2). The dashed-line represents the survival intercept obtained from survival-growth functions and general linearized mixed effect models. Lighter colors (e.g. yellow) represent a greater relative contribution of vital rates to the population growth rate. Values across the diagonal represent contributions from survival, those above the diagonal represent contributions from sexual reproduction and those below the diagonal represent contributions from growth and vegetative reproduction.

survival-growth of larger size lianas in the ayahuasca population experiencing increased harvest pressure (treatment 2) which led to a 24.7% (λ = 0.987 vs. λ1 = 0.74; Figure5) population growth rate reduction retrospectively. There was a greater relative contribution of survival-growth of smaller size classes between (1-3mm, log), including vegetative reproductive individuals, to the population growth rate (λ) in the ayahuasca population experiencing increased harvest pressure (Figure 5). This indicates that the higher rate of clonal production in this population attenuated the rate of population decline but not enough to offset the reduced survival-growth of larger size-classes in the population (Figure 5).

DISCUSSION

This paper has described the use of IPMs in ethnobiological contexts which can guide an understanding of the potential for sustainable harvest of ayahuasca [*Banisteriopsis caapi* (Spruce ex. Griseb.) C.V. Morton] in harvested ecosystems. In doing so, we have provided details on the development of an IPM, subsequent analyses and their use for the first rigorous study on the effects of harvest on ayahuasca in a localized region of the Peruvian Amazon basin. We are

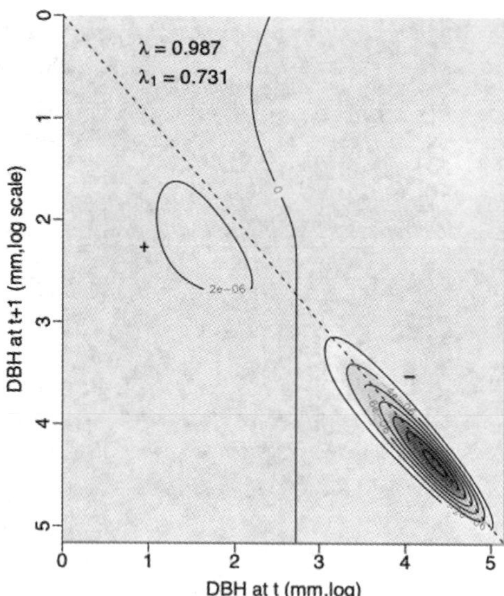

Fig. 5 LTRE contributions of ayahuasca (*B. caapi)* lianas experiencing increased vs. less harvest pressure. Darker colors represent life-history transitions that make greater contributions to higher λ values observed for the ayahuasca population experiencing less harvest pressure (treatment 1). Lighter colors represent life-history transitions that make greater contributions to higher λ values observed for the ayahuasca population experiencing increased harvest pressure (treatment 2). Values across the diagonal represent contributions from survival-growth, and those below the diagonal represent contributions from growth and clonal reproduction.

optimistic that we have provided other researchers the methodologies necessary to directly assess the ecological effects of harvest on ayahuasca liana populations and encourage the use of these approaches presented here to aid in the development of sustainable harvest plans for ayahuasca.

Overall, we have shown that demographic functions for ayahuasca, *B. caapi,* under the effect of harvest are important to consider for sustainable management approaches. Our results indicate that there was no significant negative effect of harvest on survival of lianas in the *B. caapi* population experiencing less harvest pressure. Conversely, we found increased harvest intensity had a significant negative effect on the probability of ayahuasca liana survival in the *B. caapi* population experiencing increased harvest pressure. Small-to-intermediate size lianas < 2.5mm, log scale had a greater probability of survival (Figure 2b) under the effect of harvest compared to large size lianas (>2.5 mm log scale). Given most harvested lianas in both ayahuasca populations were of larger size classes (Coe and Gaoue 2023, unpublished data) we expect the significant effect of harvest on liana survival is due to the increased harvest pressure as a result of supply and demand chains linked to the globalization, commercialization and widespread production and use of ayahuasca brew.

Our results suggest that increased harvest pressure can significantly affect population dynamics of ayahuasca (*B. caapi*). While the population of lianas experiencing less harvest pressure was projected to increase over the long-term compared to the population experiencing increased harvest pressure which was shown to be in decline ($\lambda < 1$), both populations were projected to decline in the short-term. This highlights that long-term projections should be interpreted with caution, especially since there was an overall uncharacteristic decrease in harvest pressure of 31% between the treatments over the census period and because management plans are generally designed and implemented over the short-term. While LTRE's revealed there was greater survival-growth of larger size-class lianas in the ayahausca population experiencing less harvest pressure (treatment 1) which offset the reduction (23.6%) of the population growth rate in response to harvest retrospectively (λ1 = 0.796 vs. λ = 1.032), harvest by reducing the survival-growth of larger size-classes of lianas led to a 25.6% reduction of the population growth rate of the ayahuasca population experiencing increased harvest pressure (treatment 2) (Figure 5).

We found intermediate to larger size classes of lianas had a higher probability of reproducing clonally (Figure 3b) which may be an indirect effect of harvest as there were fewer seedlings (n= 18) produced than clones (n=54) in response to harvest. Because harvest had a significant effect on the number of clones produced, this finding warrants further investigation. We found the probability of fruiting was size-dependent where larger size lianas, 3mm, log ≥, had a greater probability of reproducing sexually (Figure 3a). Given larger size lianas were shown to experience greater mortality rates with increasing harvest intensity in the both ayahuasca populations (Figure 2b) and there were fewer seedlings produced than clones in this study, future research investigating if there is a life-history trade-off where clonal reproduction is favored rather than seedling production (see for exaample Silvertown et al. 1993) in response to harvest is essential to understanding not only the demographic responses of ayahuasca (*B. caapi*) to harvest in natural habitats, but also possible patterns and processes surrounding life history strategies and genetic variability of this species in a modern context. In general, lianas are considered clonal species that periodically reproduce sexually (Ledo and Schnitzer 2014). It is also well known that ayahuasca lianas can be vegetatively propagated with ease and much of the native range of *B. caapi* and its widespread use throughout the Amazon basin has been speculated to be established with the aid of Indigenous Amerindian people through trade routes and migration patterns (Gates 1982; Torres and Fitzpatrick 2018). Therefore, if growers including Indigenous peoples and local communities and agroforestry cultivators (e.g. União do Vegetal, Santo Daime), are currently relying primarily on clonal and vegetative propagation rather than seed, it is unclear whether not ayahuasca populations may experience reduction in fitness due to the loss of heterozygosity at certain alleles over time (see for example Eckert and Barret 1993). This may or may not be the case because nature tends to find a way as seen in some asexually reproducing species where random mutations may occur to allow for fitness and gene-flow over time (Honnay and Bossuyt 2005). However, the loss in genetic diversity of ayahuasca could directly contribute to the species becoming threatened and is a factor often underestimated or completely overlooked by the IUCN Red List (Garner, Hoban, and Luikart 2020). Though it is expected that overall liana reproduction and abundance are expected to increase as a result of future climate regimes (Vogado et al. 2022), the long and short-term effects of harvest on liana sexual vs. asexual reproduction life history tradeoffs and genetic diversity in this context are less understood. As such, these demographic responses of ayahuasca to varying levels of harvest intensity warrant further investigations.

We have highlighted the importance of elasticity analysis in determining vital rates that are likely critical for implementing management approaches of *B. caapi* and subsequently the sustainable development of ayahuasca. Our elasticity analysis has shown that survival of mature ayahuasca lianas are important for the persistence of the ayahuasca populations in the short-term (Figure 4a; Figure 4b). This finding is supported by prior research that has demonstrated survival of long-lived individuals of certain lifeforms such as trees and lianas often have a greater relative importance to the contribution of the population growth rate (λ) compared to short-lived species such as perennials (Franco and Silvertown 2004; de Campos Franci et al. 2016). Although it is expected that the survival of long-lived species is likely to play a more central role in population persistence and the relative contribution to the long-term population growth rate (λ) (Franco and Silvertown, 2004; Silvertown et al., 1993), we are unaware of any study investigating the transient (short-term) elasticity patterns of lianas, moreover, ayahuasca (*B. caapi*) in response to harvest. Interestingly, in our study the contribution of survival of mature ayahuasca vines to the short-term population grow rate (λ) were similar under both harvest treatments (Figure 4a; Figure 4b). Given it has been cautioned, long-term elasticity analysis may not always adequately describe the relative importance of vital rate life stage contributions to the short-term population growth rate (λ) (Bialic-Murphy, Gaoue, and Kawelo 2017; Gaoue 2016; Haridas and Tuljapurkar 2007; Wong and Ticktin 2015), we suggest future research investigating both the short and long-term elasticity patterns of ayahuasca is critical to understanding ayahuasca population responses to harvest and for the development of sound management plans for this culturally and economically important plant species.

To date, we are unaware of any other study on the population dynamics of ayahuasca (*B. caapi*) in response to harvest which indicates this area of research in population ecology or ethnobiology is understudied (Schmidt et al. 2011; Ticktin 2004) and may be driven in part because lianas are often viewed ecologically as structural parasites (Phillips et al. 2002) despite their overall importance in ecosystem dynamics (Schnitzer 2015) and to cultural communities worldwide (Guadagnin and Gravato 2013). Therefore, future studies on the demography of ayahuasca lianas in response to harvest are needed and warrant considerable efforts to address growing sustainability concerns in the Peruvian Amazon basin. Our research indicates that the short-term population dynamics of *Banisteriopsis caapi* (Spruce ex. Griseb.) C.V. Morton vary as a function of size in response to harvest where larger size-classes significantly contributed to vital rate functions both prospectively and retrospectively (Figure 4a; Figure 4b; Figure 5). Given larger size-class lianas were more likely to experience greater harvest pressure and mortality because they were often preferentially selected for the production of ayahuasca brew, approaches towards sustainable ayahuasca liana harvest and production should consider novel management strategies to offset the reduction of survival-growth of larger lianas with increasing harvest pressure and intensity. While syncretic religious groups including the União do Vegetal and Santo Daime have become pioneers in developing agroforestry strategies to manage ayahuasca production (see for example Thevenin and Sambuichi 2020) where ayahuasca source plants (*B. caapi* (Spruce ex. Griseb.) C.V. Morton and *P. viridis* Ruiz & Pav.) have been planted in the Brazilian Amazon and in the United States in efforts to satisfy considerable ayahuasca use in a religious context (Tupper 2009), in some cases, wild ayahuasca harvest by these groups continues and it is clear there have yet to be any rigorous studies and empirical evidence to support whether or not these cultivation efforts are ecologically sound and can provide enough ayahuasca over the long-term. To date, cultivated *B. caapi* lianas have been shown to contain lower concentrations of β-carbolines compared to native ayahuasca lianas (Santos et al. 2020). Therefore, further research is needed to understand the ecological drivers of differences in secondary chemistry composition between native and cultivated B. caapi and whether or not increased harvest intensity may result from either native B. caapi lianas being preferentially selected for due to greater alkaloid content or greater harvested biomass of cultivated B. caapi lianas needed for the potentiation of DMT (dimethyltryptamine) in ayahuasca brew.

Though our study was the first to directly assess the effects of harvest on ayahuasca from an ethnobiological and a conservation perspective, the results we have presented here were obtained from our IPM with a census interval of 2 years. Therefore, long-term studies (>3-5 years) will greatly advance our understanding on the demographic responses of ayahuasca to increasing harvest pressure and intensity over time (Doak, Goss, and Morris 2005). Future research should also include both transient (short-term) and stochastic models rather than solely using deterministic models in order to uncover population-level patterns in response to abiotic and biotic variability over both the short- and long-term. Additionally, developing a deeper understanding of local people and Indigenous community knowledge of ayahuasca management is essential for sustainable development and collaborative efforts. This is critically important because Indigenous peoples and local communities are significant stakeholders in ayahuasca production and ancestral lands and in many cases they have advanced knowledge of their environment and know how to successfully manage these species at a local level (Berkes, Colding, and Folke 2000; Pretty et al. 2009; Gadgil et al. 2001; Colding and Folke 2001; Turner, Ignace, and Ignace 2000; Athayde et al. 2021). Given the globalization of ayahuasca continues with expected increased harvest pressures of ayahuasca source plants over time (e.g. Tupper 2009), collaborative efforts involving both Indigenous people and local community knowledge of species management and ecosystem dynamics will likely be essential to advancing our collective understanding of ayahuasca harvest sustainability (Fernández-llamazares et al. 2022).

In our study, there were several notable harvesting methods that warrant further investigation. For example, it was not uncommon to discover collateral damage of ayahuasca host trees that had been cut down in order for harvesters to gain greater access to a single ayahuasca liana for its bark and stem (Figure 6a). This may negatively alter ecosystem dynamics by reducing overall tree biodiversity and total carbon sequestration while increasing atmospheric Co_2 levels and shifts in functional ecosystem composition in tropical ecosystems (Chapin III et al. 2000; de Campos Franci et al. 2016; Phillips et al. 2002). On one hand, ayahuasca can be selective for certain host trees (Coe and Gaoue 2023, unpublished data) and the overall persistence of liana populations may vary due to host tree dependence at certain life-history stages (larger size classes) and favorable resource availability and climatic conditions across ontogeny (de Campos Franci et al. 2016; Schnitzer and Bongers 2002). Therefore, the loss of companion trees may negatively influence the demographic responses of ayahuasca following harvest by increasing regeneration time driven by the reduction of tree community composition (available host trees) and resource availability (see for example de Campos Franci et al. 2016); especially if conditions are such that host tree disturbance does not result in increased light availability at the forest canopy (Schnitzer and Bongers 2002). Further, the population growth rate of lianas has been shown to be greater in areas with an increased density of larger size host trees (de Campos Franci et al. 2016) indicating that the loss of these companion trees may also result in population decline. On the other hand, lianas are known to respond favorably to disturbance-induced increased light and resource availability due to tree falls which can also lead to overall increased ayahuasca growth rates and liana density in tropical ecosystems (Phillips et al. 2002; Schnitzer and Bongers 2002; Schnitzer et al.

2014). Therefore, a greater understanding of host tree compatibility and demographic responses of ayahuasca to host tree disturbance across life-history and in varying eco- (fragmented forests, disturbed areas vs. old growth forests) and climatic- regions will be informative in understanding how such harvesting practices may positively or negatively alter ecosystem dynamics and which practices are favorable for sustainable ayahuasca harvest.

Another harvesting method noted in our study involved replanting (propagation) of small sections of an intermediate-to-larger size class ayahuasca liana that had been harvested previously in effort to facilitate regeneration following harvest (Figure 6b); which differs from harvested lianas where new shoots emerge from a common root system (Figure 6c). It is important to consider how these local harvesting and management practices affect ayahuasca liana regeneration time following harvest. Although overall liana density and reproduction is expected to increase in response to projected increase in atmospheric CO_2, climate-induced drought, and anthropogenic disturbance (Vogado et al. 2022; Schnitzer et al. 2014), the persistence of ayahuasca liana populations will also significantly depend on the demographic responses to increased harvest and intensity over the short- and long-term. Future studies should seek to understand differences in regeneration time to maturity between new shoots emerging from a common root system of harvested lianas, new seedlings, clonal ramets, and propagation techniques involving replanted stem bark in differing climate zones and eco-regions to understand which conditions and management techniques are favorable for increased ayahuasca growth rates and regeneration over time.

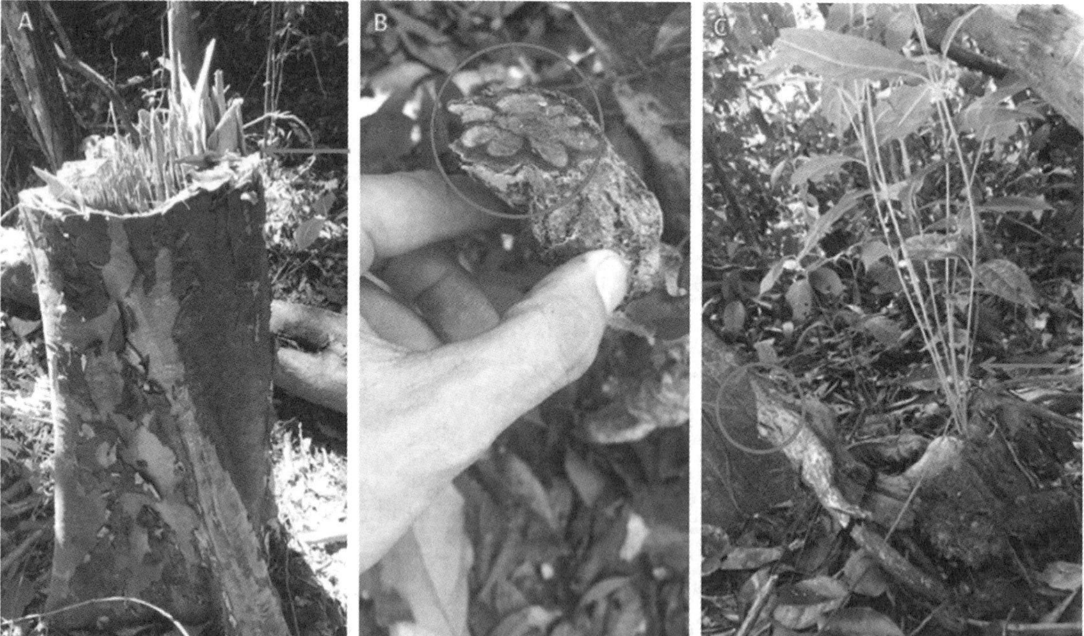

Fig. 6 (A-C) Localized harvesting practices. (a) a cut host or companion tree, (b) harvested stem of *B. caapi* that was selectively propagated, (c) ayahuasca shoots emerging from a common root-system of a harvested adult in the Peruvian Amazon basin.

THE FUTURE OF AYAHUASCA: A POTENTIAL PATH FORWARD

In closing, we highlight a preliminary conceptualization of the sustainable development of ayahuasca involving some of the primary stakeholders and key elements of consideration within four domains including ecological, cultural, social and economic (Figure 7). We acknowledge that this work in progress has yet to be exhaustive. Our intention here is to spark the catalyst of thoughtful consideration on how future collaborations involving an integration of scientific knowledge combined with Indigenous people and local community knowledge (including stakeholder knowledge), for the co-production of knowledge, can inform *woven science* frameworks (a.k.a. two-eyed seeing) for the sustainable development of ayahuasca production and help ensure ayahuasca source plant species persistence and sustainable harvest over time. Some of the key stakeholders represented include syncretic religious groups (churches), growers, harvesters, producers, ayahuasca centers, exporters and various ayahuasca practitioners including but not limited to local people and Indigenous communities, Indigenous and Mestizo shamanic practitioners and ayahuasca researchers under the understanding that these stakeholders may overlap. We are optimistic that with greater knowledge on the ecology and demography of ayahuasca source plants informed by IPM along with local knowledge on growing and harvesting practices, an interconnected web of knowledge from these various stakeholders can inform sustainable ayahausca production. Key considerations within the four domains of sustainable ayahuasca production are as follows:

Ecological

An essential consideration is that ayahuasca brew is a plant-derived decoction that is dependent on the stability of social and ecological systems. Given, the numerous threats to the biological, cultural, linguistic and chemical diversity of the Amazon basin including land-use changes, climate change, deforestation, mining, logging and land-grabs (Carrero et al. 2022; Athayde et al. 2021; Finer et al. 2008; Davis 2003; Gorenflo et al. 2012), a logical path forward on the roadmap for sustainable ayahuasca production should include investigations on whether or not local and commercial ayahuasca harvest and production is ecologically sustainable. Additionally, rigorous studies on the genetic diversity of ayahuasca and possible ayahuasca liana varieties are needed. Considerable efforts to ensure that ancestral lands of Indigenous peoples and local communities are protected along with the ayahuasca source plants *in situ* are essential for the persistence of local medicinal plant knowledge and these species in their natural habitat. Further, the development of an ayahuasca sustainability guide informed by local management practices and IPM's will prove useful in facilitating resiliency of both social and ecological systems by reinforcing local knowledge and collaborative species management.

Economic

A key consideration within this domain of sustainable ayahuasca production is the development of a fair market price for both the ayahuasca liana and ayahuasca brew including reasonable living wages for growers, harvesters, and producers, etc. Given that the globalized use of ayahuasca is expected to continue as a result of the growing number of studies that have demonstrated its therapeutic potential in contemporary medicine (Tupper 2009; Kuypers et al. 2016; Morales-García et al. 2017; McKenna and Riba 2016), numerous ayahuasca retreat centers in Peru (Fotiou 2016) and popularization in the media (Brabec de Mori 2021; Tupper 2009), increased global demand is certain. Aside from ayahuasca churches who primarily use the ayahuasca brew as a sacrament in religious contexts and do not receive monetary gain for its consumption, numerous stakeholders depend on ayahuasca liana harvest and ayahuasca brew production for not only local livelihoods but also revenue streams generated from globalized use by Westerners in Peruvian cities and the exportation of concentrated ayahuasca brew to other parts of the world. It has become well-known that ayahuasca centers in Peru around Iquitos and Pucallpa and the Urubamba Valley hold retreats for people from countries all over the world. Therefore, another logical step forward is to encourage incentives for sustainably sourced ayahuasca rooted in fair trade agreements between stakeholders (i.e. growers, producers, centers, etc.). Further, if any natural products are developed from the ayahuasca brew or source plants, then it is reasonable to consider novel approaches toward commercial profit sharing for Indigenous peoples and local communities whose knowledge has undoubtedly benefited ayahuasca users.

Cultural

While ayahuasca has primarily been used among numerous Indigenous Amerindian societies from Pre-Colombian times until the latter part of the 20th century (Luna 1986; McKenna 2005), it is clear that it has become a global phenomenon over the last fifty years. For many Amerindian societies, ayahuasca has historically and still continues to be an integral part of their material and non-material elements of culture including their world views, rituals, rites of passage, divination, artistic expression, music, healing practices, subsistence strategies, etc. (Luna and White 2017; Reichel-Dolmatoff 1971; Brabec de Mori 2012b). As such, ayahuasca is undeniably culturally important with widespread uses that have expanded beyond traditional Amerindian use in the last several decades where ayahuasca can now be found numerous countries throughout the world and is often consumed by a variety of traditional Indigenous, Mestizo, neo-shamanic, and recreational users in an array of contexts (Brabec de Mori 2021; Winkelman 2005; Fotiou 2016).

Additionally, within the last fifty years ayahuasca has become a religious sacrament among ayahuasca religious groups and more recently has been declared as part of the National Cultural Heritage of Peru (Feeney and Labate 2015; Tupper 2009). A direction forward is to ensure that the sustainable production of ayahuasca is culturally acceptable for both producers and consumers. Therefore, a greater understanding on how and whether or not sustainably sourced ayahuasca can affirm cultural heritage and support biocultural resilience is needed.

Social

An important consideration for the development of sustainable ayahuasca production is the empowerment of Indigenous peoples and local communities of the Amazon basin. Within this consideration, as supported by the Declaration of Belem, are the inseparable links between biological and cultural diversity including the acknowledgement of Indigenous peoples and local communities as significant knowledge holders of intellectual property (IP) directly linked to the ayahuasca brew including its source and admixture plants (Athayde et al. 2021; Tupper 2009) with rights to their ancestral lands and equitable compensation for sharing this knowledge and any natural products developed from it (Cox 2001). It is also important to consider if a road map toward sustainable ayahuasca production would be more efficient with collaborations between growers and ayahuasca producers and how this could be adequately facilitated. In addition, the development of ayahuasca sustainability programs and educational tools guided by local management practices and IPM's could help to reinforce traditional local knowledge while providing opportunities for collaborations among stakeholders and reciprocal knowledge exchange which will advance our global understanding of ayahuasca sustainability.

In moving forward with the development of sustainable ayahuasca production, it is important to consider the global impact of ayahuasca harvest driven by stakeholder ayahuasca consumption. It is clear very little effort has been made to assess the effect of harvest of ayahuasca source plants in both natural and agroforestry systems despite growing concerns for sustainability and reports of ayahuasca (*B. caapi*) shortages around Peruvian ayahuasca tourist cities (e.g. Iquitos and Pucallpa) in the mainstream media. Therefore, we strongly encourage rigorous studies on the effect of harvest on ayahuasca source plants across a range of eco-regions and habitats to facilitate a greater understanding on whether the current rates of harvest across the Amazon basin and elsewhere are sustainable for future generations and if current ayahuasca agroforestry efforts are ecologically sound and provide adequate attenuation of wild ayahuasca harvest over both the short and long-term. Further, studies aiming to understand the significance of ethnotaxonomic varieties of ayahuasca (see de Oliveira et al. 2021; Santos et al. 2020) have yet to provide unequivocal support for whether or not they are definitively unique taxa from *Banisteriopsis caapi* (Spruce ex. Griseb.) C.

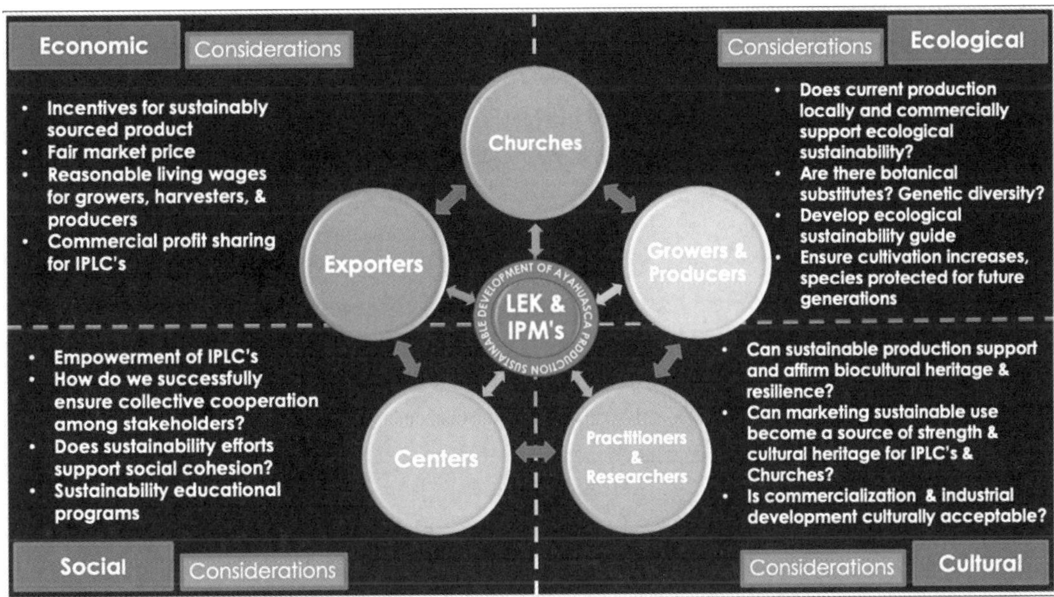

Fig. 7 Conceptualization of the sustainable development of ayahuasca. Spheres represent primary stakeholders and an interconnected web of knowledge informed by IPMs coupled with Indigenous people and local community knowledge of species management. Key elements of consideration are highlighted within four domains including ecological, cultural, social and economic (rectangles).

V. Morton, chemotypes or ecotypes of the same species (Gates 1982), or the same species exhibiting phenotypic plasticity under different abiotic or biotic conditions. Though ethnotaxonomic varieties of *B. caapi* have been described locally based on various morphological features (e.g. swollen nodes) and have been found to exhibit differences in alkaloid composition between cultivated vs. native varieties (Santos et al. 2020), rigorous taxonomic and genetic investigations on ethnotaxonomic varieties are lacking. The identification of other Malpighiaceae lianas traditionally used in the preparation of ayahuasca may provide valuable insights on understanding ethnotaxonomy and the various morphological characters and possible differences in secondary chemistry composition that differentiate these species or varieties from *B. caapi*. However, it remains unclear if the predicted use of these species in lieu of *B. caapi* would significantly alleviate any ayahuasca liana harvest pressure given that aside from the clear identification of separate species or varieties by taxonomists, presumably these species are already being preferentially selected for ayahuasca harvest and production by various stakeholders. Given that other Malpighiaceae lianas potentially used in ayahuasca production would undoubtedly be closely related evolutionarily, it is expected that these species would also have similar life-histories, regeneration time to maturity and demographic responses to harvest (Enright, Franco, and Silvertown 1995; Silvertown et al. 1993; Franco and Silvertown 2004) and likely experience increased harvest pressures and intensities with the increased globalization of ayahuasca over time. While stakeholders including Indigenous peoples and local communities often decide the quantity, the location of and when to harvest based on their understanding of the responses of these plants to previous harvest (Berkes, Colding, and Folke 2000; Turner, Ignace, and Ignace 2000; Gaoue, Horvitz, and Ticktin 2011), in certain contexts where access to resources is highly competitive and driven by economic interests or subsistence needs, decisions about whether and how much to harvest may result in harvest intensity and frequency beyond thresholds stakeholders themselves would consider sustainable (Gaoue, Horvitz, and Ticktin 2011). Therefore, the future of ayahuasca sustainability warrants considerable research and attention by all stakeholders.

Finally, as part of these considerations mentioned above, it is important to acknowledge that ayahuasca use is an integral part of living and dynamic cross-cultural ways of being liked to sociocultural systems where many stakeholders that consume ayahuasca whether for personal or spiritual growth, rites of passage, divination, religious beliefs, healing and diagnosing illnesses, etc. hold a deep appreciation for ayahuasca beyond economic benefits resulting from globalization. As such, the use of ayahuasca is often associated with a sense of maintaining social taboos and dietary proscriptions (e.g. dieta, samá) as a form of reciprocity (Brabec de Mori 2021; McKenna, Luna, and Towers. 1995; Luna 1984a) between the ayahuasca consumer and ayahuasca source and other teacher plants. Perhaps in this context, similar social taboos or rationale could be adopted by stakeholders to include a responsibility of reciprocity rooted in sustainable ayahuasca harvest and production alike other traditional adaptive resource management strategies (see for example Berkes, Colding, and Folke 2000; Colding and Folke 2001) and those used in managing ritual and sacred plants (Quiroz and van Andel 2015).

Whether or not current rates of ayahuasca harvest in the Amazon basin are sustainable, it is clear that the current threats to the biocultural diversity (e.g. deforestation, logging, mining, land grabs etc.) of the Amazon basin are unwaning and are likely contributing to significant compounding effects were losses of species' native ranges and ancestral lands of cultural communities are unprecedented (Carrero et al. 2022; Athayde et al. 2021). These factors along with the increased harvest of ayahuasca lianas as a result of globalized use may contribute to species decline over the long-term. Therefore, time is of the essence and the opportunity to learn how to respectfully manage ayahuasca production while laying the appropriate foundations for species protection and the protection of Indigenous peoples and local community ancestral lands must not slip through our fingertips because there is much at stake beyond the revenue streams of commercialization, subsistence, and local livelihoods. Entire ways of living and being are undeniably at risk and in many cases being forced out of existence at a rate beyond a given culture's capacity for adaptation (Davis 2004, 2003) and the loss of ayahuasca source plants and overall biological and cultural diversity of the Amazon basin are no exception. A way to help ensure that these diverse ways of being and ways of knowing inspired by the interconnection between the human experience and ayahuasca source plants remain, is to advance our understanding on how ayahuasca source plants respond to increasing harvest pressures over time. This will help ensure a continued dialog of reverence. We are hopeful that the methods, insights from fieldwork, and preliminary conceptualization of sustainable ayahausca production highlighted in this paper help to provide a deeper understanding of not only the ecology and demography of *Banisteriopsis caapi* (Spruce ex. Griseb.) C.V. Morton but also provide inspiration for future research and a preliminary road map forward for fruitful collaborations between stakeholders.

ACKNOWLEDGEMENTS

We would like to thank The McKenna Academy of Natural Philosophy and the other organizers of the Ethnopharmacological Search for Psychoactive Drugs III conference for their support and inclusion of this work in the proceedings. We would like to thank the Shipibo-Konibo collaborators for sharing their knowledge, their time, hospitality, and for supporting this research, volunteer's and fellow researchers at *Alianza Arkana* NGO for their fieldwork contributions. A special thanks to Paul Roberts, Laura Dev, Marcos Urquia Maynas, Orestes Rengifo Cauper, Migueas Panduro, Elias Mahua Campos, Neyda Cairuna, Karal Vikat, Hannes Reineker, Diego Villegas, Manuela Mahua Ahuanari, Gilberto Mahua Ochavano, Feliciano Lopez Panduro, Alberto Barbaran Cauper and Brian Robert Best for their field work support and to Juan Celidonio Ruiz Macedo for his integral works in plant identification and taxonomy. We are grateful for comments on an earlier version of the manuscript from Tamara Ticktin, Christine Beaule, Mark Merlin, Dennis McKenna, Luis Eduardo Luna, and two anonymous reviewers.

Data availability statement

The data generated and analyzed for the current study are available in the DRYAD repository

Authors' contributions

MAC and OGG conceived of the idea for the paper and outlined and structured its content. MAC collected and analyzed the data with contribution from OGG. MAC wrote the first draft of the manuscript with additional edits from OGG. All authors read and approved the final manuscript.

BIBLIOGRAPHY

Albuquerque, Ulysses Paulino, Luiz Vital Fernandes Cruz Cunha, Reinaldo Farias Paiva Lucena, and Rômulo Romeu Nobrega Alves. 2014. *Methods and Techniques in Ethnobiology and Ethnoecology*. Edited by Ulysses Paulino Albuquerque, Luiz Vital Fernandes Cruz Cunha, Reinaldo Farias Paiva Lucena, and Rômulo Romeu Nobrega Alves. Springer New York.

Albuquerque, Ulysses Paulino, and Natalia Hanazaki. 2009. "Five Problems in Current Ethnobotanical Research—and Some Suggestions for Strengthening Them." *Human Ecology* 37 (5): 653–61.

Albuquerque, Ulysses Paulino, Marcelo Alves Ramos, Washington Soares Ferreira Júnior, and Patrícia Muniz De Medeiros. 2017. *Ethnobotany for Beginners*. Springer International Publishing.

Alexiades, Miguel N., and Jennie Wood Sheldon. 1996. *Selected Guidelines for Ethnobotanical Research: A Field Manual*. The New York Botanical Garden, Bronx, New York.

Athayde, Simone, Glenn Shepard, Thiago M Cardoso, Hein van der Voort, Stanford Zent, Martha Cecilia Rosero-Peña, Angélica Almeyda Zambrano, Gasodá Wawaeitxapôh Suruí, and Daniel M Larrea-Alcazar. 2021. "Chapter 10: Critical Interconnections between the Cultural and Biological Diversity of Amazonian Peoples and Ecosystems." *Amazon Assessment Report 2021*. https://doi.org/10.55161/iobu4861.

Bates, Douglas, Martin Maechler, Ben Bolker, and Steve Walker. 2015. "Fitting Linear Mixed-Effects Models Using Lme4." *Journal of Statistical Software* 67 (1): 1–48.

Berkes, Fikret, Johan Colding, and Carl Folke. 2000. "Rediscovery of Traditional Ecological Knowledge as Adaptive Management." *Ecological Applications* 10 (5): 1251–62.

Bialic-Murphy, Lalasia, Orou G. Gaoue, and Kapua Kawelo. 2017. "Microhabitat Heterogeneity and a Non-Native Avian Frugivore Drive the Population Dynamics of an Island Endemic Shrub, Cyrtandra Dentata." *Journal of Applied Ecology* 54 (5): 1469–77. https://doi.org/10.1111/1365-2664.12868.

Bialic-Murphy, Lalasia, Tiffany M. Knight, Kapua Kawelo, and Orou G. Gaoue. 2022. "The Disconnect Between Short- and Long-Term Population Projections for Plant Reintroductions." *Frontiers in Conservation Science* 2 (January): 1–10. https://doi.org/10.3389/fcosc.2021.814863.

Brabec de Mori, Bernd. 2012a. "A Medium of Magical Power : How to Do Things with Voices in the Western Amazon." In *Zakharine, Dmitri and Meise, Nils (Eds.): 'Electrified Voices. Medial, Socio-Historical and Cultural Aspects of Voice Transmission*, 379–401. Göttingen: V&R unipress.

Brabec de Mori, Bernd. 2012b. "About Magical Singing, Sonic Perspectives, Ambient Multinatures, and the Conscious Experience." Indiana 29 (29): 73–101.

Brabec de Mori, Bernd. 2021. "The Power of Social Attribution: Perspectives on the Healing Efficacy of Ayahuasca." Frontiers in Psychology 12 (October). https://doi.org/10.3389/fpsyg.2021.748131.

Campos Franci, Luciana de, Jacob Nabe-Nielsen, Jens Christian Svenning, and Fernando Roberto Martins. 2016. "Short-Term Spatial Variation in the Demography of a Common Neotropical Liana Is Shaped by Tree Community Structure and Light Availability." Plant Ecology 217 (10): 1273–90. https://doi.org/10.1007/s11258-016-0655-0.

Carrero, Gabriel Cardoso, Robert Tovey Walker, Cynthia Suzanne Simmons, and Philip Martin Fearnside. 2022. "Land Grabbing in the Brazilian Amazon: Stealing Public Land with Government Approval." Land Use Policy, no. April: 106133. https://doi.org/10.1016/j.landusepol.2022.106133.

Casimiro, Lavado, Waldo Sven Labat, David Ronchail, Josyane Espinoza, Jhan Carlo Guyot, and Jean Loup. 2013. "Trends in Rainfall and Temperature in the Peruvian Amazon-Andes Basin over the Last 40years (1965-2007)." Hydrological Processes 27 (20): 2944–57. https://doi.org/10.1002/hyp.9418.

Caswell, Hal. 2000. "Prospecitve and Retrospective Perturbation Analyses : Their Roles in Conservation Biology." Ecology 81 (3): 619–27.

Chapin III, F. S., E.S. Zavaleta, V.T. Eviner, R.L. Naylor, P.M. Vitousek, H.L. Reynolds, D.U. Hooper, et al. 2000. "Consequences of Changing Biodiversity." Nature 405 (6783): 234–42. https://doi.org/10.12944/cwe.10.special-issue1.63.

Coe, Michael A., and Orou G. Gaoue. 2023. "Increased clonal growth in heavily harvested ecosystems failed to rescue ayahuasca lianas from decline in the Peruvian Amazon rainforest. *Journal of Applied Ecology*, 60(10), 2105-2117.

Colding, Johan, and Carl Folke. 2001. "Social Taboos:'Invisible' Systems of Local Resource Management and Biological Conservation." *Ecological Applications* 11 (2): 584–600.

Cox, Paul Alan. 2001. "Ensuring Equitable Benefits: The Falealupo Covenant and the Isolation of Anti-Viral Drug Prostratin from a Samoan Medicinal Plant." *Pharmaceutical Biology* 39 (1): 33–40. https://doi.org/10.1076/phbi.39.s1.33.0001.

Crawley, Michael J. 2013. *The R Book.* John Wiley & Sons. https://doi.org/10.1037/023990.

Davis, Wade. 1996. *One River: Explorations and Discoveries in the Amazon Rain Forest.* Simon and Shuster.

Davis, Wade. 2003. "Dreams from Endangered Cultures." In *TED Conferences.*

Davis, Wade. 2004. *The Lost Amazon: The Photographic Journey of Richard Evans Schultes.* San Fancisco: Chronicle Books.

Doak, Daniel F., Kevin Goss, and William F. Morris. 2005. "Understanding and Predicting the Effects of Sparse Data on Demographic Analyses." *Ecology* 86 (5): 1154–63.

Easterling, Michael R., Stephen P. Ellner, and Philip M. Dixon. 2000. "Size-Specific Sensitivity: Applying a New Structured Population Model." *Ecology.* https://doi.org/10.1890/0012-9658(2000)081[0694:SSSAAN]2.0.CO;2.

Eckert, Christopher G ., and Spencer C . H . Barret. 1993. "Clonal Reproduction and Patterns of Genotypic Diversity in Decodon Verticillatus (Lythraceae)." *American Journal of Botany* 80 (10): 1175–82.

Ellner, Stephen P., and Mark Rees. 2006. "Integral Projection Models for Species with Complex Demography." *The American Naturalist* 167 (3): 410–28. https://doi.org/10.1086/499438.

Enright, NJ, Miguel Franco, and J Silvertown. 1995. "Comparing Plant Life Histories Using Elasticity Analysis: The Importance of Life Span and the Number of Life-Cycle Stages." *Oecologia.* http://link.springer.com/article/10.1007/BF00365565.

Feeney, Kevin, and Beatriz Caiuby Labate. 2015. "The Expansion of Brazilian Ayahuasca Religions: Law, Culture and Locality." In *Prohibition, Religious Freedom, and Human Rights: Regulating Traditional Drug Use,* 110–30. Springer, Berlin, Heidelberg. https://doi.org/10.1007/978-3-642-40957-8.

Fernández-llamazares, Authors, Chelsey Geralda, S Eduardo, Álvaro Fernández-llamazares, Dana Lepofsky, Ken Lertzman, Chelsey Geralda Armstrong, et al. 2022. "Scientists ' Warning to Humanity on Threats to Indigenous and Local Knowledge Systems." *Journal of Ethnobiology* 41 (2): 144–69.

Finer, Matt, Clinton N. Jenkins, Stuart L. Pimm, Brian Keane, and Carl Ross. 2008. "Oil and Gas Projects in the Western Amazon: Threats to Wilderness, Biodiversity, and Indigenous Peoples." *PLoS ONE* 3 (8). https://doi.org/10.1371/journal.pone.0002932.

Fotiou, Evgenia. 2016. "The Globalization of Ayahuasca Shamanism and the Erasure of Indigenous Shamanism." *Anthropology of Consciousness* 27 (2): 151–79. https://doi.org/10.1111/anoc.12056.

Fox, Gordon A., and Jessica Gurevitch. 2000. "Population Numbers Count: Tools for near-Term Demographic Analysis." *American Naturalist* 156 (3): 242–56. https://doi.org/10.1086/303387.

Franco, Miguel, and Jonathan Silvertown. 2004. "A Comparative Demography of Plants Based upon Elasticities of Vital Rates." *Ecology* 85 (02): 531–38.

Gadgil, Madhav., Per. Olsson, Fikret Berkes, and Carl. Folke. 2001. "Exploring the Role of Local Ecological Knowledge in Ecosystem Management: Three Case Studies." In *Navigating Social-Ecological Systems,* 189–209. Cambridge University Press, New York.

Gaoue, Orou G. 2016. "Transient Dynamics Reveal the Importance of Early Life Survival to the Response of a Tropical Tree to Harvest." *Journal of Applied Ecology* 53 (1): 112–19. https://doi.org/10.1111/1365-2664.12553.

Gaoue, Orou G., Michael A. Coe, Matthew Bond, Georgia. Hart, Barnabas. C. Seyler, and Heather McMillen. 2017. "Theories and Major Hypotheses in Ethnobotany." *Economic Botany* 71 (3): 269–87. https://doi.org/10.1007/s12231-017-9389-8.

Gaoue, Orou G., Carol C. Horvitz, and Tamara Ticktin. 2011. "Non-Timber Forest Product Harvest in Variable Environments: Modeling the Effect of Harvesting as a Stochastic Sequence." *Ecological Applications* 21 (5): 1604–16. https://doi.org/10.1890/10-0422.1.

Gaoue, Orou G., Jacob Moutouama, Michael A. Coe, Matthew Bond, Elizabeth Green, Nadejda Sero, Bezeng Bezeng, and Kowiyou Yessoufou. 2021. "Methodological Advances for Hypothesis-Driven Ethnobotany." *Biological Reviews.*

Gaoue, Orou G., Lawren Sack, and Tamara Ticktin. 2011. "Human Impacts on Leaf Economics in Heterogeneous Landscapes: The Effect of Harvesting Non-Timber Forest Products from African Mahogany across Habitats and Climates." *Journal of Applied Ecology* 48 (4): 844–52. https://doi.org/10.1111/j.1365-2664.2011.01977.x.

Garner, Brittany A., Sean Hoban, and Gordon Luikart. 2020. "IUCN Red List and the Value of Integrating Genetics." *Conservation Genetics* 21 (5): 795–801. https://doi.org/10.1007/s10592-020-01301-6.

Gates, Bronwen. 1982. "Banisteriopsis, Diplopterys (Malpighiaceae) Author." *Flora Neotropica* 30: 1–237.

Gorenflo, L. J., Suzanne Romaine, Russell A. Mittermeier, and Kristen Walker-Painemilla. 2012. "Co-Occurrence of Linguistic and Biological Diversity in Biodiversity Hotspots and High Biodiversity Wilderness Areas." *Proceedings of the National Academy of Sciences of the United States of America* 109 (21): 8032–37. https://doi.org/10.1073/pnas.1117511109.

Grob, Charles S., Dennis J. McKenna, James C. Callaway, Glacus S. Brito, Edison S. Neves, Guilherme Oberlaender, Oswaldo L. Saide, et al. 1996. "Human Psychopharmacology of Hoasca, a Plant Hallucinogen Used in Ritual Context in Brazil." *Journal of Nervous and Mental Disease* 184 (2): 86–94. https://doi.org/10.1097/00005053-199602000-00004.

Guadagnin, Demetrio Luis, and Isabel Cristina Gravato. 2013. "Ethnobotany, Availability, and Use of Lianas by the Kaingang People in Suburban Forests in Southern Brazil." *Economic Botany* 67 (4): 350–62. https://doi.org/10.1007/s12231-013-9249-0.

Haridas, C. V., and Shripad Tuljapurkar. 2007. "Time, Transients and Elasticity." *Ecology Letters* 10 (12): 1143–53. https://doi.org/10.1111/j.1461-0248.2007.01108.x.

Hoffman, Bruce, and Timothy Gallaher. 2007. "Importance Indices in Ethnobotany." *Ethnobotany Research and Applications* 5 (December): 201–18.

Honnay, Olivier, and Beatrijs Bossuyt. 2005. "Prolonged Clonal Growth: Escape Route or Route to Extinction?" Oikos 108 (2): 427–32. https://doi.org/10.1111/j.0030-1299.2005.13569.x.

Hurrell, Julio Alberto, and Ulysses Paulino Albuquerque. 2012. "Is Ethnobotany an Ecological Science ? Steps towards a Complex Ethnobotany." *Ethnobiology and Conservation* 1 (4): 1–16.

Koons, David N., James B. Grand, Bertram Zinner, and Robert F. Rockwell. 2005. "Transient Population Dynamics: Relations to Life History and Initial Population State." *Ecological Modelling* 185 (2–4): 283–97. https://doi.org/10.1016/j.ecolmodel.2004.12.011.

Kroon, Hans De, Jan Van Groenendael, and Johan Ehrlén. 2000. "Elasticities: A Review of Methods and Model Limitations." *Ecology* 81 (3): 607–18.

Kuypers, K. P.C., J. Riba, M. de la Fuente Revenga, S. Barker, E. L. Theunissen, and J. G. Ramaekers. 2016. "Ayahuasca Enhances Creative Divergent Thinking While Decreasing Conventional Convergent Thinking." *Psychopharmacology* 233 (18): 3395–3403. https://doi.org/10.1007/s00213-016-4377-8.

Ledo, Alicia, and Stefan A. Schnitzer. 2014. "Disturbance and Clonal Reproduction Determine Liana Distribution and Maintain Liana Diversity in a Tropical Forest." *Ecology* 95 (8): 2169–78. https://doi.org/10.1890/13-1775.1.

Luna, Luis Eduardo., and Steven F. White. 2017. *Ayahuasca Reader: Encounters with the Amazon's Sacred Vine.* Synergetic Press.

Luna, Luis Eduardo. 1984a. "The Concept of Plants as Teachers among Four Mestizo Shamans of Iquitos, Northeastern Peru." *Journal of Ethnopharmacology* 11 (2): 135–56. https://doi.org/10.1016/0378-8741(84)90036-9.

Luna, Luis Eduardo. 1984b. "The Healing Practices of a Peruvian Shaman." *Ethnopharmacology* 11 (2): 123–33.

Luna, Luis Eduardo. 1986. *Vegetalismo: Shamanism among the Mestizo Population of the Peruvian Amazon*. Almqvist & Wiksell International.

Maffi, Luisa. 2002. "Endangered Languages, Endangered Knowledge." *International Social Science Journal* 54 (173): 385–93. https://doi.org/10.1111/1468-2451.00390.

Maffi, Luisa. 2005. "Linguistic, Cultural, and Biological Diversity." *Annual Review of Anthropology* 34 (1): 599–617. https://doi.org/10.1146/annurev.anthro.34.081804.120437.

McKenna, Dennis J. 2004. "Clinical Investigations of the Therapeutic Potential of Ayahuasca: Rationale and Regulatory Challenges." *Pharmacology and Therapeutics* 102 (2): 111–29. https://doi.org/10.1016/j.pharmthera.2004.03.002.

McKenna, Dennis J. 2005. "Ayahuasca and Human Destiny." *Journal of Psychoactive Drugs* 37 (2): 231–34. https://doi.org/10.1080/02791072.2005.10399805.

McKenna, Dennis J., Luis Eduardo Luna, and George H. N. Towers. 1995. "Biodynamic Constituents in Ayahuasca Admixture Plants: An Uninvestigated Folk Pharmacopoeia." In *Ethnobotany: Evolution of a Discipline*, 349–61.

McKenna, Dennis J., and Jordi Riba. 2016. "New World Tryptamine Hallucinogens and the Neuroscience of Ayahuasca." In *Behavioral Neurobiology of Psychedelic Drugs*, 283–311. Springer, Berlin, Heidelberg. https://doi.org/10.1007/7854.

Morales-García, Jose A., Mario De La Fuente Revenga, Sandra Alonso-Gil, María Isabel Rodríguez-Franco, Amanda

Feilding, Ana Perez-Castillo, and Jordi Riba. 2017. "The Alkaloids of *Banisteriopsis Caapi*, the Plant Source of the Amazonian Hallucinogen Ayahuasca, Stimulate Adult Neurogenesis in Vitro." *Scientific Reports* 7 (1): 1–13. https://doi.org/10.1038/s41598-017-05407-9.

Narby, Jeremy, and Rafael Chanchari Pizuri. 2021. *Plant Teachers: Ayahuasca, Tobacco, and the Pursuit of Knowledge*. New World Library.

Oliveira, Regina Célia de, Júlia Sonsin-Oliveira, Thaís Aparecida Coelho dos Santos, Marcelo Simas e Silva, Christopher William Fagg, and Renata Sebastiani. 2021. "Lectotypification of *Banisteriopsis Caapi* and B. Quitensis (Malpighiaceae), Names Associated with an Important Ingredient of Ayahuasca." *Taxon* 70 (1): 185–88. https://doi.org/10.1002/tax.12407.

Osório, Flávia L. de, Rafael F. Sanches, Ligia R. Macedo, Rafael G. dos Santos, João P. Maia-De-Oliveira, Lauro Wichert-Ana, Draulio B. de Araujo, Jordi Riba, José A. Crippa, and Jaime E. Hallak. 2015. "Antidepressant Effects of a Single Dose of Ayahuasca in Patients with Recurrent Depression: A Preliminary Report." *Revista Brasileira de Psiquiatria* 37 (1): 13–20. https://doi.org/10.1590/1516-4446-2014-1496.

Phillips, Oliver, and Alwyn H. Gentry. 1993. "The Useful Plants of Tambopata, Peru: I. Statistical Hypotheses Tests with a New Quantitative Technique." *Economic Botany* 47 (1): 15–32.

Phillips, Oliver, Rodolfo Vésquez Martínez, Luzmila Arroyo, Timothy R. Baker, Timothy Killeen, Simon L. Lewis, Yadvinder Malhi, et al. 2002. "Increasing Dominance of Large Lianas in Amazonian Forests." *Nature* 418 (6899): 770–74. https://doi.org/10.1038/nature00926.

Pinard, Michelle. 1993. "Impacts of Stem Harvesting on Populations of Iriartea Deltoidea (Palmae) in an Extractive Reserve in Acre , Brazil." *Biotropica* 25 (1): 2–14.

Pretty, Jules, Bill Adams, Fikret Berkes, Simone Ferreira De Athayde, Nigel Dudley, Eugene Hunn, Luisa Maffi, et al. 2009. "The Intersections of Biological Diversity and Cultural Diversity: Towards Integration." *Conservation and Society* 7 (2): 100–112. https://doi.org/10.4103/0972-4923.58642.

Quiroz, Diana, and Tinde van Andel. 2015. "Evidence of a Link between Taboos and Sacrifices and Resource Scarcity of Ritual Plants." *Journal of Ethnobiology and Ethnomedicine* 11 (1). https://doi.org/10.1186/1746-4269-11-5.

R Development Core Team. 2019. "R: A Language and Environment for Statistical Computing." http://www.r-project.org.

Rees, Mark, and Stephen P. Ellner. 2009. "Integral Projection Models for Populations in Temporally Varying Environments." *Ecological Society of America* 79 (4): 575–94.

Reichel-Dolmatoff, Gerardo. 1971. *Amazonian Cosmos: The Sexual and Religious Symbolism of the Tukano Indians*. University of Chicago Press.

Sampaio, Maurício Bonesso, and Flavio Antonio Maës dos Santos. 2015. "Harvesting of Palm Fruits Can Be Ecologically Sustainable: A Case of Buriti (Mauritia Flexuosa; Arecaceae) in Central Brazil." In *Ecological Sustainability for Non-Timber Forest Products*, 87–103. Routledge.

Santos, Beatriz Werneck Lopes, Regina Célia de Oliveira, Julia Sonsin-Oliveira, Christopher William Fagg, José Beethoven Figueiredo Barbosa, and Eloisa Dutra Caldas. 2020. "Biodiversity of β-Carboline Profile of *Banisteriopsis Caapi* and Ayahuasca, a Plant and a Brew with Neuropharmacological Potential." *Plants* 9 (7): 1–14. https://doi.org/10.3390/plants9070870.

Schmidt, Isabel B., Isabel B. Figueiredo, and Tamara Ticktin. 2015. "Sustainability of Golden Grass Flower Stalk Harvesting in the Brazilian Savanna." In *Ecological Sustainability for Non-Timber Forest Products: Dynamics and Case Studies of Harvesting*, 199–214. Routledge.

Schmidt, Isabel B., Lisa Mandle, Tamara Ticktin, and Orou G. Gaoue. 2011. "What Do Matrix Population Models Reveal about the Sustainability of Non-Timber Forest Product Harvest?" *Journal of Applied Ecology* 48 (4): 815–26. https://doi.org/10.1111/j.1365-2664.2011.01999.x.

Schnitzer, Stefan A. 2015. "The Contribution of Lianas to Forest Ecology, Diversity, and Dynamics." In *Biodiversity of Lianas*, 149–60. Springer, Cham.

Schnitzer, Stefan A., Geertje Van Der Heijden, Joseph Mascaro, and Walter P. Carson. 2014. "Lianas in Gaps Reduce Carbon Accumulation in a Tropical Forest." *Ecology* 95 (11): 3008–17. https://doi.org/10.1890/13-1718.1.

Schnitzer, Stefan A., Suzanne Rutishauser, and Salomón Aguilar. 2008. "Supplemental Protocol for Liana Censuses." *Forest Ecology and Management* 255 (3–4): 1044–49. https://doi.org/10.1016/j.foreco.2007.10.012.

Schnitzer, Stefan A, and Frans Bongers. 2002. "The Ecology of Lianas and Their Role in Forests." *Trends in Ecology & Evolution* 17 (5): 223–30.

Schultes, Richard Evans, Albert Hofmann, and Christian Rätsch. 2001. *Plants of the Gods: Their Sacred, Healing, and Hallucinogenic Powers*. Rochester, VT: Healing Arts Press,.

Silvertown, Jonathan, Miguel Franco, Irene Pisanty, and Ana Mendoza. 1993. "Comparative Plant Demography—Relative Importance of Life-Cycle Components to the Finite Rate of Increase in Woody and Herbaceous Perennials." *The Journal of Ecology* 81 (3): 465. https://doi.org/10.2307/2261525.

Stott, Iain, Stuart Townley, and David James Hodgson. 2011. "A Framework for Studying Transient Dynamics of Population Projection Matrix Models." *Ecology Letters* 14 (9): 959–70. https://doi.org/10.1111/j.1461-0248.2011.01659.x.

Stubben, Chris, and Brook Milligan. 2007. "Estimating and Analyzing Demographic Models." *Journal Of Statistical Software* 22 (11): 1–23. https://doi.org/10.18637/jss.v022.i11"https://doi.org/10.18637/jss.v022.i11.

Suárez Álvarez, Carlos and Jerónimo Mazarrasa. 2023. International Center for Ethnobotanical Education, Research and Service (ICEERS) Executive Summary: Global Ayahuasca Consumption & Reported Deaths. 1-24

Thevenin, Julien Marius Reis, and Regina Helena Rosa Sambuichi. 2020. "Phytogeography and Floristics of the Arbor Component in União Do Vegetal Territories Intended for the Cultivation of *Banisteriopsis Caapi* and *Psychotria Viridis* in Rondônia." *RAEGA—O Espaco Geografico Em Analise* 49: 42–63. https://doi.org/10.5380/raega.v49i0.67208.

Ticktin, Tamara. 2004. "The Ecological Implications of Harvesting Non-Timber Forest Products." *Journal of Applied Ecology* 41 (1): 11–21. https://doi.org/10.1111/j.1365-2664.2004.00859.x.

Torres, Constantino Manuel, and S. M. Fitzpatrick. 2018. "The Origins of the Ayahuasca/Yagé Concept: An Inquiry into the Synergy between Dimethyltryptamine and Beta-Carbolines." In *Ancient Psychoactive Substances. Scott Fitzpatrick, Ed.*, 234–64. Gainesville: University Press of Florida.

Tupper, KW. 2009. "Ayahuasca Healing beyond the Amazon: The Globalization of a Traditional Indigenous Entheogenic Practice." *Global Networks: A Journal of Transnational Affairs* 9 (1): 117–36.

Turner, Nancy J., Marianne Boelscher Ignace, and Ronald Ignace. 2000. "Traditional Ecological Knowledge and Wisdom of Aboriginal Peoples in British Columbia." *Ecological Society of America* 10 (5): 1275–87.

Vandebroek, Ina, Andrea Pieroni, John Richard Stepp, Natalia Hanazaki, Ana Ladio, Rômulo Romeu Nóbrega Alves, David Picking, et al. 2020. "Reshaping the Future of Ethnobiology Research after the COVID-19 Pandemic." *Nature Plants* 6 (7): 723–30. https://doi.org/10.1038/s41477-020-0691-6.

Vogado, Nara O., Jayden E. Engert, Tore L. Linde, Mason J. Campbell, William F. Laurance, and Michael J. Liddell. 2022. "Climate Change Affects Reproductive Phenology in Lianas of Australia's Wet Tropics." *Frontiers in Forests and Global Change* 5 (June): 1–11. https://doi.org/10.3389/ffgc.2022.787950.

Winkelman, Michael. 2005. "Drug Tourism or Spiritual Healing? Ayahuasca Seekers in Amazonia." *Journal of Psychoactive Drugs* 37 (2): 209–18. https://doi.org/10.1080/02791072.2005.10399803.

Wong, Tamara M, and Tamara Ticktin. 2015. "Using Population Dynamics Modelling to Evaluate Potential Success of Restoration: A Case Study of a Hawaiian Vine in a Changing Climate." *Environmental Conservation* 42 (1): 20–30.

Zapata, Thirza Ruiz, and Mary T. Kalin Arroyo. 1978. "Plant Reproductive Ecology of a Secondary Deciduous Tropical Forest in Venezuela." *Biotropica* 10 (1): 221–30.

Sociosphere

Psychoactive Substances, Institutions, Law & Policy

Integration of Ceremonial Plant Practices Outside the Countries of Origin: Blessing or Curse?

Jerónimo Mazarrasa

Social Innovation Director for ICEERS | Founding member of Plantaforma (Platform for the Defense of Ayahuasca in Spain)

> *"There simply aren't enough plants, shamans, payés, taitas, padrinhos and mestres in all of the jungle to attend to all the people all over the world who could potentially want to seek healing from ayahuasca, to name just one sacred medicine that is under pressure."*
>
> —Jerónimo Mazarrasa

This essay is a thought piece on the integration of ceremonial plant practices outside of the countries of origin, and what lessons they might bring to today's psychedelic science.

What I am about to describe are the results of a 20-year reflection on ceremonial plant use, particularly ayahuasca, outside of its countries of origin.* The encounter between traditional indigenous medicines and Western societies is a complex topic. In this piece, I won't attempt to list or establish objective facts. Instead, I will try to arrive at a certain *truth* or essence that seems to stand beneath things. To do this, I'll be using stories, metaphors, and polarities. These tools, which are much older than the scientific method, don't provide accurate descriptions of reality. Rather, they are simplifications that can help us hold complex realities and think about them from different perspectives, knowing that one should never confuse the map with the territory.

I will start with a story. I've been told that it reappears in different shapes in many cultures, and yet, like all proper myths, it is always current and always true.

At the beginning of time, at the time of the First People, the Gods gave the People a Gift. This Gift was very powerful, but it came with a catch. It was neither good nor bad; it could be either, depending on the relationship that the people established with the gift. If the gift was

---

* This paper focuses on the integration of ceremonial plant practices outside of the countries of origin, due to space considerations doesn't address the essential discussion of this how affects the cultures of origin themselves. The paper "When Your Friends are the Problem: Plant Medicines, Commercialization, and Biocultural Conservation" by Andrea Langlois and I, in this ESPD55 edition tackles these issues and should be regarded as complementary to this paper.

approached with reverence and wisdom, it would bestow great blessings on the people. If the gift was approached with disrespect or with ignorance, the Gift would turn into a curse causing great harm and destruction.

The Gift was an open possibility, even a test, a sort of mirror, that reflected back and amplified whatever was put in front of it, good or bad, wise or ignorant.

What was the Gift? That changes in different versions of the myth, it could be fire in all its forms, or it could be the combustion engine or nuclear power. The Gift could also be artificial intelligence. It could also be the coca plant, tobacco, ayahuasca or any other sacred plant. Each of them could be a blessing or a curse.

This myth is, of course, a metaphor for all powerful things. Fire, considered the first technology, can be a blessing or a curse depending on whether it is used to prepare a nourishing meal, or to destroy a forest. Medicines are another type of technology where the same tension applies. This is clearly embodied in the Greek word *pharmakon*, which means both *medicine and poison*. Not one or the other, but both, medicine *and* poison, the same word for both things. The Greeks seemed to know something we often forget. There is no difference between medicines and poisons, it's a matter of dosage. All medicines can kill if the dose is high enough. It only takes a couple of boxes of aspirin to create an ulcer that goes on to be lethal. At the same time, most poisons can be medicinal if the dose is low enough. Chemo and radio therapies for cancer are examples of poisons we use to treat illness.

The myth of the Gift is more than a metaphor about certain technologies; it speaks to us about a certain truth, not just about powerful things, but about the types of relationships that we establish with them. It does so by presenting us with a polarity: Will it be a blessing or a curse? The answer will depend on us.

This polarity is a good lens through which to think about many things—medicines, power, relationships, life. It's a good map, but it's not the truth. Life is not either/or. Life is a continuum where parts of the blessing and parts of the curse are always present in some measure. This myth helps us think about things that in reality are not black or white, but stand in the broad continuum of grays between them.

With that said, I want to bring us back to ethnobotanicals, to look at them through this metaphor.

Tobacco is the king of American shamanic inebriants. It is widely used all over North and South America. It is smoked, inhaled, drunk, licked, chewed. In the Indigenous cultures where it's used, it's considered a medicine and a teacher, a living being and a spirit. Tobacco teaches strength, it teaches wisdom, it teaches clarity. It's a tool for prayer, and helps humans live better. Like the Makuna educator Maximiliano Garcia said: "Tobacco is the very essence of life, it is like the sensitivity that exists within a human body, which enables us to better understand, to accept things with wisdom, to reject things with wisdom, and to be able to live better in the territory".* In Indigenous cultures, tobacco has largely been a blessing. Yet, in the 500 years since Europeans

* UNESCO. "Traditional Knowledge of the Jaguar Shamans of Yuruparí," November 22, 2011. 4:15 to 4:27, http://about:blank"https://www.youtube.com/watch?v=CqWoosEGy2Q

first came into contact with tobacco, it has become the leading cause of preventable death worldwide. How did we get here?

Indigenous people would say that we didn't respect tobacco, or the spirit of tobacco. That we treated it not as living being, but as a thing, or rather, as a *product*; we disrespected tobacco, and it took revenge on us. It became a curse rather than a blessing—a poison instead of a medicine.

A similar case is the coca plant. For the cultures that have had the longest relationships with coca it is the leaf of life, a superfood, a tool for social cohesion, a blessing. The entire structure of the Kogi, Makuna or Huitoto cultures, not to mention the Incas, is impossible to understand without the role that coca plays. When we look at Colombia's Kogi, the Yurupari cultures of the Vaupés, or the Huitoto *mambeadero*,* we find a plant that is loved and respected. It is a plant with more calcium than cow's milk, and a plant that gives strength when one is tired and at high altitudes. In community gatherings coca gives the ability to listen intently, and to speak calmly. It is the fuel that feeds community consensus. In each of these societies, coca acts as a scaffolding around which the culture is not just held, but regularly renewed.†

When the West encountered coca, after an initial romance, we sought to ban it, and then we split into two halves. One half was cocaine, the other half was decocainized coca (leaf extract without the cocaine), which is still the secret in the secret formula of Coca Cola. Split into two halves, as cocaine or Coca Cola, the coca plant took over the world. Coca Cola is "the most-recognized brand in human history" (Elmore, 2014). Today, one can find legal Coca Cola and illegal cocaine in every country in the world. But instead of a blessing, this divided coca plant is mostly a curse for us. Rather than a superfood, Coca Cola is junk food—it rots teeth, and degrades health. And, instead of a tool for social cohesion, cocaine generally erodes our social fabric. It brings corruption, violence, and suffering. The horrors that surround cocaine's production and distribution are endless. Even a cursory look at its most "glamorous" side, the most opulent cocaine parties of the West, we find the opposite of social cohesion. We see a group of people where everyone is talking, and nobody is listening. It is almost a caricature, an inversion, of what happens in the *mambeaderos* and *casas de palabra* of Indigenous communities where individuals take turns to speak while everyone listens. Every aspect of the West's relationship with the coca plant has turned into a terrible curse. Even attempts to eradicate it through nonsensical glyphosate-spraying planes have brought nothing but terrible toxic pollution, and now a unique breed of glyphosate-resistant coca plants (Davis, 2004). Now, every sprayed plant dies, except the coca!

How did we bring this curse onto ourselves? We know what Indigenous people might say .‡

---

* Mambe is "Coca powder that is obtained after roasting, grinding, and sifting process out of coca leaves and ashes, which has healing and nutritional properties, in addition to the sacred power that is granted to it by the Colombian indigenous people", "What Is Mambe | IGI Global". Accessed April 20th, 2023 https://www.igi-global.com/dictionary/mambe/81820

† To learn more about coca see the papers "The therapeutic potential of coca" by Dr Andrew Weil and "Coca: The Divine Leaf of Immortality" by Professor Wade Davis in this ESPD55 edition.

‡ Kogi mamo Jacinto Zarabata does an excellent job commenting on this topic in this video. Arwikoka. "¿Por Qué Atentan Contra La Coca?," May 17, 2011. Accessed April 20th, 2023, https://www.youtube.com/watch?v=BrIzQKbPF_4.

CUSTOMS VS PRODUCTS

What stands out in the stories of tobacco and coca is that although the plants are the same, our relationship to them can be very different from the cultures from which they originate. For example, we normally would say "the way these plants are used is very different," and even that verb, *to use*, expresses something powerful about how we relate to these plants.

Shamanic relationships to tobacco have to do with accessing certain realms of knowledge, with healing, with renewing the culture and building social cohesion in collective rituals. Similarly, coca is chewed as a source of nourishment, as a tool for being more productive at work, and as fuel to build community consensus. There is a particular set of customs associated with these relationships, and these customs mostly revolve around increasing personal and collective well-being.

On the other hand, the use of tobacco and coca that has evolved in the West is very different. Although they also include some customs and rituals, the uses are mostly to do with consumption, with individual satisfaction, with escape, and with the buzz and rush of personal desire. Almost no medicinal, healing, or spiritual activity in the West has included tobacco or coca. Even though both tobacco and coca first entered Western countries as medicines, they have not ended up as such.

I'm speaking in polarities because it is a useful lens, not because they are absolute truths. We can also find examples of negative, individualistic, destructive relationships to tobacco and coca in Indigenous communities, and we could probably find some positive, prosocial examples of tobacco and coca use in Western contexts. This is not about establishing a polarity as crude as "all traditional use is cultural and good", and "all Western use is commercial and bad". Instead, I'm trying to point out a contrast, which is real, and can be quite stark, in the way the same plants can be medicines or poisons in different cultures. The same plants can be a blessing or a curse, or tools for liberation or enslavement. They can be a scaffolding for building cultures, or solvents that will undermine people and weaken communities. This is the Gift from the Gods that the myth points to.

Another way to look at this particular issue is to think of it in terms of customs vs products. What happens when a psychoactive plant is stripped of its custom, and becomes a product for another culture? The myth states that the harms go up and the benefits go down. We get more of the curse, instead of the blessing.

PROHIBITION

Many of my anti-prohibitionist peers would quickly point out that the violence, corruption, and toxic poisoning associated with the cocaine trade are the results of a wrong-headed drug war. I agree with them. However, I cannot help but notice that at least two of the curses that I've discussed—Coca-Cola and tobacco—are fully legal, regulated products, and this hasn't been enough to make our use of them anywhere near as beneficial as the traditional use seems to be.

So, prohibition and the war on drugs are a terrible problem, have had terrible consequences, and need to stop. But the curse seems to hold, whether they are prohibited or legalized. It might well be that in a post-prohibition world many of the curses would still be present in the now-legal coca products, like many of the curses are present today in our legal tobacco. I do not believe

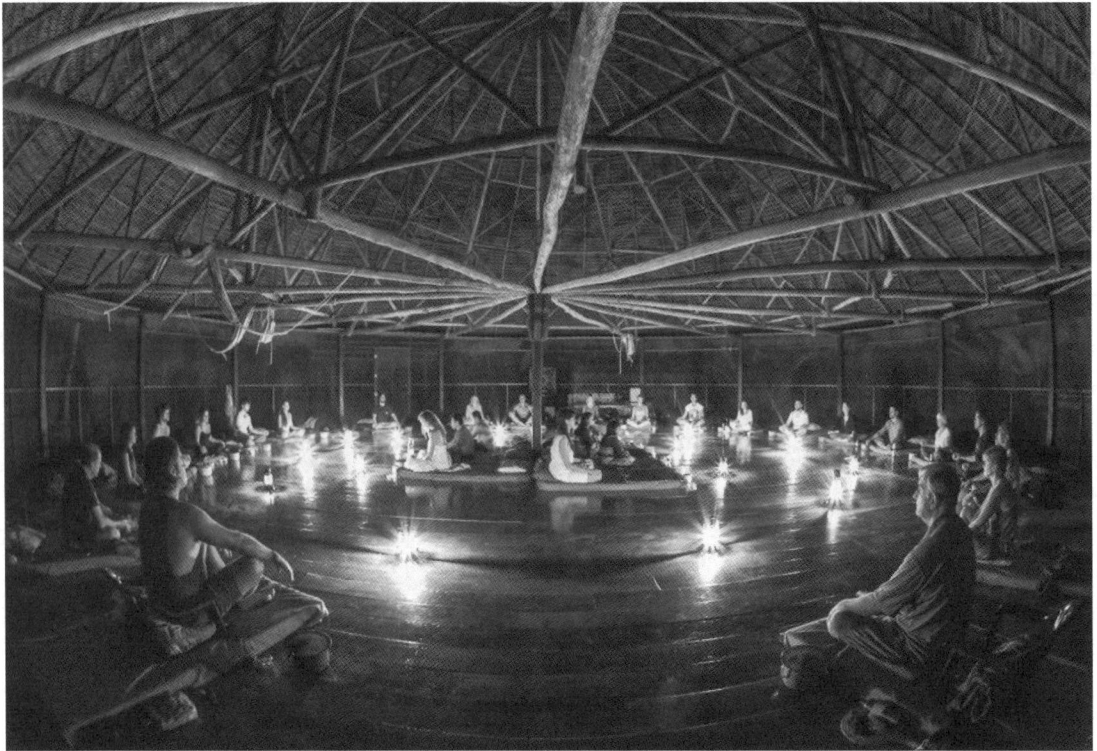

Fig.1 Temple of the way of light: Ayahuasca healing retreat center ©.

ending prohibition would be the end of all our problems with psychoactive plants, only the end of the problems directly related to prohibition.

Ethan Nadelmann says that "if one wants to imagine what a future capitalist industry of recreational drugs could look like in a post-prohibition world one only has to look at the current food industry, and their fully legal but still predatory practices" (Quinones, 2022). Our food is legally laced with additives, sugar, fats, and flavor enhancers in order to increase consumption and raise benefits. It is the nature of evolved capitalism to grow by trying to sell us more. When we add powerful substances, legal or not, to the mix, we see the emergence of perverse dynamics that are poison to people and communities, but still make sense from a business profit perspective. The recent opioid crisis in the US is an example of how a fully legal, fully regulated, pharmaceutical company (Purdue) can lose its way, when blinded by the incredible profits that stand on the other side.

But let's get back to the plants.

THE CASE OF AYAHUASCA

Figure 1 is a photo of an ayahuasca ceremony. Is it taking place in Peru or 20 kilometers from where you are? If it were not for the wooden roof of the maloca, it may be hard to tell—and this is precisely the point. In a Western ayahuasca ceremony, a group gathers to drink ayahuasca, while guided by people who have more experience and training, who gauge the dose, and are responsible for what happens to everybody during the night. These people will perform some sort of ceremonial act that contains, accompanies and modulates the experience of the participants and usually music is a part of it. If we were to describe a traditional Amazonian ayahuasca ceremony, understanding the term "traditional" widely, from Indigenous use to the Brazilian ayahuasca religions, every one of the things I mentioned, from a guide who gauges the dose to the presence of a ceremonial act, would be the same.

There is something very particular, even historical, happening in the West that is not obvious at first sight. In the past 500 years many sacred plants from the Americas have gone global. I've described the examples of tobacco and coca, but there's also Maria Sabina's sacred mushrooms, Peyote, San Pedro, and even cocoa. Not once in those 500 years did the way the West related to these plants resemble the original uses... not until ayahuasca. Ceremonial ayahuasca use marks the first time in this 500-year history that a sacred plant has traveled outside the Americas with some of its associated ritual still attached. Ayahuasca is mostly arriving to the West as a custom.

Again, I want to be careful with polarities or exaggerations. Western ayahuasca circles are in many ways different from traditional Amazonian rituals. Yet, there is a certain essence, a skeleton if you will, of the Amazonian practices that is still recognizable. There is something in the way that ayahuasca is being globalized that reaches back to the original cultures. Through this, by staying connected to the original customs, I'd argue that we're managing to stay a little bit closer to the blessing and a little bit further from the curse that we have seen with the other psychoactive plants that left the Americas.

So, on the one hand we have a long 500-year history of Amerindian sacred plants being put to mediocre (or appalling) use by Western societies. On the other hand, we seem to be facing an opportunity, a break in the 500-year-old pattern, in the form of what's happening with ceremonial ayahuasca use in the West.

What will the future of ayahuasca outside of the Amazon look like? I've been engaged with this question for the better part of a decade, and it's something I've been actively working on as leader of a project within ICEERS.* This project engages diverse ceremonial plant communities worldwide to co-create a detailed vision of the future integration of ayahuasca practices outside of the countries of origin

To think about the future integration of psychedelics into our societies is to try to imagine something that has never happened. One way that futurists and other experts approach the problem of how to imagine something that has not happened yet is by creating a range of possible future scenarios. I will present two possible models of the future of psychedelics.

---

* ICEERS is The International Center for Ethnobotanical Education, Research, and Service. A non-profit organization dedicated to transforming society's relationship with psychoactive plants. They do this by engaging with some of the fundamental issues resulting from the globalization of ayahuasca, iboga, and other ethnobotanicals. "Our vision is that of a future where these practices are integrated and valued parts of society—where every individual and each community is granted the right to pursue healing and self-empowerment, where indigenous cultures are respected, and where bridges are built between traditional knowledge and science." More information can be found at www.iceers.org.

They embody yet another polarity, one that is already present today. They highlight the tension between the medicalized use model and the community practices model.

A FUTURE MODEL FOR THE MEDICALIZATION PATH

Imagine a large space with many small cubicles. In each of them there is a bed. In that bed there is a person laying down. Each of them has been given a pharmaceutical psychedelic. They have a mask over their eyes and headphones over their ears. A number of sensors measure several biomarkers, and this data is fed in real time to an artificial intelligence program that keeps track of the patient's state. Another AI uses some of that data to generate a customized musical playlist that will adapt to the patient's emotions. Individuals are alone in their cubicles as they experience the effects of the psychedelic, they're being watched over by the AI program. They are also being monitored through a camera that connects to a control room where a few humans are looking at hundreds of video feeds. When somebody is beginning to have a difficult time, an alarm goes off and an intervention team is activated who inject, with minimum physical contact, an antidote to immediately bring the psychedelic experience to an end. When the person comes out of the experience, after a quick check up, they will go back home on the same day.

In the following weeks, an AI chatbot on their phone provides follow-up and integration. It will ask: "How do you feel?" It will do this several times a day. This lets machines track the patient's state, using a variety of data sources, the app polling, the chatbot, phone health measures, etc. When people seem to be having some trouble integrating the experience, another alarm will light up and this will trigger additional interventions, some involving people.

A version of this model, individualized, medicalized, built for scale, light on people and heavily reliant on technology, is already on its way. There are many startups developing all the technologies I have described, from the automated playlists to the mobile phone-based AI tracking and integration. They argue, and it might be true, that this is the only economically feasible way to integrate psychedelics into existing healthcare systems. Since psychedelic experiences (and their integration) are long, and both human presence and human care are among the costliest expenses of any business, the logical solution is to try to do as much as possible with machines instead of humans.

I think the existence in the future of something resembling this vision is pretty much inevitable. It is the obvious end point of our current business logic. Certainly, the psychedelic medicine of the future will also include offerings that are much more luxurious, classy, and full of human attention ...available to those who can afford it. My point is that if one looks at the models emerging from today's psychedelic industry, we can see a linear progression to what tomorrow's psychedelic medicine will look like. It will look like today's healthcare industry, plus a psychedelic offering.

A FUTURE MODEL FOR THE COMMUNITY SPACES PATH

Now let's imagine a different space, a community space, or rather a set of spaces, because community practices are as diverse as communities themselves. Some of these spaces will be in cities; some will be in nature. Some spaces will be as small as someone's apartment; some will be as large as a temple. The activities that will take place in these spaces will also be diverse. Some activities could be called therapeutic, but the space will not be a clinic- not exactly. Some activities could be called spiritual or religious, but the space will not always be a church- not exactly. Some spaces will have activities that could be called "education for adults", but the curriculum will be neither academic nor technical. Instead, people will be learning something that's closer to "How to Live". How to live with themselves, with each other, with their community, and with the world at large. Most of these spaces will offer a combination of all three aspects, therapeutic, spiritual and educational, in different degrees.

People will go to these community spaces when their lives are getting complicated or confusing, when they need a break, or clarity, or wayfinding. None of these reasons are necessarily medical conditions, that's why these places are not medical clinics. Yet, these are the main reasons why psychedelics have historically been used by humans. Reasons closer to what happens in the transition between life stages, when we have to let go of something, when we give birth to something, when something is stuck, when we need to grow, or repair something that was damaged, usually a connection, with ourselves, our lives, each other, with our culture, or the world at large. These are spaces of reconciliation.

Ceremonial plant practices will be part of many of these reconciliations, but the plants are just a part of it, because what are underlying these spaces are *relationships*. The key is not just that people are having a psychedelic experience, but rather that people are being held by other people as they undergo a transformation. Because life evolves through difficult times by strong relationships, and even the powerful transformative experiences that we can have as individuals need to be witnessed and sustained by others in order to be fully active. Individual transformation is very difficult in isolation, we need support from the environment, we need accountability, witnessing and community validation. So, what is being renewed in these spaces is not just individuals, but communities, and tapestries of human relationships.

THE PSYCHEDELIC RENAISSANCE AND THE PSYCHEDELIC ENLIGHTENMENT

So, these are the pieces of the puzzle. A Gift from the Gods stands before us. We have seen that in the societies of origin, these plants, from tobacco to coca to ayahuasca, serve very much as a blessing, not just for personal self-actualization, but also for collective or cultural self-actualization. Yet historically when those same plants, from tobacco to coca, arrived on our shores, they became more of a curse than a blessing. Prohibition has been part of the problem, but it is not the whole problem. Today's medicalization might be a necessary step forward, but it is not a complete solution, for it integrates these substances by amputating a large part of their value. Psychedelics are much more than new psychiatric medicines for our old mental health crisis. Historically, most people who have benefitted from them did not have something that our doctors today would qualify as a medical pathology. They were working on personal growth, on existential and relational issues, on meaning, on spirituality, on life choices. Are they going to be denied access? Will most of today's users need to be diagnosed with a pathology in order to legally access these substances in the future? Or worse, will life transitions now become pathologies so that medication can be prescribed for them? And, as prescription psychedelic medicines become the sole realm of medical professionals, what will happen to the traditional practitioners that do not have a medical degree but thousands of years of accumulated empirical knowledge instead? Will they now be prosecuted for practicing medicine without a license?

The last piece in this puzzle is that none of this is written in stone, what happened in the past does not need to happen in the future. This is exemplified by something unique, an exception, a singularity, that seems to be happening around ceremonial ayahuasca practices outside of the countries of origin. It shows us that it is possible for Western societies to break the 500-year-old pattern and to develop a relationship to traditional indigenous medicines that is significantly different from the ones of the past.

As we look towards the future we face another polarity, two models- one is the medicalization track. It's been called the psychedelic renaissance. It is well on its way to become a reality, and billions have already been invested in this industry. There will be psychedelic clinics in the not-so-distant future. Some, especially the most affordable ones, will have many of the features I presented above. It is almost certain that some version of this model will come to be.

So, what to do with this Gift? I would like to close with three antidotes, three stories that can serve as a starting point for people of Western cultures, particularly western biomedical cultures, to begin to understand what it is that we don't know (or we have forgotten) about working with these powerful medicines, so that they can become a blessing and not a curse. Each antidote is a parable, a story that ends with a lesson.

CUSTOMS VS PRODUCTS: THINKING IN TERMS OF SPACES

The first story is the story of coffeehouse. We imagine coffee as a product. Coffee beans toasted, ground, roasted, packed. Coffee is the fuel that moves of our working world. It is the second most traded commodity after oil. When Europeans started using coffee a cultural revolution followed, but the revolution was not in the product itself; rather, it was in the arrival of a new space and a new custom: the coffeehouse. A revolutionary new social space where people could not only drink coffee, but read newspapers and books for free, discuss ideas and engage in horizontal debates while invigorated by caffeine. In the 1700s in Oxford, coffeehouses were known as "penny universities" because for the cost of a cup of coffee one could listen to and participate in some of the most avant-garde intellectual discussions of the day. Coffeehouses brought a new custom, which opened a space of possibility that went on to became ground zero for a number of revolutionary cultural changes. The modern newspaper industry, the French Revolution, and other tectonic shifts in the last 400 years of Western culture, science and politics are unthinkable without the coffeehouse.

When cannabis activists in the Netherlands engaged the government in the 70s it was not around the cannabis plant, but around the toleration of a space. From this the coffeeshop was born, where cannabis would not only be sold but consumed. Staff could screen customers by age, educate them on cannabis varieties and effects, and oversee customers. People who had too much could be helped and given support. My point is that the Dutch administration tolerated (never fully legalized) a *space,* the coffeeshop, not just a product, cannabis.

I could name many examples from traditional cultures, from the Moroccan teahouses where Kif was smoked, to the Amazonian mambeaderos. This shows that adequate spaces foster relationships, create new customs, and this tends to maximize the benefits and minimize the harms of any substance. What is the difference between drinking in a pub and alone at home? which is more dangerous? which is less harmful? (let's skip the drinking and driving part for now). And, if the act of drinking is generally safer in a pub than drinking alone at home, then why does the current wave of cannabis dispensaries resemble a store, with racks of products, where you can enter, purchase and leave, rather than a community space where people can spend time, be educated, have some oversight, maybe even meet some other people? How would our thinking change if we tried to imagine the future of psychedelics in terms of spaces?

What if instead of thinking of regulating the plants, substances, or practices, we thought of regulating the type of *community spaces* that would minimize the harms and maximize the benefits of psychedelics? What would that regulation look like? A restaurant license involves accessibility requirements, emergency and fire regulations, hygiene in the kitchen, etc. This regulation says nothing about the décor, the music, or the menu, unless someone gets food poisoning, in which case there are clear consequences. Could this be a better model to think about the regulation of non-medical uses of psychedelics?

BEING INSPIRED VS APPROPRIATING

The second antidote is at the core of my argument. It comes in the form of two stories. The first story is an example of how societies can learn about their blind spots by engaging with other cultures. The second story is an example of how we can establish the types of relationships that turn these Gifts into more of a blessing, instead of more of a curse. Both stories exemplify the difference between appropriating and being inspired.

What is appropriation? Indigenous people all over the world have been stripped of their lands, their resources, their livelihoods, in a process that continues in the present, and is now expanding to their immaterial wealth, their traditions, their spirituality, their medicines and their knowledge. Cultural appropriation is taking what isn't ours to take, usually without permission, often by disrespectfully copying and profiting from other peoples' cultures. At its base, appropriation of shamanic practices involves confusing ritual forms with spiritual power. But since many people in psychedelic science world balk both at the word ritual and at the word spiritual, I will put this in terms they can understand, for this paper is aimed at them. Appropriating shamanic practices is a bit like thinking that by having Michael Jordan's shoes one can play like him. We know this is stupid, the quality of one's play does not stem from one's shoes, yet some people do this, they take ritual acts and objects, and copy them, thinking that's where the power is. But the power is not there. When Michael Jordan shoots a hoop, it can look like a deceptively simple gesture, yet it's taken decades to master. One could easily copy the gesture but most likely one would still miss the hoop. It is the same with ceremonial ayahuasca work, from the outside, many parts of it might look simple, but in fact they are the result of years of training, many long fasts and plant dietas, difficult initiations into a bewilderingly complex biocultural system of ancient relationships between people and plants.

One example is the *soplada*, a technique of traditional Amazonian medicine where tobacco smoke, perfumes and other liquids are blown or sprayed over different points of the patient's body. Having received many *sopladas* over the years, I can only say they are wonderfully effective. There is a notable difference before and after receiving them, especially if one has been having a difficult time. Sopladas, when done well, really work. Is there anything our future psychedelic doctors could learn from them?

I think there are many things that our doctors could not learn, even after many years, and there are also some things they could learn. For example, by observing that beyond its literal form, underneath a soplada is an *act of care*. During the psychedelic experience sometimes people will go through difficult times and they will need caring for. When one receives a soplada there is no doubt one is being cared for. Yet, a soplada is an act of care that takes a completely different form than everyday acts of support and intimacy, and so it cannot be confused with anything else.

In our world there has been for some time an ongoing debate about how much physical contact is OK in the context of psychedelic therapy. When and how should facilitators touch, hold hands or hug participants? On the one hand some participants might need this type of support and really benefit from it, on the other hand for some people these same forms of contact might be triggering, traumatic and terribly counterproductive. So, how can we support people in need while avoiding harm?

In the Amazon curanderos care for people by touching them without touching them. They touch them with their breath, with tobacco smoke, with aromas, with a leaf fan, with a feather... But that's not the humble lesson for us, that is the ritual form. The humbling lesson that indigenous knowledge can bring to non-indigenous cultures is that the psychedelic experience, being outside of everyday life, requires *a language of care that is different from the language of care of everyday life*. Psychedelic therapists will sometimes need to care for people and comfort them during the psychedelic experience, and now we know that they need to do so in a way that cannot be misinterpreted *or misused*.

So, what would that look like? How can we be inspired by sopladas without appropriating the ritual form? I will tell a second story, an example of success which hopefully gives some inspiration. It comes from groups in the US who do initiation rituals for young people. These collectives have also been dealing with the question of how can one learn from indigenous traditions? However they don't use plants, and they've been working on this issue since the 70s and therefore have a 30-to-40-year head-start on Western ceremonial plant use.

In some traditional cultures an initiation ritual can involve young people being taken from their parents' homes, and made to pass a difficult experience. This can involve spending a long period alone in the forest without food or water, sometimes being repeatedly bitten by poisonous animals. It can take many forms, but the common element is that young people are put in a situation where they need to rely on their own strength and resources to get through something very difficult. An ordeal like this process seems to provoke a growth, a maturation, and the person returns transformed.

So, these groups in the US set up to do something similar. It was relatively simple to take young people to the woods in the context of a summer camp and make them pass some sort of transformative experience that was acceptable to our Western standards. The young people were having powerful experiences, but not as transformative as they seemed to have been in indigenous cultures. The question was why not? Looking closer they saw that in traditional cultures the initiation didn't end when the kids returned from the woods. Life back in the village also reflected the changes the young people had gone through, a special song was sung, the names of the young people were changed, the group started to address them differently, or give them new roles. Again, the practices varied from culture to culture, yet each of these practices was an individual cultural answer to the same universal human question. The solution for these US groups was not to copy one or more practices from individual indigenous groups, the solution was to look at the universal human question that stood behind, and to create a new individual cultural answer for it. One way for us to phrase that question could be something like: How does one go from altered states to altered traits?

The lesson from indigenous societies is that human beings can have very powerful transformative experiences, but the staying power of these experiences depends on whether or not their environment and community reflect and acknowledge this transformation. So, instead of copying the answers of other cultures, the US groups came up with their own answer to the same universal question. At the end of the camp, when the parents picked up their children at the parking lot, they were instructed to greet them as if they were greeting a new person, someone they've never met.

"Hello" the parents would say "It is very nice to meet you. I'm looking forward to getting to know you better."

Often one cannot read, or tell, this story without feeling a surge of emotion. That's how we know something profound, a real universal human need, has been addressed. The US groups could have not learned this lesson without indigenous knowledge, yet this is a long way from cultural appropriation.

This lesson also teaches us something about clinical research, which often gives great results in the lab and less positive results when implemented in the real world. There are many factors at play, careful subject selection, controlled environment, etc. but this story points out an additional aspect, during research people are being closely witnessed in their healing by the researchers. When we lose the witnessing and support of the temporary community created between researchers and research subjects, we lose part of the effectiveness. This is not a bias, nor a problem to weed out. This is a human reality to work with.

The US groups give us an example of how we should learn from indigenous cultures, by being *inspired in a useful direction,* instead of by appropriating cultural forms from other cultures. This is how we can learn from those who have so more experience than we do, while respectfully remaining within the boundaries of each other's cultures.

THE NEED FOR COLLABORATION BETWEEN DIFFERENT SCIENCES AND KNOWLEDGES

The last story is about someone I know. A person who is a very skilled ayahuasca curandero. He is not indigenous, not even Amazonian, but he did more than two decades of apprenticeship in Perú. He does sopladas (by the way I'm not saying no else can do them- it is just that like in basketball, one has to learn the proper way). Decades of training are needed to learn sopladas, so that when one does the gesture, one actually makes the hoop.

Recently this curandero attended a psychedelic assisted therapy training because he was going to give ayahuasca to war veterans with PTSD. He was the only member of the cohort who was not a psychologist or a psychiatrist. Part of the training was to watch a number of videos where people were having very difficult or overwhelming effects. The ayahuasquero was astounded at the reactions of his fellow students. These mental health professionals were deeply uncomfortable, even afraid, at the thought that they would have to deal with a situation like that by themselves.

"Isn't there way to make it stop?" They asked. "Isn't there an antidote? What would I do if this happened to me?" They were worried. The curandero laughed as he told me "What would they do? They asked in terror, but there are a million things you can do! This the bread and butter of this work. The real measure of one's ability. If you can't deal with people having difficulties, then you can't do this work. And these future therapists they were terrified at the prospect!"

On the other end of the spectrum, most times people are relatively calm through a psychedelic experience. This also brings its own challenges. A young psychedelic therapist once confessed to me that sometimes it was incredibly boring for him to sit for hours next to someone who was lost in their experience but needed little or no help. Indigenous people also have solutions for this, but let's get back to the terror first.

I think these psychedelic therapists in training were terrified for a good reason. A person might have studied medicine for 15 years, have a psychiatry and neuroscience PhDs from an Ivy League school, and still be thoroughly unprepared to help another person through a psychedelic session. Those two PhD's might give them a very good preparation (with some additional training) to interview and screen participants, and to assess possible drug interactions, *before* the experience. The PhD's might also help (with some additional training) to talk to people *after* the experience, to help them understand and integrate what happened to them. But in terms of what happens *during* the experience, especially during complicated experiences, their PhD's will give them precious little indication on how to act.

Most (not all but *most*) Western psychotherapeutic training has to do with talking to people *after* something has happened to them, but not being with them *during* the experience. Most Western psychiatric training revolves around prescribing drugs to *reduce* a patient's symptoms, not to sit with them while their symptoms temporarily *increase*.

In terms of what happens *during* the psychedelic experiences, when symptoms might indeed increase, could it be that the better prepared person can be someone with no Western medical studies but a long apprenticeship in traditions that have been close to psychedelics for centuries? That's the first humbling lesson. The second humbling lesson is that it took them decades to get there. Can we accept this other type of science? Can we acknowledge the value of decades of individual practice embedded into centuries of accumulated empirical knowledge? And, if we can, why are medical professionals and traditional practitioners not collaborating more?

Personally, when it comes to interactions between prescription medicines and psychoactive plants, I prefer the advice of an informed pharmacologist or doctor. In terms of integrating and making sense of my psychedelic experiences, I like to talk after the session to my psychologist, who is also a psychiatrist. Would I want my ayahuasca facilitator to do my screening or my integration? No, I wouldn't. I understand that Western doctors can help me better with that. Conversely, would I want to sit in a psychedelic session facilitated by my pharmacologist or by my psychotherapist? Absolutely not, I wouldn't. They would most likely be terrible at it, even after months of training. It's common sense that my curandero is better prepared and has more experience handling what happens *during* the night.

There is a need and an opportunity for collaboration that is sadly being overlooked. A necessary cooperation between complimentary skill sets. Why are we in a mad rush to train thousands of therapists to do the before, the during and the after? Why don't we include the people who are already well trained at handling the middle part, the during? Most Western countries have very few psychedelic therapists with long-term experience. In the coming years we will need to train tens of thousands of new psychedelic therapists. That means most of the people who will receive prescription psychedelic medicines in the near future will receive them from therapists with limited to very limited working experience. At the same time, many Western countries already have a thriving ceremonial underground with many experienced facilitators. Not only are they better trained and more comfortable facilitating during the experience, they are never bored (they know how to sing!) they have experience and techniques for handling challenging effects, and they can work with whole groups at a time. These are all things, from the groups to the challenging effects, that most of the newly trained psychedelic therapists not will be comfortable with for some time.

On the other hand, the traditionally trained facilitators would also benefit from the knowledge on screening, interactions, integration, therapeutical alliance and ethical boundaries, amongst others things that medical professionals can bring to the table both before and after the experience. My own friend, the curandero, also told me he learned many useful things in the PTSD training.

In terms of turning the gift of psychedelics into more of a blessing for our cultures, many (not all) but many people in the psychedelic science world would benefit from a dose of humility when considering cultures that are more experienced than their own. Some traditional cultures have hundreds and even thousands of years of more progress in terms of developing successful relationships to what we call psychedelics.

Furthermore, we can only see our blind spots with the help of others. We don't know what we don't know, and we can't know that we don't know it, because we don't know we don't know it. This is the reason why mental health professionals have supervisors. Similarly, we can only see our cultural blind spots with the help of other cultures. Let other cultures be a source of inspiration. They present individual cultural answers to universal human questions. If we can focus on the universal questions, while approaching other cultures with humility and respect, we can learn so much from them without taking what was never ours to take.

And last but not least, psychedelic medicine people and ceremonial plant people need each other. They have complimentary needs and gift, and more collaboration would benefit the doctors, the facilitators, their patients, and society at large.

I call this collaboration the psychedelic enlightenment, because historically, after the renaissance, came the enlightenment.

THE PSYCHEDELIC ENLIGHTENMENT

As we know, the psychedelic renaissance is mostly pharmaceutical-based, mostly for people with a medical diagnosis, mostly prescribed by doctors, and hopefully covered by insurance. It will probably take place in for-profit clinics that will perform individual treatments.

The psychedelic enlightenment should complement and complete the above, filling the gaps that can't be covered by medicalization, which are many. The psychedelic enlightenment will be mostly plant-based, mostly for life transitions and other non-medical issues, and mostly facilitated by collaboration between traditional practitioners and Western care professionals. The setting will mostly look like collective rituals and will take place in community spaces. Often these spaces will be based on non-profit business models. This will be out of virtue, but also out of necessity. It might well be that that the level of care and human attention necessary to work with altered states of consciousness does not make for profitable, scalable business models.* People will operate these new spaces from a position of service. It is no coincidence that in traditional societies, this work is considered sacred. Even atheists understand that there is a part of every human being that is very intimate, profound, and valuable, a part of us that we guard, that we don't share easily, a part that is not for show, nor for sale, a part that is, in that sense, sacred. That's the part that psychedelics tend to touch. This is not like selling sunglasses, or aspirin, or spa circuits, and it should never be.

The psychedelic enlightenment incorporates indigenous knowledge, and integrates the lesson that in order for transformative experiences to really be transformative, they not only need to be integrated by the person, they also need to be integrated by a community who will witness and acknowledge that the transformation has taken place. Without the validation that comes from the community, even the most powerful inner experiences will quickly erode, and lose their power to transform our lives.

The bridge between today's psychedelic renaissance and tomorrow's psychedelic enlightenment will start to be built when the new Western psychedelic doctors begin to collaborate with traditional practitioners, each doing what they are trained to do best.

The psychedelic enlightenment is not a dream, in South American countries this is a reality that has been quietly growing for decades. In my work I have met dozens of examples of medical doctors and psychologists working in close collaboration with indigenous doctors and plant medicine facilitators and each doing what they do best. Outside of South America I've visited communities that after their encounter with indigenous plant medicines have been inspired to develop new relationships to their local plants, to their territory and their own traditions. This is already happening, though not many people in the English speaking world know about it. The psychedelic enlightenment is a name for a wish, a wish for a renaissance in relationships. A wish

* This is a summary of what I have observed in the past few years advising a number of startups. The psychedelic clinic or retreat center business model doesn't seem to work monetarily unless a) you are mostly treating wealthy people paying high prices or b) you are treating first world customers while paying third world operation costs and salaries. In other words, it will not scale unless your customers are wealthy, you compromise the level of care, or you go for non-profit community models. However, this is a separate topic for another paper.

for a day in which these plants can be as important, as respected, as beneficial and as much of a blessing for our cultures as they are for the cultures of origin.

On a final note, often in my work people often talk to me about "psychedelic exceptionalism".* This always makes me think that the ceremonial plant practices that I focus my work on must be *the exception to the exception*. They are so small, compared to the large psychedelic ecosystem. So why did I pick this particular focus?

I did it because I believe ceremonial plant practices are a keystone species† inside the larger psychedelic ecosystem. When a keystone species (even if it's small in numbers) goes extinct, the whole ecosystem takes a dive. Ceremonial plant practices are still persecuted today. Their survival is not at all guaranteed by the current psychedelic renaissance, in fact it is quite the opposite. Yet I know that if we lose them, the psychedelic ecosystem will lose a lot more than just that piece.

So, I chose to make this exception to the exception my life's work, because I know the myth of the Gift of the Gods, like all proper myths, is always current and always true. If as a culture we can figure out how to turn this Gift of the Gods into more of a blessing than a curse, then maybe, just maybe, we can learn to get other Gifts from the Gods right as well. This is a skill we will desperately need in these accelerating times. However, this is something we will never be able do by ourselves. We will always need others, other people, other cultures, other states of consciousness, to help us see our blind spots.

A FINAL NOTE

I would like to thank everyone who has contributed ideas, support and comments to this piece. The list is long, Andrea Langlois, Hattie Wells, my colleagues at ICEERS, the many amazing people I've met on this path, and the plants and traditions who have accompanied me in this twenty-year inner and outer exploration. I specially want to thank Dennis McKenna and the rest of the ESPD55 staff, researchers, and participants. When I started on this path two decades ago, I could never imagine I would end up in a book in the company of so many people I've looked up to and continue to admire today. In a more traditional context, I would address many of my fellow authors in this book as "aunt" or "uncle", not because of family ties, but as a sign of deference and deep respect.

On a personal note, I will confess it's been very difficult for me to write this piece. For many months now most of my mental space has been occupied not with plants, but pondering relationships, and how hard it is to establish right relationships with others (any others! human or not).

* "Psychedelic exceptionalism describes an ideology that claims psychedelics should be privileged for reform, but other purportedly more harmful drugs, like heroin and cocaine, should remain prohibited." For a more nuanced discussion of this false dichotomy see. "The Myth of Psychedelic Exceptionalism." (Marlan, 2021).

† A keystone species is a species that helps define an entire ecosystem. Keystone species have a dominant influence on their natural environment, relative to their abundance. The concept was founded by zoologist Robert T. Paine in 1969. They play a vital role in maintaining the structure of an ecosystem, and affect many other organisms in an ecological community. For example, keystone species can influence the types of species and population sizes in an ecosystem. Without the keystone species the ecosystem would be drastically different or even cease to exist altogether.

Recently I met someone who, in two years, taught me more about my blind spots than ayahuasca had taught me in the previous twenty. This is a very tall statement, yet it's the truth. It's been an enormously humbling lesson on what I didn't know I didn't know. I think my indigenous friends would agree that while the plants can teach a lot, when one meets the right companion, well…

Therefore, I would like to close with a thought that's been keeping me up at night. The most important things we will ever learn will be learned in relationship. These encounters are also Gifts from the Gods. They can turn into blessings that flower in our lives, descend into curses that take us down, or can hang somewhere in between. The choices we make, and how we handle them, are our school of being alive. They are how we learn *how to live*.

So, this goes, in gratitude, and in love, to all those companions, human and not, who have taught me and continue to teach me so much.

BIBLIOGRAPHY

Davis, Joshua. 2004. "The Mystery of the Coca Plant That Wouldn't Die." *WIRED*, November 1, 2004. https://www.wired.com/2004/11/columbia/.

Elmore, Bartow J. 2014. *Citizen Coke: The Making of Coca-Cola Capitalism*. W. W. Norton & Company.

Marlan, D. (2021) *The myth of psychedelic exceptionalism*, *Bill of Health*. Available at: https://blog.petrieflom.law.harvard.edu/2021/03/24/psychedelic-exceptionalism-drug-policy/ (Accessed: 31 May 2023).

Quinones, Sam. 2022. "Sam Quinones on the Rise of Fentanyl & P2P Methamphetamine" Interview by Ethan Nadelmann.

When Your Friends Are the Problem: Plant Medicines, Commercialization, and Biocultural Conservation

Andrea Langlois, MA, and Jeronimo Mazarrasa

Former Director of Engagement, ICEERS | Former Conservation Committee member, Indigenous Medicine Conservation Fund advisor

Social Innovation Director for ICEERS | Founding member of Plantaforma (Platform for the Defense of Ayahuasca in Spain)

> *"A huge wave of interest in traditional plant medicines is building, a wave so big it might go beyond what the fragile cultures and ecosystems of origin can sustain."*
>
> —Andrea Langlois

This essay shares insights on the unintended impacts of the globalization of psychoactive plants and fungi and suggests antidotes to extractivism.

INTRODUCTION

Plant medicines, such as ayahuasca, iboga, and mushrooms are quickly becoming the friends of many—with medicine spaces opening around the world, and more articles in popular and academic publications than anyone could hope to read in a week. Yet the increasing popularity of these medicines that were introduced to modern culture by Indigenous and traditional people does not come without consequences. Some medicines, such as peyote, the Sonoran Desert Toad, and iboga, are at a tipping point, where overharvesting is threatening their biological sustainability, while others are seeing the hallmarks of their culture (such as songs, textiles, rituals) becoming "fashion" for the masses. These tensions are important to examine as we move towards a world where medicines that are considered sacred to many are on their way to becoming spiritual and medical products. The central question posed in this chapter is this: What happens when rituals become products? Or, said in another way, what happens when your friends become the problem?

Globally, we are in a new time and place—a moment wherein these kinds of plants and fungi have traveled so far from their places of origin and across the globe so quickly. In the early days of Western research and writing about psychoactive plants and fungi, it was ethnobotanists and anthropologists who were the ones seeking understanding. As Merlin Sheldrake points out, the discipline of ethnobotany "makes cultural ways of knowing its scientific subject. Consequently, ethnobotanists must learn about plants through people, and aren't able to conceal their interactions with indigenous informants and other ethnobotanists." (Sheldrake 2020). Through their eyes, reading early descriptions of what they learned from Indigenous Peoples, we experience a curiosity and desire to understand the places and roles of ethnobotanicals within their ecosystems and particularly with the humans around them. These interactions, particularly due to the powerful effects of these ethnobotanicals, created intricate threads of human culture, which themselves were woven into a tapestry of interconnectedness, relationship, and balance with the ecosystem itself. The plants and those who worked with them engaged in generations-long dances of master-apprentice relations, of interdependence, and dialogue. Art, song, textiles, culture, architecture, relationships with the waters, mountains, ancestors, and complex traditional medicine systems are what make up the origins of what in today's psychedelic renaissance are reduced to a singular plant, "active component," or effect.

The revival of the Ethnopharmacologic Search for Psychoactive Drugs symposium in 2017, and again in 2022, reminds us of this history. Of the curiosity that was embedded in understanding the Indigenous and botanical origins of plants and fungi. During what is now being called the "psychedelic renaissance," the revival of this curiosity, wonder, and awe is needed more than ever, so that we do not get carried away with the tide of pharmaceutical and corporate interests and growth in spiritual tourism, biopiracy, and appropriation of practices.

As plants travel from the places where relationships with them have been stewarded for hundreds, if not thousands of years, to new contexts, there are both opportunities and challenges. This chapter is inspired by what we have learned by working on the ground in an international non-governmental organization called ICEERS (International Centre for Ethnobotanical Education, Research and Service), which was founded in 2009 and has since been operating in the liminal spaces between drug policy, human rights, legal defense, psychedelic movements, Indigenous rights, and emerging grassroots practices. We will explore some of the undesired impacts of Western interest in traditional plant and fungi medicines and propose antidotes towards a vision of a future that does more than reproduce colonial patterns of cooptation and extractivism.

LET'S START WITH A STORY...

Once upon a time there was a wild cactus that was traditionally used by people in Mexico to make a very special drink. The cactus was called agave and this drink was called Mezcal. One day, about a decade ago, Mezcal was discovered by people in faraway lands—people like us. Before you know it, bars and mixologists in the West began to promote mezcal as an artisanal drink, and *mezcalerias* popped up in big cities very far from the Mexican home of agave.

Production of this drink grew and grew as its popularity expanded; big companies got into the business and exports rose. Between 2013 and 2017, the exports of Mezcal quadrupled to 2.7 million liters a year. Two years later, this figure doubled again, reaching 5.8 million liters a year. Within seven years, production multiplied by six.

We're talking about a beverage that was made from a plant that only grows in the wild and takes years to grow. You can imagine what might happen when demand for something that grows slowly in the wild is multiplied by six. The agave cacti themselves began disappearing, facing pressures of overharvesting, and the 100 other species (from butterflies to bats) that depend on agave were seriously impacted. Small scale producers faced being pushed out of the market and losing their livelihoods as the industry began to cultivate agave in monocrops that were then plagued by illness. When the boom started, it felt like a great chance and a great opportunity for small scale producers. But the real costs of this popularity only became apparent many years later. This is what happens when your friends become the problem.

WHAT HAPPENS WHEN A CUSTOM BECOMES A PRODUCT?

Often the downsides of popularity are not seen until it's too late. With Mezcal, it was not only agave that was impacted by overharvesting, but other species in its ecosystem (such as pollinators) were as well. When production expanded, after the wild agave was nearly gone, cultivation began, forests were cut down to plant monocrops of agave using cloned cacti rather than biodiverse seeds, destroying complex ecosystems for cash crops. The cloned plants started to get sick. The high volumes of wood needed to cook the agave drew heavily on local energy resources. Wastewater and pulp clogged local waterways. Local family businesses struggled to keep up with demand while availability of wild cacti dwindled.

Eventually the crisis with the supply of wild agave pushed locals and big businesses to address sustainability issues, or face the complete collapse of their industry. Solutions included creating a system for tracing agave plants, which is now in place, and a push to ban wild harvesting. Biological diversity conservation measures have been explored, such as seed saving and cross-pollination between species. But it taxes about 30 years for an agave cactus to grow, and the pressures on water and wood supplies also need to be addressed, as well as the disposal of acidic waste products. The new traceability requirements were challenging to small producers, who now had layers of paperwork to deal with. Progress is happening slowly, you can now buy Mezcal that is considered more sustainable, and there is now a market for sustainable, family-crafted mezcal. It looks like the path for Mezcal is somewhat back on track, although populations of the cactus in the wild may have been irreversibly impacted. This is a story of how unaware actions lead to devastations, and efforts being put in place to put things right.

PSYCHOACTIVE PLANTS AND FUNGI IN A GLOBALIZED CONTEXT

When we turn to the growing popularity of psychoactive flora, fauna, and funga,* we see a similar story. For plants like iboga and peyote, the increased demand has led to unprecedented pressure on wild populations. Iboga appears on the IUCN Red List as "of least concern," yet population counts in the forests of Gabon and the Congo Basin have not been conducted and reports of increased sales on the international black market are growing. Peyote, on the other hand, has been listed as "vulnerable," and its decline in the wild has raised concerns and led to several

* We are using the word funga purposefully—as it was revived at the conference, along with a request by Guiliana Furci and the Fungi Foundation that it be given its place alongside flora and fauna. It is a recent term considered to be needed to simplify conservation and educational projects. Thank you to Guilana Furci and the Fungi Foundation for introducing us to this term. Learn more about their work at: https://www.ffungi.org/.

conservation efforts, most notably by the Indigenous Peyote Conservation Initiative. The *Incilius alvarius* toad of the Sonoran Desert (which was previously known by *Bufo alvarius,* or simply bufo) has also been significantly impacted by climate change and poaching. Several organizations and Indigenous leaders have asked the psychedelic community to not engage in practices with *I. alvarius,* instead pointing to synthetic 5-MeO-DMT as an alternative (ICEERS, 2022).

Plants have been traded (as well as stolen) since time immemorial, with unforeseen impacts. In the case of tea and coffee, as Michael Pollan outlines in his new book *This is Your Mind on Plants,* when powerful psychoactive substances, such as cacao, tea and coffee, enter new cultures, the impact can be significant and, at times, only really understood in retrospect. He writes: "The kind of magical thinking that alcohol sponsored in the medieval mind began to yield to a new spirit of rationalism and, a bit later, Enlightenment thinking. … To see, lucidly, 'the reality of things:' this was, in a nutshell, the rationalist project. Coffee became, along with the microscope, telescope and the pen, one of its indispensable tools" (Pollan, 2021). Caffeine has been the drug of choice in the capitalist era, fueling productivity and alongside it slavery and colonization needed to establish the global coffee industry (Pollan, 2021). If coffee and tea had such an impact on shaping culture and mindsets, how might the future be shaped by the current popularization of ceremonial plant use, microdosing and the mainstreaming of psychedelic therapy? As explored by Paul Stamets in this volume, perhaps the neurogenisis offered by mushrooms is exactly what is needed at this time in history for the evolution Homo sapiens need at this time.* Or, if they are simply turned into a commodity, perhaps the story of "few benefit at the cost of many" will be reproduced.

It's too early to know. When it comes to plant concoctions, such as ayahuasca, it may be many decades before we truly understand the impacts that they will have on our cultures and societies and what impact turning them into commodities will have on their places and cultures of origin. Yet, we can see a few clues. Ayahuasca has expanded its reach to dozens of countries around the globe, and has also inspired a spiritual tourism industry in South America, particularly in Peru. If we look at what happened to agave with the increasing commodification of Mezcal, can we see the writing of what is in store for this Amazonian brew and its source plants?

Living in an age of globalized digital capitalism means that flora, fauna or funga that pique the interest of humans can become popular almost overnight.[5] With the "psychedelic renaissance" hitting a fierce pace, there are dozens of articles published daily on a myriad of topics and a multitude of new business ventures launching. Looking at google analytics data on ayahuasca shows an exponential growth in interest in ayahuasca in the last 10 years, that is 50 years after the publication of William S. Burroughs and Allen Ginsberg's *Yagé Letters*, a chronicle of Burroughs' search for the mysterious brew in the early 1950s. In June 2021, the keyword "ayahuasca" was

* See our paper "Revisiting the McKenna Stone Ape "Theory" and the ever evolving case of its plausibility for stimulating neurogeneration" by Paul Stamets for more insights on this topic.

searched for 380,000 times in Google, with the top searches coming from the USA (90.5K), Great Britain (33K), Canada (22.2K), Spain (22.2K), and the Netherlands (18.1K).*

What we see here is an exponential growth in interest in ayahuasca; as internet search trends provide a small window into the growth in popularity. It also shows how quickly interest can grow in something new that is finding its way into pop culture, books, and those seeking a new experience or healing. The Internet makes it possible for us to see this trend, but also offers the insight that the genie is out of the bottle—there appears to be no turning back when it comes to the growth of communities drinking ayahuasca globally. How did this medicine, this experience that can be quite intense physically and emotionally, become so popular?† It is not the psychoactive ethnobotanical that anyone expected to gain notoriety. As Wade Davis eloquently shared to the audience of the 2019 World Ayahuasca Conference in Girona, Spain: "If you had asked me back in 1974 to name the South American entheogen that would have caught the wind of the zeitgeist 50 years later … I have to confess that *yagé* would not have topped the list." Yet, in the growing search for spirituality outside the dominant institutions of religions, it seems these experiences offer a direct experience, often in community, that people are yearning for.

Extraction of resources from the Amazon has a long history linked to colonization, and currently the threats to the lungs of the plant loom large, as deforestation, cattle ranging, mining and oil extraction threaten Indigenous communities and their ways of life, as they are connected profoundly to their territories. Although Wade Davis was the one to document some of the impacts of rubber extraction from the Amazon in the late 1800s and early 1900s in his book *One River*, as the quote above illustrates, he did not predict that what were once hubs for the rubber boom, cities such as Iquitos, are now the heart of spiritual retreat centers. One could ask whether they are a form of spiritual extractivism that is the equivalent to ranching, mining, and old extraction. Ayahuasca is the latest in a long list of extraction of knowledge and materials from the Amazon. Yet, it isn't only the brew that has traveled, but the rituals and ceremony styles as well, which makes ayahuasca unique as an "export."

Although in the past 500 years many sacred plants from the Americas have traveled to the West, from tobacco to Maria Sabina's sacred mushrooms. It is the first time in history that a sacred plant from the Americas travels together with its associated ritual, or custom. What we're seeing is the custom, not the product‡ that is becoming equally popularized. There is something in the way that ayahuasca is being globalized that remains entwined with its original cultures. Through this, by staying connected to the customs, the rituals, we're managing to get a little bit

* Search conducted June 2021. Google Trends is a search trends feature that shows how frequently a given search term is entered into Google's search engine relative to the site's total search volume over a given period of time. There is a correlation between the increase in searches for the word "ayahuasca" (and other close spellings) worldwide and with the search in the following countries: the USA, Great Britain, Canada, Spain and the Netherlands.

† Dennis McKenna commented on the question posed "I think it is because our culture is spiritually bereft. People long for genuine spiritual experience; organized religion is often a hollowed-out shell that no longer provides genuine spiritual succor. We can't blame people for wanting this- we all seek that. The problems come when you co-opt spiritual traditions."

‡ Read more about this topic in our paper "Blessing or curse? The integration of ceremonial plant practices outside countries of origin" by Jerónimo Mazarrasa.

more of the blessing and a little bit less of the curse that can come associated with these plants when they are taken out of their original contexts.*

GLOBALIZATION OF CEREMONY: THE BAD NEWS

Yet, it's important to problematize the rising interest in this sacred medicine and rituals—that research is showing can help conditions such as treatment resistant depression, grief, and addiction—because as with everything, popularity comes with downsides. Like with most trends, the downsides are first witnessed at the source. Riccardo Vitale, advisor to the Indigenous-led organization the Union of Indigenous Yagé Doctors of the Colombian Amazon (UMIYAC), articulates the impacts of the commercialization of yagé on the traditional communities in Colombia's Putumayo region:

> *"Community members are increasingly deserting yagé ceremonies because of the presence of paying foreigners in their village malokas. There is a growing trend of improvisers who leave their communities and try their luck as self-appointed 'taitas,' selling marketable versions of 'traditional practices' this creates internal strife, resentment and divisions. There is proliferation in the region of spiritual tourism, healing centers and ayahuasca schools, controlled by foreign capitals. Community disputes and divisions arise when curacas engage in unequal business transactions with urban and foreign new-age entrepreneurs."*

Interest in participating in Indigenous-led ceremonies leads to imbalances in communities. As foreigners arrive and offer to pay for ceremonies, a "trade" in culture and healing (for money) is established, which has the consequence of creating divisions within communities as individuals benefit, and can result in drawing traditional healers away from their community-oriented service and into foreign owned retreat centers. The list of impacts is long—from the disruption of local practices, to the introduction of money for services, and the proliferation of self-appointed ceremony leaders who may not have adequate training nor the blessing of their communities. Following the 4th Indigenous Ayahuasca Conference, held in Brazil in 2022, those who gathered released a historic declaration that calls for the protection of Territories of Life in the Amazon and the ethics of sharing Indigenous medicines (Prime, 2022).

In Peru, the country with the highest number of ayahuasca retreat centers, the jungle cities of Iquitos and Pucallpa now have dozens of retreat centres (Suárez Álvarez, n.d.-b). These centers receive thousands of tourists and have driven increased harvesting of the vine, and as the journalist Carlos Suarez has documented in his multimedia book on ayahuasca, the vine has become a "cash crop" that is being harvested before maturity (typically over 7 years), which puts pressure on wild ecosystems (Suárez Álvarez, n.d.-b). And, while the influx of tourism and income may

* Dennis McKenna commented "Because ayahuasca is difficult to dissociate from its cultural context, it is more respected. That may help people wake up to the threats facing it and want to help protect and preserve both the plants but also the traditions. We should not be blind to the possibly that in this way, ayahuasca has the potential to transform global consciousness, to help heal not only individual souls, but the soul of our species. This is why in my opinion we need to seek ways to share it with the world while protecting it and respecting the traditions."

be welcomed as it can create jobs for locals, it also creates a dependency on external resources for local economies (Fotiou, 2016). This dependency was exposed during the early days of the 2020 Covid pandemic; the individuals and communities who depended on this income were hit hard as tourism halted suddenly, with retreat centers closing, some of which never reopened, with locals losing access to work (ICEERS, 2021). Those who made a living shipping medicine around the world also found themselves without buyers as communities internationally were forced to stop hosting ceremonies due to lock-downs and other government measures aimed at quelling the pandemic (ICEERS, 2021b). This economic hardship was poignant and revealing of this global financial interdependence, which was very slightly abated through crowdfunding efforts to send funds to communities and families.

Anecdotal reports and more on the ground explorations are also showing that while the ayahuasca vine is not being pushed to the brink of extinction, as with some sacred plants, it is being overharvested in the areas of hundreds of kilometers around concentrations of retreat centers, such as in the Loreto and Ucayali departments of Peru (Kilham, 2018). Furthermore, it is not only ayahuasca and chacruna that are sought but other plants and ceremonial objects, such as carved items, embroidered textiles and beadwork, as well as more troubling items such as animal teeth. A study published in the journal *Conservation Science and Practice* documented evidence of a growing trade in jaguar body parts across Latin America, particularly in Brazil, Bolivia, Suriname, Costa Rica, and Peru. The study authors postulate that commercialized ayahuasca tourism may be an undervalued contributor to the trade in jaguar parts, which are marketed to ayahuasca "tourists" or sold for use in Traditional Chinese Medicine (Braczkowski et al., 2019b).

It is important to note that the "trade" of ayahuasca, notably the export and import has led to numerous arrests and seizures, as ayahuasca and other plants (from iboga to San Pedro) are getting caught in the nets of drug control. While we won't go into detail about this here, it is important to note that the increasing number of seizures of ayahuasca, in particular, is troubling in that countless packages of ethnobotanical plants are being confiscated and destroyed worldwide (McAllister, 2021). This adds to the pressures on plants in the wild, when they are harvested only to be destroyed because of the international drug control regime.

ANTIDOTES TO EXTRACTIVISM

When ICEERS was founded, over 13 years ago, most of our work had to do with what we considered to be the "enemies" of the plants—the people who were making plants illegal, the drug war. For many years, most of our work focused on educating policy makers, judges, and other drug policy sectors on the value of these plants and practices. In the last five years, however, we began to realize that the friends of the plants can also be a problem, when there's too many of them. The popularity of these sacred medicines can lead to extractivism, over harvesting, and the erosion of their cultures of origin. The rest of this chapter is dedicated to exploring antidotes to runaway trends that are pushing traditional medicines and cultures to the tipping point in their places of origin. The greatest hope for these ethnobotanical practices is that they may have the ability to wake us up to our connection to life. We are facing the sixth mass extinction—can we ensure that relationships with these plants, animals and fungi are based in respect and forge a new way forward where we are reconnected to something bigger than ourselves? We can reframe the possibility as our greatest opportunity—to allow ourselves to be changed by our interactions with these plants and fungi, and to look at how a "consumer" approach can be disrupted through actions that seek to repair the past and to open, through dialogue and curiosity, to collectively finding a new way that is worthy of these sacred gifts.

BIOCULTURAL CONSERVATION

Biocultural conservation is an approach to sustainability and regeneration that acknowledges that the diversity of life is made up not only of the diversity of plants and animal species, habitats, and ecosystems found on the planet, but also of the diversity of human cultures and languages. When applied to the ecosystems of ethnobotanical flora, fauna, and funga, this means that measures are taken to ensure that the cultures and ecosystems thrive together. It's a much-cited statistic that at less than 5% of the world's population, Indigenous people protect 80% of global *biodiversity* (Raygorodetsky, 2021)—this points to the fact that healthy relationships with territory and land may be at the root of healthy cycles of reciprocity between humans and their environments. The diversity of life is made up not only of the diversity of plants and animal species, habitats, and ecosystems found on the planet, but also of the diversity of human cultures and languages. We have co-evolved as a part of nature. Over time people have adapted to their local environments while drawing material and spiritual sustenance from it. Through this mutual adaptation, human communities have developed thousands of languages and cultures, with distinctive ways of seeing, knowing, doing and speaking (Terralingua, 2022). This "ethnosphere," to use a concept articulated by Wade Davis, is the richness of the human experience on earth—the cumulative total of thoughts, beliefs, myths and inspirations brought into being by humans since the dawn of our existence.

As Imika Tarirú, Leader of the Tubú Hummurimassä people reminds us—it is the relationship with medicine-holders that turns plants into medicines. He says: "Is it the plants of knowledge that bring healing or is it the integral perspective of the healers (wise ones) and their deep study that has the capacity to turn it into medicine?"* When it comes to ethnobotanical medicines, it's about the threads of relationship between cultures, humans and medicine plants—who are all within the web of life. Different people and different cultures have developed unique relationships with what are sometimes called 'teacher plants' or 'master plants'—which evolved into keystone species that support evolution, adaptation, resiliency. If we look to some of the cultures that have relationships with ayahuasca, peyote, and iboga, for example, we also can see strengths and ways of knowing that have supported resistance to and recovery from the pressures of colonization. Looking through the lens of biocultural conservation requires stepping back and seeing the forest (the context, cosmovisions, and cultures in which they are embedded), not just the trees (i.e., the medicines themselves).

This lens is critical for our path forward. It's incredible that our interactions with these

* Imika Tarirú, Leader of the Tubú Hummurimassä people via Claude Guislain, interviewed by Andrea Langlois, 19 May 2022.

plants and fungi can (although not always) support greater nature-connectedness, reverence for life, and wonder with the natural world. The health of humans and cultures is interconnected with the health of the territories in which we live.* Thus, it is increasingly important to protect these traditional practices as they are essential in supporting communities to heal and to engage in territory (i.e., ecosystem) protection. And, it is critical to say—that protecting the plants and communities of these original territories of life need to be guided by local peoples and not "saved" so that dominant cultures can benefit from extracting them.

This is where the concept of "right relationship" comes into play—the idea speaks to a core understanding of interconnectedness and a recognition that all of our actions must have the inability to compartmentalize. Being in "right relationship" is a way of talking about living in a sustainable, balanced, harmonious, and loving way with all living beings and with all of nature. When considering how we approach the integration of ethnobotanicals into new contexts, it's essential to also ensure that newly developing rituals, uses and customs don't deplete traditional resources, including the plants, toads or fungi in the wild, and that we listen to the desires, needs, and perspectives of traditional knowledge holders. Being in right relationship incorporates a "do no harm" approach wherein new practices (whether ceremonial or clinical) should be measured to ascertain whether they will cause harm to any of the ecosystems they are a part of.

RECONCILIATION AND REPARATIONS

An important step to regaining balance, there may be reparations that need to be made and a process of reconciliation undertaken. Reconciliation refers to efforts made to address the harms caused by various policies and programs of colonization. Reparations are broadly understood as compensation given for an abuse or injury. Unfortunately, the current "renaissance" brings with it a shadowy history—not only linked to the colonization of countries such as Mexico, Gabon, and Amazonian countries, but also linked to the events surrounding what is often called the "discovery" of these medicines by Westerners.

The story of Maria Sabina serves as an entry point to untangling what this means. When Gordon and Valentina Wasson traveled to Mexico to search out the traditional mushroom healers, what happened as a result couldn't have been known to them or to Maria Sabina, who permitted Gordon Wasson to participate in a traditional ceremony. Likely their intentions were not to cause harm, yet over 60 years later we can look back with hindsight. As Wasson himself reflected: "As a consequence of my articles published in *Life Magazine*, a mob of thrill-seekers struck over Huautla de Jimenez… hippies and tourists altering and corrupting the lifestyle of what used to be an idyllic indigenous town" (Vidriales & Ovies, 2018). After the famous *Life Magazine* article was published, Maria Sabina faced multiple and many negative consequences.

This story is well documented by Konstantine Gerber and colleagues who look at it within the light of the intellectual property claims and patents being sought in the 2020s. "Within two years of the story's publishing, psilocin and psilocybin, the main active compounds in the mush-

* Comment from Dennis McKenna "This is the essence of symbiosis, what is happening with these plants and our species is a cultural process but it is also a co-evolutionary process."

rooms, were isolated, characterized, synthesized and named by Swiss chemist Albert Hofmann at the Sandoz pharmaceutical company. Sandoz quickly patented the extraction procedure and a method for 'therapeutic tranquilization,' marketing pills under the trade name Indocybin" (Gerber et al., 2021b). While Hofmann and Sandoz were setting the stage for what has become a "gold rush" for patents and commercialization of therapeutic uses of psilocybin, the Mazatec people of Mexico have experienced what can only be called "a story of extraction, cultural appropriation, bioprospecting, and colonization" (Gerber et al., 2021b).

After this exposé, Maria Sabina faced multiple personal tragedies—she was jailed briefly, her house was burned down and throngs of the first generation of psychedelic tourists began to flood into Huautla de Jimenez. What were sacred rituals quietly guarded for generations became commodities and even though today Maria Sabina has been given the status of mushroom and psychedelic cultural icon, it is all too clear that the costs to her, her community and culture have been high. Can this wrong be righted? With 60 years of time that has passed since this original act of blind theft, and the proliferation of synthetic psilocybin, how can we trace steps back to come into right relationship with the Mazatec people, sacred mushrooms, and the land?

It's not a clear path of how we can walk the path of reconciliation with Mazatec Peoples without causing more harm. Yet that does not mean that it is not worth exploring how to honor the mycelial networks of mushroom and culture that led to modern hopes for healing depression and spiritual journeying. Reparations can take the shape of benefit sharing, ensuring equitable access to therapies for BIPOC people and other marginalized groups, and of remembering to acknowledge the origins of the knowledge upon which patent claims are now being made. As Konstantin Gerber and co-authors remind us—there are "a number of international treaties asserting indigenous rights to their intangible cultural heritage"—how might they be applied to ensure adequate reparations are made to the Mazatec people?

An example of an initiative that is guided by and motivated by deep listening on this topic is the Indigenous Medicine Conservation Fund, a high impact strategic fund created to ensure that Indigenous communities and organizations can succeed in their own biocultural conservation efforts. Working around five keystone medicines, including mushrooms, where they are engaging with Mazatec people in a process of deep listening to understand how this generation of medicine people, leaders, and families articulate ways in which reparations, reconciliation, and benefit sharing might be transformed from concepts into community-serving actions.

BENEFIT SHARING

Benefit sharing is also a concept and framework that encourages the sharing of financial and other benefits that are being generated from the growing industry of psychedelic retreats and medicines. There are several avenues for benefit sharing, one of which is the Nagoya Protocol on Access to Genetic Resources and the Fair and Equitable Sharing of Benefits Arising from their Utilization, which is a global agreement that implements the access and benefit-sharing obligations of the Convention on Biological Diversity. The Nagoya protocol sets out core obligations for signatories to take measures in relation to access to genetic resources, benefit-sharing and compliance. It came into force in 2014 and has been signed by over 50 countries (including

Gabon, the UK and the EU). Ultimately the protocol is a mechanism for indigenous and local peoples to benefit from the use of their community's resources, which includes knowledge as well as "genetic" (i.e. plant or animal) materials, and that consent has been sought prior.

The sharing of benefits could come in the form of the payment of royalties, research collaborations, joint ownership of intellectual property rights, or preferential access for the provider country to any medicine derived from genetic resources and associated traditional knowledge: preferential rates to purchase medicine. These are a few examples. The most notable application of the Nagoya protocol is in South Africa, where Khoi and San entered into a benefit sharing agreement around the rooibos tea (Nordling, 2019). As of this writing, processes are underway for the exportation of iboga from Gabon in alignment with the Nagoya protocol, which means that it will be the first ever psychoactive plant medicine legally exported with benefits going directly to communities.

The foundational efforts of the organization Blessings Of The Forest (BOTF) are what has led to this groundbreaking moment internationally, which will bring recognition and benefits to local people in Gabon through government regulations implementing the Nagoya protocol. BOTF funds and technically supports community-based permaculture agroforestry projects with iboga as the anchor plant surrounded by additional useful plants. BOTF also develops Income Generating Activities (beekeeping, handicrafts, tourism, cultural promotion...) while waiting for the maturation and commercialization of the cultivated iboga. The iboga that is sold will go to international clients who are then responsible for communicating back to the communities about how it was used and any knowledge derived (for example research findings). It is a full-circle example of how traditional knowledge can be respected and local communities provided an opportunity to contribute to healing for people in other countries with their medicines and to receive much needed resources to fund local projects.

REGENERATIVE CULTIVATION

To return to the story of agave, a critical lesson was how quickly overharvesting of the cacti led to a serious imbalance in local ecosystems. Many of the places that are the wild sources of medicines (from peyote, to toad, ayahuasca and iboga) are areas that are also under threat from climate change, deforestation, and extraction oil and gas—pressures that threaten the ecosystems above and beyond the harvesting of the plants or toads themselves. Indigenous and local communities in many parts of the world are struggling to protect territories of life with high levels of biodiversity—territories that are the lifeblood and health of their communities and that contribute to balance for us all. The rainforests of the Amazon and of Gabon are noted as being the lungs and the heart of our blue planet.

Within this context, ethnobotanical plants, fungi and animals are what is known as "keystone species"—an organism that helps define an entire ecosystem. Like the keystone at the top of a stone arch, which if removed would collapse the whole structure, without a keystone species, the ecosystem would be dramatically different or cease to exist altogether. Traditional medicines, such as iboga, ayahuasca, and peyote, are keystone medicines in that they play a pillar role within cultural and natural ecosystems. Their conservation is therefore of critical importance both from a biological as well as a cultural perspective. Overharvesting, destruction of habitat (such as forests and desert ecosystems) must be halted in these areas of high importance. Conservation of land under indigenous and local stewardship is of importance, as is the halting of poaching of these keystone species from their natural habitats.

Regeneration of these ecosystems is another path forward—and this can include reforestation efforts and domestic cultivation of medicinal plants so that wild harvest is reduced. Communities in Gabon, as noted above, are creating agroforestry permaculture initiatives where they are growing iboga alongside other useful medicine and food crops. In the Amazon, for example, the ayahuasca churches (such as the Santo Daime and União do Vegetal) have cultivation programs to ensure that ayahuasca and chacruna are available to their communities, while also seeking to regenerate forests. In the Sonoran Desert, Yacqui peoples are concerned about the damage that toad harvesting is having on local populations, as well as the pressures of climate change. The synthetic drug 5-MeO-DMT has been heralded as an alternative to the Sonoran Desert Toad for people wanting to work with this medicine.

For communities sourcing medicine, regenerative sourcing is a high-level value. Communities need to be ready to have the conversation about where their medicine has come from, whether it was harvested in a good way, and to understand if the exchange has been fair.

SOLIDARITY AND RECIPROCITY

To live in reciprocity is to live in relationship (kinship) with all things. If you use something, you must repay it back in some manner. There is the understanding that no action is isolated; every action executed contributes either positively or negatively to the interconnected web of life and thus, it is our responsibility to always act with this knowledge and with respect to the sanctity of life. As Edgar Villenueva says, "No one is just a giver or a taker; we're all both at some point in our lives. This also reflects a cyclical dynamic, as opposed to a one-off, one-way relationship" (Villanueva, 2021).

Reciprocity—returning the gift as Robin Wall Kimmerer calls it—is not just good manners; it is how the biophysical world works (Kimmerer, 2022b). Balance in ecological systems arises from negative feedback loops, from cycles of giving and taking. Yet when it comes to practices, such as those with ayahuasca, over the last decade there has clearly been more "taking" by non-indigenous people than "giving." Commenting on how many ayahuasca drinkers say that their time in the jungle has changed their lives, Narby asked the provocative question: "What did the Amazonians who attended to them get out of it? Perhaps some payment, but probably nothing quite so life-changing" (Narby, J., 2019). According to Narby, undoing this imbalance and making our relations with Amazonian people more reciprocal is the "work of a lifetime" (Narby, J., 2019).

In the psychedelic space, it has become fashionable to talk about "giving back" to the original stewards of this medicine and of "sacred reciprocity." While the intentions towards these discourses may be good, the rhetoric has been quickly slipping into a type of "greenwashing" or, as some call it, "tie-dyeing." Reciprocal cycles in nature are not directly transactional; they are not tit-for-tat exchanges, but rather based on a trust in the greater system and its favoring of balance.

We caution, therefore, against shallow use of the term reciprocity and point to a deepening of understanding of what it truly means to be in reciprocity with the Earth and all its beings seen and unseen. Moving towards balance with the Indigenous peoples who have stewarded practices and relationships with plants and fungi requires giving before taking, carrying out acts of repair, and acting in solidarity—all of which require deep listening. For example, peoples of the Amazon may benefit from financial support, yet what in many cases is urgently needed are acts of solidarity to support the defense of traditional territories from extractive industries. In countries like Colombia, Indigenous leaders' lives are under threat.

Acts of reciprocity must consider how benefit sharing is being done on a larger scale (i.e., with companies in the space) and also is something that can be addressed as an individual who is interested in or engages in practices with plant and fungi medicines. As Alnoor Ladha and Rene Suša articulate so well in their article about the psychedelic renaissance and colonialism: "A responsible and accountable engagement with sacred plants and medicines is not about self-realization, self-aggrandization, self-creation, self-expression, self-validation or anything else that may be the devotional goal of Western well-being. It is more about getting over ourselves, our ideas of what constitutes the self, of where we end and someone or something else begins." (Ladha, 2022). If we engage in this way, which is less about self-development and more about seeking our place in the grand ecosystem of life, about how to be accountable, and to give more than we take, then the psychedelic "revolution" may indeed become worthy of that name.

CONCLUSION

In the words of Robin Wall Kimmerer: "Reciprocity among parts of the living Earth produces equilibrium, in which life as we know it can flourish. When the gift is in motion, it can last forever." (R. Kimmerer, 2022). The most important question, therefore, for the future of plant medicines in a globalizing world is this—how do we keep the gift in motion? While the mainstream public and governments still have a way to go in understanding what treasures ethnobotanical plants are, there are many of us who are not from the cultures where these practices originate that are aware of the potential that these plant/fungi relationships offer. We wouldn't be the first to suggest that the time could not be riper for more humans to wake up to the possibility that psychoactive plants and fungi can help us at the critical time in human history, where we face eco-anxiety and grief, and mental health challenges associated with life giving natural processes are out of balance. Alongside the incredible importance of honoring and standing in solidarity with Indigenous peoples in protecting territories of life, we have the opportunity to ensure that these gifts (ayahuasca, iboga, mushrooms, and more) are not hoarded, not turned into products, not extracted for the benefit of few. We have the opportunity to ensure that the gift stays in motion.

ACKNOWLEDGEMENTS

Gratitude to the teams at ICEERS and the Indigenous Medicine Conservation Fund, and all those who have contributed perspectives and help, as well as Hattie Wells, Riccardo Vitale, Imika Tarirú, Skye Selway, and the plants and mushrooms.

BIBLIOGRAPHY

Braczkowski, A., Ruzo, A., Sanchez, F., Castagnino, R., Brown, C., Guynup, S., Winter, S., Gandy, D., & O'Bryan, C. J. (2019a). The ayahuasca tourism boom: An undervalued demand driver for jaguar body parts? *Conservation Science and Practice*, *1*(12). https://doi.org/10.1111/csp2.126

Braczkowski, A., Ruzo, A., Sanchez, F., Castagnino, R., Brown, C., Guynup, S., Winter, S., Gandy, D., & O'Bryan, C. J. (2019b). The ayahuasca tourism boom: An undervalued demand driver for jaguar body parts? *Conservation Science and Practice*, *1*(12). https://doi.org/10.1111/csp2.126

Fotiou, E. (2016). The Globalization of Ayahuasca Shamanism and the Erasure of Indigenous Shamanism. *Anthropology of Consciousness*, *27*(2), 151–179. https://doi.org/10.1111/anoc.12056

Gerber, K., Flores, I. G., Ruiz, A. C., Ali, I., Ginsberg, N. L., & Schenberg, E. E. (2021a). Ethical Concerns about Psilocybin Intellectual Property. *ACS Pharmacology & Translational Science*, *4*(2), 573–577. https://doi.org/10.1021/acsptsci.0c00171

Gerber, K., Flores, I. G., Ruiz, A. C., Ali, I., Ginsberg, N. L., & Schenberg, E. E. (2021b). Ethical Concerns about Psilocybin Intellectual Property. *ACS Pharmacology & Translational Science*, *4*(2), 573–577. https://doi.org/10.1021/acsptsci.0c00171

ICEERS. (2021a). How Ayahuasca Communities Are Adapting during the Pandemic. *ICEERS*. https://www.iceers.org/how-ayahuasca-communities-adapting-pandemic/

ICEERS. (2021b). Plant Medicine Sourcing in Changing Times. *ICEERS*. https://www.iceers.org/plant-medicine-sourcing-in-changing-times/

ICEERS. (2022). Bufo Toad (Incilius alvarius): Basic Info. *ICEERS*. https://www.iceers.org/incilius-alvarius-basic-info/

Kilham, C. (2018). *Ayahuasca Vine Cultivation and Harvesting in the Peruvian Amazon | Medicine Hunter*. https://www.medicinehunter.com/chris-kilham-medicine-hunter-field-report-ayahuasca-vine-cultivation-and-harvesting-peruvian-amazon

Kimmerer, B. R. W. (2022a). The Serviceberry. *Emergence Magazine*. https://emergencemagazine.org/essay/the-serviceberry/

Kimmerer, R. (2022). Returning the Gift. Center for Humans and Nature. https://humansandnature.org/earth-ethic-robin-kimmerer/

Ladha, A. (2022). Why the “Psychedelic Renaissance” is just Colonialism by Another Name. *DoubleBlind Mag*. https://doubleblindmag.com/colonialism-by-another-name/

McAllister, S., Esq. (2021). Ayahuasca FOIA Requests Reveal Increased Ayahuasca Seizures, Lack of Due Process and Government Secrecy. *Chacruna*. https://chacruna.net/ayahusca_religious_freedom_information_act_church_of_the_eagle_and_condor/

Narby, J. (2019, February 8). *Confessions of a White Vampire | Jeremy Narby | Granta*. Granta. https://granta.com/confessions-of-a-white-vampire/

Narby, J. (2019, September 23). *My life as a white vampire: Gringos, Amazonnians and the antidote of reciprocity* (video). ICEERS. https://www.youtube.com/watch?v=jAGdBhi1pZw

Nature, C. F. H. A. (2022). Returning the Gift. *Center for Humans and Nature*. https://humansandnature.org/earth-ethic-robin-kimmerer/

Nordling, L. (2019). Rooibos tea profits will be shared with Indigenous communities in landmark agreement. *Nature*, *575*(7781), 19–20. https://doi.org/10.1038/d41586-019-03374-x

Pollan, M. (2021, August 12). The invisible addiction: is it time to give up caffeine? *The Guardian*. https://www.theguardian.com/food/2021/jul/06/caffeine-coffee-tea-invisible-addiction-is-it-time-to-give-up

Prime, G. (2022, October 27). Declaration from the 4th Ayahuasca Indigenous Conference. *Medium*. https://medium.com/@gordianprime/declaration-from-the-4th-ayahuasca-indigenous-conference-d44a5518dc96

Raygorodetsky, G. (2021, May 4). Indigenous peoples defend Earth's biodiversity—but they're in danger. *Environment*. https://www.nationalgeographic.com/environment/article/can-indigenous-land-stewardship-protect-biodiversity-

Sheldrake, M. (2020). The 'enigma' of Richard Schultes, Amazonian hallucinogenic plants, and the limits of ethnobotany. *Social Studies of Science*, *50*(3), 345–376. https://doi.org/10.1177/0306312720920362

Suárez Álvarez, C. (n.d.). *Ayahuasca, Iquitos and Monster Voräx*. http://www.ayahuascaiquitos.com/en/

Terralingua. (2022, June 5). *What Is Biocultural Diversity?* https://terralingua.org/what-we-do/what-is-biocultural-diversity/

Vidriales, A. L., & Ovies, D. H. (2018). Psychedelic tourism in Mexico, a thriving trend. *PASOS Revista De Turismo Y Patrimonio Cultural*, *16*(4), 1037–1050. https://doi.org/10.25145/j.pasos.2018.16.072

Villanueva, E. (2021). *Decolonizing Wealth: Indigenous Wisdom to Heal Divides and Restore* (2nd ed.). Berrett-Koehler Publishers.

Intellectual Property Rights Issues in Community-Based Participatory Research: The Case of the Sucumbíos Cofán Yagé (Ayahuasca)

David F. Rodriguez-Mora, Doctoral Candidate

Ethnobotanist | Environmental Anthropologist | PhD student at the University of Texas at San Antonio

> *"Intellectual Property Rights (IPRs) are rights endowed and enforced by juridical institutions to protect a person's exclusive use of a legally endorsed creation. They encompass patents, trademarks, copyrights, and trade secrets. While IPRs' eligibility criteria comprehensively assess the suitability of a postulated invention for legal rights, they favor general knowledge over Indigenous Local Knowledge (ILK) creations and often disregard ILK contributions to general knowledge creations."* —David F. Rodriguez-Mora

This paper shares invaluable insights on engaging in ethical research practices with Indigenous people, where benefit sharing, protection, and common social justice goals are prioritized.

How do we rectify a system that so brilliantly serves its intended purpose?

—Dorothy E. Roberts

ABSTRACT

Community-Based Participatory Research (CBPR) offers a holistic framework for designing, implementing, and evaluating research collaborations in ethnobotany and ethnopharmacology. Through a collaborative and integrative methodological approach, CBPR renders high-quality data that strengthens research partnerships and contributes to social justice. Importantly, an open attitude to assess the research throughout its course enables the research partners to identify and address underlying issues formerly unrecognized. In this paper, I narrate the co-creation of my community-based ethnobotanical research partnership with the Sucumbíos Cofáns in southwestern Colombia. Initially, we centered our collaboration on the ethnobotanical assessment of the diversity of their Yagé—a.k.a., Ayahuasca—lianas growing in the wild, and the collection of stem cuttings for the community's restoration efforts. Nevertheless, as the project advanced, significant tension emerged regarding handling the research results and the legal and political implications of publishing our study. To address this problem, I evaluated the publication risks of our ethnobotanical study in light of the global Intellectual Property Rights (IPRs) regime. I determined that the current IPRs prevent the protection of the Sucumbíos Cofáns' self-determination and sovereignty rights regarding their Yagé Traditional Knowledge (TK). On the one hand, the legal circumscription of IPRs allows the granting of individual patents on the application and use of innovations based on collective Yagé plants TK. Consequently, these laws disregard the contributions and basic human rights of Indigenous groups who use Yagé—i.e., *Yageceros*. On the other hand, ethnobotanical and ethnopharmacological research has been used as a commodification tool of Indigenous *Yageceros*, their TK, and their territories. By addressing the IPRs challenges exposed through our research partnership, I exemplify how CBPR guided our work towards achieving common social justice goals. I argue that CBPR may help scholars in ethnobotany and ethnopharmacology (among other disciplines) to better direct their work towards resolving important issues in their research partnership and their work's legal and political implications. Finally, I suggest potential orientations in our research and practice to question the ongoing use of ethnobotany and ethnopharmacology as a commodification tool of TK. My goal is that this case study inspires the discussion and reformulation of the current IPRs for boosting the collective innovative potential of our biocultural heritage, implementing adequate mechanisms that include marginalized communities' epistemological and ontological commitments.

THE COFÁNS: A NATION AT RISK

The Cofáns are an Indigenous nation of fewer than 6000 people, whose ancestral territory spans southwestern Colombia and northeastern Ecuador (Cepek, 2012; Fundación Z.I.O.-A'i, 2012; Stocks et al. 2020). Despite the scanty data regarding the Cofáns before pre-Conquest times, particularly in the Colombian territory, they were estimated to have been between 15,000–70,000 inhabitants, occupying a geographical range far into the Andean valleys (Cepek, 2012; Friede, 1952). Although they resisted Inca subjugation attempts, including Huayna Capac (Davis, 2014), in the late fifteenth and early sixteen centuries, their oral histories mainly suggest hostile relations with Tukanoan and other Amazonian groups (Borman, 2009; Robinson, 1979). Through the "cinnamon" expedition of Captain Gonzalo Díaz de Pineda in the sixteenth century, the Cofáns were displaced from the Andes to the alluvial gold deposits of the Aguarico for mining exploitation and enslavement (Cepek, 2012; Davis, 2014). Over 400 years, the Cofáns settled in the Andes-Amazon territory, resisting the Spaniard military and Jesuit and Capuchin missionaries, and survived devastating epidemics, including measles and tuberculosis (Borman, 2009; Cabodevilla, 1996; Cepek, 2012; Davis, 2014; Friede, 1952; Kohn, 2002; Robinson, 1979). Furthermore, they endured enslavement and exploitation through harvesting of non-timber forest products —e.g., the quena tree bark for treating malaria and rubber for the automobile and the World War II military defense industry (the Amazon Rubber Boom) (Cepek, 2012; Davis, 2014; Mongua Calderón, 2020). Since the mid-twentieth century, their territory's primary legal economic sectors has included oil extraction, mining, and cattle ranching (Plotkin et al., 2017).

In Colombia, the Cofáns and their territory have also been significantly impacted by narcotrafficking, particularly in the past four decades (Fundación Z.I.O.-A'i, 2012), as a side effect of the cocaine consumption frenzy demanded by the Global North's underground market and the prohibitionist laws that govern it. These issues have been at the center of the internal armed conflict that has killed between 120,000–800,000 Colombians between 1985–2018 (Ganem Maloof, 2022). After the signing of the Colombian peace accord in 2016 (Paz, 2016), the armed conflict has been drastically reduced, but it is by no means over. Colombia is not only the number one country in orchid and bird diversity but is also number one in environmental and social leaders murdered. Since the signing of the peace accord, over 1000 leaders have been killed (González Perafán, 2022). In 2022 alone, every one to two days, one leader was murdered in cold blood, 30% of whom belonged to Indigenous populations (Defensoría del Pueblo, 2022). This accounts for almost half of the total number of world human rights activists assassinated in 2022 (Frontline Defenders, 2022). This data exposes the increased vulnerability of Indigenous people in Colombia, as their population roughly totals ~4% (Minsalud, 2020). The lives of environmental, social, and political Cofán leaders have also been taken away in such massacres.

The Cofáns have been praised by explorers, such as Richard Evans Schultes and his protégés Wade Davis, Mark Plotkin, and Homer Pinkley, and the ethnographer Michael Cepek, for their sophisticated knowledge about the environment and medicinal plants. Other than the Yagé* drink, their Traditional Knowledge (TK) legacy includes the concoction of *curare*, a complex plant-based hunting poison, which often includes species in the genera *Chrondrodendron* or *Strychnos*. It is used to hunt wild game through accurately aimed, silent, deadly palm darts skillfully rocketed through a blowgun. Another stimulant drink is called *yoco*, and is made from the outer bark of the *Paullinia yoco* R.E.Schult. & Killip liana. It alleviates hunger, which was useful for their first 4-5 hours of morning fieldwork, and has roughly twenty times the caffeine content of a cup of coffee. There is also the powerful and extremely dangerous psychoactive drink, *va'u*, which comprises trees in the genus *Brugmansia* and is used for advanced shamanic training, including shapeshifting (Cepek, 2012; 2018; Davis & Schultes, 2004; Davis, 2014). Schultes noticed that the Cofáns had the highest number of shamans per population size and described them as acutely intelligent, with imposing personalities, helpful, and willing to share their knowledge with respectful, interested naturalists (Davis, 2014; Plotkin et al., 2017). Pinkley (personal communication, April, 2021) also remarked on the Cofáns' distinct sense of humor, which made his doctoral dissertation fieldwork one the most delightful chapters of his life. Among the Cofáns, he identified for the first time in Western botany the common Yagé admixture *Psychotria viridis* Ruiz & Pav., from the coffee family, and the hunting poison *Ocotea venenosa* Korterm. & Pinkley, from the avocado and cinnamon family (Pinkley, 1973).

The Cofáns self-identify as forest people and guardians of the forest, a claim supported by GIS data revealing that they have maintained 80% of the forest land cover as opposed to the mere 20% held by adjacent mestizo communities (Stocks et al., 2020). Currently, the Colombian Cofáns only have 4% of their ancestral territory legally entitled to them, as the remaining 96% has been taken over by the forces of "colonialism," "development," and "free trade" in just 40–60

* I capitalize Yagé to acknowledge the agency, personhood, and power recognized to this being by the Sucumbíos Cofáns in their everyday speech.

years span of oil and agricultural exploitation (Stocks et al., 2020). These "economic" waves have disrupted and degraded the fragile rainforest ecology and the TK upon which the Cofáns have relied for subsistence. The Cofáns speak A'ingae; a language isolate (Hengeveld & Fischer, 2018), the single language within its language family (Campbell, 2010), with 40% of its vocabulary estimated to deal with forest ecology (Borman, 1976; Borman pers. comm. as cited in Stocks et al., 2020). The Colombia-Ecuador border reflects a linguistic divide, with one A'ingae dialect predominant on either side, yet mutually intelligible (Cepek, 2012). About 20% of the Colombian Cofáns speak A'ingae fluently, most of whom are elders over 60 years old (Fundación Z.I.O.-A'i, 2012). Thus, with the further erosion of the Cofán territory, culture, and language, humanity could be losing a unique understanding of their relationship with the rainforest and its medicines in the upcoming years and decades, further dwindling our species' global capacity to respond to the challenges of the ensuing century.

THE YAGÉ CONCEPT

Yagé is a term of unknown origin used in Colombia, Ecuador, and Perú by several Indigenous nations in the Amazon basin, including the Cofáns. Ayahuasca, instead, is a word derived from the northern Quechua, the lingua franca of the pre-Columbian peoples of the Amazon and Andes of northern Peru, Ecuador, and southern Colombia (Highpine, 2012). Ayahuasca means "vine with a soul," a term more frequently used by the Indigenous nations of Peru, Ecuador, Bolivia, and Brazil (Highpine, 2012). Yagé—also spelled Yaje and Yajé—is synonymous with Ayahuasca and encompasses a series of lianas in the family Malpighiaceae. However, the most well-known and employed species by Amazonian and Andean communities is *Banisteriopsis caapi* (Spruce ex Griseb.) C.V.Morton (Torres, 2017). The term Yagé also comprises of the concoctions brewed from the stems of these lianas and the shamanic ritual in which these drinks are ingested. It has been argued that Yagé shamanism has been in practice for several centuries and possibly since pre-Columbian times (Tupper, 2006; Brabec de Mori, 2011; Samorini, 2014; Samorini, 2015; Torres, 2018; Samorini, 2019a; Samorini, 2019b; Brabec de Mori, 2020).

The Yagé ritual is generally presided over by an experienced practitioner who must have endured extensive training and is widely acknowledged by their affiliated community—particularly elder *Taitas* (see below), community authorities, and relatives (Zuluaga, 2000). Yagé practitioners are recognized with "titles" according to their level of expertise working with Yagé (Zuluaga, 2000). Currently, the most widespread title in the lower Putumayo is *Taita*, which means "father" in Quechua, and is a word extensively adopted with that meaning into Spanish usage in Latin America. Elder *Taitas* —*Taitas* mayores in Spanish—are the most advanced practitioners working with Yagé, and are amply endorsed by their communities. *Taita* is synonymous with *curaca* —a.k.a, *curaga*; from the Quechua *Kukara*, a term used for Indigenous Andean leaders who mediated between colonial officials, deities and their communities (Cepek, 2023; Szeminski, 1987)—, traditional medics, and Yagé Indigenous medics (Zuluaga, 2000; see also Cepek, 2023; Jutte, 2000). Like fathers, *Taitas* teach, guide, and reprimand their students (Zuluaga, 2000). Some practitioners who are not as advanced in Yagé shamanism as *Taitas*, but who have made substantial progress in their shamanic training, are also authorized to preside over Yagé ceremonies, provide the drink, and even heal patients. They are called *Seguidores* [of a *Taita*], which means followers in Spanish. In some communities, to practice shamanism one must always be supervised by an elder *Taita* (Zuluaga, 2000). Finally, those who are either beginning or at an intermediate stage in their training, but who are not yet allowed to provide the drink or heal patients, are referred to as apprentices (Zuluaga, 2000).

Alternatively, however, there is an ample and rich vocabulary in A'ingae of several terms used to address a shaman or an apprentice, which allude to their potential attributes. For instance, derived from the verbs *atesuye* (to learn/to know)—e.g., *atesu'cho* (one who has learned)—and átteye (to see)—e.g., *áttepa canse'cho a'i* (one whose seeing is central to their life) (Cepek, 2023). Also there are terms derived from the nouns *coco*—a.k.a., *cuco, cucu, cocoya,* or *cucuya* (devil, demon, or malevolent supernatural entity)—e.g., *coco a'i* (demon people)—and *davu* (the Cofán shamanism's dart-like projectiles)—e.g., *davu'pa* (a possessor of davu), to name a few (Cepek, 2018; 2023). The wide range of meanings for the words that describe Yagé practitioners suggests different geographically situated, sociocultural, historical, and generational perspectives of Yagé shamanism.

Additionally, due to the cultural spread and scientific advancements surrounding Yagé, primarily in the past half-century, there has been an exponential rise in the number of travelers seeking to drink the Yagé brew and experience the ritual, resulting in a phenomenon known as Yagé tourism (Tupper, 2006; Fotiou ,2019). This term describes the tourism and trade surrounding the Yagé plant, drink, and ritual (Tupper, 2006; Fotiou, 2019), and is condemned by some comunidades *Yageceras* (communities that use Yagé) as one of the elements that sap the strength of the plant (Jutte, 2016; Zuluaga, 2000). Hundreds of thousands of users are estimated to participate yearly in Yagé ceremonies worldwide, especially in South America (Tófoli, 2019). Moreover, new religious and nonreligious instituciones *Yageceras* (institutions that use Yagé) and practices have emerged worldwide—i.e., *neoayahuasquero* groups (Labate, 2000), further increasing the number of Yagé ceremony participants. These groups use Yagé within a broad range of cultural and ritual traditions—from Indigenous to Christian, Hindu, and Islamic practices, to name a few (Tófoli, 2019). Brazil alone had roughly 50,000–150,000 domestic Yagé users estimated in 2019 (Tófoli, 2019). Such phenomena are interesting and alarming, as the conservation status of the non-cultivated Yagé lianas is yet to be evaluated. At the same time, their estimated native range in the Amazon basin rapidly dwindles.

THE YAGÉ ENIGMA

Yagé is a research topic that has been vastly explored by anthropologists, ethnobotanists, taxonomists, phytochemists, and, more recently, physicians and psychiatrists. This scholarly inquiry has been ongoing for over 170 years and continues to grow. Multiple Yagé species have been mentioned in the literature throughout this time. Despite the lack of evident morphological differences, Indigenous people have been known by ethnobotanists for their ability to recognize many types of Yagé lianas on the spot. Such a skill troubled and inspired the 20th-century explorer Schultes to extensively address this taxonomic enigma (Schultes 1954; 1957; 1963; 1972; 1975; 1976; 1982; Schultes, R. E., & Raffauf, 1990; 1992; Schultes et al., 2001; Sheldrake, 2020). Yet it was not until 1986 that Brownen Gates, a student of William Anderson (a renowned world Malpighiaceae authority), resolved many taxonomic problems associated with the reported Yagé lianas, narrowing their circumscription to four species: *B. caapi*, *Banisteriopsis muricata* (Cav.) Cuatrec., *Callaeum antifebrile* (Griseb.) D.M.Johnson, and *Tetrapterys styloptera* A.Juss (Gates, 1982; 1986). While the use of *B. caapi* has been regarded as ubiquitous throughout the Amazon basin, the use of the other three lianas has only been confirmed in one or a few locations each (Anderson, 2001; Gates, 1986). Because of that use disparity, while *B. caapi* is commonly referred to in the literature as the Yagé liana, the other species are Malpighiaceous Yagé analogues.*

In 1990, Schultes reported another Malpighiaceous Yagé analogue among the Karapaná Indigenous people in the Vaupés region of Colombia, the species *Tetrapterys mucronata* Cav (Schultes & Raffauf, 1990). Three decades passed until a group of Brazilian scholars revealed two new Malpighiaceous Yagé analogues: *Banisteriopsis laevifolia* (A.Juss.) B.Gates and *Diplopterys pubipetala* (A.Juss.) W.R.Anderson & C.Davis (Nagamine-Pinheiro et al., 2021; de Oliveira et al., 2023). This was the first time a species in the genus *Diplopterys* had been reported as a Malpighiaceous Yagé analogue. Yet analyzing the Yagé enigma through an ethnographic framework, M. L. Cepek (personal communication, March 19, 2023) suggests that *curagas* are taught each Yagé type by the supernatural Yagé "owners". They encounter these in the *ccusi'pa*—the shaman's "expansive and connecting body/space, the web of collective agency" where shamanistic work takes place. In English it is vaguely translated as "[Yagé] drunkness" (Cepek, 2023). Based on over two decades of anthropological and shamanic epistemological research with the Ecuadorian Cofáns, shaman Cesario Lucitante explains, "For example, you drink a certain kind of Yagé, you encounter a certain people, and they tell you, "We're the Jaguar People." Hence, you know that the yaje you drank was "ttesi yaje" [jaguar Yagé]" (M. L. Cepek, personal communication, March 19, 2023). These recent findings suggest that Schultes's Yagé enigma is far from over.

To further complicate this, the Yagé drink is not only made with either *B. caapi* or the mentioned Malpighiaceous Yagé analogues but it usually — not always (Beyer, 2010)— also incorporates at least one additional ingredient out of three plants regarded as Yagé admixtures. Two of these plants are also Malpighiaceous species: *Diplopterys cabrerana* (Cuatrec.) B.Gates and *Diplopterys* cf. *longialata* (Nied.) W.R.Anderson & C.Davis. Locally known as *chagropanga*, *Yagé-oko*, or *pinta*, they are employed primarily by communities that use the term Yagé in Colombia and Ecuador (Gates, 1986; Torres, 2017). The other species is *Psychotria viridis*, a member of the coffee family (Rubiaceae). Locally known as *pinta* or *opirito*, it is mainly used by communities that use the term Ayahuasca in the Amazon basin of Peru and Brazil (Torres, 2017). Yet the Yagé brew's complexity does not end here, as over a hundred other plants have been reported to be added to the concoction during its preparation, which vary depending on the community and shaman's practice (Rätsch, 2005; Schultes & Raffauf, 1990; 1992; Schultes et al. 2001). There are also plants that are not used directly in the drink preparation as Yagé admixtures but are also worked with during the Yagé ritual. Notably, tobacco (*Nicotiana tabacum* L. and *Nicotiana rustica* L.) is smoked and employed for spiritual purposes. Furthermore, *ñome'mbas* (perfumes) (Pinkley,

* Lianas that belong to the family Malpighiaceae and are less known but culturally used in the same way than the species *Banisteriopsis caapi*.

1973)—better known as *riegos* or *fluidos* in Spanish—are plant-based aromatic tinctures that are rubbed on the skin and inhaled during the ritual, for protection and to harmonize the "drunkenness." Thus, it is apparent that we are just scratching the surface regarding our understanding of this diverse practice, right at a time when the Andean-Amazonian heirs of these shamanic ontologies and epistemologies are increasingly facing rapid cultural transformations.

COMMUNITY-BASED PARTICIPATORY RESEARCH AND THE YAGÉ ENIGMA AMONG THE SUCUMBÍOS COFÁNS

In January 2019, during a Yagé ceremony presided over by *Taita* Alejandro,* I met a leader from his community, Pedro, who invited me to speak with all the community authorities and evaluate my interest in establishing a research collaboration. On my first visit to the community, over a period of five days, we had three meetings with the local authorities. Right from our first meeting, they mentioned how they were tired of self-interested outsiders who sought to take something from them, leaving little contribution behind. The Cofáns agreed they would help fulfill partnership commitments, and that I would have a chance to reciprocate. During this first meeting, I introduced myself and my ethnobotanical research experiences, expressing my interest in potentially studying their wild edible species in their protected territory. As their protocol has it when consulting about community affairs, each session was followed by a Yagé ceremony (Vargas Roncancio & Rodriguez-Mora, 2024). During the ceremonies, the community members and I continued getting to know each other, discussing potential ideas for establishing a Community-Based Participatory Research (CBPR) partnership (Strand et al., 2003). By the end of this visit, the authorities asked me to pursue a project to help them restore the crops and populations of the Yagé lianas, which they argue had been diminished as collateral damage of the glyphosate spraying promoted by the Plan Colombia and War on Drugs policies (Peterson, 2002; Sherret, 2005; Matthews, 2014; Rodríguez, 2016).

In this preliminary visit, the Cofáns shared with me that they grew at least eight types of Yagé lianas, which I presumed corresponded to the species *B. caapi*. Under the guidance of my mentors during my Master of Science in plant biology studies, I reviewed the literature on whether the purported diversity of *B. caapi* had ever been evaluated to correspond to a rank above form or cultivar. Additionally, I searched whether the Cofán Yagé types had ever been identified as *B. caapi* subspecies or other species—i.e., Malpighiaceous Yagé analogues. The literature on the Cofáns only reports *B. caapi* as the Cofán Yagé liana (Pinkley, 1973; Robinson, 1976; Schultes & Raffauf, 1990; 1992; Cerón, 1995), without any reference to Yagé analogues. However, multiple Yagé liana types have been mentioned and considered cultural variants of *B. caapi* (Jütte, 2016). On the one hand, the *pildé* Yagé liana has been referred to as a Yagé type that the Cofáns received from the Afro-Colombian people and communities coming from the Pacific coast of Colombia, and the *tena* Yagé—a.k.a., Napo yaje (M. L. Cepek, personal communication, March 19, 2023)—liana as a variant brought from Tena, Ecuador (Jütte, 2016). On the other hand, the *Hilberio* and *Piranga* Yagé liana types are claimed to be from two powerful shamans who had those names

* I have used fictitious names for the research participants mentioned in this paper to protect their identity.

(Jütte, 2016). It has been documented that the Cofáns recognize cultivated and wild* Yagé lianas. While the cultivated types are purportedly potent and less delicate to work with, the wild ones are the most powerful but also the most demanding to work with (Jütte, 2016). However, no systematic studies have thus far documented voucher specimens that would enable assessing these reported Cofán Yagé liana types. Despite the scanty botanical data about each of these Cofán Yagé liana types, to the best of my knowledge, they have been assumed to be *B. caapi*. As pointed out by de Oliveira et al. (2018), this informational gap is prevalent among the overall Yagé lianas reported in the literature. Given their morphological variability in the thickness of the main stem, the thickness and color of the stem fibers, and the presence or absence of a winged leaf stem and nodes in the stems with variable sizes, their accurate botanical assessment has been difficult to achieve (de Araújo et al., 2016; de Oliveira et al., 2018; Gates, 1986; Rodd, 2008; Sonsin et al., 2016). This issue is further exacerbated by the lack of mature stems collections, which are instrumental in the taxonomic determination of the lianas (de Oliveira et al., 2018). Regarding the Yagé admixtures, the aforementioned have also been cited to be used by the Cofáns, namely *D. cabrerana*, *D.* cf. *longialata*, and *P. viridis* (Pinkley, 1973; Schultes & Raffauf, 1990; 1992; Cerón, 1995).

In the latest revision for the genus *Banisteriopsis*, Gates (1982) considered the cultural types of *B. caapi* to be "chemical variants," vegetatively propagated by stem cuttings. Yet more data is needed to back up this assertion, and it warrants further investigation. Thus, I wondered if this "chemical variants understanding" was robust among the multiple *B. caapi* types reported in the literature. And if the "chemical variants" held for the cultivated varieties, do they also hold for the ones considered wild? Since the Sucumbíos Cofáns reported during my preliminary visit that their eight Yagé liana types also grew in the wild, without human intervention, I sought to combine my aim to address the Yagé enigma in their territory with their request to support their Yagé restoration efforts. Thus, I proposed for our collaboration to assess the ethnobotanical, taxonomic, and ecological diversity of the wild Yagé lianas at their protected territory, collecting stem cuttings of the encountered individual lianas at the forest canopy to be provided to the Cofáns in support of their restoration endeavors. At their protected territory, I aimed to evaluate the following null hypothesis: there is no correlation between the Cofán classification of their wild Yagé liana types and the lianas' diversity analyses, and there are no significantly distinct entities of *B. caapi* at a rank above form or cultivar. Before returning to the field, my project was reviewed by an Institutional Review Board (IRB) and I became acquainted with the code of ethics of the International Society of Ethnobiology (2006).

Upon my return to the Cofán community in June 2019, I met with the Cofán authorities, their proposed participants in the study, and the overall community members. We had been

* I use this term in this paper to illustrate the Cofán's distinction between their cultivated Yagé plants (*Yagé cultivado*), and their Yagé plants found in non-cultivated areas, or areas which have been intervened with either currently or in recent generations (*Yagé silvestre*). Yet upon further inquiring about the provenance of the "wild" Yagé plants, elders express that they may have been planted either by past Cofán generations or by the invisible people of the forest (*los invisibles*) (see also Vargas Roncancio & Rodriguez-Mora, 2024). M. L. Cepek has encountered the same understanding about the "wild" Yagé —*tsampi'su yaje* (forest Yagé)—origin among the Ecuadorian Cofáns (personal communication, March 19, 2023)

discussing my research proposal over the phone and had arranged basic logistics to go to their protected territory. However, with the active engagement of the community, we carried out a participatory mapping exercise, created a detailed research plan, and signed a research agreement. Five male participants, recognized for their shamanic knowledge and expertise, were appointed by the Cofán authorities to work on our research collaboration. Each of them independently led between one and two expeditions to their protected territory, for five to seven days, looking for their wild Yagé liana types. When a liana was found, I conducted a semi-informal interview with the accompanying participant (Martin, 2010). I asked questions about their ethnobotanical and ethnoecological relationship with the plant, such as their uses and preparations, when they first learned about the plant, where it grows, how prominent its occurrence in the landscape is, etc. Additionally, I inquired about the Cofán classification of each individual liana and the characteristics that enabled their identification. Furthermore, I documented twelve ecological features in the field, including altitude, plant community type, and human disturbances. Moreover, I collected at least three voucher specimens—including the mature stems (I was cautious not to harm the lianas)—and morphological data that could be lost after the plants were dried (e.g., flower color and leaf smell). Most voucher specimens were collected after the five expeditions led by the research participants, given the time-consuming task of employing tree climbing techniques to reach their leaves, flowers, and fruits in the canopy and emergent layer of the forest where these organs grow—between 72–131 ft (22–40 m) above the forest floor. It is worth emphasizing that I documented the participant's description of the lianas in detail, so that I could contrast this data with the lianas' morphological assessment using taxonomic keys and flower dissections under the stereoscope, and type herbarium specimens.

When I returned to the Cofán community from the fieldwork at their protected territory, some community members expressed concern about our collaboration. Given that my research methods encompassed voucher specimen collections and the use of microphones to record the research participants' interviews, some community members worried that the project was becoming a layer of surveillance or that I could exploit their TK and Yagé plants. Yet, fortunately, in the subsequent community meeting, I explained in detail the importance of collecting voucher specimens and recording the elders' interviews to identify the plants through Western botanical methods and accurately cross-reference the plants with the elders' knowledge. I also committed to amply discussing the study data and results, including derivative publication opportunities, for them to decide whether to/what to publish. Similarly, throughout the remaining four—out of eight (8) in total—community meetings in our study, I continued to transparently and openly answer any questions from the Cofáns, as we continued to strengthen our mutual trust. Through these community meetings, I became increasingly aware that working with the Cofáns as a mestizo graduate student, studying in a US institution entailed entering into asymmetrical power relationships. This understanding has made me engage in critical self-reflection throughout my research and practice, and I earnestly seek to contribute to the achievement of the Cofán's social justice goals.

Surprisingly, through the analysis of the collected data, the morphological evidence enabled me to conclude that the wild Cofán Yagé liana types include more than one Malpighiaceous species, none of which corresponds to *B. caapi*. Although this study was completed in May 2021, an audiovisual summary,* showcasing the general results of the study was publicly displayed for the first time at the Ethnopharmacological Search for Psychoactive Drugs 55 (ESPD55) conference once the Cofáns authorized its disclosure. The specific results of this work were embargoed until May 2025, respecting the Cofáns' request to further discuss the implications of these findings, which enabled them to make an informed decision regarding publications. Given their colonial history and the ongoing commodification and exploitation of Yagé TK, the Cofáns hold a reserved and protective stance towards publishing their TK. Sympathizing with their position, I apply TallBear's (2014) "standing with" concept, remaining open to being altered in my approach to knowledge and critically self-reflecting on the implications of our collaboration. Thus, integrating anthropology and ethnobotany, I assessed Intellectural Property Rights (IPRs) as a potential underlying issue that could direct our research toward a more decolonial analysis. Consequently, I sought to address the risks of publishing our study results (Smith, 2021), particularly regarding potential eventual patents that may disenfranchise the Cofáns from their right to direct the relationship between people and their Yagé lianas and territory.

Although I was the principal investigator in this research, my work was co-created, discussed, guided, and assessed with the active participation of the Sucumbíos Cofáns. While few members of the community speak A'ingae fluently, everyone is fluent in Spanish, my native tongue. Since my cultural perspective is tied to Latino, Colombian, Bogotanian, mestizo, and more recently, Northern perspectives on plant-human relations and the law, acknowledging the difference in perspective in relation to the Cofáns is critical. Although as a Colombian, I am not an outsider in the country, as a Bogotanian mestizo, I am an outsider in the Cofán territory. Consequently, I do not speak as a representative of the Cofáns in my work. I have been raised in a middle-class-mestizo-Colombian family and I am aware of the many unearned privileges I have. As a graduate student in a US institution, I recognize that my privileged education enables me to analyze Indigenous plant-human relations and the potential impacts between IPRs and our study findings, but only through a limited cultural perspective. In my research, I frequently engage in critical reflexivity to evaluate whether my work may inadvertently harm my research partners; for example, by perpetuating colonizing and exploitative research. I aim to be perceived by the Cofáns as a community ally, eager to contribute to achieving the Cofáns' social justice goals, while respecting, learning, and celebrating the Cofán biocultural legacy. I aim for my Cofán colleagues to clearly recognize the value I place upon their ontological and epistemological commitments, and the critical stance I take on the positivist and Cartesian perspectives of the Western academic hegemony. Yet my positionality as an outsider is unavoidable since my perspectives and interpretations are informed through formal academies. Thus, I have made a concerted effort to listen carefully to the active feedback provided by my Cofán colleagues in our community meetings and throughout our study, to identify and address underlying issues in our collaboration.

INTELLECTUAL PROPERTY RIGHTS FOR WHOM?

Property is the codification of a social relation between owner and non-owner. While material

* An audiovisual summary of this work can be found on YouTube under the entry "La Diversidad de Yagé (a.k.a. Ayahuasca) entre los Cofanes de Sucumbíos (Colombia)"— https://youtu.be/qat7JwyXmuI.

property rights ensure material holding, IPRs ensure intellectual withholding. Although material property is rivalrous and competitive in the market, intellectual property is generally non-rivalrous. But by artificially creating information scarcity, ideas foster competition, generate market advantages, become competitive and obtain a price. The deliberate fictitious creation of information scarcity commodifies ideas into ownership for the granting of legal benefits (May & Sell, 2006). On the one hand, public action prevents the rise of material property prices. On the other hand, the artificial scarcity of IPRs ensures the rise of ideas prices (Plant, 1934). Thus, IPRs constitute "a forceful form of social power" where innovation rights undermine nonowner rights, regardless of social cost (Anawalt, 2003). IPRs are temporary rights with three core benefits: "rent for use, compensation for loss, and payment for transfer" (May & Sell, 2006). They incentivize individual effort, protection, resource allocation efficiency, innovation, and reward. Yet paradoxically, without counteracting measures, excessive property rights and monopoly abuses suppress innovation (May & Sell, 2006). Patents are IPRs of industrial ideas granted on the basis of novelty, non-obviousness, and industrial applicability.

Intellectual property approximations were applied in Greece through poetry, Alexandria through texts, the Roman Empire through oil lamps and texts, and in the authorship reporting of Jewish orators (Carson, 1999). During the Middle Ages, guild trademarks became prevalent, conferring market advantages that benefited the local economy (May & Sell, 2006). To justify trademarks, monopoly producers may have appealed to quality, reliability, and the suppression of competition (Paster, 1969). There is no certainty about the first official patent. Still, the 1416 patent for Ser Franciscus Petri stands as the earliest record, which conferred him exclusionary rights by the Grand Council of Venice for a device that turned wool into felt (Sichelman & O'Connor, 2012). While there is no evidence that Petri was the device inventor, he received the patent because it gave him proprietary advantages in Venice (Sichelman & O'Connor, 2012). A decade later, Filippo Brunelleschi was also given special privileges for designing a vessel, Il Badalone, which was intended to transport marble for constructing the Dome of Florence (Prager,1946). Operating within the Florentine territory and lasting three years, this innovation set the patent precedents of novelty, scope, and temporality.

In 1474, the ideas about owning knowledge and information were formalized in the Venetian statute. This was the first generalized law that intended to favor creativity and industrial development. At this stage in the development of IPRs, there was already a practical view of the balance between private benefits and public welfare, with the government fostering competitive advantages and economic organization (May & Sell, 2006). In 1624 and 1710, the Statute of Monopolies and the Act of Anne established the modern patent and copyright laws in England, followed by the development of intellectual property institutions (Macfarlane, 1978). In the eighteenth century, IPRs notions spread in continental Europe—especially in France—where they were used to build economic relations within the growing capitalist system. In 1883, a multilateral treaty was signed at the Paris Convention for the Protection of Industrial Property.

In the twentieth century, patent cartels dominated the interwar period and after WWII, the US promoted an economic order based on multilateralism, freedom, democracy, and competition (Porter, 1999). But given the limitations of patent enforcement at the time, these years were characterized by distrust toward patents (May & Sell, 2006). Through the 1951 Patent Act, the

US government increased patent protection, clarified their withholding right, and launched the blocking patent—i.e., the granting of a right to exclude others from using an invention (May & Sell, 2006). By the end of the twentieth century, an IPRs global regime was established: The Agreement on Trade Related Aspects of Intellectual Property Rights (TRIPS). This treaty has been criticized as an Anglo-Saxon legal discourse that reflects US ways of thinking about the law, imposing a singularized notion of property that considers "the capitalist market as the only solution to political economic problems" (Burch, 1995; May & Sell, 2006; Sell, 2003). By promoting a neo-liberal agenda, Shiva (2016) argues that TRIPS frames IPRs as "a prescription for a monoculture of knowledge."

During the last decades of the twentieth century, scientific advancements in genetics and chemistry guided the developments in biotechnology IPRs. Three different governance mechanisms deal with this area: TRIPS, the Convention on Biological Diversity (CBD), and the International Union for the Protection of New Varieties of Plants (UPOV) (Code, 2015; Secretariat, 1992; World Trade Organization, 1994). In contrast with TRIPS' multilateralism, the CBD recognizes natural resources' sovereignty rights, communal knowledge rights, and the consented application of traditional practices (Secretariat, 1992). While these mechanisms claim to exclude patentability from plants, animals, and biological processes, they enforce plant varieties' patent protection and fail to protect the commodification of bioresources. Shiva (2000) argues that by manipulating language, life forms and TK are redefined as "biotechnological inventions," patenting life and marginalized people's knowledge through the imposition of the Global North's law. Despite multiple petitions by economically disadvantaged countries calling for an amendment of the TRIPS Agreement "to demand patent applicants to disclose the genetic resource origin and TK used, and to demonstrate prior informed consent and fair and equitable benefit sharing," the US and Europe have refused to implement these measures (Shiva, 2000; World Trade Organization, 2008).

IPRs may be the central issue of our current and future political economy (May & Sell, 2006). Yet rather than universal, natural, or inevitable mandates, IPRs are politically situated, contested, contingent, and continuous ideas. They reflect the horse-trading history between private benefits vs. public welfare, protection vs. exclusion, and competition vs. dissemination (May & Sell, 2006). Far from a neutral and technical assessment of the social benefits created by IPRs, their historical agenda has been shaped by political interest. For instance, the intentional creation of new markets through the politics of property and competition (Fligstein, 1996; May & Sell, 2006). IPRs represent singular universalizing laws, reminiscent of the modern Cartesian substance ontology. Here, reality is conceived as a phenomenon that divides the world into matter and thought to explain the material world fully (Descartes, 2017). This ontology holds that matter is stable or static and will act following its inherent properties. Intellectual Property Rights (IPRs) separate and superimpose humans from other life forms and things, arbitrarily granting the former the right to possess, control, and profit from the latter.

IPRs privilege general knowledge appropriated by powerful economic groups over TK. Moreover, IPRs often disregard TK contributions to the creation of general knowledge. Despite the broad recognition of TK's value, Western institutions still deem TK as 'unscientific' or as a common heritage. These notions are employed by IPRs institutions to justify their reluctance to recognize and confer IPRs to TK (Brush, 1993; Shiva, 2016). It is claimed that, unlike general knowledge, TK exhibits problems with its precise differentiation, group identity, legal status, and the establishment of well-developed markets (Brush, 1993). Furthermore, IPRs are also complicated and expensive to obtain, monitor, enforce, and preserve. Thus, whether inadvertently or not, powerful economic groups' creations in industrialized countries have been historically favored to the detriment of Indigenous peoples' innovations and knowledge contributions, especially in developing nations (Brush, 1993; Shiva, 2016). The prevailing circumscription of IPRs diminishes the political power of historically marginalized people, such as the Cofáns. These laws effectively disenfranchise people from their TK rights, not only regarding the use and management of their knowledge, but also the enforcement of their ontological commitments. Although several national and international protocols advocate for the protection of the sovereignty and self-determination rights of historically marginalized groups (e.g., Indigenous and Tribal Peoples Convention No. 169, The Rio Declaration on Environment and Development, and The Nagoya Protocol) (Declaration, 1992; International Labor Organization, 1989; Secretariat, 2011), their enforcement is limited and cannot override TRIPS' IPRs global regime. Consequently, despite current intergovernmental efforts, a potential derivative patent from a third party using the results of the ethnobotanical research presented here would be very problematic. Such a patent would legally protect the patent holders instead of holding them accountable for, say, asking for consent or sharing benefits with the Cofáns.

YAGÉ'S SUSCEPTIBILITY TO BIOPIRACY

In the past few decades, the number of studies scientifically validating the medicinal value of *B. caapi* has proliferated. Particularly, its potential use in the treatment of psychological and neurodegenerative disorders (Rommelspacher 1981, Samoylenko et al. 2010, Brierley & Davidson 2012, Frecska et al. 2016, Coe & McKenna 2017, Lawn et al. 2017, Franquesa et al. 2018, Hamill et al. 2019). Additionally, growing scientific evidence has validated an extraordinary broad-spectrum role of the main active principles of *B. caapi* (Millard 2017, Patel et al. 2012), the ß-carboline alkaloids harmine and harmaline (Barriga-Villalba 1925, Deulofeu 1967, Rivier & Lindgren 1972, Callaway et al. 1999, Callaway et al. 2005). Other than their monoamine oxidase inhibitory (MAOI) activity (McKenna et al. 1984, Callaway 2005, Morales et al. 2017), these alkaloids also exhibit anticancer, antitumor, antiviral, antimicrobial, antiparasitic, anti-senescence, anti-diabetic, antidepressant, osteogenic, neurogenic, and neuroprotective effects (McKenna & Towers 1981, Di Giorgio et al. 2004, Splettstoesser 2005, Moura et al. 2007, Rosenkranz & Wink 2008, Brahmbhatt 2010, Neenah 2010, Patel et al. 2012, Alomar et al. 2013, Zhao & Wink 2013, Chen 2015, Quintana et al. 2016, Millard 2017). Furthermore, the advancements in the biochemical understanding of these, as well as related alkaloids, have been pivotal in the design and development of bioactive compounds for the treatment of an array of diseases and medical conditions, as varied as cancer and sexual dysfunction (Cao et al. 2007, Bayih et *al.* 2016, Sharma et al. 2016, Pagano et al. 2017, Dai et al. 2018). Other constituents of *B. caapi* have also been found to exert beneficial biochemical effects, such as the antioxidant ability of the proanthocyanidins, epicatechin, and procyanidin B2 (Wang et al. 2010).

Given the potential medical applications of *B. caapi* and its active principles, numerous pending and some already granted patents have been developed to date concerning this species. As the Centro de Estudios para la Justicia Social Tierra Digna (2020) demonstrate, ethnobotanical and ethnopharmacological Yagé studies have been fundamental to these patent developments. According to the patent databases PATENTSCOPE and USPTO, as of October 2019, thirty-eight patent applications were associated with the entry "*Banisteriopsis caapi*," eight of which have already been approved and granted (Centro de Estudios para la Justicia Social Tierra Digna, 2020). Some relevant examples include the well-known Banisteriopsis caapi (CV) "Da Vine" patent by Loren Miller, which claimed "novelty" in a "developed" Yagé variety. This patent appears current after being revoked once—when it was challenged for biopiracy of Indigenous Amazonian knowledge—and re-granted back in 2001 (Centro de Estudios para la Justicia Social Tierra Digna, 2020). Yet, after being re-granted, the patent was virtually useless, as it only protected Miller's "rights" to the derivative lianas propagated from his specimen (Beyer, 2010). The other seven patents constitute biochemical "innovations," primarily for medicinal applications encompassing psychological, psychiatric, and physical ailments (Centro de Estudios para la Justicia Social Tierra Digna, 2020). But the most egregious case is the synthetic ayahuasca patent by Herkenroth Thomas. Granted in 2018, this patent protects pharmaceutical innovations in the preparation of extracts containing the active principles of *B. caapi* and *P. viridis*, or *B. caapi* and *D. cabrerana* (Centro de Estudios para la Justicia Social Tierra Digna, 2020). Importantly, most of the eight current patents are owned by people in the Global North. This suggests that the ethnobotanical and ethnopharmacological Yagé research has been used as a commodifying tool of Amazonian Indigenous peoples, their TK, and their territories.

The Centro de Estudios para la Justicia Social Tierra Digna (2020) further characterizes the *modus operandi* of states, companies, and scientific communities involved in pharmacological patent development. According to this research group, these actors create centralized databases of bioprospecting candidate species, modify local policies to privilege the free trade of target biological and genetic resources, and employ such resources to advance their own scientific research, develop derivative patents, and commercialize products (Centro de Estudios para la Justicia Social Tierra Digna, 2020). Depending on the level of "innovation," it could be argued that not all Yagé-related patents constitute biopiracy. However, disregarding the crucial contributions of Amazonian communities, without which the patents could have never been realized, socially and economically excludes these historically marginalized groups. Consequently, I suggest this issue may be constituting an affront to their undermined IPRs. Moreover, many Indigenous comunidades *Yageceras* remain oblivious to the sophisticated scientific advancements in understanding and commodifying the Yagé active compounds and the granted and pending patents. These issues suggest that the search for psychoactive plants, fungi and natural products has been instrumental in increasing the Yagé susceptibility to biopiracy.

LEVERAGING INTELLECTUAL PROPERTY RIGHTS ISSUES IN ETHNOBOTANY AND ETHNOPHARMACOLOGY THROUGH COMMUNITY-BASED PARTICIPATORY RESEARCH

Privileging Western epistemologies and ways of knowing is a pervasive research orientation applied across many nations worldwide, including universities in the US and Colombia. In my ethnobotanical partnership with the Sucumbíos Cofáns, I became increasingly aware that the TK I was documenting could be superseded by Western science and by derivative technological developments. Accordingly, bioprospecting and technological innovations that emerge from ethnobotanical and ethnopharmacological studies often disregard the voice of the original knowledge holders, without whom such innovations would not have been possible. These problems are further exacerbated through IPRs laws, which privilege individual general knowledge innovations over TK. As IPRs deem TK as common collective knowledge that lacks established markets, the Sucumbíos Cofán TK documented in our collaboration does not qualify for IPRs. While at the national and international levels, the mandates of multiple states and the United Nations advocate for protecting TK and benefit-sharing concerning biological and genetic resources, their enforcement is precarious. This situation, coupled with the high cost of fighting legal battles to challenge individual IPRs derivative from TK, leaves original knowledge holders at odds with powerful economic groups profiting from TK (May & Sell, 2006; Shiva, 2000; 2016). As they stand, IPRs constitute an axiological norm that disregards TK. By serving the disenfranchisement of marginalized communities from their sovereignty and self-determination rights (Saito, 2020), these laws perpetuate bioprospecting social injustices.

Similarly, using ethnobotanical and ethnopharmacological research as a tool for the profit of powerful economic groups, at the expense of marginalized communities' TK, calls into question our research approach and practice as well as our institutions thinking (Atalay, 2012; Mogstad & Tse, 2018; Smith, 2021). We must reconceptualize our practice, questioning the service that our work and actions pay to legitimate the settler state. Research is often subordinated to the researcher and institutions' career agendas, regardless of the community's legal mandates about the use, management, commodification, and commercialization of their TK. Yet CBPR reminds us to see independent sovereigns in our partner communities instead of informants of our work. Consequently, before the dissemination of research results, it is key for researchers to amply discuss with their partner communities the potential risk associated with their knowledge publication. Moreover, the community's right to decide the use, access, management, and eventual profit that may derive from their knowledge should be acknowledged in the research publications. But most importantly, we must address the legal and political implications of our research. I suggest that, at the very least, scholars should disclose in their publications the IPR challenges for their community research partners. Ideally, we should strive to foster dialogues among the stakeholders involved in the legal and political applications of our work, aiming to help in the protection of our partner's TK and territories. This is especially relevant for the Yagé lianas, as they are cultural keystone species used for healing and protecting the forest.

Rather than uncritically accepting IPRs, researchers can aid in the evaluation and reformulation of these laws and direct their efforts toward social justice goals sought in CBPR collaborations. Decolonizing our research may require leveraging the pluralization of ontology beyond our practice, transcending Western metaphysical categories and assumptions in our laws and politics, and taking people's otherness seriously (Latour, 2012; Smith, 2021; Viveiros de Castro, 2004). For instance, the everyday and long-term use of Yagé as a protocol by the Sucumbíos Cofáns needs deep understanding and sensitivity. This includes discussing the Yagé-related IPRs, as well as better understanding the Yagé-human relations and their potential. This demands the long, slow, and continuous engagement of the multiple stakeholders at play, and would include dialogues with elder shamans in ceremonial contexts and under the effect and guidance of Yagé (see also Vargas Roncancio & Rodriguez-Mora, 2024). May & Sell (2005) argue that establishing IPRs as defined by the TRIPS settlement resulted from the conjunction of technological, legal/political, and philosophical developments in the history of modern capitalism. Thus, while the current TRIPS treaty favors powerful economic groups, the authors' historical analysis suggests that contesting the agreement could reverse its extreme measures. Archer (1995) argues that affected agents must organize themselves collectively to engage in political processes that may lead to effectively sharing their common interests and leveraging the desired changes. While this approach may be "Western" in orientation, it encourages researchers to promote collective action in academia, beyond individualistic gain. Scholars may also strive to foster spaces where "technical expertise, political power, and access to resources and the institutions they wish to change" are gathered (May & Sell 2005).

Finally, it is crucial to transcend the scope of our work in our practice and institutions' thinking, striving to extend our efforts to earnestly respect our historically marginalized partner communities. For example, by supporting their grass-roots initiatives to reduce inequality and leverage self-determination (Atalay, 2012; Saito, 2020). Through this approach, we can open our minds to conceptualizing and learning alternative possibilities of sociopolitical and economic organization and reciprocal ways to relate to one another and our environment. CBPR may expose the constraints of our worldviews and extant law and enable us to understand racial justice better (Saito, 2020). As we face global climate change and the sixth mass extinction, we can be instrumental in voicing the importance of the legal codes of Indigenous people and the enforcement of their fundamental rights, freedom, dignity, reconstitution, and reparations. It is time to evaluate whether there is a lack of will to legally recognize that the Yagé drink and Yagé shamanism, and not only their patented commodified "innovations," hold an outstanding potential to heal and safeguard our imperiled ethnosphere and biosphere. Lastly, as suggested by Shiva (2016), recognizing the regenerative life force in our relations may be the leading agency that can guide us into a new era of more equitable political economics, as is yet to be seen by the law.

ACKNOWLEDGEMENTS

I want to express my deep gratitude, appreciation, and admiration to the Yagé lianas, their associated entities, and the Sucumbíos Cofáns. To my mentors, Drs. Lauren Raz, Jillian De Gezelle, Alexander Krings, Adrian Smith, Michael Cepek, Miguel Rojas-Sotelo, and Rafael Felipe de Almeida, for their trust, rigorousness, and dedicated guidance. To my beloved relatives, Stephanie Smith and Carlina Mora, for their unconditional support and ample love. To my colleagues, Dr. Michael Coe, for his example and encouragement to further my research, Dr. Iván Vargas Roncancio, for his continuous support, guidance, and feedback throughout my research, and Miguel Duarte, for his pertinent feedback on previous versions of this manuscript. To my brother Camilo Rodríguez, whose transformation inspired me to experience the Yagé ritual. To Rebecca Lazarou for her wholehearted support and patience during the making of this paper.

To Annette Badenhorst for her decisive leadership and kind generosity, which encouraged me to deepen my work. And to Dr. Dennis Mckenna, the Mckenna Academy, and Nicholas and Dinah Shaftesbury for bringing the ESPD55 Conference to fruition.

BIBLIOGRAPHY

Anawalt, Howard C. 2003. "International Intellectual Property, Progress, and the Rule of Law." *Santa Clara Computer and High Technology Law Journal* 19, no. 2: 383–405.

Anderson, W. R. (2001). Malpighiaceae. In Berry, P. E., Yatskievych, K., & BK (Ed.) HOLST. (1995). *Flora of the Venezuelan Guayana* (Vol. 1, pp. 161-191). St. Louis: Missouri Botanical Garden.

Archer, M. (1995). Realist Social Theory: The Morphogenetic Approach. Cambridge: Cambridge University Press.

Assembly, U. G. (2012). Convention on the Prevention and Punishment of the Crime of Genocide (1948). *United Nations, Treaty Series, 78.*

Atalay, S. (2012). Community-based archaeology: Research with, by, and for indigenous and local communities. Univ of California Press.

Barriga-Villalba, A. M. (1925). Yajeine. A new alkaloid. *Journal of the Society of Chemistry and Industry* Vol. 44: 205-207.

Bell, D. (1991). Racial realism. *Conn. L. Rev., 24,* 363.

Beyer, S. V. (2010). Singing to the plants: A guide to mestizo shamanism in the upper Amazon. UNM Press.

Brabec de Mori, B. (2011). Tracing hallucinations. Contributing to a critical ethnohistory of ayahuasca usage in the Peruvian Amazon. Beatriz C. Labate & Henrik Jungaberle (éd.), The Internationalization of Ayahuasca, Zürich, LIT-Verlag, 23-47.

Brabec de Mori, B. (2020). Is Ayahuasca Possibly Less than Five Hundred Years Old? Retrieved on February 05th, 2021, from https://chacruna.net/is-ayahuasca-possibly-less-than-five-hundred-years-old/

Borman, M. B. 1976. Vocabulario cofán: Cofán-castellano, castellano-cofán. Vocabularios indígenas 19. Quito: Instituto Lingüístico de Verano (Summer Institute of Linguistics).

Borman, R. B. 2009. "A History of the Río Cofanes Territory." In Rapid Inventory No. 21: Ecuador: Cabeceres Cofanes-Chingual, ed. C. Vriesendorp, William S.

Brush, S. B. (1993). Indigenous knowledge of biological resources and intellectual property rights: the role of anthropology. *American Anthropologist, 95*(3), 653-671.

Brierley, D. I., & Davidson, C. (2012). Developments in harmine pharmacology—Implications for ayahuasca use and drug-dependence treatment. Progress in neuro-psychopharmacology and biological psychiatry, 39(2), 263-272.

Burch, Kurt. 1995. "Intellectual Property Rights and the Culture of Global Liberalism." Science Communication 17, no. 2 (December): 214–232.

Cabodevilla, M. M. (1996). Coca: La región y su historia. Pompeya, Ecuador: CICAME.

Callaway, J. C. (1999). Phytochemistry and neuropharmacology of ayahuasca. Ayahuasca, R. Metzner, Thunder's mouth press, New York. pp-259-261.

Callaway, J. C. (2005). Various alkaloid profiles in decoctions of Banisteriopsis caapi. *Journal of Psychoactive Drugs,* 37(2), 151-155.

Callaway, J. C., Brito, G. S., & Neves, E. S. (2005). Phytochemical analyses of Banisteriopsis caapi and *Psychotria viridis.* Journal of psychoactive drugs, 37(2), 145-150.

Campbell, L. (2010, August). Language Isolates and Their History, or, What's Weird, Anyway?. In Annual Meeting of the Berkeley Linguistics Society (Vol. 36, No. 1, pp. 16-31).

Carson, Anne. 1999. Economy of the Unlost. Princeton, NJ: Princeton University Press.

Centro de Estudios para la Justicia Social Tierra Digna. (2020) Plantas sagradas y conocimientos ancestrales de la Amazonia: los riesgos de las patentes de la ayahuasca y de la sangre de dragó. Tierra Digna.

Cepek, M. L. (2012). A future for Amazonia. In A Future for Amazonia. University of Texas Press.

Cepek, M. L. (2018). Life in oil: Cofán survival in the petroleum fields of Amazonia. University of Texas Press.

Cepek, M. L. (2023). "Perceptions, Relations, and Possessions: The Expansive Body as the Foundation of Cofán Shamanic Epistemology." In Barret, C., Cepek, M., Quintanilla, P., Fabiano, E., and Machery, E. (Eds), *Southern Epistemologies: Knowledge, Wisdom and Understanding in the Andes and Western Amazon (Volume II),* Chicago: HAU Books.

Cerón, C. E. (1995). Etnobiología de los Cofanes de Dureno. Publicaciones del Museo Ecuatoreano de Ciencias Naturales Serie: Monografia Ano, 10(3).

Code, U. P. O. V. (2015). International Union for the protection of new varieties of plants.

Coe, M. A., & McKenna, D. J. (2017). The therapeutic potential of Ayahuasca. In Evidence-based herbal and nutritional treatments for anxiety in psychiatric disorders (pp. 123-137). Springer.

Cham. Degnen, C. (2018). Cross-cultural perspectives on personhood and the life course. Basingstoke: Palgrave Macmillan.

Fundación, Z. I. O.-A'i. (2012). Plan de salvaguarda pueblo cofán.

Davis, W., & Schultes, R. (2004). The lost Amazon: the photographic journey of Richard Evans Schultes. Chronicle Books.

Davis, W. (2014). One river: Explorations and discoveries in the Amazon rain forest. Random House.

de Araújo, T.A., Dos Passos, J.M., Behrens, C.S.B, Fagg, C.W., Oliveira, J.S., Oliveira, R.C, Gomes, S.M. (2016). *Leaf Anatomy Distinguishes the Ayahuasca Lianas "Caupuri" and "Tucunacá" (Banisteriopsis caapi,* Malpighiaceae*).* Retrieved on July 22, 2020 from https://dtihost.sfo2.digitaloceanspaces.com/sbotanicab/67CNBot/resAnexo1-1370-1488-844fbd1093cb7520a5ae8cd2163f0d3e.pdf

de Oliveira, R.C., Fagg, C.W, Labate, B., & Sonsin, J.O. (2018). *The Urgent Need to Review the Botanical Classification of the Ayahuasca Vine.* Retrieved on July 22, 2020, from https://chacruna.net/urgent-botanical-classification-ayahuasca/

de Oliveira, R. C., Behrens, C. S., Nagamine-Pinheiro, N., Fagg, C. W., e Silva, M. S., Martins-Silva, T., & Sonsin-Oliveira, J. (2023). Ethnobotany and Wood Anatomy of Banisteriopsis caapi Ethnotaxa and Diplopterys cf. pubipetala, Components of Ayahuasca in Brazilian Rituals. Economic Botany, 1-30.

Declaration, R. (1992). Report of the United Nations conference on environment and development. *The Rio Declaration on Environment and Development 1992.*

Defensoría del Pueblo (2022). Entre enero y julio de este año han sido asesinados 122 líderes sociales y personas defensoras de DD. HH. *).* Retrieved on December 30, 2022 from https://www.defensoria.gov.co/-/entre-enero-y-julio-de-este-a%C3%B1o-han-sido-asesinados-122-l%C3%ADderes-sociales-y-personas-defensoras-de-dd.-hh.

Descartes, R. (2017) "Principles of philosophy." *Copyright© Jonathan Bennett.*

Deulofeu, V. (1967). Chemical compounds isolated from Banisteriopsis and related species. In Efron, D.H., Holmstedt, B., & Kline, N.S. (Eds), *Ethnopharmacologic Search for Psychoactive Drugs* (pp. 393-402).Fligstein, Neil. 1996. "Markets as Politics: A Political-Cultural Approach to Market Institutions." American Sociological Review 61, no. 4 (August): 656– 673.

Franquesa, A., Sainz-Cort, A., Gandy, S., Soler, J., Alcázar-Córcoles, M. Á., & Bouso, J. C. (2018). Psychological variables implied in the therapeutic effect of ayahuasca: A contextual approach. Psychiatry research, 264, 334-339.

Frecska, E., Bokor, P., & Winkelman, M. (2016). The therapeutic potentials of ayahuasca: possible effects against various diseases of civilization. Frontiers in Pharmacology, 7, 35.

Friede, J. (1952, August). Los Cofán: Una tribu de la Alta Amazonía Colombiana. In Proceedings of the thirtieth International Congress of Americanists. Cambridge MA.

Frontline Defenders (2022). Global Analysis 2022.

Fotiou, E. (2019). Technologies of the Body in Contemporary Ayahuasca Shamanism in the Peruvian Amazon: Implications for Future Research. Human Ecology, 1-7.

Ganem Maloof, K. (2022). Hay futuro si hay verdad: informe final, convocatoria a la paz grande.

Gates, B. (1982). Banisteriopsis, Diplopterys (Malpighiaceae). Flora Neotropica, 30, 1-237.

Gates, B. (1986). La taxonomía de las malpigiáceas utilizadas en el brebaje del ayahuasca. América Indígena, 46(1), 49-72.

Hamill, J., Hallak, J., Dursun, S. M., & Baker, G. (2019). Ayahuasca: psychological and physiologic effects, pharmacology and potential uses in addiction and mental illness. Current neuropharmacology, 17(2), 108-128.

Hengeveld, K., & Fischer, R. (2018). Cofánngae (Cofán/Cofán) operators. Open Linguistics, 4(1), 328-355.

Higuita, A. (2011). Historia de conflicto Pueblo Cofán. Proyecto Mitigación de conflictos interétnicos territoriales en Colombia: Protección de los derechos de las comunidades rurales al territorio y a los recursos 2009-2011. Mesa Permanente del Pueblo Cofán.

Highpine, G. (2012). Unraveling the Mystery of the Origin of Ayahuasca. *Núcleo de Estudos Interdisciplinares sobre Psicoativos (NEIP)[Internet].*

International Labour Organization. (1989) Indigenous and Tribal Peoples Convention, C169, 27 June 1989, C169. Retrieved on April 20, 2023 from https://www.refworld.org/docid/3ddb6d514.html

International Society of Ethnobiology (2006). International Society of Ethnobiology Code of Ethics (with 2008 additions).

Jütte, M. (2016). Reisende im Strom der Zeit: zum Yagé (Ayahuasca)--Gebrauch der kolumbianischen Cofán (Vol. 64). LIT Verlag Münster.

Kohn, E. (2002). "Infidels, Virgins, and the Black-Robed Priest: A Backwoods History of Ecuador's Montaña Region." Ethnohistory 49(3):545–582.

Kostylo, J. (2010). From gunpowder to print: The common origins of copyright and patent. *Privilege and Property*, 21.

Labate, B. (2000). A reinvenção do uso da ayahuasca nos centros urbanos. Dissertação de Mestrado apresentada ao Programa de Pós-Graduação em Antropologia Social do IFCH. Unicamp.

Latour, B. (2012). We have never been modern. Harvard university press.

Lawn, W., Hallak, J. E., Crippa, J. A., Dos Santos, R., Porffy, L., Barratt, M. J., ... & Morgan, C. J. (2017). Well-being, problematic alcohol consumption and acute subjective drug effects in past-year ayahuasca users: a large, international, self-selecting online survey. Scientific Reports, 7(1), 1-10.

Martin, G. J. (2010). Ethnobotany: a methods manual. Routledge. May, C., & Sell, S. K. (2006). Intellectual property rights: A critical history (p. 37). Boulder: Lynne Rienner Publishers.

Matthews, G. (2014). Aerial Spray Drift–Consequences of Spraying Small Droplets of Herbicide. Outlooks on Pest Management, 25(4), 279-283.

May, C., & Sell, S. K. (2006). Intellectual property rights: A critical history (p. 37). Boulder: Lynne Rienner Publishers.

Millard, D. (2017). Broad Spectrum Roles of Harmine in Ayahuasca. In Prance, S.G., McKenna, D.J., De Loenen, B., & Davis, W. (Eds), *Ethnopharmacologic Search for Psychoactive Drugs* (pp. 82-94). Synergetic Press.

Minsalud. (2020). Boletines poblacionales: Población Indígena Corte a Diciembre de 2019. Gobierno de Colombia. Retrieved on December 30, 2022 from https://www.minsalud.gov.co/sites/rid/Lists/BibliotecaDigital/RIDE/DE/PS/boletines-poblacionales-poblacion-indigena.pdf

Mogstad, H., & Tse, L. S. (2018). Decolonizing Anthropology: Reflections from Cambridge. *The Cambridge Journal of Anthropology*, *36*(2), 53-72.

Mongua-Calderón, C. (2018). Caucho, frontera, indígenas e historia regional: un análisis historiográfico de la época del caucho en el Putumayo-Aguarico (Colombia). Boletín de Antropología Universidad de Antioquia, 33(55), 15-34.

Mongua Calderón, C. (2020). Fronteras, poder político y economía gomífera en el Putumayo-Aguarico: más allá de la marginalidad y el aislamiento, 1845-1900. Historia Crítica, (76), 49-71.

Nader, H. (Ed.). (2004). The Book of Privileges Issued to Christopher Columbus by King Fernando and Queen Isabel 1492-1502 (Vol. 2). Wipf and Stock Publishers.

Nagamine-Pinheiro, N., Fagg, C. W., Gomes, S. M., Oliveira, R. C., & Sonsin-Oliveira, J. (2021). Vegetative anatomy, morphology and histochemistry of three species of Malpighiaceae used in analogues of the Amazonian psychoactive beverage Ayahuasca. Flora, 275, 151760.

Pagden, A. (2018). The School of Salamanca, the Requerimiento, and the Papal Donation of Alexander VI. *Codex*, *7*(37), 3.

Paster, Benjamin G. 1969. "Trademarks—Their Early History." The Trademark Reporter 59: 551–572

Patel, K., Gadewar, M., Tripathi, R., Prasad, S. K., & Patel, D. K. (2012). A review on medicinal importance, pharmacological activity and bioanalytical aspects of beta-carboline alkaloid "Harmine". Asian Pacific journal of tropical biomedicine, 2(8), 660-664.

Paz, A. C. "Acuerdo Final para la Terminación del Conflicto y la Construcción de una Paz Estable y Duradera." *Gobierno Nacional de Colombia* (2016).

Perafán, L. G. (2022). #PARENLAMASACRE. Instituto de Estudios para el Desarrollo y la Paz (Indepaz). Retrieved on December 30, 2022 from https://indepaz.org.co/parenlamasacre/

Peterson, S. (2002). People and ecosystems in Colombia: Casualties of the drug war. The Independent Review, 6(3), 427-440.

Pinkley, H. V. (1973). The ethno-ecology of the Kofan Indians (Doctoral dissertation, Harvard University).

Plant, Arnold. 1934. "The Economic Theory Concerning Patents for Inventions." Economica 1 (February): 30–51.

Plotkin, M. J., Hettler, B., & Davis, W. (2017). Viva Schultes—A Retrospective. In Prance, S.G., McKenna, D.J., De Loenen, B., & Davis, W. (Eds), *Ethnopharmacologic Search for Psychoactive Drugs* (pp. 95-119). Synergetic Press.

Porter, Tony. 1999. "Hegemony and the Private Governance of International Industries." In C. Cutler, V. Haufler, and T. Porter, eds., Private Authority and International Affairs, 257–282. Albany: State University of New York Press.

Prager, F. D. (1946). Brunelleschi's patent. J. Pat. Off. Soc'y, 28, 109. Rätsch, C. (2005). The encyclopedia of psychoactive plants: ethnopharmacology and its applications. Simon and Schuster.

Rivier, L., & Lindgren, J. E. (1972). "Ayahuasca," the South American hallucinogenic drink: An ethnobotanical and chemical investigation. Economic Botany, 26(2), 101-129.

Roberts, D. E. (2007). Constructing a criminal justice system free of racial bias: An abolitionist framework. *Colum. Hum. Rts. L. Rev.*, *39*, 261.

Robinson, S. S. (1979). *Toward An Understanding of Kofan Shamanism*. Cornell University.

Rodd, R. (2008). Reassessing the cultural and psychopharmacological significance of Banisteriopsis caapi: preparation, classification and use among the Piaroa of Southern Venezuela. Journal of psychoactive drugs, 40(3), 301-307.

Rodríguez, G.A. (2016). Una decisión tardía. Semana Sostenible. Revista Semana. Retrieved on July 22, 2020 from URL https://sostenibilidadpruebas.semana.com/opinion/articulo/una-decision-tardia/34500

Rodriguez-Mora, D. F. (2021). La Diversidad del Yagé (a.k.a. Ayahuasca) y Otras Plantas Usadas en la Espiritualidad y el Chamanismo Cofán, Jardines de Sucumbíos, Colombia. Manuscrito en preparación. Tesis de Maestría. Universidad Estatal de Carolina del Norte.

Rommelspacher, H. (1981). The β-Carbolines (Harmanes)-A New Class of Endogenous Compounds. Pharmacopsychiatry, 14(04), 117-125.

Samorini, G. (2014). Aspectos y problemas de la arqueología de las drogas sudamericanas. Cultura y Droga, 19(21), 13-34.

Samorini, G. (2015). Acerca de la presencia de beta-carbolinas en tejidos biológicos de los hallazgos arqueológicos sudamericanos.

Samorini, G. (2019a). The oldest archaeological data evidencing the relationship of Homo sapiens with psychoactive plants: A worldwide overview. *Journal of Psychedelic Studies*, 3(2), 63-80.

Samorini, G. (2019b). Fake News About Ayahuasca's Archaeological Antiquity. Retrieved on February 05, 2021 from URL https://chacruna.net/fake-news-about-ayahuascas-archaeological-antiquity/

Samoylenko, V., Rahman, M. M., Tekwani, B. L., Tripathi, L. M., Wang, Y. H., Khan, S. I., ... & Muhammad, I. (2010). *Banisteriopsis caapi*, a unique combination of MAO inhibitory and antioxidative constituents for the activities relevant to neurodegenerative disorders and Parkinson's disease. Journal of ethnopharmacology, 127(2), 357-367.

Schultes, R. E. (1954). PLANTAE AUSTRO-AMERICANAE IX: PLANTARUM NOVARUM VEL NOTABILIUM NOTAE DIVERSAE. Botanical Museum Leaflets, Harvard University, 16(8), 179-228.

Schultes, R. E. (1957). The identity of the malpighiaceous narcotics of South America. Botanical Museum Leaflets, Harvard University, 18(1), 1-56.

Schultes RE (1963) Botanical sources of the new world narcotics. The Psychedelic Review 1: 147–166.

Schultes RE (1972) De plantis toxicariis e mundo novo tropicale commentationes X: New data on the malpighiaceous narcotics of South America. Botanical Museum Leaflets, Harvard University 23(3): 137–14

Schultes, R. E. (1975). De plantis toxicariis e Mundo Novo tropicale commentationes XIII. Notes on poisonous or medicinal malpighiaceous species of the Amazon. Botanical Museum Leaflets, Harvard University Vol. 24: 128, t. xxvii, Fig. 2.

Schultes RE (1976) Richard Spruce and the ethnobotany of the northwest Amazon. Rhodora 78(813): 65–72.

Schultes RE (1982) The beta-carboline hallucinogens of South America. *Journal of Psychoactive Drugs* 14(3): 205–220.

Schultes, R. E., & Raffauf, R. F. (1990). The healing forest: medicinal and toxic plants of the Northwest Amazonia. Dioscorides Press.

Schultes, R. E., & Raffauf, R. F. (1992). Vine of the soul: medicine men, their plants and rituals in the Colombian Amazonia. Synergetic Press Inc.

Schultes, R. E., Hofmann, A., & Ratsch, C. (2001). Plants of the Gods: Their sacred, healing, and hallucinogenic powers, revised edition. Healing Arts Press.

Secretariat, C. B. D. (1992). Convention on biological diversity. In *Convention on biological diversity*.

Secretariat, C. B. D. (2011). Nagoya Protocol on access to genetic resources and the fair and equitable sharing of benefits arising from their utilization to the convention on biological diversity: text and annex. UN.

Sell, S.K. (2003). Private Power, Public Law. The Globalisation of Intellectual Property Rights. Cambridge: Cambridge University Press

Sheldrake, M. (2020). The 'enigma'of Richard Schultes, Amazonian hallucinogenic plants, and the limits of ethnobotany. Social Studies of Science, 50(3), 345-376.

Sherret, L. (2005). Futility in action: coca fumigation in Colombia. *Journal of Drug Issues*, 35(1), 151-168.

Shiva, V. (2000). North-South Conflicts in Intellectual Property Rights. Peace Review, 12(4), 501-508.

Shiva, V. (2007). Bioprospecting as sophisticated biopiracy. Signs: *Journal of Women in Culture and Society*, 32(2), 307-313.

Shiva, V. (2016). Biopiracy: The plunder of nature and knowledge. North Atlantic Books.

Sichelman, T., & O'Connor, S. (2012). Patents as promoters of competition: the guild origins of patent law in the Venetian Republic. San Diego L. Rev., 49, 1267.

Sismondo, C. (2022). A Canadian psychedelic drug company has created medical grade ayahuasca. Toronto Star.

Smith, L. T. (2021). Decolonizing methodologies: Research and Indigenous Peoples. Bloomsbury Publishing.

Sonsin, J.O., Bezerra, G.B., Behrens, C.S.B, Gomes, S.M., Fagg, C.W., & Oliveira, R.C. (2016). *Wood Anatomical Distinction of Lianas (Banisteriopsis caapi) (Spruce ex Griseb.) Morton (Mapigiaceae)) Used in Ritualistic Ceremonial of Ayahuasca*. (2016). Retrieved on July 22, 2020, from https://dtihost.sfo2.digitaloceanspaces.com/sbotanicab/67CNBot/resAnexo1-1095-1274-4e295c601776730e823dbcd2e1a774e9.pdf

Stocks, A., Reyes, M. R., & Rios-Franco, C. A. (2020). GIS and the A'i of Colombia: Reserves, Resguardos and the Future. In Indigenous Studies: Breakthroughs in Research and Practice (pp. 711-734). IGI Global.

Strand, K. J., Cutforth, N., Stoecker, R., Marullo, S., & Donohue, P. (2003). Community-based research and higher education: Principles and practices. John Wiley & Sons.

Szeminski, Jan. 1987. "Why Kill the Spaniard? New Perspectives on Andean Insurrectionary Ideology in the 18th Century." In Resistance, Rebellion, and Consciousness in the Andean Peasant World, 18th to 20th Centuries. S. J. Stern, ed. Madison: University of Wisconsin Press.

TallBear, K. (2014). Standing with and speaking as faith: A feminist-indigenous approach to inquiry. *Journal of Research Practice*, 10(2), N17-N17.

Torres, C. M. (2017). From beer to tobacco: A probable prehistory of ayahuasca and Yagé. In Prance, S.G., McKenna, D.J., De Loenen, B., & Davis, W. (Eds), *Ethnopharmacologic Search for Psychoactive Drugs* (pp. 36-54). Synergetic Press.

Torres, C. M. (2018). The Origins of the Ayahuasca/Yagé Concept. An Inquiry into the Synergy between Dimethyltryptamine and Beta-Carbolines. In Ancient psychoactive substances. University Press of Florida.

Tupper, K. W. (2006). The globalization of ayahuasca: Harm reduction or benefit maximization?. *International Journal of Drug Policy*, 19(4), 297-303.

Valderrama, D. F., & Pérez, Á. L. (2004). Manual botánico para el reconocimiento ambiental y cultura de Ukumari Kankhe. Instituto de Investigación de Recursos Biológicos Alexander von Humboldt y Fundación Zio A'i..

Vargas Roncancio, I. D., & Rodriguez-Mora, D. F. (2024). The making of an ethnobotanical research agreement in Southern Colombia: Yagé, invisible people and the law of the place. In I. D. Vargas Roncancio (Ed.), *Law, Humans and Plants in the Andes-Amazon: The Lawness of Life*. Routledge.

Viveiros de Castro, E. (2004). Perspectivismo e multinaturalismo na América indígena. O que nos faz pensar, 14(18), 225-254.

World Trade Organization. (1994, April 15). Agreement on Trade-Related Aspects of Intellectual Property Rights (unamended). Retrieved on April 21, 2023 from https://www.wto.org/english/docs_e/legal_e/27-trips_01_e.htm

World Trade Organization. (2008, November). TRIPS: REVIEWS, ARTICLE 27.3(B) AND RELATED ISSUES. Retrieved on April 20, 2023 from https://www.wto.org/english/tratop_e/trips_e/art27_3b_background_e.htm#:~:text=Article%2027.3(b)%2C%20explained,cover%20all%20fields%20of%20technology.

Zuluaga, G. (2000). El pensamiento de los mayores. Código de Ética de la Medicina Indígena del Piedemonte Amazónico Colombiano. UMIYAC.

Psychedelics, Patents and the Future of Psychedelic Medicine

Carey Turnbull

President Heffter Institute

> *"There are three primary ways to achieve legal safe access to psychedelic plants, drugs, and experiences. None of them are easy, quick, or inexpensive."* —Carey Turnbull

In this essay Carey Turnbull shares the complexities of the legal frameworks which both support and prohibit psychedelic medicines.

HOW DOES REGULATION WORK?

There are three primary ways to achieve legal and safe access to psychedelic plants, fungi, drugs and experiences. These are the right to religious freedom, legislative changes resulting in decriminalization or legalization, including those resulting from ballot initiatives, and the FDA approval process for new prescription drugs. None of these are easy, quick or inexpensive. The FDA path stands out among the three given the costs, complexity and timeframes involved in bringing new drugs to market. Given the degree to which this third pathway has become the focus on much of the current activity in psychedelics, it is not surprising that the current topic of discussion has become an opportunity and has occurred as a result of complications created by regulatory awards of monopoly.

Typically, we attempt to prohibit monopolies in our economic system. The US Department of Justice seeks to break up corporations with excessive market dominance because they are not in the public interest, whether that be the example of big oil in the early 20th century or discussions regarding Big Tech in the present era. Disproportionate market share equates to excessive pricing power, and in the extreme represents monopoly power requiring government intervention. The exceptions to the rule of prohibiting monopolies are rare. One, for instance, is the electricity business, which operates under a regulatory model based on an understanding that having a single electricity provider—one set of wires, one power generating station etc,- is useful in producing power economically. When an electricity business is awarded a monopoly, it is controlled by a public utility commission. Every six months the resident utility must go to the commission and present their costs—fuel, operation of a generating station, wire maintenance etc. The public utility commission adjusts electricity rates on a quarterly or biannual basis based upon these costs, using a cost-plus formula that allows the electricity provider to make a reasonable profit while controlling prices for consumers. Here we have an example of a monopoly but a carefully controlled one.

Another example is the pharmaceutical industry which is, under specific circumstances, given awards of monopoly. There are three levels to the pharma trade. On the top-level, regulations encourage the formation of capital pools to incentivize the risky and expensive search for novel or more effective treatments for various medical indications. Regulations encourage this by awarding exclusivity for a limited number of years to firms that succeed. No harm, no foul there. There's some tension around cost and we in America don't want to have to go to Canada or Mexico to get our meds. So, the second level comes 10 or so years later, when an award for a novel invention runs out of monopoly protection. Then generic firms compete to be high-quality low-cost providers. These firms can also be billion dollar publicly traded firms. Again, not necessarily any harm or foul there. The third level in the pharma trade is represented by, for instance, the Gates Foundation. In 1950s, a vaccine for polio was invented. Originally there was an award of a monopoly allowing the developer of the vaccine to realize profits for the work they had done in developing it. Polio was eventually eradicated in the developed world but some years later the Gates Foundation recognized that there were still small pockets of Polio in Pakistan and Africa so they began to give the vaccine away for free.

So what do we do with psychedelic drugs like psilocybin, a naturally occurring molecule to which no potential provider or manufacturer can claim status as the inventor? It is my view that psilocybin should be somewhere between levels two and three. Firms can aspire to be a generic provider, or like the Usona Institute, which is advancing psilocybin through the FDA process as a treatment for depression, and give it away for free.

FREEDOM TO OPERATE AND HOW PATENTING WORKS

I started an organization called Freedom to Operate (FTO). Freedom to Operate is a term of art in the field of intellectual property law and refers to the ability to develop and market products without legal liabilities to third parties who claim intellectual property rights in those products. FTO was formed primarily for the advancement of science and education, specifically to support and facilitate science and research in the public interest and for public benefit. FTO expects its primary method for doing so will be to challenge certain patent rights which are improperly claimed and which, therefore, inappropriately discourage or prevent other individuals and organizations from engaging in research and innovation in the public interest and for the public benefit. There's an important public policy interest in invalidating bad patents, those which were mistakenly issued by, for instance, the US Patent and Trademark Office, and in promoting free competition that does not infringe on validly granted patents and other intellectual property. Issued patents are presumed valid and so operate to discourage investment by others into the same or similar subject matter. The public is benefited when incorrectly issued patents are challenged. There is a strong federal policy favoring free competition, permitting third parties to challenge the validity of issued patents without first being accused of infringement.

Before further detailing the work of FTO, it is worth briefly touching on the difference between intellectual property and tangible real property. Real property—the best example is tangible property you can hold in your hand—you can stand on it, you can build a house on it. It's known as real estate because it represents the real or tangible part of your personal estate, of your personal property. And then there's intellectual property, property that can't be held in the hand. I will give two examples of intellectual property and how it can be used or misused. I'll start with the example of Paul McCartney who wrote the song *Lucy in the Sky with Diamonds*. Songs are registered at ASCAP, the American Society for Composers, Authors and Publishers. Paul McCartney having written it then records it. Paul McCartney has the rights to the song that he wrote. Now let's say someone else came along later and said, "hey, I wrote a great song and it's called *Lucy in the Sky with Diamonds* and here's how it goes", then hums ASCAP a bar or two. If the person behind the desk wasn't a Beatles fan and had never heard of the song, they would probably register it with the ASCAP stamp. What's going to happen next is when Paul McCartney hears about that he's going to go to ASCAP and say, "hey, that's prior art, I actually wrote that quite some time ago." And he may have to go to some lengths to prove that, say by showing an example of his singing the song beforehand. So, there's one example of intellectual property and the use and misuse of intellectual property laws.

A second example of use and misuse of intellectual property laws occurred some time ago when we became aware that Compass Pathways had filed a patent on psilocybin. The patent's title indicated it was meant to cover psilocybin, it's method of manufacture, it's polymorphs and uses. When a patent is filed, the patent applicant is usually given a year or so during which the contents behind the title are kept secret, to give the patent holder, who ostensibly invented something new, a year and a half head-start with their invention. So, we had to wait a year or so in order to get a full look at what was being claimed. Our assumption was that the likelihood of this being what it said was rather slim and that it was more likely that somebody made some little improvement for instance to the method of manufacture. Something that added some value that they wanted to benefit from in terms of the intellectual property rights to such an innovation. But when it came out it did appear that they were attempting to patent psilocybin, its methods of manufacture, it's polymorphs and use. However, if you look at the written opinion of the International Searching Authority, which operates under the Patent Cooperation Treaty, they conclude that the claimed patent included no inventive steps.* They say, actually we looked this up and Paul McCartney of The Beatles wrote this, or in this particular case, Albert Hoffman did this in 1963. And going back to 1958, he was the first person to isolate the psychoactive molecule in the psilocybin mushroom that had been brought back from Mexico by Gordon Wasson. Gordon had given it to a few people to try to see how this could possibly be creating this experience. Somebody must have put two and two together that it seemed kind of like that LSD that Sandoz has been distributing. So, Wasson sent it to Sandoz, and Albert Hofmann was able to isolate the psychoactive molecule and show how to make it in a lab.

When you make psilocybin in the lab, you end up with a solution. After you get that molecule in a solution, you next dry that carefully, slowly, under very controlled conditions, and you end up with a powder, and that powder takes the form of a salt, and the salt is called a polymorph.

* Written Opinion of the International Searching Authority, Patent Cooperation Treaty, International Patent Application No. PCT/IB2018/057811, Patent Applicate, Compass Pathways Limited

Now I'm not a chemist so I had no idea what a polymorph was, and I had to ask. The easiest way to understand this, as my best education was in kindergarten, like most of us, and in kindergarten, we were told that when a raindrop freezes into a snowflake they make an infinite number of patterns. Every snowflake is different. That may be a child's fairytale-I doubt that there are that many, but when you take a solution of a simple molecule made in a beaker and you dry it, you end up with a powder that crystalizes into a salt pattern. Typically, there are less than a half dozen forms any molecule can take as a very structured pattern, and those are its polymorphs.

When you look for a place to register a patent it's not uncommon to venue shop, to go to a place where it's going to be easy to get your patent approved. If you go to South Africa, the policy is most patents asked for is stamped approved. The assumption is that if it's not a novel invention, someone is going to fight it out in court. They do a little bit more searching in Europe. Apparently, the firm looking on behalf of the Compass patent got it stamped approved. The European Patent Office made some observations that narrowed it to the polymorph claim.

You can imagine that if someone said I'm going to patent insulin, Merck or whoever owns the patent and makes billions of dollars a year would immediately say we're going to invalidate that patent. I assume the idea here was people in the patent office had never heard the word psilocybin. We can get this approved and then we have a means to exclude potential competitors. Now we have the problem of who's now going to complain about that? Now looking at the idea that the last element of the claim standing here is the polymorph. The rest of it they recognized was not unique, but the polymorph claim seems to have some teeth in it. I said to my patent attorney, "what might we do about that?" Because I don't know: is that a novel polymorph or is it not?" And he said, "Well, the way to find that out is let's get a sample of psilocybin that predates their patent application". To do that it has to be psilocybin with a forensic trail because you're going to be looking at submitting your findings in a legal proceeding. We asked the places that would have psilocybin, the universities that have been researching it for some time. Largely those are people who have had a long relationship with Heffter Research Institute, who did the academic work on psilocybin. We got psilocybin samples from, say, a dozen or so universities. We also got a sample from the National Institute of Drug Abuse, and the DEA. We also reached out through various channels to Sandoz, who still had a bottle of theirs from 1963. We ended up with about a dozen samples of psilocybin with a forensic trail that predated the Compass patent application. At that point we needed to get to know more about how to test them. Psilocybin is a schedule one drug, so the maker has a scheduling license, and it gets shipped to the university which has to get a schedule one license and a DEA license. So, these samples have a clear forensic trail. The one we ended up using was made by Dave Nichols, a storied psychopharmacologist—one of the world's experts on the psychopharmacology of psychedelics, and a founding member of Heffter. It was made by Dave with his DEA license, had been shipped to Johns Hopkins University and used by Roland Griffiths to conduct research. So, there we have a forensic trail, and we've got a look at what this is. One of the people we bumped into when looking for psilocybin samples was a researcher in Scandinavia. When we began to investigate the polymorph, chemists told us this is a very rarefied corner of chemistry and first said, "you need to find a physical chemist." And a physical chemist said, "this spins beyond me, it's more rarefied. You need a crystallographer, someone who knows how these simple molecules form themselves into patterns." One psilocybin researcher in Scandinavia said, "actually I have a friend and he is the chair of the Nobel Prize chemistry committee.", and so that seemed unimpeachable. When you get in front of a patent court, you get into a situation where expert testimony can become "he said, she said". My guy says it's true, your guy says it's not. We felt the chair of the Nobel Prize chemistry committee would be unimpeachable. At that point you need to be because this is so specialized that not only wouldn't a patent officer understand it, whoever is considering the legal proceedings will not be able to understand it. At this point we were looking for evidence you could put into a court and we thought, what better evidence than a peer reviewed paper. Because rather than getting one person's expert testimony that says "yes, it is", and another expert testimony says "no, it's not", you're relying on someone whose duty it is to pass judgement on the facts. It was not a chemist, nor a physical chemist, nor crystallographer, but a journal of crystallographers. This particular peer reviewed journal probably has a publication list of about 1000 but they're the world's experts.

For academic papers or books I read the opening paragraph and the final paragraph, and I feel like that tells me everything I need to know in between. I'm going to share the first paragraph of the peer reviewed published psilocybin paper. "Psilocybin is a zwitterionic tryptamine natural product found in numerous species of fungi known for their psychoactive properties. Following its structural elucidation and chemical synthesis in 1959, purified synthetic psilocybin has been evaluated in clinical trials and has shown promise in the treatment of various mental health disorders. In a recent process-scale crystallization investigation, three crystalline forms of psilocybin were repeatedly observed: Hydrate A, Polymorph A, and Polymorph B. The crystal structure for Hydrate A was solved previously by single-crystal X-ray diffraction. This article presents new crystal structure solutions for the two anhydrates, Polymorphs A and B, based on Rietveld refinement using laboratory and synchrotron X-ray diffraction data, and density functional theory (DFT) calculations. Utilizing the three solved structures, an investigation was conducted via Rietveld method (RM) based quantitative phase analysis (QPA) to estimate the contribution of the three different forms in powder X-ray diffraction (PXRD) patterns provided by different sources of bulk psilocybin produced between 1963 and 2021" (Sherwood et al., 2022). Over the last 57 years, each of these samples quantitatively reflects one or more of the hydrate and anhydrate polymorphs. In addition to quantitatively evaluating the composition of each sample, this article evaluates correlations between the crystal forms present, corresponding process methods, sample age, and storage conditions. Furthermore, revision is recommended on characterizations in recently granted patents that include descriptions of crystalline psilocybin inappropriately reported as a single-phase 'isostructural variant.' Rietveld refinement demonstrated that the claimed material was composed of approximately 81% Polymorph A and 19% Polymorph B, both of which have been identified in historical samples. In this article, we show conclusively that all published data can be explained in terms of three well-defined forms of psilocybin and that no additional forms are needed to explain the diffraction patterns." (Sherwood et al., 2022).

No human being has ever seen a molecule because a molecule is smaller than a wavelength of light. And there's no such thing as magnifying it to a point where the human eye can see one, so you use what's called x-ray powder diffraction. Take the salt and they shoot X rays through it, and what you get is not a picture but a unique pattern, provided in this instance from different sources of psilocybin produced between 1963 and 2021. A more precise way to do it now is by contracting to use a particle accelerator like the Argonne National Laboratory just outside Chicago. There are only a half dozen of these in the world, each the size 5 football fields and created at a cost of billions of dollars. It was made available to us by Sven Leiden who is on the Nobel Prize chemistry committee. He told us the older way to do this was by using x-ray powder diffraction, XRPD. The more precise way to do it now is by using a particle accelerator, aka an atom smasher. It was constructed under the design and operation of, and is funded by, the Department of Energy and it assists the nuclear research community in examining radioactive samples as a high energy x-ray microscope. The modern way to look at a polymorph is to use one of these devices. Instead of a swarm of electrons moving through an object (aka an x-raymachine) and creating a picture, it is a single electron at a time therefor creating an extremely precise picture of the object—in this case of molecules arranged in a crystal pattern, or polymorph. It was when we had asked for the psilocybin sample from the universities that someone at a university in Europe said they knew someone who can get an even better more definitive picture of the molecule and it's polymorphs, Sven Lidin, the Nobel Prize Chemistry Chair. Sven lit up with the idea that we would take a psilocybin molecule, or a psilocybin polymorph, and put it into the particle accelerator, and definitively identify the shape of the polymorph that no human eye has ever, or will ever see. Because a molecule is smaller than a wavelength of light. And which x-ray powder diffraction, XRPD, can identify, but not as well as it can be identified by this method. I'm not sure to this day whether he lit up because he's a psychonaut, or because he's a science geek. You can't pay your way onto these machines, you need credentials. Sven ended up being one of the authors on the FTO peer reviewed psilocybin crystallography paper. So, we have this peer reviewed paper reviewed by the chair of the Nobel Prize Committee, and it's conclusion of structure determination, using the synchrotron that's at the Argonne National Lab. The analysis indicated the three most commonly encountered crystalline forms of psilocybin obtained from routine synthesis and that one or more of the three phases were identified in all 24 psilocybin samples evaluated. And most importantly the paper concluded that the polymorph being claimed by Compass as an invention is in fact a mixture of previously identified polymorphs rather than something new or innovative.

What Freedom To Operate wants is of important public policy interest in invalidating bad patents, those which were mistakenly issued by the US Patent and Trademark Office. I'm not opposed to Big Pharma and awards of monopoly, because they encourage the formation of capital pools to do what's necessary in the pursuit of new or better treatments for patients. However, synthetic psilocybin has been around for many decades—how to make it, its methods of manufacture and now yes, it's polymorphs and its uses have been known for decades. This doesn't mean that generic manufacturers won't make fortunes competing to be the high-quality low-priced providers of psilocybin to the human race. Fortunes will be made. Manufacture, distribution, provision of care, these are all big businesses.

Having said that, let me transition to two other things. These are the things that move out of this problem of patents. First is the US Food and Drug Administration writing to the USPTO.*

* U.S. Food and Drug Administration letter to the U.S. Patent and Trademark Office, dated September 12, 2021. Issued pursuant to Execuive Order 14036.

They write pursuant to executive order in the hope of furthering developing the FDAs engagement with the USPTO to help ensure that the patent system, while incentivizing innovation, does not also cause unjustified delay in generic drug and biosimilar competition beyond that reasonably contemplated by applicable law. This executive order instructs the Secretary of Health and Human Services through the commissioner of the FDA, to write a letter to the undersecretary of Commerce for intellectual property, and director of the USPTO enumerating and describing any relevant concerns of the FDA, namely bringing more drug competition to the market and addressing the high cost of medicines by improving access to affordable medicine as a top priority the administration, the Department of Health and Human Services and the FDA. The FDA does not have a direct role in how drugs are priced, however, the FDA plays an indirect role in holding down prices by bringing efficiencies to drug development and review process and promoting robust competition for established drugs. It has nothing to do with psychedelics. This is about Big Pharma, and Big Pharma has been given the right to monopolies, but we know that monopolies are very unusual in our system. So, here's the FDA and US Patent Office attempting to get involved in Big Pharma in general and the tendency to patent and how those patents impact prices and patient access.

The other thing I'd like to reference is a paper from the Harvard Law Review on patents and psychedelics. This relates to the paper we just saw between the FDA and the USPTO asking how we can work with the pharmaceutical industry to encourage competition. I'll start here, "In the past two decades, pioneering research has rekindled interest in the therapeutic use of psychedelic substances such as psilocybin, ibogaine, and dimethyltryptamine (DMT). Indigenous communities have used them for centuries, and researchers studied them in the 1950s and '60s. However, most psychedelics were banned in the '70s, when President Nixon launched the U.S. war on drugs. Fifty years later, rising rates of mental illness, substance use, and suicide are prompting researchers to revisit psychedelics, and some have gained permission to study them in limited quantities. Clinical trials are producing promising results, creating enthusiasm for commercializing and patenting psychedelics" (Marks & Cohen, 2021c).

This essay analyzes the ethical, legal, and social implications of patenting these controversial substances. Patents on psychedelics raise unique concerns associated with their unusual qualities, history, and regulation. Because they were criminalized for decades, the U.S. Patent and Trademark Office (PTO) lacks personnel with expertise in the field, rendering more questionable the quality of its evaluation of psychedelic patents. Moreover, because Indigenous communities pioneered many aspects of modern psychedelic therapies, their patenting by Western corporations may promote biopiracy, the exploitation of Indigenous knowledge without compensation. Importantly, control of psychedelics by a small number of companies may stifle innovation and reduce access to these therapies. The essay presents proposals to reduce the risk of biopiracy and the issuance of unwarranted psychedelic patents. Potential solutions include the implementation of psychedelic patent pledges, the creation of psychedelic prior art repositories, and the tightening of patentability requirements for novel drug therapies. The essay concludes that ultimately, due to their importance to the advancement of science and public health, it may be appropriate to view psychedelics as tools of scientific discovery, eligible only for limited patent protection." (Marks & Cohen, 2021c).

This was written by bioethics law professors at Harvard Law School. The paper concludes as follows:

"Psychedelics may represent a paradigm shift for mental healthcare and the most promising solution to the mental health crisis. However, if a small number of companies secure wide swaths of intellectual property early on, then the beneficial impact of that shift may be blunted.

In this essay we have set out a series of proposals for discouraging unwarranted patents in the psychedelics field, some radical, some less so. It is essential to have these conversations now, while the industry remains in its nascent stage. The political economy is such that once new players become large enough, they will have an outsized influence over potential changes to the law, especially those that threaten their dominant positions." (Marks & Cohen, 2021c).

BIBLIOGRAPHY

Marks, M., & Cohen, I. (2021c). Patents on Psychedelics: The Next Legal Battlefront of Drug Development. *Social Science Research Network*. https://doi.org/10.2139/ssrn.3948757

Sherwood, A. M., Kargbo, R. B., Kaylo, K. W., Cozzi, N. V., Meisenheimer, P., & Kaduk, J. A. (2022). Psilocybin: crystal structure solutions enable phase analysis of prior art and recently patented examples. *Structural Chemistry*, 78(1), 36–55. https://doi.org/10.1107/s2053229621013164

Psychedelics and the Prevention of Interpersonal Violence: The Role of Emotional Regulation

Michelle St. Pierre, PhD, and Zach Walsh, PhD

Postdoctoral Research Fellow at The University of British Columbia

Professor of Psychology at The University of British Columbia | Clinical psychologist

"The past decade has seen growing empirical support for third-wave behavior therapies that share mechanisms of action with psychedelic experiences such as enhancing mindfulness, decentering, emotion regulation, and distress tolerance." —MICHELLE ST. PIERRE

This paper explores research on psychedelics as a tool for reducing interpersonal violence.

INTRODUCTION

The resumption of psychedelic research in recent decades has focused primarily on the therapeutic potential of psychedelic-assisted therapies (PAT) for treating internalizing problems such as depression, anxiety, and trauma-related disorders. However, research conducted prior to the tightening of restrictions in the late 1960s, also examined the externalizing spectrum of psychopathology, with particular attention to aggressive and antisocial behavior (Krueger et al. 2005). As work on internalizing problems continues to yield promising results, it is timely to further consider the application of PAT in addressing antisocial and aggressive behavior. In this chapter, we provide a narrative review of research on psychedelics, aggression, and antisociality, outline potential mechanisms of therapeutic action, and propose a framework for the clinical application of PAT to externalizing problems, with a specific focus on interpersonal aggression.

INTERNALIZING VS EXTERNALIZING

Humans are emotional beings who require sophisticated coping strategies to manage the range of intense emotions experienced over a lifetime. Difficulties with emotion regulation often manifest as either internalizing or externalizing patterns. Internalizing reflects inward responses to stress, such as depression, anxiety, withdrawal, or self-harm. Externalizing reflects outward responses, characterized by impulsivity and antisocial behavior (Eisenberg et al. 2001). According to the Diagnostic and Statistical Manual of Mental Disorders, Fifth Edition (DSM-5), externalizing behaviors "violate the rights of others or bring the individual into significant conflict with societal norms or authority figures" (American Psychiatric Association 2013, p. 461). Common externalizing outcomes include interpersonal aggression, property crime, and problematic substance use.

Among the most problematic externalizing behaviors are violent crimes, particularly intimate partner violence (IPV). IPV, sometimes referred to as domestic violence, is defined as physical, sexual, or psychological abuse by an intimate partner (Coker et al. 2002) and is one of the most common forms of interpersonal violence. The World Health Organization estimates that 30% of women in heterosexual relationships have experienced IPV (WHO 2013). Although less studied, men are also affected (Walsh et al. 2010) with about 34% reporting lifetime IPV (Smith et al. 2014). IPV has far-reaching consequences, including increased risk of mental health problems and future violence among children exposed in the home (Forke et al. 2018). Identifying risk factors and developing effective interventions for IPV is a critical public health priority.

Reviews of the literature reveal a robust positive relationship between certain forms of substance use and aggression. For example, stimulant use—such as methamphetamine and cocaine—has been consistently linked to violence (Forke et al. 2018; Ernst et al. 2008), and alcohol use has been extensively shown to increase the risk of both perpetrating and experiencing IPV (Foran and O'Leary 2008). In contrast, the relationship between other psychoactive substances and aggression remains somewhat obscure. Research examining the effects of cannabis and psychedelics on aggression is mixed, with evidence suggesting both potential risk and protective effects (Moore and Stuart 2005; Smith et al. 2014; Walsh et al. 2017; Feingold, Kerr, and Capaldi 2008). Reviews on the topic have concluded that there is insufficient evidence to establish a link between psychedelic use and violence (Boles and Miotto 2003; Hoaken and Stewart 2003).

PSYCHEDELICS AND EXTERNALIZING—EARLY EVIDENCE

Recent research on the therapeutic potential of psychedelics has largely focused on internalizing problems, such as anxiety (e.g., Yu et al. 2021), and traumatic stress (e.g., Khan et al. 2022). However, evidence from the pre-prohibition era of psychedelic research suggests that psychedelic use may also reduce criminal and aggressive behaviors. This association is particularly promising, given that many interventions aimed at reducing criminality have shown limited effectiveness (Alper 2018; Yukhnenko, Sridhar, and Fazel 2020).

Although empirical research on the effects of psychedelic use on criminality and violence remains limited (for a review see Holoyda 2020), three experimental studies from the 1960s stand out. The earliest of these examined the effects of psychedelics on 10 treatment-resistant sexual offenders who participated in LSD-assisted group psychotherapy sessions. Tenenbaum reported that LSD contributed to in behavioral improvements and changes in personality. Specifically, nine participants demonstrated increased empathy, insight, communication, and treatment engagement (Tenenbaum 1961).

Shortly after Tenenbaum's study, another experimental investigation examined the potential of LSD-assisted therapy to rehabilitate male criminal offenders deemed "incurable" (Arendsen-

Hein 1963, p. 101). Participants followed individualized treatment plans in which LSD was administered weekly or biweekly over 10 to 20 weeks depending on their clinical progress. Each psychedelic session was accompanied by a group therapeutic discussion on the day of treatment, followed by individual therapy sessions in subsequent days. Non-LSD group therapy was held twice weekly. Arendsen-Hein observed "functional changes in the personality" and suggested that LSD could mobilize "the process of mental growth in many criminal patients" (Arendsen-Hein 1963, p. 106), including shifts in values, behavioral improvements, confrontation of repressed emotions, and insights into the relationship between current circumstances and past experiences (Neitzke-Spruill 2020).

The final and most prominent pre-prohibition study was conducted by pioneering scientist and drug policy activist Dr. Timothy Leary and colleagues in the Concord Prison Experiment (1961-1963), which assessed the effect of psilocybin-assisted psychotherapy on criminal recidivism among male inmates, the majority serving time for violent offenses (Leary et al. 1965). The 32 participants, most nearing parole, attended group therapy twice weekly for six weeks, including two sessions involving psilocybin administration. Departing from the dominant medical framework, Leary and colleagues collaborated with the inmates emphasizing their intrinsic capacity for change. Prior to the psilocybin sessions, participants were encouraged "to plan and initiate their own personality change programs" (Leary et al. 1965, p. 63), and follow-up group meetings and reflective writing facilitated integration of the psychedelic experience.

Leary initially reported that psilocybin-assisted therapy reduced recidivism for new crimes and reincarceration. However, a 34-year follow-using official criminal records found no long-term impact on recidivism rates (Doblin 1998). Despite this, Leary maintained that psychedelics had the potential to reduce violent behavior.

A recent reanalysis of the Concord study focused on acute changes rather than long-term criminal outcomes. Neitzke-Spruill (2020), conducted a qualitative content analysis of 72 psychedelic session reports from 29 participants, including four sessions that combined mescaline with psilocybin. Common themes included changes in emotion, perception, social interaction, and self-knowledge. Participants frequently described increased self-awareness, self-reflection, and dissociation from the self, imagining post-release identities committed to behavioral change.

Unfortunately, these acute characterological changes did not translate into reduced criminal behavior in post-release environments. Leary argued that criminogenic contexts—such as limited housing, employment, and social support—undermined the maintenance of positive effects, noting that "a support system is really needed" (Doblin 1998, p. 424). Neitzke-Spruill (2020, p. 1) similarly emphasized that social environments can constrain the ability to enact meaningful behavioral change. Methodological limitations—including small sample sizes, variations in set and setting, and the use of jails or medical facilities that may attenuate psychedelic effects—likely also muted the observed impact of psychedelic-assisted therapy (Metzner and Leary, n.d.). These factors highlight the complex interplay between individual therapeutic experiences and broader structural conditions that influence criminal behavior.

PYSCHEDELICS AND EXTERNALIZING—NEW DEVELOPMENTS

Criminality

Contemporary research provides growing support for the idea that psychedelics may reduce criminal recidivism and violence. In one of the first epidemiological studies linking psychedelics to criminal behavior, Hendricks and colleagues examined 25,622 individuals with a prior felony conviction under community supervision in the United States (Hendricks et al. 2014). Hallucinogen use was coded according to DSM classifications, including hallucinogen abuse and hallucinogen use disorder (HUD). The DSM category is broad, encompassing phenylalkylamines (e.g., mescaline and MDMA), indoleamines (e.g., psilocybin and DMT), ergolines (e.g., LSD and morning glory seeds), and phenethylamines (e.g., 25I-NBOMe). Hendricks and colleagues found that a HUD diagnosis was associated with a reduced probability of supervision failure (OR = 0.60), in stark contrast to cannabis use disorder (OR = 1.68), cocaine use disorder (OR = 2.24), alcohol use disorder (OR = 1.11), opiate use disorder (OR = 1.41), or amphetamine use disorder (OR = 1.33), which all significantly increased the likelihood of supervision failure. While suggestive, these results must be interpreted cautiously due to the observational design, which precludes causal conclusions.

In a subsequent study, Hendricks and colleagues (Hendricks et al. 2018). examined the association between classic psychedelic use and criminal behavior among over 480,000 adult using 13 years (2002-2014) of National Survey on Drug Use and Health data (2002-2014). Lifetime psychedelic use was coded as positive if participants reported ever using ayahuasca, DMT, LSD, mescaline, peyote or San Pedro, or psilocybin-containing mushrooms. Lifetime psychedelic use was associated with reduced odds of criminal behavior, including 27% lower odds of past-year larceny/theft, 22% lower odds of arrest for a property crime, 18% lower odds of arrest for a violent crime, and 12% lower odds of past-year assault. By contrast, lifetime use of other illicit substances was generally associated with increased odds of criminal behavior. These findings were extended in a replication study analyzing 2015–2019 survey data, which again found that a history of psychedelic use was associated with lower odds of past-year arrest (Jones and Nock 2022), suggesting protective effects in the general population as well as forensic samples.

Intimate Partner Violence

In addition to broader effects on criminal behavior, psychedelics may specifically attenuate intimate partner violence (IPV). A 2016 study from our research group examined whether prior hallucinogen use was associated with a reduced IPV recidivism after prison release (Walsh et al. 2016). This longitudinal study included 302 male inmates (M age = 26) diagnosed with a substance use disorder, serving sentences of one year or less, with 72% incarcerated for violent crimes. Hallucinogen use was assessed through interviews and coded in two ways: any lifetime use (endorsed by about half of the participants) and the lifetime presence of a DSM-IV hallucinogen use disorder (endorsed by 13%), a proxy for more frequent use.

Survival analyses examined time from release (0–118 months) to IPV recidivism. Lifetime hallucinogen use was associated with lower IPV rates: 27% of hallucinogen users were rearrested (mean survival time = 63 months, SE = 2.25) versus 42% of non-users (mean survival time = 55 months, SE = 2.65). The effect was even stronger among individuals with a HUD: only 14% were rearrested for IPV, compared to 35% of those without HUD (Figure 1), indicating a notable protective association between hallucinogen use and IPV recidivism.

This research provides evidence that hallucinogen use is associated with reduced criminality and violence among individuals involved in the criminal justice system. However, the extent to which hallucinogen use may protect against IPV perpetration in community members remains unclear. College students, in particular, experience some of the highest rates of IPV. A recent survey found that 52% of female college students reported at least one episode of IPV in their lifetime, with 12% experiencing IPV in the preceding semester (Fantasia, Sutherland, and Hutchinson 2018).

The transition to college is a distinctive developmental period. Many students are living outside their parents' homes for the first time, facing increased academic and interpersonal stressors, and encountering greater access to substances, including alcohol. College years are also associated

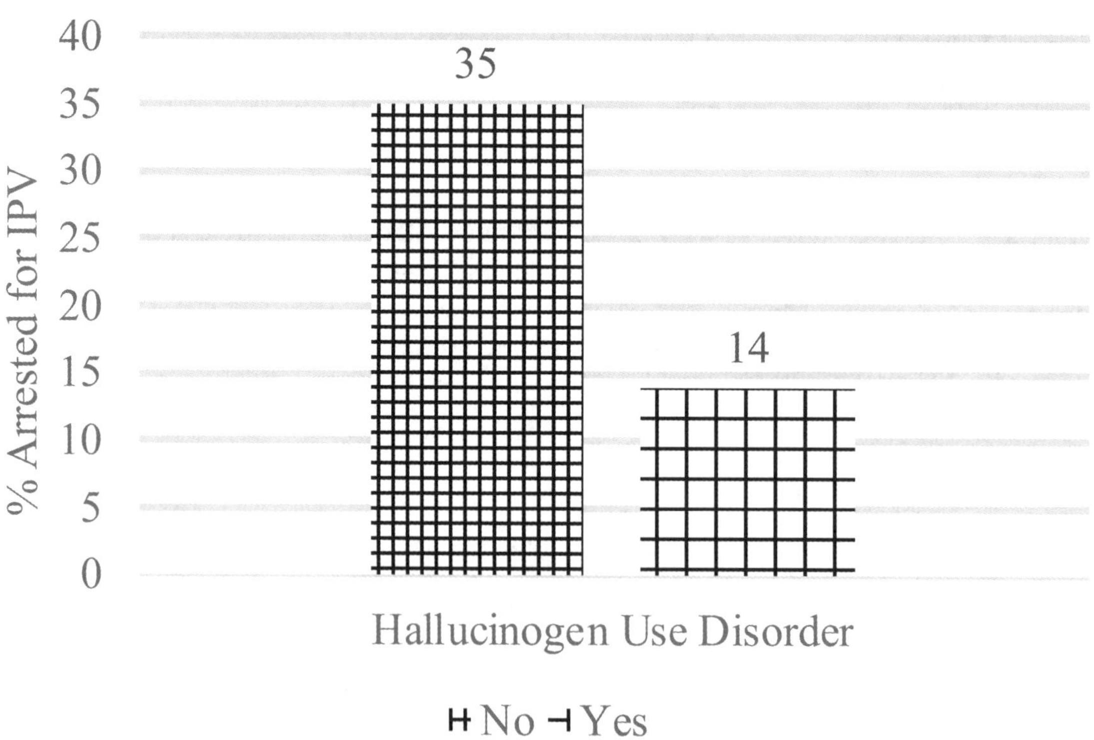

Fig. 1 Percentage of Males Rearrested for IPV.

with the highest rates of drinking compared to any other periods across the lifespan (Johnston et al. 2007). The combination of elevated IPV and substance use rates made this population particularly salient for our research.

In a study designed to examine the prevalence and mechanisms underlying the association between psychedelic use and IPV, we surveyed university students and other community members (*N* = 1266, 62% female, *M* age = 23) about lifetime psychedelic use (i.e., if they ever used LSD and/or psilocybin mushrooms), IPV, and other outcomes of interest. Lifetime psychedelic use was reported by 32%, and 11% reported past-year IPV. Among men, those with a lifetime history of psychedelic use were roughly half as likely to report intimate partner violence perpetration compared to non-users (5.1% vs 10.0%; see Figure 2). This protective effect was not observed among female respondents.

Emotion regulation difficulties were a primary target in our effort to understand the mechanisms psychedelic use and IPV. Poor emotion regulation is associated with increased mental health problems, antisocial behaviour, and potentially violence, and may be modifiable through psychedelic use. Experimental studies have demonstrated that psilocybin administration reduces amygdala reactivity during emotion processing (Kraehenmann et al. 2015), and can acutely shift

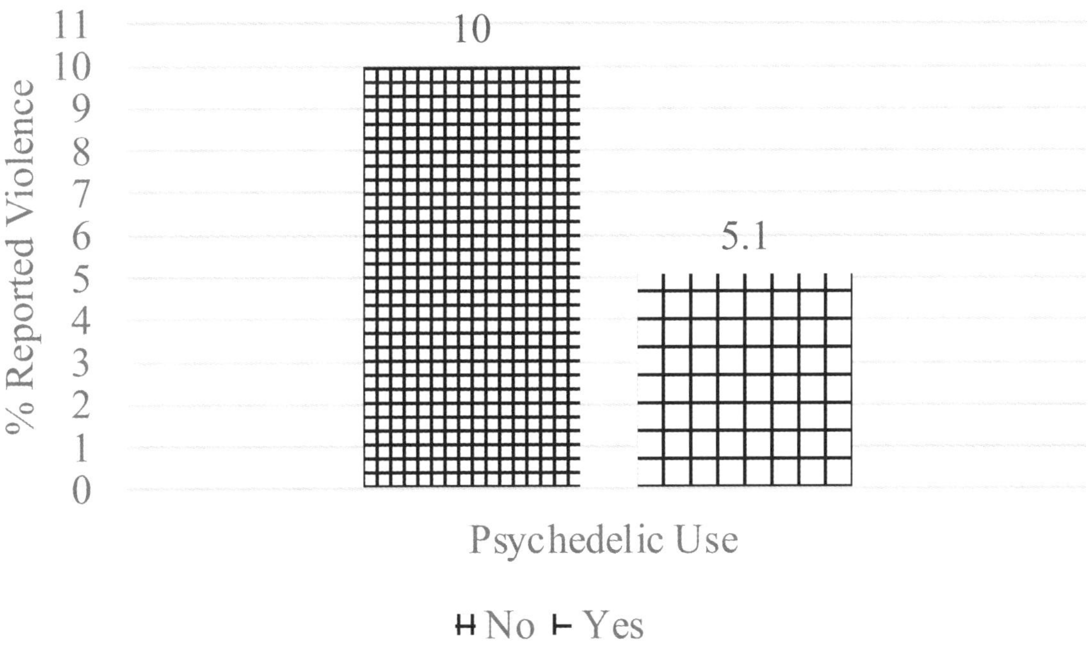

Fig. 2 Lower Rates of Intimate Partner Violence Among Men That Used Psychedelics.

negative emotional biases towards positive ones (Kraehenmann et al. 2016). Psychedelic use has been proposed to facilitate mindfulness, emotional integration and psychological flexibility (A. Watts 1968; Walsh &Thiessen, 2018; Gallimore and Strassman 2016), all key features of therapies developed to address emotional dysregulation (Hayes 2004; Hayes et al. 2006; Linehan 1993).

Consistent with this theoretical framework, male psychedelic users reported fewer difficulties with emotion regulation ($b = -0.12$, $SE = 0.05$, $p < 0.05$) compared to non-users. Perpetrators of IPV exhibited greater emotion regulation difficulties ($b = 0.19$, $SE = 0.05$ $p < 0.01$). When emotion regulation was included in the model, the negative association between psychedelic use and IPV ($b = -0.11$, $SE = 0.04$, $p < 0.05$) was attenuated ($b = -0.09$, $SE = 0.04$, $p > 0.05$), suggesting a potential mediating effect (see Figure 3). Although the data are cross-sectional and causal direction cannot be inferred, these findings provide preliminary evidence that emotion regulation may help explain the protective effects of psychedelic use against IPV.

Note. (a) Psychedelic use is associated with reduced IPV perpetration among men; (b) psychedelic use is hypothesized to exert an indirect effect on IPV through emotion regulation. * = $p < 0.05$, ** = $p < 0.01$.

The findings from both studies of psychedelic use and IPV (Walsh et al., 2016, Thiessen et al., 2018) were consistent in direction and magnitude, collectively providing an encouraging signal regarding the potential of psychedelics to reduce IPV across correctional and community samples of men. Moreover, the evidence that emotion regulation mediates the relationship between psychedelic use and IPV suggests that psychedelic-induced modulation of emotional responses (Kraehenmann et al. 2015; 2016; Preller et al. 2015) may persist beyond the acute psychedelic effects of the substances. However, these contemporary studies were observational and assessed naturalistic psychedelic use, which occurred across diverse settings and with varied intentions.

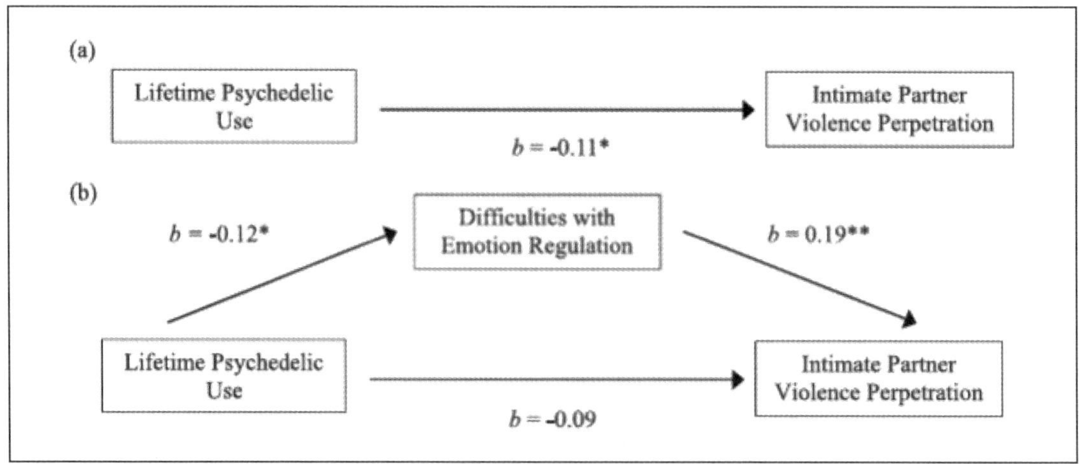

Fig. 3 Emotion Regulation Mediates the Association Between Psychedelic Use and Intimate Partner Violence.

Recent research has examined mental health outcomes of recreational psychedelic according to three broad categories of intention—self-expansion, social/recreational, and coping with negative affect—alongside setting, and post-use integration (St Arnaud and Sharpe 2022). This work demonstrated that psychedelic use can either enhance or diminish mental health depending on those contextual factors, often referred to as set and setting, which have long been recognized as profoundly influencing both the experience and outcomes of psychedelic use. Accordingly, it is plausible that intentional, well-integrated psychedelic use could produce even more pronounced protective effects than those observed in these naturalistic studies.

Approaches to Psychedelic Assisted Psychotherapy to Address Externalizing Disorders

As interest in PAT continues to rise, determining which therapeutic interventions maximize its healing potential for specific conditions has become a research priority. Matching specific modalities to particular conditions, as well as identifying transdiagnostic mechanisms, will be key to optimizing PAT. A comprehensive discussion of potential approaches is beyond the scope of this review and has been addressed elsewhere (Garcia-Romeu and Richards 2018; Yaden et al. 2022).

With regard to interventions aimed at mitigating interpersonal violence, evidence for the moderating role of emotion regulation suggests potential benefits of behavioral therapies that focus on developing these skills. Research from our group has highlighted the synergies between psychedelics and third-wave CBT approaches (Walsh 2017; Walsh and Thiessen 2018). In a narrative review, we focused on three of the most extensively studied third-wave therapies—Acceptance and Commitment Therapy (ACT; Hayes et al. 1999), Dialectical Behavior Therapy (DBT; Linehan 1993), and Mindfulness Based Cognitive Therapy (MBCT; Segal, Williams, and Teasdale 2002). These approaches informed by contemplative spiritual practices, share potential mechanisms including enhanced mindfulness, decentering, emotion regulation, psychological flexibility, and distress tolerance. Subsequent efforts to manualize PAT have drawn heavily from these interventions (Guss, Krause, and Sloshower 2020; R. Watts 2021). Developing these skills during preparatory sessions may help establish the psychological 'set,' a factor proposed to enhance the likelihood of positive psychedelic experiences (i.e., set and setting; Hartogsohn 2017). Yaden and colleagues (2022) further argue for the use of a default therapeutic framework in mainstream American and European contexts, noting that cognitive-behavioral approaches minimize cultural insensitivity, make few speculative assumptions about the nature of the mind and reality, and have the largest empirical support for safety and effectiveness outside of psychedelic therapy.

CONCLUSION

In this narrative review, we present converging evidence suggesting that classic psychedelics may have protective effects against violent and criminal behavior. Individually, each study reviewed here has limitations that complicate interpretation. Nonetheless, collectively, these methodologically diverse studies—including small interventional trials with incarcerated individuals, epidemiological studies of the general U.S. population, prospective studies of forensic populations, and cross-sectional investigations of university students—consistently point to a protective effect of psychedelic use. This convergence is particularly striking given its contrast with the well-documented criminogenic effects of widely used substances such as alcohol and stimulants.

This discrepancy challenges the ongoing stigmatization and criminalization of psychedelics and problematizes their inclusion in the broad "war-on-drugs" classification. Rather than causing harm, psychedelics combined with appropriate psychotherapeutic support may hold potential as tools for reducing violence and criminal behavior. Building on the pioneering work of Dr. Leary and his colleagues, future research should refine best practices for integrating psychedelics with specific psychotherapeutic interventions to protect and improve the lives of individuals affected by violence and crime.

BIBLIOGRAPHY

Alper, Mariel. 2018. "2018 Update on Prisoner Recidivism: A 9-Year Follow-up Period (2005-2014)."
Alper, Mariel. 2018. "2018 Update on Prisoner Recidivism: A 9-Year Follow-up Period (2005-2014)."
American Psychiatric Association. 2013. *Diagnostic and Statistical Manual of Mental Disorders. Arlington*. https://doi.org/10.1176/appi.books.9780890425596.744053.

Arendsen-Hein, G. W. 1963. "LSD in the Treatment of Criminal Psychopaths." In *Hallucinogenic Drugs and Their Psychotherapeutic Use*, edited by R. W. Crocket, R. A. Sandison, and A Walk, 101–6. H. K. Lewis & Co.

Boles, Sharon M., and Karen Miotto. 2003. "Substance Abuse and Violence: A Review of the Literature." *Aggression and Violent Behavior* 8 (2): 155–74. https://doi.org/10.1016/S1359-1789(01)00057-X.

Coker, Ann L., Keith E. Davis, Ileana Arias, Sujata Desai, Maureen Sanderson, Heather M. Brandt, and Paige H. Smith. 2002. "Physical and Mental Health Effects of Intimate Partner Violence for Men and Women." *American Journal of Preventive Medicine* 23 (4): 260–68. https://doi.org/10.1016/s0749-3797(02)00514-7.

Doblin, R. 1998. "Dr. Leary's Concord Prison Experiment: A 34-Year Follow-up Study." *Journal of Psychoactive Drugs* 30 (4): 419–26. https://doi.org/10.1080/02791072.1998.10399715.

Eisenberg, N., A. Cumberland, T. L. Spinrad, R. A. Fabes, S. A. Shepard, M. Reiser, B. C. Murphy, S. H. Losoya, and I. K. Guthrie. 2001. "The Relations of Regulation and Emotionality to Children's Externalizing and Internalizing Problem Behavior." *Child Development* 72 (4): 1112–34. https://doi.org/10.1111/1467-8624.00337.

Ernst, Amy A., Steven J. Weiss, Shannon Enright-Smith, Elizabeth Hilton, and Emily C. Byrd. 2008. "Perpetrators of Intimate Partner Violence Use Significantly More Methamphetamine, Cocaine, and Alcohol than Victims: A Report by Victims." *The American Journal of Emergency Medicine* 26 (5): 592–96. https://doi.org/10.1016/j.ajem.2007.09.015.

Fantasia, Heidi Collins, Melissa A. Sutherland, and M. Katherine Hutchinson. 2018. "Lifetime and Recent Experiences of Violence Among College Women." *Journal of Forensic Nursing* 14 (4): 190–97. https://doi.org/10.1097/JFN.0000000000000211.

Feingold, Alan, David C. R. Kerr, and Deborah M. Capaldi. 2008. "Associations of Substance Use Problems with Intimate Partner Violence for At-Risk Men in Long-Term Relationships." *Journal of Family Psychology : JFP : Journal of the Division of Family Psychology of the American Psychological Association (Division 43)* 22 (3): 429–38. https://doi.org/10.1037/0893-3200.22.3.429.

Foran, Heather M., and K. Daniel O'Leary. 2008. "Alcohol and Intimate Partner Violence: A Meta-Analytic Review." *Clinical Psychology Review* 28 (7): 1222–34. https://doi.org/10.1016/j.cpr.2008.05.001.

Forke, Christine M., Rachel K. Myers, Joel A. Fein, Marina Catallozzi, A. Russell Localio, Douglas J. Wiebe, and Jeane Ann Grisso. 2018. "Witnessing Intimate Partner Violence as a Child: How Boys and Girls Model Their Parents' Behaviors in Adolescence." *Child Abuse & Neglect* 84 (October): 241–52. https://doi.org/10.1016/j.chiabu.2018.07.031.

Gallimore, Andrew R., and Rick J. Strassman. 2016. "A Model for the Application of Target-Controlled Intravenous Infusion for a Prolonged Immersive DMT Psychedelic Experience." *Frontiers in Pharmacology* 7. https://www.frontiersin.org/articles/10.3389/fphar.2016.00211.

Garcia-Romeu, Albert, and William A. Richards. 2018. "Current Perspectives on Psychedelic Therapy: Use of Serotonergic Hallucinogens in Clinical Interventions." *International Review of Psychiatry (Abingdon, England)* 30 (4): 291–316. https://doi.org/10.1080/09540261.2018.1486289.

Guss, Jeffrey, Robert Krause, and Jordan Sloshower. 2020. "The Yale Manual for Psilocybin-Assisted Therapy of Depression (Using Acceptance and Commitment Therapy as a Therapeutic Frame)." PsyArXiv. https://doi.org/10.31234/osf.io/u6v9y.

Hartogsohn, Ido. 2017. "Constructing Drug Effects: A History of Set and Setting." *Drug Science, Policy and Law* 3 (January): 205032451668332–205032451668332. https://doi.org/10.1177/2050324516683325.

Hayes, Steven C. 2004. "Acceptance and Commitment Therapy, Relational Frame Theory, and the Third Wave of Behavioral and Cognitive Therapies." *Behavior Therapy* 35 (4): 639–65. https://doi.org/10.1016/S0005-7894(04)80013-3.

Hayes, Steven C., Jason B. Luoma, Frank W. Bond, Akihiko Masuda, and Jason Lillis. 2006. "Acceptance and Commitment Therapy: Model, Processes and Outcomes." *Behaviour Research and Therapy* 44 (1): 1–25. https://doi.org/10.1016/j.brat.2005.06.006.

Hendricks, Peter S., C. Brendan Clark, Matthew W. Johnson, Kevin R. Fontaine, and Karen L. Cropsey. 2014. "Hallucinogen Use Predicts Reduced Recidivism among Substance-Involved Offenders under Community Corrections Supervision." *Journal of Psychopharmacology (Oxford, England)* 28 (1): 62–66. https://doi.org/10.1177/0269881113513851.

Hendricks, Peter S, Michael Scott Crawford, Karen L Cropsey, Heith Copes, N Wiles Sweat, Zach Walsh, and Gregory Pavela. 2018. "The Relationships of Classic Psychedelic Use with Criminal Behavior in the United States Adult Population." *Journal of Psychopharmacology* 32 (1): 37–48. https://doi.org/10.1177/0269881117735685.

Hoaken, Peter N. S., and Sherry H. Stewart. 2003. "Drugs of Abuse and the Elicitation of Human Aggressive Behavior." *Addictive Behaviors* 28 (9): 1533–54. https://doi.org/10.1016/j.addbeh.2003.08.033.

Holoyda, Brian. 2020. "The Psychedelic Renaissance and Its Forensic Implications." *The Journal of the American Academy of Psychiatry and the Law* 48 (1): 11. https://doi.org/DOI:10.29158/JAAPL.003917-20.

Johnston, L D, P M O'Malley, J G Bachman, and J E Schulenberg. 2007. "Monitoring the Future National Survey Results on Drug Use, 1975-2006 Volume II." NIH Publication No. 07-6206. Bethesda, MD: National Institute on Drug Abuse.

Jones, Grant M., and Matthew K. Nock. 2022. "Exploring Protective Associations between the Use of Classic Psychedelics and Cocaine Use Disorder: A Population-Based Survey Study." *Scientific Reports* 12 (1): 2574. https://doi.org/10.1038/s41598-022-06580-2.

Khan, Amanda J., Ellen Bradley, Aoife O'Donovan, and Joshua Woolley. 2022. "Psilocybin for Trauma-Related Disorders." In *Disruptive Psychopharmacology*, edited by Frederick S. Barrett and Katrin H. Preller, 319–32. Current Topics in Behavioral Neurosciences. Cham: Springer International Publishing. https://doi.org/10.1007/7854_2022_366.

Kilgore, J. 2015. *Understanding Mass Incarceration*. The New Press. https://thenewpress.com/books/understanding-mass-incarceration.

Kraehenmann, Rainer, Katrin H. Preller, Milan Scheidegger, Thomas Pokorny, Oliver G. Bosch, Erich Seifritz, and Franz X. Vollenweider. 2015. "Psilocybin-Induced Decrease in Amygdala Reactivity Correlates with Enhanced Positive Mood in Healthy Volunteers." *Biological Psychiatry* 78 (8): 572–81. https://doi.org/10.1016/j.biopsych.2014.04.010.

Kraehenmann, Rainer, André Schmidt, Karl Friston, Katrin H. Preller, Erich Seifritz, and Franz X. Vollenweider. 2016. "The Mixed Serotonin Receptor Agonist Psilocybin Reduces Threat-Induced Modulation of Amygdala Connectivity." *NeuroImage. Clinical* 11: 53–60. https://doi.org/10.1016/j.nicl.2015.08.009.

Krueger, Robert F., Kristian E. Markon, Christopher J. Patrick, and William G. Iacono. 2005. "Externalizing Psychopathology in Adulthood: A Dimensional-Spectrum Conceptualization and Its Implications for DSM-V." *Journal of Abnormal Psychology* 114 (4): 537.

Linehan, M. 1993. *Skills Training Manual for Treating Borderline Personality Disorder.* New York: The Guilford Press. https://psycnet.apa.org/record/1995-98090-000.

Metzner, Ralph, and Timothy Leary. n.d. "On Programming Psychdelic Experiences." *Psychedelic Review*, 4–19.

Moore, Todd M., and Gregory L. Stuart. 2005. "A Review of the Literature on Masculinity and Partner Violence." *Psychology of Men & Masculinity* 6: 46–61. https://doi.org/10.1037/1524-9220.6.1.46.

Neitzke-Spruill, Logan. 2020. "Race as a Component of Set and Setting: How Experiences of Race Can Influence Psychedelic Experiences." *Journal of Psychedelic Studies* 4 (1): 51–60. https://doi.org/10.1556/2054.2019.022.

Preller, K.H., T. Pokorny, R. Krähenmann, I. Dziobek, P. Stämpfli, and F.X. Vollenweider. 2015. "The Effect of 5-HT2A/1a Agonist Treatment On Social Cognition, Empathy, and Social Decision-Making." *European Psychiatry* 30 (March): 22. https://doi.org/10.1016/S0924-9338(15)30017-1.

Segal, Zindel V., J. Mark G. Williams, and John D. Teasdale. 2002. *Mindfulness-Based Cognitive Therapy for Depression: A New Approach to Preventing Relapse*. Mindfulness-Based Cognitive Therapy for Depression: A New Approach to Preventing Relapse. New York, NY, US: Guilford Press.

Smith, Philip H., Gregory G. Homish, R. Lorraine Collins, Gary A. Giovino, Helene R. White, and Kenneth E. Leonard. 2014. "Couples' Marijuana Use Is Inversely Related to Their Intimate Partner Violence over the First Nine Years of Marriage." *Psychology of Addictive Behaviors : Journal of the Society of Psychologists in Addictive Behaviors* 28 (3): 734–42. https://doi.org/10.1037/a0037302.

St Arnaud, Kevin O., and Donald Sharpe. 2022. "Contextual Parameters Associated with Positive and Negative Mental Health in Recreational Psychedelic Users." *Journal of Psychoactive Drugs*, February, 1–10. https://doi.org/10.1080/02791072.2022.2039815.

Tenenbaum, B. 1961. "Group Therapy with LSD-25. (A Preliminary Report)." *Diseases of the Nervous System* 22 (August): 459–62.

Timothy, Leary, Metzner Ralph, Presnell Madison, Weil Gunther, Schwitzgebel Ralph, and Kinne Sara. 1965. "A New Behavior Change Program Using Psilocybin." *Psychotherapy: Theory, Research & Practice* 2: 61–72. https://doi.org/10.1037/h0088612.

Walsh, Zach, dir. 2017. *Psychedelic Therapy & Third Wave Behaviorism: Prevention of Interpersonal Violence*. Psychedelic Science. Oakland, California. https://www.youtube.com/watch?v=SywINXoGIPE.

Walsh, Zach, Raul Gonzalez, Kim Crosby, Michelle S. Thiessen, Chris Carroll, and Marcel O. Bonn-Miller. 2017. "Medical Cannabis and Mental Health: A Guided Systematic Review." *Clinical Psychology Review*. https://doi.org/10.1016/j.cpr.2016.10.002.

Walsh, Zach, Peter S Hendricks, Stephanie Smith, David S Kosson, Michelle S Thiessen, Philippe Lucas, and Marc T Swogger. 2016. "Hallucinogen Use and Intimate Partner Violence: Prospective Evidence Consistent with Protective Effects among Men with Histories of Problematic Substance Use." *Journal of Psychopharmacology*. https://doi.org/10.1177/0269881116642538.

Walsh, Zach, Marc T. Swogger, Brian P. O'Connor, Yael Chatav Schonbrun, M. Tracie Shea, and Gregory L. Stuart. 2010. "Subtypes of Partner Violence Perpetrators among Male and Female Psychiatric Patients." *Journal of Abnormal Psychology* 119: 563–74. https://doi.org/10.1037/a0019858.

Walsh, Zach, and Michelle S. Thiessen. 2018. "Psychedelics and the New Behaviourism: Considering the Integration of Third-Wave Behaviour Therapies with Psychedelic-Assisted Therapy." *International Review of Psychiatry (Abingdon, England)* 30 (4): 343–49. https://doi.org/10.1080/09540261.2018.1474088.

Watts, Alan. 1968. "Psychedelics and Religious Experience." *California Law Review* 56 (1): 74–85. https://doi.org/10.2307/3479497.

Watts, Rosalind. 2021. "Psilocybin for Depression: The ACE Model Manual." https://doi.org/10.31234/osf.io/5x2bu.

WHO. 2013. "Global and Regional Estimates of Violence against Women: Prevalence and Health Effects of Intimate Partner Violence and Non-Partner Sexual Violence." Geneva: WHO.

Yaden, David B., Dylan Earp, Marianna Graziosi, Dara Friedman-Wheeler, Jason B. Luoma, and Matthew W. Johnson. 2022. "Psychedelics and Psychotherapy: Cognitive-Behavioral Approaches as Default." *Frontiers in Psychology* 13: 873279. https://doi.org/10.3389/fpsyg.2022.873279.

Yu, Chia-Ling, Fu-Chi Yang, Szu-Nian Yang, Ping-Tao Tseng, Brendon Stubbs, Ta-Chuan Yeh, Chih-Wei Hsu, Dian-Jeng Li, and Chih-Sung Liang. 2021. "Psilocybin for End-of-Life Anxiety Symptoms: A Systematic Review and Meta-Analysis." *Psychiatry Investigation* 18 (10): 958–67. https://doi.org/10.30773/pi.2021.0209.

Yukhnenko, Denis, Shivpriya Sridhar, and Seena Fazel. 2020. "A Systematic Review of Criminal Recidivism Rates Worldwide: 3-Year Update." *Wellcome Open Research* 4 (November): 28. https://doi.org/10.12688/wellcomeopenres.14970.3.

Where We Are, and Where This Might All Be Going

Wade Davis, PhD

Professor of Anthropology | BC Leadership Chair in Cultures and Ecosystems at Risk at the University of British Columbia | Ethnobotanist | Author | Filmmaker

> *"I'm very proud and happy to say that I wouldn't write the way I write, I wouldn't think the way I think, I wouldn't treat gay people the way I treat gay people, I wouldn't treat women the way I treat women, I wouldn't understand the power and resonance of biology- of nature itself, if I hadn't taken psychedelics."* —WADE DAVIS

In these final moving words, Wade Davis speaks to the importance, value and hope for the future of the psychedelic and ethnobotanical renaissance.

It's truly an honour to have been invited to share a few thoughts to help wind up this amazing gathering, these few magical days. An event that is but one manifestation of a global movement dedicated to the power and promise of sacred plants, a resurgence of research and passion that is both profoundly hopeful and long overdue.

Often I'm asked, as no doubt you are, whether I'm optimistic about the fate of the world. I am, and as a father, I must be. I've always thought of pessimism as an indulgence, despair an insult to the imagination, orthodoxy the enemy of invention. Do what needs to be done, my father always said, and only then ask whether it was possible or even permissible. He was an eternal optimist.

Optimism is in short supply these days. We live in challenging times, the spectre of climate change, the covid crisis, the war in Ukraine. But truth be told, what generation has ever been born into a world free of troubles? My parents and grandparents endured two world wars and the Great Depression. Many of us came of age in a decade marked by assassinations, haunted by the prospect of nuclear war, with cities aflame and a distant and endless war in Viet Nam.

But we also lived through glorious events that will be spoken about 10,000 years from now. Christmas Eve 1968, when Apollo emerged from the dark side of the moon to reveal for the first time in human history not a moonrise or a sunrise but the earth itself ascendant, a small and fragile sphere of life, a blue planet, floating in the velvet void of space.

Like a great wave of hope, this energy of illumination, only made possible by the brilliance of science, spread everywhere. Almost immediately we began to think in new ways. When I was a boy just getting people to stop throwing garbage out of a car window was a great environmental victory. No one spoke of the biosphere or biodiversity; now these terms are part of the vocabulary of school children.

In little more than a generation, women have gone from the kitchen to the boardroom, gay men and women from the closet to the altar, people of colour from the woodshed to the White House. What's not to love about a world capable of such scientific genius, such cultural capacity for change and renewal?

And yet, even as we celebrate this remarkable transformation, a shift in awareness and consciousness that had, among many wonders, the Beatles going from *She Loves You* to *Tomorrow Never Knows* in three years, a key ingredient in the recipe of social change remains overlooked, expunged from the record, at least until now.

I'm referring, of course, to the millions of young men and women, and no small number of elders, in all corners of the world, who found themselves prostrate before the gates of awe having taken a psychedelic.

Sometimes when giving a talk, one I've delivered more than once, a part of me hovers above the podium, looking down, listening to my own words. I find myself asking how on earth did that little boy raised in that modest family in an ordinary suburb of Montreal come to have such ideas, to think such thoughts?

How do any of us become the adults that we are, moving toward the end of lives forged by experience, but invariably inspired by serendipity?

To be sure, I suffered as a youth from what Baudelaire called the great malady, horror of home. I was drawn to anthropology at least in part because I wanted to leave a world, my world, that I had come to see as being problematic—in terms of the environment, social and racial justice, treatment of women and gay men and women.

Simply put, I sought escape from a middle class world of monotony in the hope that I might find in distant places the means to rediscover and celebrate the enchantment of being human. Many of my generation, including many in this room, shared this yearning for raw and authentic experience.

Jim Whittaker, the first American to reach the summit of Everest, famously said that if you're not living on the edge when young, you're taking up too much space. Our departed friend and brother, Terence McKenna, spoke of the great secret of the sages; jump off a cliff, and you land not on rocks but on a feather bed. The world exists to lift you up, not put you down.

I did live on the edge when young, and most certainly jumped off many a cliff. Tim Plowman once quipped that my entire vocabulary at twenty was limited to a single word, yes.

I also benefited from a fine education, made possible by a wonderful father who spent half of his savings to send me to Harvard, knowing full well that every day I was there could only widen the gap between us.

Within weeks of arriving in campus, just as I was discovering this completely new world of knowledge, psychedelics cracked open the sky, flinging wide the windows of the mystic. From that moment, Harvard and these sacred medicines went hand in hand, as if part of a single pedagogy.

I wouldn't speak as I do, write as I do, see the world, understand culture, or embrace nature as I do, had I not taken psychedelics. Back in the day our parents tried to warn us: "Don't take these drugs, you'll never come back the same." They didn't understand that not coming back the same was the entire point of the exercise.

Let me share one other revelation of science, the moon shot of this generation, a voyage of discovery not into space but into the very fiber of our beings. Nothing in our lifetimes has done more to liberate humanity from the petty hatreds and tyrannies that have haunted us since the dawn of awareness.

Science has affirmed the intuitions of all the poets and saints who have through the ages perceived humanity as a single interconnected whole. The genetic endowment of humanity is indeed a continuum. Biologically, race is an utter fiction. We truly are brothers and sisters, all descendants of common ancestors, including those who walked out of Africa some 65,000 years ago and carried the human spirit to every corner of the habitable world.

But here's the important thing. If humans are cut from the same genetic cloth, then all cultures share the same genius, the same mental acuity, the same raw intellectual genius. How this is expressed is simply a matter of choice and adaptive imperatives. There is no hierarchy of culture, no evolutionary rankings. That old Victorian notion that humans progressed from the savage to the barbarian to the civilized of the Strand in London, has been exposed as but a false conceit of the 19th Century, as irrelevant to our lives today as the conviction of the clergymen that the earth is but 6000 years old. In a stunning affirmation of the human spirit, science has confirmed that all of humanity is as one.

The other peoples of the world are not failed attempts at being modern, let alone failed attempts to be us. Every culture is a unique answer to a fundamental question; what does it mean to be human and alive? Every culture has something to say; each deserves to be heard, just as none has a monopoly on the route to the divine.

My father wasn't a religious man, but he used to say that there's good and evil in the world, take your side and get on with it. There was great wisdom in this. Good and evil march side by side, and our job is to put our shoulders to the wheel of justice, knowing always, as Martin Luther King said, that the arc of history bends towards righteousness, towards the good. And that's what it's all about. Coming together, as we have over these last days, leaning into the right side of history, pushing the wheel of life forward for the benefit of all. That's what this movement is all about.

As we bring this wonderful conference to a close, I'd like to reflect on something that has come up time and again over the last days, in our presentations and conversations, in our thoughts as we've strolled around this beautiful land. I'm referring to the notion of the sacred.

As a young boy I prayed every night, hands together, elbows perched on the sill of a bedroom window open to the winter air, eyes wide to the stars sparkling through the branches of the giant elm trees that in those years still thrived in the neighborhoods of old Quebec. I conversed with a God whose presence could be felt, and whose spiritual authority and omnipotence I accepted as an act of faith.

My parents, broken by the war, rarely saw the inside of a church. So, from the age of six, I dutifully set off every Sunday on my own, and continued to do so without fail for five years: I still have the gold pin with the silver cross that rewarded my attendance record. Like a pilgrim at the gates of a great cathedral, I didn't attend service to worship the building; I went there to be in the presence of God. For a long time, he was always to be found. But, as the years went by and I learned more and more about the world, there came a day when he simply failed to show. I never again entered a church as a Christian believer.

When, years later, I returned to that small community as an adult, what astonished me most was to realize how small my universe had been and how intimately I had known it. Every blade of grass resonated with a story. Shadows marked the ground where trees had fallen in my absence. Innovations and new construction I took as personal insults, violations of something sacred that lay at the confluence of landscape and memory.

What I felt so powerfully in that moment was not nostalgia but rather a connection to the actual force that for all of those years had propelled my spiritual yearning, a numinous energy that, thanks to a brilliant writer and close friend, Shefa Siegel, I now recognize as being the essence of the sacred, the invisible presence that the French philosopher Henry Corbin described as the imaginal, a suprasensory dimension that transcends religion, a space of intuition and revelation impossible to describe yet accessible to those in every culture who perceive the world, as Corbin wrote, "through the eyes of the heart".

My longings as a child, I realized, had not been of a religious nature, at least not in a formal sense; I'd been looking for a path that embraced the mystic among the multitudes, the promise of all people in all places through all time who had found peace and comfort in their pursuit of the divine. I came to see God as but the product of our desires. Our spirit and imagination transform an edifice of stone into a sacred space. A shrine is sanctified by the legacy of all those who have come before, with their hopes, fears, promises and prayers. Relics, icons, chalices and crosses, all simple objects crafted from wood, silver, and bone, take on spiritual resonance only over time, like old tools, warm from decades of human touch.

Sacrifice means to make sacred, and if the idea of the sacred is as old as humanity itself, as Shefa's mentor, anthropologist Roy Rappaport suggests, then the sacred can never be divorced from human agency. We dream the sacred into being. Ritual is the ground from which it springs. The sacred becomes manifest through the enactment of rituals that summon the spirit and give form to the divine.

In Jerusalem, as the Jewish people water the Western Wall with their tears and melt the stone with their kisses, they achieve spiritual clarity and purpose as God's eternal nation, his chosen people.

In Haiti, the waterfall at Saut D'eau is the home of Damballah-Wedo, the serpent god, repository of spiritual wisdom and the source of the falling waters. When the first rains fell, a rainbow, Ayida Wedo, was reflected. Damballah fell in love with Ayida, and their love entwined them in a cosmic helix from which all creation was fertilized. Every summer, over three days in July, as many as 15,000 pilgrims, all devotees of the *lwa*, the spirits of the Vodoun pantheon, make their way to the sacred site. One need only touch the water to feel its grace, and for some it is enough to dip into the shallow silvery pools. But most go directly to the cascades, men and women, old and young, baring their breasts and scrambling up the wet slippery bedrock that rises in a series of steps toward the base of the falls. Merely to submit to the waters is to open oneself to Damballah, and at any one time at the base of the waterfall in the shadow of the rainbow, there are a hundred or more pilgrims possessed by the spirit, slithering across the wet rocks.

For most of the year the Sinakara Valley in the southern Andes of Peru is home only to solitary shepherds and their flocks. But for three days between the feast of the Ascension and Corpus Christi, as the Pleiades re-emerge in the night sky, as many as 40,000 pilgrims converge at the base of the mountain to take part in the Qoyllur Rit'I, the Star Snow Festival. Some arrive on foot, some by mule, and others in open trucks and buses. The pilgrims make their way up a trail that climbs for seven miles, a route marked by altars and cairns, the stations of the cross, where men and women pause to pray and make offerings. Each pilgrim carries a bundle of small stones, a symbolic burden of sin to be lightened one by one as the valley comes near.

It falls upon ritual specialists, the *pablitos*, to perform the most dangerous and solemn act of the Qoyllur Rit'i. Like Christ himself, they shoulder a terrible burden, carrying the crosses from their village churches up the flanks to the icefields of the Colquepunku, where they implant them in the snow to be charged by the energy of the mountain and the earth. Then, before dawn on the morning of the third day, roped together by whips, they climb back to the ice to retrieve the crosses as, far below, thousands of pilgrims kneel in silent prayer. All eyes are on the summit, in homage to the *apus*, the mountain deities.

As the sun comes up, the crosses come down and make their way on the backs of the pilgrims through the Sinakara and out through the pass, into the trucks that will bring them back to the villages. The men also carry from the mountain small blocks of ice, which completes the devotional cycle: The people go to the mountain; the essence of the mountain returns to the villages to bring fertility to the fields, well-being to the families, health to the animals. Pilgrimage through sacred geography, homage to the gods, becomes a collective prayer for the cultural survival of the entire pan-Andean world.

When the first humans reached the shores of Australia, they went walking, establishing in time more than ten thousand clan territories, independent homelands all bound together by the Songlines, the tracks followed by the primordial ancestors who, in the time of the Rainbow Serpent, sang the world into being. As Aboriginal people today trace the Songlines and chant the stories of the first dawning, they enter the Dreamtime, which is neither a dream nor a measure of the passage of time. It is the very realm of the ancestors, a parallel universe where the ordinary laws of time, space, and motion do not apply, where past, future, and present merge into one.

To walk the Songlines is to become part of the ongoing creation of the world, a place that both exists and is still being formed. Thus, the Aborigines are not merely attached to the earth, they are essential to its existence. Without the land they would die. But without the people, the earth would wither. Should the rituals stop, the voices fall silent, all would be lost. Everything on earth is held together by the Songlines, just as everything is subordinate to the Dreaming, which is constant but ever changing. Every landmark is wedded to a memory of its origins, and yet always in the process of being born. Every animal and object resonate with the pulse of an ancient event, while still being dreamed into being. The land is encoded with everything that has ever been, everything that ever will be, in every dimension of reality. The world is perfect, though constantly being reimagined and renewed. To walk the land and honor the Songlines is to engage in a constant act of affirmation, an endless dance of creation.

All of India is one vast mandala of the sacred. For two thousand years the landscape of the entire subcontinent has been defined and given meaning by the power of myth, narrative and pilgrimage. On any given day there are tens of millions on the move, making their way step by step through a living landscape of mountains, rivers, forests, and villages, all elaborately linked to the legends of the Hindu gods. Every place has its story, as Diana Eck writes, and every story has its place. What the pilgrims ultimately seek are points of illumination, sacred destinations known as *tirthas*, fords or crossing places charged with power and purity where heaven and earth come together, sometimes to meet, allowing the devotee to cross over the river of *samsara* to reach the far shore of liberation. India is a land of ten thousand *tirthas*.

The most profound cultural insight of the Barasana and Makuna, whose lives unfold in the forests of the Colombian Amazon, is the realization that plants and animals are but people in another dimension of reality. Mythology infuses land and life with meaning. Ritual reinforces the norms that drive social behavior, encoding expectations and behaviors essential to survival in the forest. There is no separation between nature and culture. Without the forest and the rivers, humans would perish. But without people, the natural world would have no order or meaning. All would be chaos. Maintaining the flow of generative energy, fomenting reciprocity among all forms of life, is the duty of the shaman, who is neither priest nor physician; he is a diplomat in constant dialogue with the spirit realm, with all the responsibilities of a nuclear engineer who must, if necessary, enter the heart of the reactor and reprogram the world. The shaman moves with ease through mystical dimensions unseen by ordinary eyes but familiar to the Barasana and Makuna, who say that they see with their minds. In ritual ceremonies that embrace the entire community, the men come together to ingest *yagé*, a powerful potion that serves as a portal to the divine. As they don the ritual regalia, the yellow corona of pure thought, the white egret plumes of the rain, they literally become the ancestors, reliving their mythic journeys, alighting on all the sacred sites, transcending every form, becoming as if a single pulse of pure energy flowing through all of creation.

To this day, the peoples of the Sierra Nevada, the Kogis, Wiwas, and Arhuacos, remain true to their ancient laws, the moral ecological and divine dictates of the Great Mother, the Madre Creadora, and they are still led and inspired by a ritual priesthood known as the *mamos*. In their cosmic scheme people are vital, for it is only through the human heart and imagination that the Madre Creadora may become manifest. For the people of the Sierra Nevada, humans are not the problem but the solution. They call themselves the Elder Brothers. We who threaten the Earth through our ignorance of the sacred law are dismissed as the Younger Brothers. They believe and acknowledge explicitly that they are the guardians of the world, that their prayers and rituals literally maintain the cosmic and ecological balance of the planet. For generations, they have watched in horror as outsiders have violated the Madre Creadora, tearing down the forests that are the skin and fabric of her body and poisoning the rivers, the actual veins and arteries of her life. "We know," Jaison concluded, "so much more about life than the Younger Brothers. We never destroy a river, for to do so would be to destroy ourselves."

The Arhuacos make no distinction between the water found within the human body and what exists outside it. "Our blood that flows through our veins," a young woman once told me, "is no different from the water that flows through the arteries of life, the rivers of the land." They see a direct relationship between urine, blood, saliva, tears, and the water of a river, a lake, a wetland, a lagoon. And in this, they are undoubtedly correct. Humans are born of water, a cocoon of comfort in a mother's womb. As infants, our bodies are almost exclusively liquid. Even as adults, only a third of our being has solidity. Compress our bones, ligaments, muscles, and sinew, extract the platelets and cells from our blood, and the rest of us, nearly two-thirds of our weight, stripped clean and rinsed, would flow as easily as a river to the sea.

Alex Jack, a Gitksan elder and guide who passed away in 1999, was 43 before he had sustained contact with the settler society. He did not come from a tradition of literacy. His soul had not been crushed in the residential schools. He was a hunter and his very vocabulary was inspired by the sounds of the wild. Just as we can hear the voice of a character when we read a novel, he could hear the voices of animals.

When Alex told a story he did so in a way that the listener actually witnessed and experienced the essence of the tale, entering the narrative and becoming transfixed by all the syllables of nature. Every telling was a moment of renewal, a chance to engage in the very dance of the universe.

Alex never spoke ill of the wind. When he hunted he spoke to the prey by name with praise and admiration. His grandmother was Cree, possessed of the medicine power, certain that language had been a gift to humans from the animals. As a Carrier elder told the great anthropologist Diamond Jenness: *We know what the animals do, what are their needs. We were taught by the animals themselves. The priests say we lie but we know better. The white man writes everything down in a book so that it will not be forgotten; but our ancestors married animals, learned all their ways and passed on this knowledge from one generation to another.*

I once asked Alex how long the cycle of tales was. It was a question Alex had put to his own father many years before. To find out, they had put on snowshoes in March month, a time of good ice, and set out to walk the length of Bear Lake, a distance of some forty miles. "All the way there," Alex recalled, "and all the way back, and the story not half way done." Here was a beautiful notion. To measure the length of such a saga, it was not enough to use a time piece. You had to walk the land, telling the tale as you moved across a sacred landscape that the myth both honoured and inspired.

Each of these stories, these cultural anecdotes if you will, is rooted in place, the product of a particular way of thinking, an unique vision of life itself. But they all express a common impulse, a fundamental human desire to engage not death but life as it is, the invisible forces that lie all around us, the realm of the imaginal in the here and now. Death, of course, is the great mystery, the edge beyond which life as we know it ends and wonder begins. How a culture comes to terms with the inexorable separation that death implies invariably determines its religious worldview. Stripped to the bone, most religious longings and traditions come down to a simple desire to wrestle with eternity and come out on top. The pursuit and embrace of the sacred, by contrast, has nothing to do with death; it is all about life.

The sacred is eternal, reaching far into the past, shining as a beacon to the future. It is everywhere and nowhere. What is sacred can never be diluted or compromised, coopted, or copied, commodified, or made sordid through commerce and greed. Sensed if never seen, elusive and mysterious by its very nature, the sacred may lie beyond our reach, yet there is comfort just in knowing that such a radiant presence may one day be encountered. The clock is not ticking. No force exists that can rob us of its promise. The traveler today walks the same spiritual ground as the pilgrim of old. As Shefa Siegel reminds us, Freya Stark crossed the desert in search of lands and peoples where "the miraculous is not yet separated from everyday life." Patrick Leigh Fermor witnessed the efficacy of prayer whilst living in a remote Benedictine monastery perched on a rocky summit in Greece. It had little to do with religion, he concluded. Prayer's power to heal was the product of desire. "No matter how often we declare sacred experiences to be unverifiable", wrote the anthropologist Clifford Geertz, "it does not stop people everywhere from having them."

When I was a boy, still in the thrall of my Christian faith, my father, without being unkind, gently dismissed religion as wishful thinking; every church, he quipped, ought to have a billboard outside with the cautionary words "important, if true." Perhaps he was right. But the pursuit of the sacred, as I discovered long ago, has nothing to do with religion. It is not concerned with what lies beyond death; it makes, in fact, no claims to anything at all. The sacred embodies and radiates the glory of what exists in this moment, on this blue jewel of a planet. In his book, *The Origin of Avarice*, Shefa Siegel cites a wonderful few lines from D.H. Lawrence. "Before the Buddha or Jesus spoke", writes Lawrence, "the nightingale sang, and long after the words of Jesus and Buddha are gone, the nightingale will still sing." The goal of the pilgrim, he adds, is to become as if a bird "dissolved in the sky, yet filling heaven and earth with song." Passing through the sky, leaving no trace, at one with the sacred.

Index

D

N

O

P